Thieme

Handbook of Spine Surgery

Third Edition

Ali A. Baaj, MD
Professor of Neurosurgery and Chief of Spine Surgery
Department of Neurosurgery
University of Arizona, College of Medicine
Phoenix, Arizona, USA

Praveen V. Mummaneni, MD, MBA
Joan O'Reilly Distinguished Professor and Vice Chair
Department of Neurological Surgery
University of California, San Francisco
San Francisco, California, USA

Juan S. Uribe, MD, FAANS
Professor and Vice Chair, Chief of Division of Spinal Disorders;
Volker K. H. Sonntag Chair of Spine Research
Department of Neurological Surgery
Barrow Neurological Institute
Phoenix, Arizona, USA

Alexander R. Vaccaro, MD, PhD, MBA
President of Rothman Orthopedic Institute
Chair of Orthopaedic Surgery at Thomas Jefferson University
Department of Orthopaedic Spine
Rothman Orthopaedic Institute at Thomas Jefferson University Hospital
Philadelphia, Pennsylvania, USA

Mark S. Greenberg, MD, FAANS
Associate Professor
Neurosurgery Residency Training Program Director
Department of Neurosurgery and Brain Repair
University of South Florida Morsani College of Medicine
Tampa, Florida, USA

233 Illustrations

Thieme
New York • Stuttgart • Delhi • Rio de Janeiro

Library of Congress Cataloging-in-Publication Data is available with the publisher.

Illustrators: Illustrations and colorizations created by Graeme Chambers at Illumina Medical Illustration Ltd, and by Birck Cox. Artwork © Thieme

Thieme Publishers New York
333 Seventh Avenue, 18th Floor
New York, NY 10001, USA
www.thieme.com
+1 800 782 3488, customerservice@thieme.com

Cover design: © Thieme
Cover image source: Cover illustration created by Graeme Chambers at Illumina Medical Illustration Ltd. / © Thieme
Typesetting by TNQ Tech Private Limited, India

Printed in USA By King Printing Co., Inc. 5 4 3 2

DOI: 10.1055/b000001054

ISBN: 978-1-68420-554-7

Also available as an e-book:
eISBN (PDF): 978-1-68420-677-3
eISBN (epub): 978-1-68420-678-0

Important note: Medicine is an ever-changing science undergoing continual development. Research and clinical experience are continually expanding our knowledge, in particular our knowledge of proper treatment and drug therapy. Insofar as this book mentions any dosage or application, readers may rest assured that the authors, editors, and publishers have made every effort to ensure that such references are in accordance with **the state of knowledge at the time of production of the book**.

Nevertheless, this does not involve, imply, or express any guarantee or responsibility on the part of the publishers in respect to any dosage instructions and forms of applications stated in the book. **Every user is requested to examine carefully** the manufacturers' leaflets accompanying each drug and to check, if necessary, in consultation with a physician or specialist, whether the dosage schedules mentioned therein or the contraindications stated by the manufacturers differ from the statements made in the present book. Such examination is particularly important with drugs that are either rarely used or have been newly released on the market. Every dosage schedule or every form of application used is entirely at the user's own risk and responsibility. The authors and publishers request every user to report to the publishers any discrepancies or inaccuracies noticed. If errors in this work are found after publication, errata will be posted at www.thieme.com on the product description page.

Some of the product names, patents, and registered designs referred to in this book are in fact registered trademarks or proprietary names even though specific reference to this fact is not always made in the text. Therefore, the appearance of a name without designation as proprietary is not to be construed as a representation by the publisher that it is in the public domain.

Thieme addresses people of all gender identities equally. We encourage our authors to use gender-neutral or gender-equal expressions wherever the context allows.

FSC
www.fsc.org
100%
Paper from well-managed forests
FSC® C103101

To my wife, Gabriela, and to my children, Hannah and Joseph, for your unwavering love and support.

Ali A. Baaj, MD

For my wife and my children, thank you for all your love and support.
For the medical students, residents, and fellows whom I have had the pleasure of training.

Praveen V. Mummaneni, MD, MBA

To my wife Catalina, my son Sebastian and my daughter Camila for their unconditional love and support.

Juan S. Uribe, MD, FAANS

My ability to function as a surgeon and educator, and contribute to this wonderful handbook, is only possible through the unconditional love and support of my wife Lauren and children, Alex Jr, Juliana, Christian, and Mia.

Alexander R. Vaccaro, MD, PhD, MBA

I dedicate this work to my father, Louis Greenberg, who has guided me throughout life with integrity, wisdom, and humor.

Mark S. Greenberg, MD, FAANS

Contents

III: Spinal Pathology

IV: Surgical Techniques

Videos

Video 35.1: Endoscopic endonasal dens resection.

Video 46.1: Freehand thoracic screw placement.

Video 50.1: MIS retropleural thoracic diskectomy. (No Audio.)

Video 52.1: Open microdiscectomy. (No Audio.)

Video 54.1: Endoscopic lumbar surgery. (No Audio.)

Foreword

It is 8 PM on a Thursday evening. I just finished my last case of the day after a very busy week. I have a difficult case scheduled tomorrow requiring a technique which I haven't used in a while. I need to review before that case, but I'm tired and have little time or desire to do that. How often have you found yourself in that situation? What you need then is a brief, condensed summary of everything you need to know for that case. Or as detective Joe Friday on *Dragnet* would say, "Just the facts ma'am."

The *Handbook of Spine Surgery*, now in its third edition, is exactly that compendium. Presented in a bullet point format, you get relevant anatomy, indications for the procedure, advantages of the technique, preoperative imaging, step-by-step technique description, common complications, considerations specific to individual patients, expected outcome, surgical tips and pearls, and the answers to common questions. Critically, these can all be read and digested in 10 minutes. Something you can do even on a Thursday night when you're tired.

This handbook covers all spine surgical anatomy and procedures commonly performed. It is completely up-to-date, even including very newly described techniques. Each chapter is authored by surgeons with known expertise in the area about which they are writing, creating a virtual "who's who" of spine surgery. As a result, this handbook is a "must have" for every surgeon, fellow, resident, and medical student pursuing spine surgery as a career. Drs. Baaj, Mummaneni, Uribe, Vaccaro, and Greenberg are to be congratulated on contributing an important text to spine surgery. Thank them for enabling you to enjoy that Thursday night...

Richard G. Fessler, MD, PhD
Professor
Department of Neurosurgery
Rush University Medical Center
Chicago, Illinois, USA

Foreword

It was once said that more important than the **incision** is the **decision**. Although this is quite true and workup and evaluation of the spinal patient in the clinic are critically important, the surgical techniques and ancillary tools we use to perform those techniques have become increasingly complicated in recent years. Our diagnostic capabilities have improved and our knowledge of outcomes and what interventions work well is challenging in spinal surgery, and knowledge in this regard has also evolved significantly. With less invasive techniques becoming quite common and more accessible, it remains incredibly important that our trainees and practitioners early in practice still understand the basics and anatomical concepts related to spinal pathology.

In this book, Dr. Baaj and contributors have created a truly comprehensive approach to spinal pathologies and their treatment. What I am particularly enamored by is the full extent to which the reader is going to be able to understand the anatomy, the tools in the perioperative diagnosis and the treatment and after-treatment of spinal disease, the particulars related to each pathology, and the technical perils for performing the surgery. The book is divided into four parts with the first part being the basic anatomy. Part II relates to all the tools we use for diagnosis including physical examination, electrodiagnosis, imaging, etc. Also included are the tools for improving safety in spinal surgery such as neuromonitoring and the tools to use after surgery during recovery. Part III is based specifically on various common spinal pathologies and physiologic problems such as congenital, trauma, infection, tumor, degenerative disease, radiculopathy, myelopathy, deformity, and spondylar arthropathies. Finally, Part IV delves into the exact techniques and how to perform these techniques that are important for performance of spinal surgery.

It is obvious after reading the above that the book is one of the most comprehensive treatises on spinal pathology. In one stop we can learn the anatomy, the pathology, the techniques both for diagnosis and treatment, and the pitfalls associated with all of the above. I congratulate the authors on delivering for us a comprehensive text that will help those who are students of spinal surgery, as well as practitioners who are attempting to take care of our challenging patients.

Todd J. Albert, MD
Surgeon-in-Chief Emeritus
Hospital for Special Surgery
Professor of Orthopaedics
Weill Cornell Medical College
New York, New York, USA

Preface

We are thrilled to present the third edition of the *Handbook of Spine Surgery*. We are grateful to all contributors as once again we were able to compile a comprehensive yet practical handbook on pathology and techniques in modern spine surgery. In this new edition, we secured additional global leaders in spine surgery as authors to offer diverse content that appeals to a wider audience. As with prior editions, we maintained the highly popular bullet format with key pearls and common clinical questions for each chapter. We are excited to have included new chapters on popular and emerging topics like spine endoscopy, robotics, and single-position surgery to name a few. We similarly ensured that core chapters on topics such as trauma, degenerative disease, deformity, and tumors continue to be thorough and clinically pertinent. We are confident that this text will continue to be a valuable resource for students, trainees, and surgeons alike in the collective efforts to provide exceptional care to our patients with spinal diseases.

Ali A. Baaj, MD
Praveen V. Mummaneni, MD, MBA
Juan S. Uribe, MD, FAANS
Alexander R. Vaccaro, MD, PhD, MBA
Mark S. Greenberg, MD, FAANS

Acknowledgments

The editors would like to thank all authors for contributing to this new text. We also thank the entire team at Thieme Publishers for the continued partnership, especially Cathrin Weinstein and Karen Edmonson.

Ali A. Baaj, MD
Praveen V. Mummaneni, MD, MBA
Juan S. Uribe, MD, FAANS
Alexander R. Vaccaro, MD, PhD, MBA
Mark S. Greenberg, MD, FAANS

Contributors

Alexander Aabedi, MD
Resident Physician
Department of Neurological Surgery
University of California, San Francisco
San Francisco, California, USA

Muhammad M. Abd-El-Barr, MD, PhD
Associate Professor
Department of Neurosurgery
Duke University Medical Center
Durham, North Carolina, USA

Ebubechi Adindu, MD
Orthopaedic Surgery Resident
Department of Surgery and Perioperative Care
University of Texas at Austin – Dell
Austin, Texas, USA

Nitin Agarwal, MD
Associate Professor;
Associate Program Director, Neurological Surgery Residency
Department of Neurological Surgery
University of Pittsburgh
Pittsburgh, Pennsylvania, USA

Pedro Aguilar-Salinas, MD
Neurosurgery Resident
Department of Neurosurgery
University of Arizona/Banner University Medical Center
Tucson, Arizona, USA

Salah A. Alakkad, MBBS, FRCSC, FACS, FAANS, DABNS
Consultant & Head
Neurospinal Surgery Unit
Johns Hopkins Aramco Healthcare
Dhahran, Saudi Arabia

Nima Alan, MD
Assistant Professor
Department of Neurological Surgery
University of California, San Francisco
San Francisco, California, USA

Ahmet Alanay, MD
Professor
Department of Orthopedics and Traumatology
Acibadem University School of Medicine
Istanbul, Turkey

Puya Alikhani, MD, FAANS
Director of Spine Division
Department of Neurosurgery and Brain Repair
USF Health;
Vice Chair
Department of Neurosurgery
Tampa General Hospital
Tampla, Florida, USA

Samuel Ammerman, BSc
Medical Student
Department of Neurosurgery
The Ohio State University
Columbus, Ohio, USA

Ivan Angelov, BA, MD Candidate
Student
Business and Economics
University of California, Los Angeles
Los Angeles, California, USA;
Baylor College of Medicine
Houston, Texas, USA

Mauricio J. Avila, MD
Assistant Professor
Department of Neurosurgery
Saint Louis University
St. Louis, Missouri, USA

Ali A. Baaj, MD
Professor of Neurosurgery and Chief of Spine Surgery
Department of Neurosurgery
University of Arizona, College of Medicine
Phoenix, Arizona, USA

Saleh Baeesa, MD, FRCSC
Professor of Neurosurgery
Department of Neurosciences
King Faisal Specialist Hospital and Research Center
Jeddah, Saudi Arabia

Edward L. Baldwin III, MD
Spine Surgeon
Department of Orthopaedic Surgery
Houston Methodist West Hospital
Houston, Texas, USA

Michelle Barrera-Arreola, MD
Clinical Researcher
Spine Clinic, Neurosurgery Department
Hospital Ángeles Centro Sur
Querétaro City, Mexico

Arnau Benet, MD, PhD
Neurosurgery Resident
Department of Neurosurgery
Barrow Neurological Institute, St. Joseph's Hospital and Medical Center
Phoenix, Arizona, USA

Stephen M. Bergin, MD, PhD
Neurosurgery Resident
Department of Neurosurgery
Duke University
Durham, North Carolina, USA

Venkat Boddapati, MD
Spine
Department of Orthopedic Surgery
Hospital for Special Surgery
New York, New York, USA

Christopher M. Bono, MD
Executive Vice Chair;
Professor of Orthopaedic Surgery
Department of Orthopaedic Surgery
Massachusetts General Hospital
Harvard Medical School
Boston, Massachusetts, USA

Jose A. Canseco, MD, PhD
Assistant Professor
Department of Orthopaedic Surgery
Rothman Institute at Thomas Jefferson University
Philadelphia, Pennsylvania, USA

Matthew T. Carr, MD
Resident Physician
Department of Neurosurgery
Icahn School of Medicine at Mount Sinai
New York, New York, USA

Eric Chalif, MD
Resident
Department of Neurosurgery
Brigham and Women's Hospital
Boston, Massachusetts, USA

Joshua Chalif, MD, PhD
Resident
Department of Neurosurgery
Brigham and Women's Hospital
Boston, Massachusetts, USA

Kelly Chamberlin, MD, MSCR
Resident Physician
Department of Neurosurgery
University of North Carolina
Chapel Hill, North Carolina, USA

Andrew K. Chan, MD
Assistant Professor;
Co-Director of Minimally Invasive Scoliosis Surgery;
Director of Neurosurgical Spine Research
Department of Neurological Surgery
Columbia University Vagelos College of Physicians and Surgeons;
Och Spine Hospital at New York-Presbyterian
New York, New York, USA

Steve W. Chang, MD
Associate Professor
Department of Neurosurgery
Barrow Neurological Institute, St. Joseph's Hospital and Medical Center
Phoenix, Arizona, USA

Dean Chou, MD
Professor and Vice Chair;
Chief, Spine Division
Department of Neurosurgery
Columbia University/Och Spine Hospital
New York, New York, USA

Timothy Chryssikos, MD, PhD
Assistant Professor
Department of Neurosurgery
University of Maryland
Baltimore, Maryland, USA

Melissa M. J. Chua, MD
Resident Physician
Department of Neurosurgery
Harvard Medical School/Brigham and Women's Hospital
Boston, Massachusetts, USA

John Clayton Clohisy Jr, MD
Assistant Professor
Department of Orthopaedic Surgery
Washington University in St. Louis
St. Louis, Missouri, USA

Ian David Connolly, MD, MS
Resident
Department of Neurosurgery
Massachusetts General Hospital
Boston, Massachusetts, USA

Jean-Valery Coumans, MD
Assistant Professor
Department of Neurosurgery
Harvard Medical School
Boston, Massachusetts, USA

Josephine Coury, MD
Resident;
Orthopedic Spine Fellow
Department of Spine Surgery
Och Spine Hospital at Columbia
New York Presbyterian
New York, New York, USA

Nader S. Dahdaleh, MD, MS
Associate Professor
Department of Neurological Surgery
Northwestern University
Chicago, Illinois, USA

Nuri Demirci, MBBS
School of Medicine
Acibadem University
Istanbul, Turkey

Rajakumar V. Deshpande, MCh
Director and Head of Department
Department of Neurosurgery
Fortis Hospitals
Bangalore, Karnataka, India

Ashish D. Diwan, MBBS, MS(Orth), DNB(Orth), FRACS, FAOrthA, PhD
Director of Spine Service and Spine Labs
Department of Orthopaedic Surgery, St George Hospital Campus
The University of New South Wales
Kogarah, Sydney, Australia

Galal A. Elsayed, MD
Assistant Professor
Department of Neurological Surgery
Weill Cornell Medicine
Och Spine at NewYork-Presbyterian
New York, New York, USA

Juan Emmerich, MD
Professor
Department of Neurosurgery
National University of La Plata
La Plata, Buenos Aires, Argentina

S. Harrison Farber, MD
Chief Resident
Department of Neurosurgery
Barrow Neurological Institute
Phoenix, Arizona, USA

Mark A. Feger, MD, PhD
Department of Orthopedic Surgery
Washington University in St. Louis
St. Louis, Missouri, USA

Brian Fiani, DO, FACOS
Neurosurgeon
Department of Neurosurgery
Mendelson Kornblum Orthopedics and Spine Specialists
Livonia, Michigan, USA

TJ Florence, MD, PhD
Resident
Department of Neurosurgery
University of California, Los Angeles
Los Angeles, California, USA

Jared Fridley, MD
Associate Professor
Department of Neurosurgery
Warren Alpert Medical School of Brown University
Providence, Rhode Island, USA

Jeff Gadsden, MD, FRCPC, FANZCA
Anesthesiologist
Department of Anesthesiology
Duke University
Durham, North Carolina, USA

Michael Galgano, MD, FAANS, FCNS
Associate Professor of Neurosurgery;
Director, Spinal Oncology & Deformity Surgery
University of North Carolina
Chapel Hill, North Carolina, USA

Marisa Gandía, MD, PhD
Neurosurgeon
Department of Neurosurgery
University Hospital La Paz
Madrid, Spain

George M. Ghobrial, MD, FAANS
Neurological Surgeon
Department of Neurological Surgery
Pikeville Medical Center
Pikeville, Kentucky, USA

Ziya Gokaslan, MD
Chairman and Neurosurgeon in Chief
Department of Neurosurgery
Brown Medical School – Rhode Island Hospital
Providence, Rhode Island, USA

Glenn A. Gonzalez, MD
Postdoctoral Research Fellow
Department of Neurological Surgery
Thomas Jefferson University Hospital
Philadelphia, Pennsylvania, USA

C. Rory Goodwin, MD, PhD
Associate Professor of Neurosurgery, Radiation Oncology, Orthopedic Surgery;
Director of Spine Oncology;
Associate Residency Program Director;
Third Year Study Program Director Neurosciences, Duke University School of Medicine;
Director of Spine Metastasis, Duke Center for Brain and Spine Metastasis
Department of Neurosurgery
Duke Cancer Institute, Duke University Medical Center
Durham, North Carolina, USA

Matthew L. Goodwin, MD, PhD, FACSM
Assistant Professor
Department of Orthopedic Surgery
Washington University School of Medicine
St. Louis, Missouri, USA

Mark S. Greenberg, MD, FAANS
Associate Professor
Neurosurgery Residency Training Program Director
Department of Neurosurgery and Brain Repair
University of South Florida, Morsani College of Medicine
Tampa, Florida, USA

Jeffrey P. Greenfield, MD, PhD
Professor of Neurological Surgery in Pediatrics
Department of Neurosurgery
Weill Cornell Medicine
New York, New York, USA

Andrew J. Grossbach, MD
Associate Clinical Professor
Department of Neurosurgery
The Ohio State University
Columbus, Ohio, USA

Dhanesh K. Gupta, MD, MBA, FASA
Professor
Department of Anesthesiology
Duke University School of Medicine
Durham, North Carolina, USA

Muhamed Hadzipasic, MD, PhD
Resident
Department of Neurosurgery
Massachusetts General Hospital
Boston, Massachusetts, USA

Sabastian Hajtovic, MD
Resident Physician
Department of Neurosurgery
North Shore University Hospital, Northwell Health
Manhasset, New York, USA

Colin B. Harris, MD
Spine Surgeon
Department of Orthopedic Surgery
Atlantic Medical Group Orthopedics, Atlantic Health System
Paramus, New Jersey, USA

James S. Harrop, MD, MSHQS, FACS
Professor, Depts of Neurological and Orthopedic Surgery;
Professor, College of Population Health;
Chief, Division of Spine and Peripheral Nerve Surgery;
Director, Enterprise Neuroscience Quality and Safety;
Neurosurgery Director of Delaware Valley SCI Center;
Professor of Public Health
Thomas Jefferson University
Philadelphia, Pennsylvania, USA

Jeremy C. Heard, MD
Research Fellow
Department of Orthopaedic Surgery
Rothman Institute at Thomas Jefferson University
Philadelphia, Pennsylvania, USA

Andrew M. Hersh, MD
Resident
Department of Neurosurgery
Johns Hopkins School of Medicine
Baltimore, Maryland, USA

Christoph Hofstetter, MD, PhD
Professor
Department of Neurological Surgery
University of Washington
Seattle, Washington, USA

Holli A. Horak, MD
Professor
Department of Neurology
University of Arizona College of Medicine – Tucson
Tucson, Arizona, USA

Brian Q. Hou, BA
Medical Student
School of Medicine
Vanderbilt University
Nashville, Tennessee, USA

Mohamad Nabih El Houshiemy, MD
Neurosurgeon
Department of Neurosurgery
American University of Beirut Medical Center
Beirut, Lebanon

Amna Hussein, MD
Research Fellow
Department of Neurosurgery
Banner University Medical Center Phoenix
University of Arizona
Phoenix, Arizona, USA

Steven W. Hwang, MD
Staff Neurosurgeon
Department of Neurosurgery
Shriners Children's Philadelphia
Philadelphia, Pennsylvania, USA

Alysha Jamieson, BA
Researcher
Department of Neurological Surgery
University of California, San Francisco
San Francisco, California, USA

Aria Jamshidi, MD
Chief Resident
Department of Neurosurgery
University of Miami/Jackson Memorial Hospital
Miami, Florida, USA

Andrew Jea, MD, MBA, MHA
Professor and Interim Chair
Department of Neurosurgery
The University of Oklahoma College of Medicine
Oklahoma City, Oklahoma, USA

Brendan F. Judy, MD
Neurosurgery Resident
Department of Neurosurgery
Johns Hopkins University School of Medicine
Baltimore, Maryland, USA

Chaitanya Prabhu K., MCh
Neurosurgeon
Department of Neurosurgery
Fortis Hospitals
Bangalore, Karnataka, India

Sarah Kawtharani, MD
Neurosurgery Resident
Department of Neurosurgery
American University of Beirut Medical Center
Beirut, Lebanon

Alexander Keister, BS
Department of Neurological Surgery
The Ohio State University College of Medicine
Columbus, Ohio, USA

Christopher K. Kepler, MD, MBA
Professor
Department of Orthopaedic Surgery
Rothman Institute at Thomas Jefferson University
Philadelphia, Pennsylvania, USA

Asham Khan, MD
Resident
Department of Neurosurgery
University at Buffalo
Williamsville, New York, USA

Cameron Kia, MD
Orthopaedic Spine Surgeon
Department of Orthopaedic Surgery
Orthopaedic Associates of Hartford, Bone and Joint Institute of Hartford Hospital
Hartford, Connecticut, USA

Han Jo Kim, MD
Professor of Orthopedic Surgery;
David B Levine, MD Endowed Chair
Department of Spine Surgery
Hospital for Special Surgery
New York, New York, USA

Eric Klineberg, MD, MS
Professor and Vice Chair;
Chief of Orthopaedic Spine Surgery;
Milton "Chip" Routt Endowed Chair of Spinal Surgery
Department of Orthopaedic Surgery
UTHealth Houston, McGovern Medical School
Houston, Texas, USA

Kevin Kwan, MD
Doctor
Department of Spine Surgery
Och Spine Hospital at Columbia New York Presbyterian
New York, New York, USA

Raj Swaroop Lavadi, MBBS
Postdoctoral Research Fellow
Department of Neurological Surgery
University of Pittsburgh School of Medicine
Pittsburgh, Pennsylvania, USA

Hai Le, MD, MPH
Associate Professor;
Spine Fellowship Program Director
Department of Orthopaedic Surgery
UC Davis Medical Center
Sacramento, California, USA

Joon Y. Lee, MD
Orland Bethel Endowed Professor
Department of Orthopedics Surgery
Division of Spinal Surgery;
Clinical Director, Ferguson Laboratory;
Executive Director, Bethel MSK Research Center
University of Pittsburgh School of Medicine
Pittsburgh, Pennsylvania, USA

Yunsoo Lee, MD
Spine Fellow
Department of Orthopaedic Surgery
Rothman Institute at Thomas Jefferson University
Philadelphia, Pennsylvania, USA

Lawrence G. Lenke, MD
Co-Director, Och Spine;
Surgeon in Chief
Department of Spine Surgery
Och Spine Hospital at Columbia New York Presbyterian
New York, New York, USA

Vijay Letchuman, MD
Resident Physician
Department of Neurological Surgery
University of California, San Francisco
San Francisco, California, USA

Allan D. Levi, MD, PhD
Professor and Chairman
Department of Neurosurgery
University of Miami
Miami, Florida, USA

Anran Li, MD
Resident
Department of Neurological Surgery
Northwestern University
Chicago, Illinois, USA

Yi Lu, MD, PhD
Associate Professor;
Spine Fellowship Program Director
Department of Neurosurgery
Harvard Medical School/Brigham and Women's Hospital
Boston, Massachusetts, USA

Joseph Maalouly, MD
Clinical Assistant Professor
Department of Orthopedic and Spine Surgery
University of Balamand
Notre dame university hospital
Jounieh, Keserwan, Lebanon

Mohamed Macki, MD, MPH
Spine Surgeon
Department of Neurological Surgery
Cleveland Clinic Foundation
Mayfield Heights, Ohio, USA

Yazid Maghrabi, MBBS, SBNS
Staff Neurosurgeon
Department of Neuroscience
King Abdelaziz Medical City, Ministry of the National Guard-Health Affairs
Jeddah, Saudi Arabia

Glen R. Manzano, MD, FAANS
Neurosurgeon
Miami, Florida, USA

Frank La Marca, MD
Neurosurgeon
Department of Neurosurgery
Henry Ford Medical Center
Jackson, Michigan, USA

Cristiano Magalhães Menezes, MD, PhD
Professor
Department of Locomotor Apparatus, School of Medicine
Federal University of Minas Gerais (UFMG)
Belo Horizonte, Brazil

Alim P. Mitha, MD, SM
Associate Professor
Department of Clinical Neurosciences
University of Calgary
Calgary, Alberta, Canada

Camilo A. Molina, MD
Assistant Professor;
Director of Spinal Deformity and Spinal Oncology
Department of Neurosurgery
Washington University School of Medicine
St. Louis, Missouri, USA

Eric Momin, MD
Neurosurgeon
Department of Neurosurgery
Intermountain Health, St. Mary's Hospital
Grand Junction, Colorado, USA

Charbel Moussalem, MD, MSc
Fellow
Department of Neurosurgery
Mayo Clinic Rochester
Rochester, Minnesota, USA

Praveen V. Mummaneni, MD, MBA
Joan O'Reilly Distinguished Professor and Vice Chair
Department of Neurological Surgery
University of California, San Francisco
San Francisco, California, USA

Mohammad Hassan A. Noureldine, MD, MSc
Resident Physician
Department of Neurosurgery and Brain Repair
University of South Florida
Tampa, Florida, USA

Jose Manuel Orenday-Barraza, MD
Resident
Department of General Surgery
University of Minnesota
Minneapolis, Minnesota, USA

Murali Krishna P., MCh
Neurosurgeon
Department of Neurosurgery
Fortis Hospitals
Bangalore, Karnataka, India

Paul Park, MD
Professor and Neurosurgeon
Department of Neurosurgery
Semmes Murphey Clinic
Memphis, Tennessee, USA

Kamakshi Patel, MD, MPH
Associate Professor
Department of Neurology
Michael DeBakey Veterans Affairs Medical Center;
Department of Neurology
Baylor College of Medicine
Houston, Texas, USA

Karan S. Patel, MD
Spine Surgeon
Department of Orthopedic Surgery
Orthopedic Partners, Hartford HealthCare
North Franklin, Connecticut, USA

Kalaventhan Pathinathan, MBBS, MD
Research Fellow
Department of Orthopaedic Surgery
St. George Hospital Campus
Sydney, New South Wales, Australia;
Consultant Orthopaedic surgeon
Department of Orthopaedics and Trauma
Base Hospital-Kalmunai
Ampara District, Sri Lanka

Anirudh Penumaka, MD, MSc
Junior Attending
Department of Neurological Surgery
The Warren Alpert Medical School, Brown University
Providence, Rhode Island, USA

Frank M. Phillips, MD
Ronald Dewald Endowed Professor of Spinal Deformities;
Spine Fellowship Director
Department of Orthopedic Surgery
Rush University Medical Center
Chicago, Illinois, USA

Woralux Phusoongnern, MD
Neurosurgeon
Chiang Mai Neurological Hospital
Chiang Mai, Thailand

Martin G. Piazza, MD
Assistant Professor
Department of Neurological Surgery
University of Pittsburgh
Medical Center
Pittsburgh, Pennsylvania, USA

John Pollina, MD
Professor
Department of Neurosurgery
University at Buffalo
Buffalo, New York, USA

Dhiraj Kumar Poonia, DNB
Neurosurgeon
Department of Neurosurgery
Fortis Hospitals
Bangalore, Karnataka, India

Esteban Quiceno
Research Fellow
Department of Neurosurgery
University at Buffalo
Buffalo, New York, USA

Javier Quillo-Olvera, MD
Spinal Neurosurgeon and
Associate Professor
Department of Neurology
Anáhuac University, Querétaro City;
Spine Clinic, Neurosurgery
Department
Hospital Ángeles Centro Sur
Querétaro City, Mexico

Javier Quillo-Reséndiz, MD
Neurosurgeon
Spine Clinic, Neurosurgery
Department
Hospital Ángeles Centro Sur
Querétaro City, Mexico

Prashanth J. Rao, MBBS, FRACS, PhD
Neurosurgeon
Department of Neurosurgery
University of New South Wales;
Neurosurgeon
Department of Neurosurgery
Norwest Private Hospital
New South Wales, Australia

Jonathan J. Rasouli, MD
Assistant Professor
Department of Neurosurgery
Northwell Health/Hosftra
University School of Medicine
Staten Island, New York, USA

Azeem A. Rehman, MD
Director of Minimally Invasive
Spine Surgery
Department of Neurosciences
Intent Medical Group
Arlington Heights, Illinois, USA

Leslie Robinson, MD, PharmD, MBA
Medical Director
Department of Neurosurgery
Enloe Health
Chico, California, USA

Miguel A. Ruiz-Cardozo, MD
Postdoctoral Research Associate
Department of Neurosurgery
Washington University in St. Louis
St. Louis, Missouri, USA

Comron Saifi, MD
Spine Surgeon
Department of Orthopedics and Sports Medicine
Houston Methodist Hospital
Houston, Texas, USA;
Associate Professor
Department of Orthopaedic Surgery
Weill Cornell Medicine Medical College
New York, New York, USA;
Adjunct Clinical Associate Professor
Department of Orthopaedic Surgery
Texas A&M University
College Station, Texas, USA

Rajiv Saigal, MD, PhD
Associate Professor
Department of Neurological Surgery
University of California, San Francisco
San Francisco, California, USA

Marlus Sérgio Borges Salomão Junior, MD
Surgeon Assistant
Department of Spine surgery
Columna Institute
Belo Horizonte, Brazil

Amer F. Samdani, MD
Chief of Surgery
Shriners Children's Philadelphia
Philadelphia, Pennsylvania, USA

Gregory D. Schroeder, MD
Department of Orthopedic Surgery
Thomas Jefferson University
Philadelphia, Pennsylvania, USA

Theodore H. Schwartz, MD
David and Ursel Barnes Professor of Minimally Invasive Neurosurgery
Department of Neurosurgery
Weill Cornell Medicine
New York, New York, USA

Cara Sedney, MD, MA
Associate Professor
Department of Neurosurgery
West Virginia University
Morgantown, West Virginia, USA

Ganesh M. Shankar, MD, PhD
Assistant Professor
Department of Neurosurgery
Massachusetts General Hospital
Boston, Massachusetts, USA

Jeremy D. Shaw, MD, MS
Associate Professor
Department of Orthopaedic Surgery
University of Pittsburgh
Pittsburgh, Pennsylvania, USA

Yong Shen, MD
Researcher
Department of Orthopedic Surgery
Columbia University Irving Medical Center
New York, New York, USA;
Resident Physician
Department of Orthopaedic Surgery
Johns Hopkins Medicine
Baltimore, Maryland, USA

John H. Shin, MD
Department of Neurosurgery
Massachusetts General Hospital
Boston, Massachusetts, USA

Quante Singleton, BS, MD
Resident physician
Department of Orthopedic Surgery
Washington University in St. Louis
Stockbridge, Georgia, USA

Ahilan Sivaganesan, MD
Department of Neurosurgery
Thomas Jefferson University
Philadelphia, Pennsylvania, USA

Sananthan Sivakanthan, MD
Resident Physician
Department of Neurological Surgery
University of Washington
Seattle, Washington, USA

Zachary A. Smith, MD
Professor with Tenure;
Vice Chair of Neurosurgery;
Vice Chair of Research;
Director of Minimally Invasive Spine Surgery;
Co-Director Neuroscience
Department of Neurosurgery
The University of Oklahoma Health Sciences Center
Oklahoma City, Oklahoma, USA

Mohamed A. R. Soliman, MD, MSc, PhD
Clinical Fellow
Department of Neurosurgery
University at Buffalo
Buffalo, New York, USA;
Associate Professor
Department of Neurosurgery
Cairo University
Cairo, Egypt

Omar Sorour, BA, MD
Researcher
Department of Neurosurgery
UCSF
San Francisco, California, USA;
Neurosurgery Resident
Tufts Medical Center
Boston, Massachusetts, USA

Jeremy Steinberger, MD
Associate Professor
Department of Neurological Surgery
Icahn School of Medicine at Mount Sinai
New York, New York, USA

Byron F. Stephens, MD, MSCI
Program Director, Orthopaedic Surgery;
Division Chief, Orthopaedic Spine Surgery;
Associate Professor of Orthopaedic Surgery and Neurosurgery
Vanderbilt University Medical Center
Nashville, Tennessee, USA

Mark Stephens, MD, MBA
Resident
Department of Neurosurgery
University of Oklahoma
Oklahoma City, Oklahoma, USA

Martina Stippler, MD
Associate Professor and Director of Neurotrauma
Department of Neurosurgery
Harvard Medical School/ BIDMC
Boston, Massachusetts, USA

Tarek P. Sunna', MD, FACS, FEBNS, FRCS
Assistant Professor
Department of Neurosurgery
American University of Beirut Medical Center
Beirut, Lebanon;
Head of Neurosurgery
Department of Neurosurgery
Aman Hospital
Doha, Qatar

David A. W. Sykes, MD
Resident Physician
Department of Neurosurgery
Weill Cornell Medical Center
New York, New York, USA

Melissa Yunting Tang, MD
Resident Physician
Department of Orthopedic Surgery
University of Pittsburgh Medical Center
Pittsburgh, Pennsylvania, USA

Khoi D. Than, MD
Professor of Neurosurgery
Department of Neurosurgery
Duke University
Durham, North Carolina, USA

Nicholas Theodore, MD, MS
Professor of Neurosurgery, Orthopaedic Surgery, and Biomedical Engineering
Department of Neurosurgery
Johns Hopkins University School of Medicine
Baltimore, Maryland, USA

Umberto Tosi, MD
Resident
Department of Neurosurgery
Weill Cornell Medicine
New York, New York, USA

Ansley Unterberger, MD
Resident
Department of Neurosurgery
Mt Sinai
New York, New York, USA

Juan S. Uribe, MD, FAANS
Professor and Vice Chair;
Chief of Division of Spinal Disorders;
Volker K. H. Sonntag Chair of Spine Research
Department of Neurological Surgery
Barrow Neurological Institute
Phoenix, Arizona, USA

Timothy D. Uschold, MD
Neurosurgeon
Department of Neurosurgery
Barrow Neurological Institute, St. Joseph's Hospital and Medical Center
Phoenix, Arizona, USA

Alexander R. Vaccaro, MD, PhD, MBA
President of Rothman Orthopedic Institute
Chair of Orthopaedic Surgery at Thomas Jefferson University
Department of Orthopaedic Spine
Rothman Orthopaedic Institute at Thomas Jefferson University Hospital
Philadelphia, Pennsylvania, USA

Juan M. Valdivia, MD
Chief of Neurosurgery
Department of Neurosurgery
BayCare Medical Group
Tampa, Florida, USA

Wilson E. Vaughan, MS
Research Fellow
Department of Orthopedic Surgery
Vanderbilt University Medical Center
Nashville, Tennessee, USA

Emiliano Vialle, MD, MSc, PhD
Head of Orthopedics;
Head of Spine Surgery
Spine Surgery Group
Cajuru Hospital, Catholic
University of Parana
Curitiba, Parana, Brazil

Joshua Vignolles-Jeong, BA
Department of Neurosurgery
The Ohio State University
Columbus, Ohio, USA

Lance Villeneuve, MD, PhD
Neurosurgery Resident Physician
Department of Neurosurgery
University of Oklahoma Health
Sciences Center
Oklahoma City, Oklahoma, USA

Jose Manuel Viñuela-Prieto, MD
Neurosurgeon
Department of Neurosurgery
Hospital Universitario La Paz
Madrid, Spain

Andrew C. Vivas, MD
Assistant Professor
Department of Neurosurgery
University of California, Los Angeles
Los Angeles, California, USA

Wyatt D. Vander Voort, MD
Resident
Department of Orthopaedic Surgery
University of California Davis
Medical Center
Sacramento, California, USA

W. Hunter Waddell, BS, MD
Orthopedic Surgery Resident
Department of Orthopedic Surgery
Vanderbilt University Medical Center
Nashville, Tennessee, USA

Michael Y. Wang, MD, MBA
Professor
Department of Neurosurgery
University of Miami
Miami, Florida, USA

James D. Whaley, MD
Orthopaedic Spine Surgeon
Department of Orthopaedic Surgery
Bon Secours Mercy Health
Greenville, South Carolina, USA

Alexandra J. White, MD, MA
Resident Physician
Department of Neurosurgery
University of California, Los Angeles
Los Angeles, California, USA

Michael D. White, MD
Neurosurgery Resident
Department of Neurosurgery
Barrow Neurological Institute and
St. Joseph's Hospital and Medical
Center
Phoenix, Arizona, USA

Joseph Wick, MD
Spine Surgeon
Department of Orthopedic Surgery
TRIA Orthopedics/Health Partners
Woodbury, Minnesota, USA

Theresa Williamson, MD, MPH
Assistant Professor
Department of Neurosurgery
Massachusetts General Hospital
Boston, Massachusetts, USA

Jean-Paul Wolinsky, MD
Professor and Vice-Chairman
Department of Neurosurgery
Northwestern University
Chicago, Illinois, USA

Grace X. Xiong, MD
Orthopaedic Spine Fellow
Department of Orthopaedic Surgery
Rothman Orthopaedic Institute/Thomas Jefferson University
Philadelphia, Pennsylvania, USA

Alexander T. Yahanda, MD
Resident
Department of Neurosurgery
Washington University School of Medicine in St. Louis
St. Louis, Missouri, USA

Michael J. Yang, MD
Resident
Department of Neurosurgery
Tufts Medical Center
Boston, Massachusetts, USA

Caglar Yilgor, MD
Associate Professor
Department of Orthopedics and Traumatology
Acibadem University School of Medicine
Istanbul, Turkey

Altug Yucekul, MD
Associate Professor
Department of Orthopedics and Traumatology
Acibadem University School of Medicine
Istanbul, Turkey

Frank J. Yuk, MD
Attending Neurosurgeon
Department of Neurosurgery
Neurosurgical Consultants
Owensboro, Kentucky, USA

Hasan Zaidi, MD
Director, Adult Deformity/Scoliosis Center;
Associate Professor
Department of Neurosurgery
Brigham and Women's Hospital
Boston, Massachusetts, USA

Xiaochun Zhao, MD
Neurosurgery Resident Physician
Department of Neurosurgery
University of Oklahoma Health Sciences Center
Oklahoma City, Oklahoma, USA

James J. Zhou, MD, PhD
Neurosurgery Resident
Department of Neurosurgery
Barrow Neurological Institute, St. Joseph's Hospital and Medical Center
Phoenix, Arizona, USA

I
Anatomy

1 Craniovertebral Junction

Nader S. Dahdaleh

Summary

The craniocervical junction is composed of two joints, the atlanto-occipital and atlantoaxial joints along with their surrounding ligamentous and muscular attachments.

Keywords: craniocervical junction, craniovertebral junction, atlas, axis

1.1 Key Points

- The craniovertebral junction (CVJ) is composed of the occiput (O), atlas (C1), and axis (C2) along with the atlantoaxial and atlantooccipital joints (**Fig. 1.1**).
- The CVJ is a very flexible junction accounting for at least 50% of the range of motion of the cervical spine in all planes. The joint orientation determines the direction of motion, and the ligaments determine the biomechanical stability of this junction (**Fig. 1.2**).

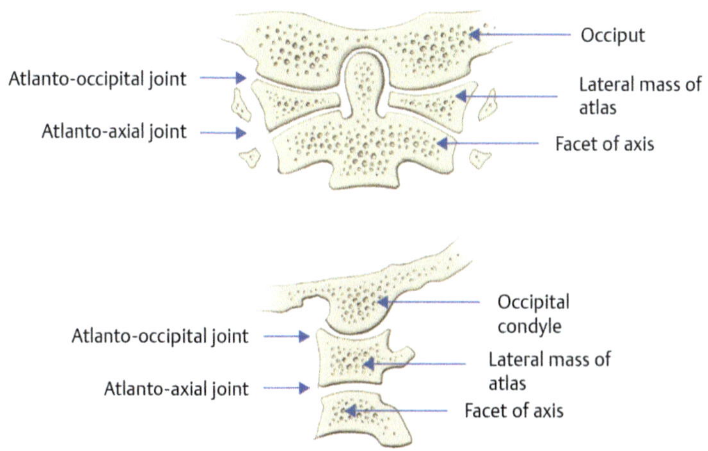

Fig. 1.1 Craniovertebral junction (CVJ) anterior (top) and lateral (bottom) views.

Motion	OC–C1	C1–2
Flexion/Extension	23°–24.5°	10.1°–22.4°
Lateral bending	3.4°–5.5°	6.7°
Axial rotation	2.4°–7.2°	23.3°–38.9°

Fig. 1.2 Craniovertebral junction (CVJ) range of motion.

1.2 Bony Anatomy

- The CVJ consists of the base of the occiput, the atlas (C1), and the axis (C2).
- The foramen magnum boundaries consist of the basion anteriorly, the opisthion posteriorly, and the occipital condyles anterolaterally.
- The atlas (C1) is composed of an anterior arch, a posterior arch, and two lateral masses (**Fig. 1.3**).
- The atlantooccipital joint is cup like in the coronal and sagittal plane allowing for flexion/extension and little axial rotation.
- The C1 anterior tubercle is the attachment site of the anterior longitudinal ligament (ALL) and the longus coli muscle.
- The vertebral artery (VA) and C1 nerve run along the superior lateral groove on C1 (sulcus arteriosus). In less than 15% of the population, the groove is roofed, forming the arcuate foramen.
- The axis (C2) consists of the body, odontoid process (dens), articulating surfaces, pedicles, pars interarticularis lamina, and large, bifid spinous process (**Fig. 1.4**).
- The atlantoaxial joint is convex in orientation allowing for axial rotation about the dens.

1.3 Neural Anatomy

- Cervical nerve roots exit above their corresponding level (e.g., the C2 nerve root exits above the C2 pedicle).
- C1 nerve root: The posterior division (suboccipital nerve) is more prominent than the anterior division. It innervates suboccipital muscles and occasionally branches to the lesser/greater occipital nerve.
- C2 nerve root: Posterior, medial (greater occipital nerve), and lateral divisions innervate suboccipital muscles and scalp from occiput to vertex. It may be sacrificed during atlantoaxial or occipitocervical fusions to enhance the exposure of the lateral mass for lateral mass screw placement and/or to access the atlantoaxial joint for direct arthrodesis.
- The lesser occipital nerve is formed by dorsal divisions of C2 and C3.

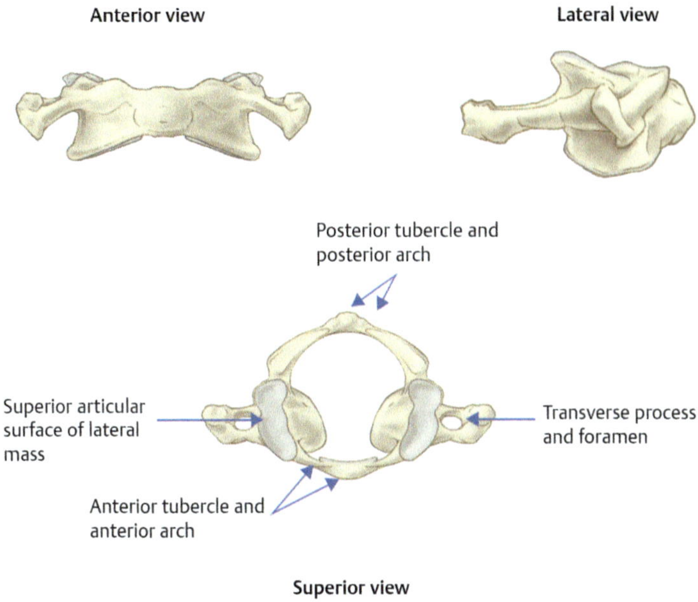

Fig. 1.3 The atlas.

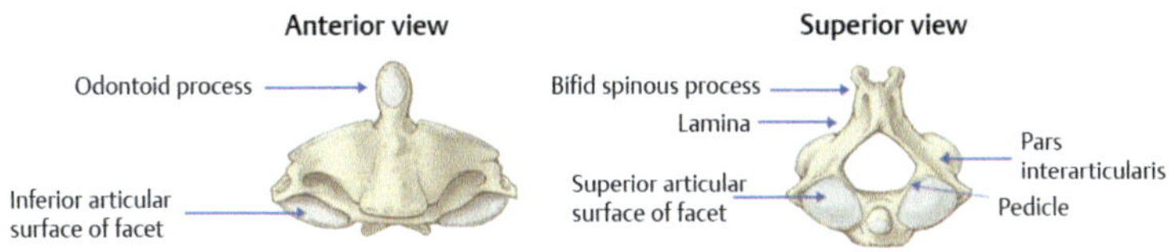

Fig. 1.4 The axis.

1.4 Vascular Anatomy

- The voluminous vertebral venous plexus that surrounds the horizontal portion of the V3 segment of the VA is encased in the suboccipital fascia. If the planes of dissection are respected, the plexus can be preemptively coagulated during exposure of the CVJ.
- The VA leaves the C2 transverse foramen (becoming V3). It takes a 45 degrees lateral projection and ascends (vertical portion of V3) into the C1 transverse foramen.

- The VA then courses medially (horizontal portion of V3) along the C1 sulcus arteriosus and then anteriorly through the atlantooccipital membrane, where it becomes intradural (beginning of V4 segment).
- Blood is supplied to the CVJ primarily through branches of the vertebral and occipital arteries.
- Blood supply to the CVJ emanate from extensions of the VA from the subaxial spine. The anterior and posterior ascending arteries branch from the VA at C2–C3, entering the vertebral column supplying the axis before anastomosing to form the apical odontoid arcade that supplies the atlas and dens.

The occipital artery completes the superior portion of the arcade.

- Lymphatic drainage of the CVJ is through retropharyngeal and deep cervical nodes.

1.5 Muscular Anatomy (Table 1.1)

- Muscular layers:
  - Superficial:
    - Trapezius.
    - Sternocleidomastoid.
  - Intermediate:
    - Splenius capitis.
  - Deep:
    - Semispinalis capitis.
  - Deepest (suboccipital muscles and triangle): The following muscles comprise the borders of the suboccipital triangle:
    - Rectus capitis posterior major and minor: Medial.
    - Obliquus capitis superior: Lateral.
    - Obliquus capitis inferior: Inferior.

1.6 Ligamentous Anatomy (Table 1.2)

The anterior ligaments can be divided into four layers. From anterior to posterior[1,2]:

- 1st layer: Atlantooccipital membrane.
- 2nd layer: Apical and alar ligaments.
- 3rd layer: Cruciate ligament (superior curx, transverse atlantal, and inferior crux).
- 4th layer: Tectorial membrane (continuation of PLL).

The biomechanical stability of the CVJ is primarily derived from its ligamentous attachments. The ligaments that contribute the most to its stability are

Table 1.1 Craniovertebral junction musculature: their attachments and modes of action

Muscle	Attachments	Action
Trapezius	Origin: Occipital bone, the ligamentum nuchae, and the spinous processes of T01–T12 Insertion: Lateral third of the clavicle and the scapula (acromion and scapular spine)	Stabilize and move the scapula
Sternocleidomastoid muscle (SCM)	Origin: Sternum, clavicle Insertion: Temporal bone (mastoid process), occipital bone	Contralateral head rotation, neck flexion
Splenius capitis	Origin: Lower half of the nuchal ligament and the spinous processes of C7–T3 vertebrae Insertion: Temporal bone (mastoid process), occipital bone	Unilaterally: Lateral bending and rotation of head to ipsilateral side Bilaterally: Extension of the head and cervical spine
Semispinalis capitis	Origin: Transverse and articular processes of C4–C7, transverse processes of T1–T6 Insertion: Between superior and inferior nuchal lines of occipital bone	Unilaterally: Lateral bending and rotation of head to ipsilateral side Extension, rotation, and lateral bending of head and cervical spine
Rectus capitis posterior major and minor	Origin: Posterior tubercle of atlas (minor), spinous process of C2 (major) Insertion: Medial part of inferior nuchal line of occipital bone	Bilateral contraction at the atlantooccipital joint: Head extension Unilateral contraction at the atlantoaxial joint: Head rotation (ipsilateral)
Obliquus capitis superior muscle of occipital bone (between superior and inferior nuchal lines)	Origin: Transverse process of atlas Insertion: Occipital bone (between superior and inferior nuchal lines)	Bilateral contraction at atlantooccipital joint: Head extension Unilateral contraction at atlantoaxial joint: Head lateral flexion (ipsilateral)

(Continued)

Table 1.1 (*Continued*)

Muscle	Attachments	Action
Obliquus capitis inferior	Origin: Spinous process and lamina of axis Insertion: Inferior aspect of the tip of the transverse process of the atlas	Rotation at the atlantoaxial joint

Table 1.2 Principal craniovertebral junction ligaments: their attachments and modes of action

Ligament	Attachments	Action
Apical	Odontoid tip (superiorly) to basion in apical cave	No significant function
Alar (paired)	Occipital–alar: Odontoid tip to occipital condyles Atlantoalar: Odontoid tip to lateral masses of atlas	Limit axial rotation and lateral bending on contralateral side and may limit anterior displacement of atlas. If transverse ligament ruptures, becomes primary ligament preventing atlantoaxial subluxation.
Cruciate	Superior: Posterior odontoid to upper clivus Inferior: Posterior odontoid to posterior surface of C2 body Transverse component: Medial tubercles of C1 lateral masses to posterior dens	Transverse component is the primary stabilizing ligament of the AAJ by keeping odontoid locked against anterior ring of C1, preventing anterior subluxation of atlas on axis. Permits axial rotation. Superior and inferior limbs offer minimal stability.
Tectorial	Posterior aspect of vertebral bodies, superiorly to IAC; continuation of PLL	Limit extension and flexion with little to no impact on stability. Prevents odontoid from compression of ventral cervical spinal cord.
ALL	Anterior aspect of vertebral bodies	Limits hyperextension, distraction.
Accessory atlantoaxial	C2 body laterally to medial C1 lateral masses	No biomechanical studies available. May mimic alar ligament function.

(Continued)

Table 1.2 (*Continued*)

Ligament	Attachments	Action
Capsular	O–C1 and C1–C2 articulating facets	Stabilizes natural motion of facet joints.
Anterior and posterior	Anterior: Anterior C1 tubercle to anterior rim of foramen magnum	AAO: May limit extension of atlantooccipital joint (AOJ). Limited studies.
		PAO: No significant role in stability.
Atlantooccipital membranes	Posterior: C1 posterior arch to posterior rim of foramen magnum	
Lateral atlantooccipital ligament	Anterolateral aspect of C1 transverse process to jugular process of occipital bone	No biomechanical studies available. May limit lateral flexion of contralateral side.
Barkow ligament	Horizontal band attaching anteromedial aspect of the occipital condyles to the attachment of the alar ligaments	May limit extension of O–C1 joint. May inhibit lateral displacement of a unilateral occipital condyle fracture. The transverse ligament must be intact for the Barkow ligament to function properly.
Atlantodental ligament	Horizontal band attaching anterior base of the dens to internal aspect of anterior arch of the atlas	Helps maintain predental space (along with transverse and alar ligaments). Limits axial rotation before alar ligaments.
		Limits posterior displacement of dens before transverse ligament.
Nuchal ligament	Cephalic extension of the supraspinous ligament extending from C7 spinous process to inion	Restricts hyperflexion of the cervical spine.

Abbreviations: AAJ, atlantoaxial joint; AAO, atlantooccipital joint; ALL, anterior longitudinal ligament; IAC, internal auditory canal; O, occiput; PAO, posterior atlantooccipital membrane; PLL, posterior longitudinal ligament.

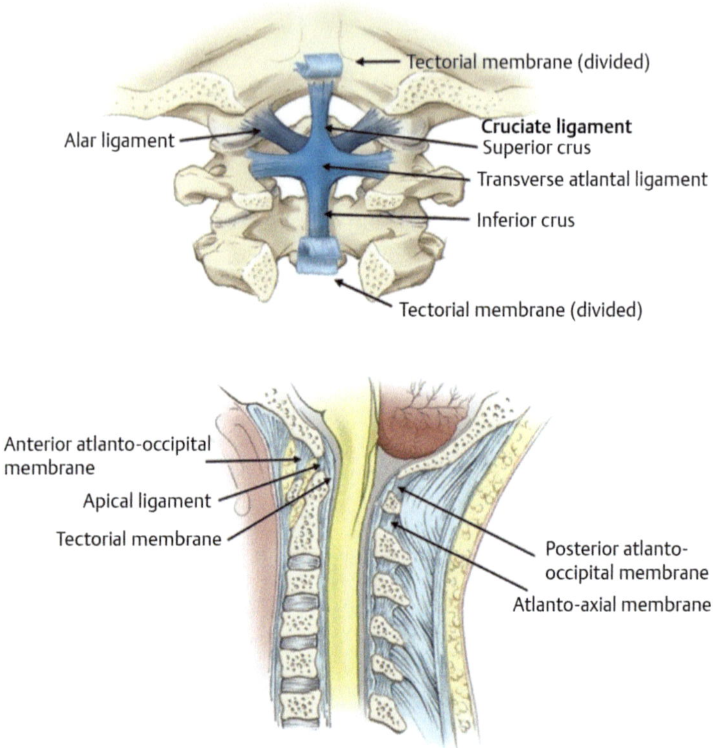

Fig. 1.5 Craniovertebral junction (CVJ) ligaments.

the paired alar ligaments which limit axial rotation and lateral bending, the transverse atlantal ligaments which limit flexion and extension of the atlantoaxial joint, and the facet capsular ligaments (**Fig. 1.5**).

1.7 Surgical Pearls

- While exposing the posterior arch of C1, monopolar cautery should be used with caution and not beyond 7 mm on both sides of the midline lateral to the posterior tubercle. Following that a dissector (Penfield number 1) is used to complete the subperiosteal dissection laterally. This is an effort to avoid heat injury to the VA coursing in the sulcus arteriosus.
- The vertebral venous plexus around C2 ganglion may cause considerable bleeding, which should not be mistaken for VA injury. Patience and the use

of hemostatic agents (e.g., Gelfoam, Floseal) are placed while exposing the other side is attempted.

- Vascular imaging such as a computed tomography angiography (CTA) or magnetic resonance angiography (MRA) is key in understanding the location, course, and dominance of the vertebral arteries.
- While placing C1 lateral mass screws, aiming at a bicortical purchase is important to improve screw pullout strength. However, the screw tip must not be more than 2 to 3 mm beyond the anterior cortex. This is in order to avoid an injury to the structures ventral to the C1 anterior arch such as the oropharynx, carotid artery, and hypoglossal nerve.

Common Clinical Questions

1. How many ossification centers C1 and C2 are formed from?
2. What forms the continuation of the posterior longitudinal ligament (PLL) at the CVJ?
3. What persistent carotid–vertebrobasilar anastomoses may be encountered in the CVJ?
4. The fourth sclerotome, the proatlas, is a precursor to which structures?

Answers to Common Clinical Questions

1. C1 is formed by the fusion of three ossification centers and C2 is formed by the fusion of four ossification centers by the age of 6 to 8 years.
2. Tectorial membrane.
3. Proatlantal intersegmental artery and persistent hypoglossal artery.
4. Anterior tubercle of clivus, apical ligament, apex of dens, occipital condyles, U-shaped part of foramen magnum, alar and cruciate ligaments, superior portion of the posterior arch, and lateral masses of the atlas.

References

1. Menezes AH, Traynelis VC. Anatomy and biomechanics of normal craniovertebral junction (a) and biomechanics of stabilization (b). Childs Nerv Syst. 2008; 24(10):1091–1100
2. Lopez AJ, Scheer JK, Leibl KE, Smith ZA, Dlouhy BJ, Dahdaleh NS. Anatomy and biomechanics of the craniovertebral junction. Neurosurg Focus. 2015; 38(4):E2

2 Cervical Spine

Ivan Angelov, Ebubechi Adindu, Woralux Phusoongnern, and Comron Saifi

Summary
The subaxial cervical spinal anatomy is critical to understand to safely navigate the neurovascular and bony anatomy during surgery. This is a common area for trauma and degenerative spinal disease, in particular. Fixation options must consider not only the bony structures and neural elements, but also the vertebral arteries. Additionally, the brachial plexus is intimately associated with the cervical spine.

Keywords: cervical spine, vertebral artery, brachial plexus

2.1 Key Points

- The subaxial cervical spine includes C3 to C7.
- The cervical spine, like the lumbar spine, normally demonstrates lordotic curvature (**Fig. 2.1**).
- Posterior instrumentation often uses lateral mass screws because the pedicles are narrower than in the thoracic and lumbar spine, increasing the risk of neurovascular injury.
- The size and volume of lateral masses decrease from the upper to lower subaxial cervical spine.
- The primary blood supply to the cervical spine is via the anterior spinal artery (ASA) and two posterior spinal arteries (PSA).

2.2 Bony Anatomy

2.2.1 Bony Landmarks

- Radiographic landmarks[1]: C3 is at the hyoid, C4 is at the thyroid cartilage, and C6 is at the cricoid cartilage.
- Palpable landmark: The anterior tubercle of the C6 transverse process (Chassaignac tubercle) is palpable.

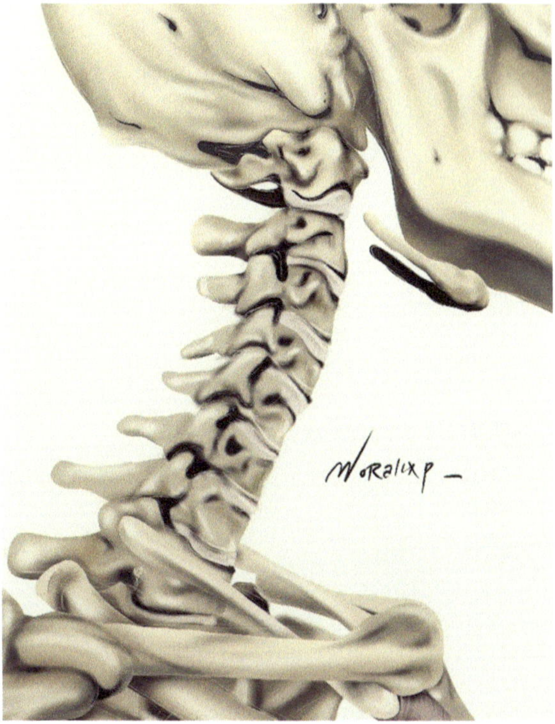

Fig. 2.1 A lateral view of the cervical spine demonstrating a lordotic curvature. (Copyright of Chiang Mai.)

2.2.2 Vertebrae Anatomy

- In the coronal plane, uncovertebral joints are noted at the anterolateral aspect of the vertebral body (**Fig. 2.2**), formed by uncinate processes of the vertebral bodies.
- Lateral masses of the subaxial spine are composed of the superior and inferior articulating processes (the facet joint).
- A lateral mass begins lateral to where the lamina and pedicle meet, helping to form the intervertebral foramen with the uncovertebral joint.
- Cervical foraminal stenosis and concurrent radiculopathy are frequently caused by degeneration of the facet or uncovertebral joints and their proximity to intervertebral foramina.
- The transverse foramen is lateral to the vertebral body and anterior to the nerve root groove.
- Anterior and posterior tubercles are noted along the transverse process.

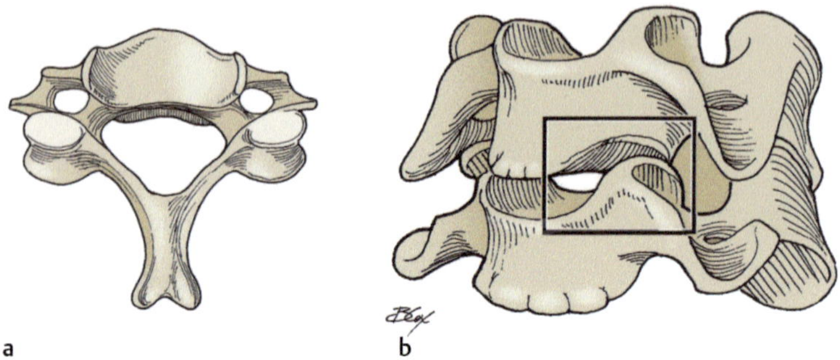

Fig. 2.2 Cervical vertebrae: (a) superior and (b) oblique views.

2.2.3 Geometric Measurements

- The spinal canal is triangular and has a greater lateral than anteroposterior (AP) dimension.
- The AP diameter of the spinal canal decreases caudally[2]: 17 mm at C3, 15 mm at C7.
- The width of vertebral body is usually 17 to 20 mm.
- Pedicles measure 5.1 to 9.5 mm in height and 3.0 to 7.5 mm in width.
- C7 is a transitional vertebra: The lateral mass is thinner and the pedicle wider than in C3 to C6.
- The normal lordotic curvature of the cervical spine is 16 to 25 degrees.[3]

2.2.4 Biomechanics and Mobility

- Biomechanical studies show maximal flexion–extension at C4/C5 and C5/C6 and maximal lateral bending at C2/C3, C3/C4, and C4/C5.
- The least mobile segment is C7/T1.
- Cervical disk herniation occurs most frequently at C5/C6 and C6/C7.

2.3 Neural Anatomy

2.3.1 Geometric Orientation

- C3 to C7 nerve roots exit above their corresponding level (e.g., C7 exits above the C7 pedicle).
- Cervical disk herniation is most frequently posterior–lateral and compresses the nerve associated with that level (e.g., C5–C6 herniation impinges on the C6 nerve).

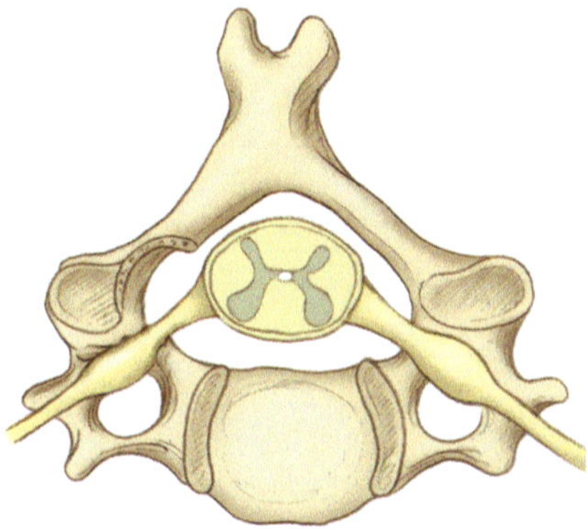

Fig. 2.3 A cervical vertebra with nerve roots exiting anterolaterally to the superior joint facet. (Reproduced with permission from Posterior Cervical Foraminotomy. In: Fessler Procedures. Thieme; 2006.)

- The C8 nerve root exits above the T1 pedicle.
- The cervical spinal cord enlarges caudally and reaches a maximal cross-sectional area at C6.
- Nerve roots enter the intervertebral foramina laterally, occupy approximately a third of the foramina, and are covered by epidural fat and venous plexus above.
- Nerve roots exit the spine at a point anterolateral to the superior joint facet (**Fig. 2.3**).

2.3.2 Cervical Plexus and Phrenic Nerve

- The cervical plexus is formed by the anterior rami of C1 to C4.
- The cervical plexus gives rise to (1) the ansa cervicalis (supplies a branch to the hypoglossal nerve and innervates the strap muscles, except for the thyrohyoid), (2) phrenic nerve (C3 to C5, but mainly C4), and (3) cutaneous nerves of the posterior head and neck.
- The phrenic nerve is formed by the anterior rami of C3 to C5 and innervates the diaphragm.

2.3.3 Brachial Plexus

- The brachial plexus is formed by the anterior rami of C5 to T1 and provides sensory and motor innervation to the upper extremity.[4]
- The brachial plexus gives rise to the (1) axillary nerve (C5 and C6 nerve roots), (2) radial nerve (C5–T1 nerve roots), (3) musculocutaneous nerve (C5–C7 nerve roots), (4) median nerve (C6–T1), and (5) ulnar nerve (C8–T1) (**Fig. 2.4**).

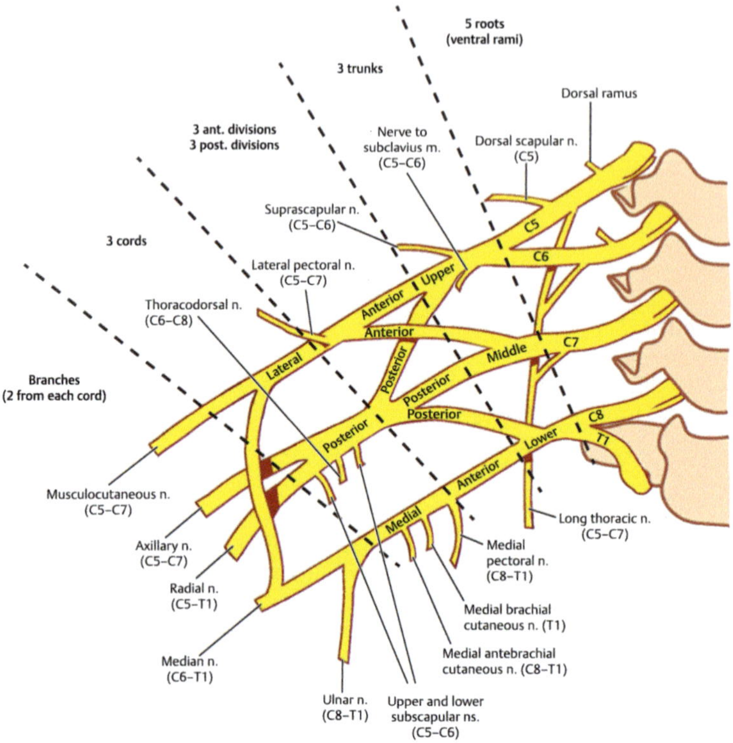

Fig. 2.4 The brachial plexus, demonstrating the relationship between the cervical nerve roots and cervical vertebrae. (Reproduced with permission from Albertstone CD, Benzel EC, Najm IM, Steinmetz M, eds. Anatomic Basis of Neurologic Diagnosis. New York, NY: Thieme; 2009.)

- Sensory and motor neurons from brachial plexus nerve roots correspond to an upper extremity dermatome and myotome respectively.
- Upper, middle, and lower trunks of the brachial plexus exit between the anterior and middle scalene muscles, cephalad and posterior to the subclavian artery as it passes posterior to the first rib.

2.3.4 Sympathetic Ganglia

- Three major sympathetic ganglia rest outside the cervical column, behind the carotid sheath: (1) The superior cervical ganglion lies along the sympathetic trunk from C1 to C4 and carries the sympathetics for the head and neck traversing along the carotid artery. (2) The middle cervical ganglion is located at C5 to C6 (also targeting the head and neck). (3) The stellate ganglion extends from C7 to T1.

2.4 Vascular Anatomy

2.4.1 Vertebral Artery Segments: V1 to V4

- Vertebral artery segments: V1 (preforaminal)—origin to transverse foramen entrance; V2 (foraminal)—C6 to C2; V3—C2 to dura; V4—intradural segment to basilar artery.
- Vertebral arteries usually originate from the subclavian artery and ascend between the anterior scalene and longus colli muscles (V1).[5]
- Vertebral arteries enter the cervical spine at the transverse foramen of C6 (V2) (**Fig. 2.5**) and travel posterior to the longus colli becoming more medial and dorsal as they move cephalad.
- The anterior spinal artery originates from the vertebral arteries just prior to the formation of the basilar artery at the pontomedullary junction (V4).
- The two posterior spinal arteries most commonly originate from the vertebral arteries but can also arise from posterior inferior cerebellar arteries (PICA).
- The anterior spinal artery and the two posterior spinal arteries enter the vertebral canal through the foramen magnum.

2.4.2 Blood Supply to Spinal Cord

- Blood supply to spinal cord includes the anterior spinal artery, the two posterior spinal arteries, and the segmental medullary arteries.
- The anterior spinal artery is found in the ventral median fissure.
- The posterior spinal arteries are found in the posterolateral sulci of the spinal cord.

2.4.3 Venous Drainage

- Venous drainage of the spinal cord includes three anterior and three posterior longitudinally running veins.
- Spinal cord is surrounded by an anterior venous plexus and a posterior venous plexus.
- The anterior venous plexus is most pronounced medial to the pedicles.

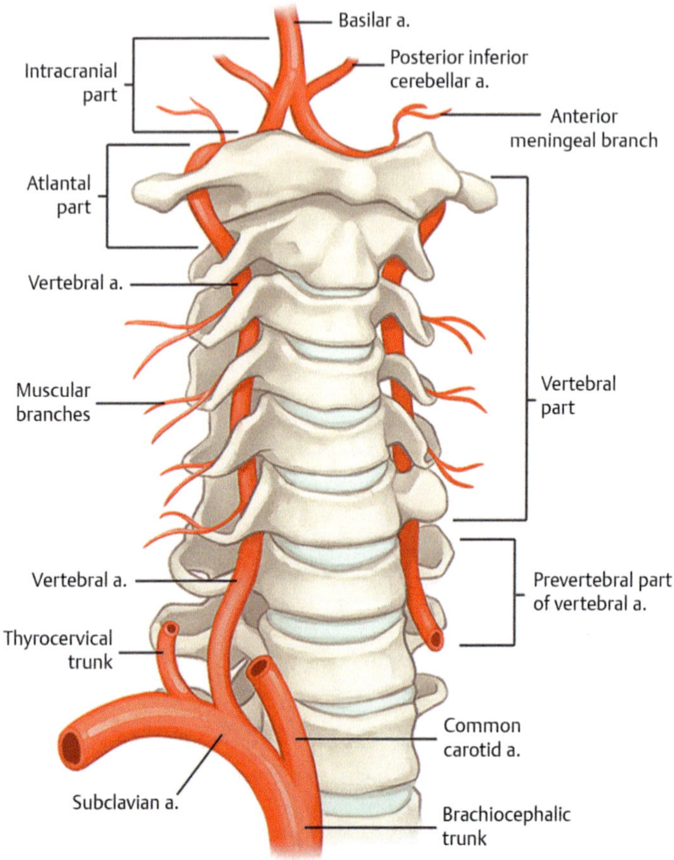

Fig. 2.5 The anatomy of the vertebral artery, emphasizing the relationship to the transverse foramina of the cervical vertebrae. (Reproduced with permission from Singh K, ed. Spine Essentials Handbook: A Bulleted Review of Anatomy, Evaluation, Imaging, Tests, and Procedures. New York, NY: Thieme; 2019.)

2.4.4 Transverse Foramen and the Vertebral Artery

- At C3 to C5, the lateralmost aspect of the transverse foramen is often anteromedial to the midpoint of the lateral mass.
- At C6 to C7, a portion of the transverse foramen is often anterior to the midpoint of the lateral mass.

2.5 Ligamentous and Muscular Anatomy

2.5.1 Ligamentous Anatomy

- The anterior longitudinal ligament covers anterior vertebral bodies, resists hyperextension, and widens as it descends.
- The posterior longitudinal ligament covers posterior vertebral bodies and resists hyperflexion.
- The interspinous and supraspinous ligaments run between adjacent spinous processes and form the ligamentum nuchae.
- The ligamentum nuchae makes up the midline avascular plane.
- The ligamentum flavum runs posteriorly to the spinal canal and connects the lamina of the sub-axial adjacent vertebra.

2.5.2 The Carotid Triangle

- The carotid triangle of the neck is an important surgical landmark for anterior approaches, formed laterally by sternocleidomastoid, superiorly by dorsal portion of the digastric, and anteriorly by omohyoid (**Fig. 2.6**).
- The carotid triangle contains the carotid sheath (common carotid artery, internal jugular vein, and vagus nerve). The artery is anteromedial, the vein is anterolateral, and the nerve runs posteriorly between the artery and vein.
- After bifurcation of the common carotid, the external branch exits the sheath, whereas the internal branch continues within.

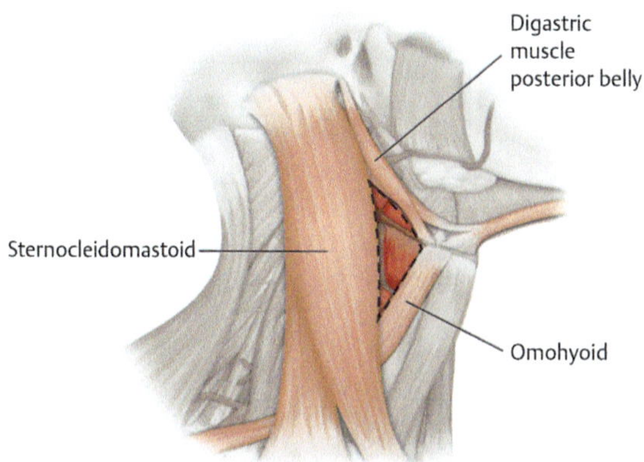

Fig. 2.6 The carotid triangle, with borders depicted. (Reproduced with permission from Kim D, Choi G, Lee S, Fessler R, eds. Endoscopic Spine Surgery, 2nd Edition. New York, NY: Thieme; 2018.)

2.5.3 Muscular Anatomy

- Longus colli muscles lie anterolateral to vertebral bodies and are elevated during anterior spinal procedures.
- Three scalene muscles lie lateral to vertebral bodies and connect vertebrae to the first two ribs.
- The anterior scalene muscle originates from the anterior tubercles of the transverse processes of C3–C6 and elevates the first rib.
- The middle scalene muscle originates between the anterior and posterior tubercles of C2–C7 and elevates the first rib.
- The anterior and middle scalene muscles form the fissure scalenorum for passage of the brachial plexus.
- The posterior scalene muscle originates from the posterior tubercles of the transverse processes of C5–C7 and elevates the second rib.
- The sternocleidomastoid muscle lies superficial to the scalene and longus colli muscles and is innervated by the spinal accessory nerve and the cervical plexus.
- The semispinalis capitis and semispinalis cervicis span the posterior aspect of the cervical spine.

2.6 Variations in Anatomy

- About 28 to 40% of patients have a prefixed brachial plexus, which involves C4–T1. In this population, C4 partially innervates the deltoid.[6]
- About 0.4 to 5% of patients have a post-fixed brachial plexus, which involves C5–T2. In this population, T2 affects hand function.[6]
- About 0.58 to 6.2% of patients have a cervical rib, which is an accessory rib stemming from C7. This may predispose to thoracic outlet syndrome due to compression of the subclavian artery and/or brachial plexus.[7]
- About 4 to 84% of patients have an accessory phrenic nerve. This nerve has variable origins, but usually arises from either the ansa cervicalis (approximately 16.5% of patients), subclavian nerve (approximately 15.8% of patients), or C5/C6 nerve roots (approximately 15.1% of patients).[8]

2.7 Surgical Pearls

- Uncovertebral joints provide several surgical landmarks: They define the lateral borders for corpectomy or diskectomy, and they define the midline for cervical plate placement.
- The Magerl technique for lateral mass screw placement is used to avoid injuring the vertebral artery or nerve root. The drill is placed 1 mm medial to the midpoint of the lateral mass and is angled 25 degrees laterally and 30 degrees superiorly.

- During anterior procedures, instruments are most safely inserted into the lateral aspect of the canal.
- During posterior cervical procedures, the patient can be placed in a slight reverse Trendelenburg position to reduce venous engorgement.
- C7 is a transitional-level vertebra. For a posterior fusion involving C7, some surgeons advocate extending the fusion to T1 to reduce adjacent-level disease.

Common Clinical Questions

1. At what level does cervical disk herniation most often occur?
2. What is the normal curvature of the cervical spine?
3. Which arteries provide the majority of blood circulation to the spinal cord?
4. What are the location and clinical significance of the vascular watershed in the cervical spine?
5. The vertebral artery travels through which transverse foramina?
6. A patient presents with pain in the cervical spine with nonlocalizable, diffuse radiation to the left upper extremity. Examination reveals weakness of left shoulder abduction from 15 to 90 degrees. MRI of the cervical spine demonstrates C3–C4 disk herniation. Why are the examination and imaging findings inconsistent?

Answers to Common Clinical Questions

1. C5/C6 and C6/C7.
2. The cervical spine normally has a lordotic curvature between 16 and 25 degrees.
3. The spinal cord is supplied by the anterior spinal artery (from the vertebral arteries), two posterior spinal arteries (from either the vertebral arteries or PICA), and segmental medullary arteries.
4. The watershed exists between the base and apex of the odontoid process. The limited blood supply between the distributions of the internal carotid artery and vertebral artery may impair healing in fractures of the odontoid process.
5. Typically, the vertebral artery travels through the transverse foramina of C1–C6. In up to 10% of patients, there may be anatomical variation in which the vertebral artery takes an atypical course. A common variation is that the vertebral artery travels through the foramen of C7. Absent, hypoplastic, triple, and open foramen are additional anatomical variations.
6. The patient most likely has a prefixed brachial plexus, an anatomical variation. The C4 nerve partially innervates the deltoid muscle in this patient.

References

1. Clark CR, Benzel EC, Currier BL, et al, eds. The Cervical Spine. 4th ed. Philadelphia, PA: Lippincott Williams & Wilkins; 2005
2. Herkowitz HN, Garfin SR, Eismont FJ, et al, eds. Rothman-Simeone: The Spine. 5th ed. Philadelphia, PA: Elsevier; 2006
3. Gore DR, Sepic SB, Gardner GM. Roentgenographic findings of the cervical spine in asymptomatic people. Spine. 1986; 11(6):521–524
4. Polcaro L, Charlick M, Daly DT. Anatomy, Head and Neck, Brachial Plexus. In: StatPearls. Treasure Island, FL: StatPearls Publishing; August 25, 2021
5. Ebraheim NA, Xu R, Yeasting RA. The location of the vertebral artery foramen and its relation to posterior lateral mass screw fixation. Spine. 1996; 21(11): 1291–1295
6. Tubbs RS, El-Zammar D, Loukas M, Cömert A, Cohen-Gadol AA. Intradural cervical root adjacent interconnections in the normal, prefixed, and postfixed brachial plexus. J Neurosurg Spine. 2009; 11(4):413–416
7. Spadliński Ł, Cecot T, Majos A, et al. The epidemiological, morphological, and clinical aspects of the cervical ribs in humans. BioMed Res Int. 2016; 2016: 8034613
8. Graves MJ, Henry BM, Hsieh WC, et al. Origin and prevalence of the accessory phrenic nerve: a meta-analysis and clinical appraisal. Clin Anat. 2017; 30(8): 1077–1082

3 Thoracic Spine

Lance Villeneuve, Xiaochun Zhao, and Zachary A. Smith

Summary
The thoracic anatomy varies widely based upon location. Furthermore, given the limited vascular supply, this area of the spinal cord can be unforgiving to manipulation. A thorough anatomic understanding is important for performing a successful surgery.

Keywords: thoracic, thoracic, artery of Adamkiewicz, ligamentous anatomy

3.1 Key Points

- Normal anatomy consists of 12 vertebral segments with ribs in the thoracic spine. However, anatomical variants consisting of 11 to 13 rib-bearing vertebral segments and/or the presence of vestigial ribs are possible.
- Rigid thoracic spinal stability is provided by the combination of spinal osteoligamentous structure and the osteoligamentous rib cage.
- Normal thoracic kyphosis ranges from 10 to 40 degrees with the kyphotic apex at T7. However, aging combined with compensatory mechanisms may exaggerate the kyphotic deformity.[1]
- Thoracic blood supply has two areas of susceptibility: the midthoracic watershed area which is vulnerable to hypotension and the lower thoracic region supplied largely by the artery of Adamkiewicz.

3.2 Bony Anatomy (Fig. 3.1 and Fig. 3.2)[2]

- The dimensions of the vertebral bodies change throughout the thoracic spine. Width and height increase linearly, in general. However, the depth of vertebral bodies increases from T1 to T7 and then remains similar from T7 to T12.[3]
- Thoracic vertebral bodies are wedge-shaped in the anterior/posterior plane resulting in the smooth kyphosis present in the thoracic spine.[1,3]
- The orientation of thoracic facets transition throughout the thoracic spine from a coronal orientation at T1 to a sagittal orientation at T12. The sagittal orientation of facets in the lower thoracic spine provides stability in flexion and extension in a similar fashion to the facets in the lumbar spine.[1,3]

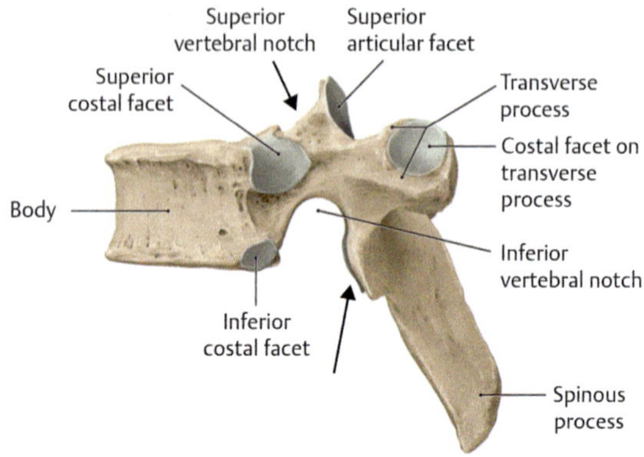

Fig. 3.1 Lateral view of thoracic vertebra. (Reproduced from Schuenke M, Schulte E, Schumacher U. THIEME Atlas of Anatomy. General Anatomy and Musculoskeletal System. 4th ed. Illustration by Voll M and Wesker K. © Thieme 2024.)

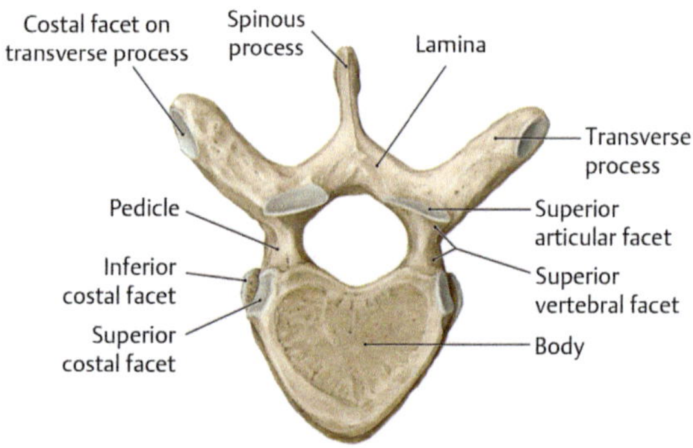

Fig. 3.2 Superior view of thoracic vertebra. (Reproduced from Schuenke M, Schulte E, Schumacher U. THIEME Atlas of Anatomy. General Anatomy and Musculoskeletal System. 4th ed. Illustration by Voll M and Wesker K. © Thieme 2024.)

- The superior articular facet is anterior and inferior to the inferior articular facet of the level above, and the facet is surrounded by a capsule. Additional repetitive friction in the facet joint can lead to a facet cyst.
- Pedicle height increases from T1 to T2, remains stable from T2 to T8, and generally increases from T8 to T12.[3]
- Pedicle width decreases from the T1 to T5 or T6, then gradually increases from T5 or T6 to T12.[1,3]

- The transverse pedicle angle (the angle from a tangential line of the intervertebral foramen to a line drawn mid-pedicle) decreases from T1 to T5, remains stable from T5 to T9, and decreases from T9 to T12.[3]
- The rostral pedicle surface is flush with superior endplate. The caudal pedicle surface insertion point on the vertebral body becomes lower as the pedicle height increases.
- The thoracic pedicle width is half to one-third of the pedicle height. Hence, pedicle width combined with the transverse pedicle angle sets the limitation on screw size during instrumentation and determines trajectory.
- Thoracic canal diameter is smallest in the midthoracic spine. The diameter of the thoracic spinal canal decreases from 20.3 mm at T1 to 15.9 mm at T5 followed by an increase to 22.3 mm at T12.[4]
- The vertebral bodies from T2 to T8 or T9 articulate with two ribs at bilateral demifacets, one superiorly and one inferiorly bilaterally. The thoracic costotransverse facets from T1 to T10 are located on the transverse process and articulate with the same-level rib at the articular tubercle of the rib (e.g., T7 rib articulates with T6 and T7 vertebral bodies at the demifacets and the T7 transverse facet).
- The T1, T10, T11, and T12 (and sometimes T9) ribs have a full facet for articulation with the corresponding vertebra.
- The 11th and 12th ribs do not articulate with the transverse processes of the vertebral body at the corresponding level.
- Due to the normal thoracic kyphosis and variations of the bony thoracic spine, miscounting vertebra is a common mistake. Utilization of multiple methods to confirm vertebral level including a marker, an intraoperative computed tomography (CT) scan, and counting vertebral levels from both the top and bottom of the thoracic area via fluoroscopy may be necessary.
- It is important to also confirm lumbar anatomy when working in the thoracic spine (e.g., confirm the number of lumbar vertebra).

3.3 Neural Anatomy

- In a normal adult, the spinal cord traverses the length of the cervical and thoracic cord. The spinal cord terminates at the conus medullaris around L1 or L2.
- During development, the spinal column grows faster than the spinal cord resulting in a discordance between the vertebral and nerve level. As such an injury in the upper thoracic vertebra will likely present as an injury of the cord in the corresponding area (e.g., T1 fracture and a T1 cord injury). However, in the lower thoracic spine, a fracture of a vertebra would result in an injury of a spinal cord that is one to two levels more caudal (e.g., a T9 fracture and a T11 spinal cord injury). However, a nerve root injury in

conjunction with a fracture will present as an injury at the appropriate level (e.g., a T9 fracture with a T9 nerve root deficit).

- Dorsal and ventral nerve roots exit the thecal sac, traverse the lateral recess, exit below the pedicle of the corresponding vertebral level (e.g., the T1 nerve root exits below the T1 pedicle), and combine in the neural foramen to form the dorsal root ganglia.
- The lateral recess, defined by the thecal sac medially and the pedicle laterally, is a site of compression due to ligamentum flavum hypertrophy or facet hypertrophy.
- The spinal cord has a ventral motor portion containing the cell bodies of lower motor neurons and a dorsal sensory portion containing the second-order sensory neurons.
- Nerves of the thoracic spine innervate the truncal and abdominal muscles with many muscles receiving innervation from multiple nerve roots.
- Sensory dermatomes overlap in the chest and abdomen. However, the T4 dermatome is roughly at the nipple line, the T6 dermatome at the base of the sternum, and the T10 dermatome at the level of the umbilicus.
- Sympathetic neurons have a preganglionic origin from the intermediolateral cell columns from T1 to L3 which coalesce into the sympathetic chain ganglia located lateral to the vertebral body bilaterally.
- The intervertebral disk is innervated by the sinuvertebral nerve. The sinuvertebral nerve is a recurrent nerve originating from the dorsal root ganglion, the spinal nerve, or the rami communicantes, which travels through the anterior portion of the neural foramina to innervate the disk above and below the corresponding nerve.[5] Facet joints are innervated by the dorsal primary ramus through the zygapophyseal nerves. These nerves together are thought to contribute to axial back pain.[6]
- Anatomical anomalies such as a tethered cord or nerve root variations may change the neural anatomy of the thoracic cord.

3.4 Vascular Anatomy

- The anterior spinal artery originates intradurally as two small branches of the vertebral artery, bilaterally, which combine at the level of the foramen magnum and travels in the anterior median fissure of the spinal cord supplying the anterior two-thirds of the spinal cord white matter.
- Paired posterior spinal arteries arise from the posterior inferior cerebellar artery (75%) or the vertebral artery (25%). Theses arteries travel in the posterior intermediate sulci of the spinal cord and supply the posterior one-third of the spinal cord white matter.
- The sulcal branches of the anterior spinal artery supply the gray matter of the spinal cord.

- The ascending cervical artery, the deep cervical artery, the intercostal arteries, the lumbar arteries, and the sacral arteries supplement the thoracic cord vasculature via radicular artery anastomoses.
- The artery of Adamkiewicz anastomoses with the anterior spinal artery at roughly T9 to L2 in 85% of people and joins from the left side in 80% of people providing the bulk of arterial supply for the lower thoracic cord. Its size is comparable to the anterior spinal artery.[1,3]
- The artery of Adamkiewicz can be visualized as a hairpin loop on an anterior/posterior angiogram. Due the variability of side and site of anastomosis, localization before large surgeries may be prudent.
- Extradural venous drainage consists of the anterior external venous plexus, the anterior internal venous plexus, the posterior internal venous plexus, and the posterior external venous plexus. The intradural venous plexus is continuous with the external plexus via the radiculomedullary veins. Venous drainage occurs radially.
- If arterial supply to the thoracic cord from the aorta is interrupted, collateral flow can come from the internal thoracic and lateral thoracic arteries, which anastomose with the posterior intercostal arteries.

3.5 Ligamentous and Muscular Anatomy (Table 3.1)

- Muscles of the thoracic spine:
  - Superficial layers:
    - Trapezius, rhomboid, and latissimus dorsi.
  - Intermediate layers:
    - Splenius cervicis, serratus posterior superior and inferior, and erector spinae (spinalis, longissimus, iliocostalis).
  - Deep layers:
    - Rotators longus and brevis, levators costarum longus and brevis, multifidus, semispinalis thoracis, and external intercostal muscles.

3.6 Surgical Pearls

- Disruption of the posterior tension band of the thoracic spine via laminectomy or during dissection can increase the risk of progressive kyphosis.
- Avoid injury to the artery of Adamkiewicz to prevent spinal cord infarction. If a surgery is near the artery, an angiogram is useful to elucidate the anatomy.

Table 3.1 Principal thoracic ligaments, the attachments, and their modes of action

Ligament	Attachments	Action
Anterior longitudinal	Ventral vertebral body and annulus	Limits extension and distraction Thickest in thoracic spine
Posterior longitudinal	Dorsal vertebral body and annulus	Limits flexion and distraction Thickest in thoracic spine
Ligamentum flavum	Lamina of adjacent vertebrae	Limits flexion
Interspinous	Spinous processes of adjacent vertebra	Limits flexion and distraction
Supraspinous	Tips of spinous processes and thoracolumbar fascia	Limits flexion and distraction
Facet capsule	Superior and inferior facets of adjacent vertebra	Supports facet joint stability
Radiate	Rib and adjacent vertebral disk space and vertebral bodies anteriorly	Stabilizes rib attachments
Superior costotransverse	The rostral rib neck and the transverse process of the vertebra one level above	Contributes to limitation of thoracic flexion, extension, lateral bending, and axial rotation
Lateral costotransverse	The apex of the transverse process to the adjacent costal tubercle	

- The area of the cord with the narrowest pedicle corresponds to the area of the cord with a tenuous vascular supply (e.g., the midthoracic area).
- Due to the limited intradural vascular supply of much of the thoracic cord, extra caution should be taken during procedures. For example, spinal cord insult from laminectomy for anterior thoracic pathology is often a result of vascular ischemia from cord retraction compressing the vascular supply.

- Lateral, posterolateral, and anterior approaches in the thoracic spine have been developed to minimize risk of cord ischemia by limiting retraction of the thoracic spinal cord. The optimal approach is determined by the localization of the herniated disk or mass and/or the presence of any calcification.
- Intraoperative navigation for pedicle screw placement is a helpful tool in the thoracic spine due to the variation in vertebra. Furthermore, it can prevent wrong-level surgery.
- Due to the rigidity of the thoracic spine, adding additional levels for fusion will not hinder mobility further. Therefore, additional levels for instrumentation and fusion can be safely included in the thoracic spine to avoid ending a fusion construct on transition point in an adult (e.g., the thoracolumbar junction, the cervicothoracic junction, or the thoracic kyphotic apex).

Common Clinical Questions

1. Pedicle screw diameter is mostly limited by the height of the thoracic pedicle. True or false?
2. Localization of the appropriate thoracic level by a single method is sufficient for surgery in the thoracic spine. True or false?
3. The artery of Adamkiewicz typically arises about the T8 level on the right. True or false?
4. The thoracolumbar junction is a transition zone. True or false?

Answers to Common Clinical Questions

1. False. Thoracic screw choice is limited by both the pedicle width and angulation. Optimizing screw choice requires an understanding of the changes of the thoracic pedicle anatomy (**Fig. 3.3**).
2. False. Due to thoracic kyphosis, miscounting vertebral levels is a real issue with anterior/posterior X-rays. We recommend using multiple methods to verify the thoracic level.
3. False. The artery of Adamkiewicz typically arises at the T9 to L2 levels. However, it enters the spinal canal from the left in 80% of people.
4. True. The thoracolumbar junction does not denote the abrupt change between two areas. Instead, it is a transition zone where the vertebra changes gradually from the thoracic to the lumbar spine.[7]

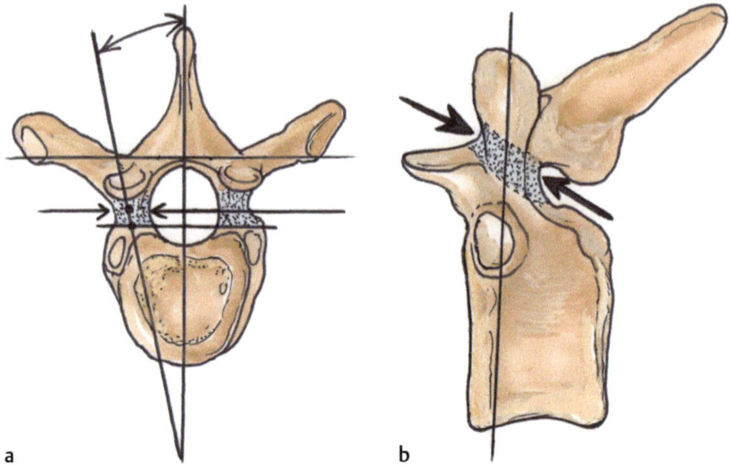

Fig. 3.3 **(a)** Anatomy of the thoracic pedicle denoting the width and angulation. **(b)** Anatomy of the thoracic pedicle demonstrating the height of the thoracic pedicle. Note the height of the thoracic pedicle is greater than the width. *Arrows* delineating height and width of pedicles. (Reproduced with permission from Fessler RG and Sekhar L, eds. Atlas of Neurosurgical Techniques: Spine and Peripheral Nerves. Thieme; 2006.)

References

1. Frempong-Boadu AK, Guiot BH. Thoracic spine anatomy and biomechanics. In: Batjer H, Loftus C, eds. Textbook of Neurological Surgery: Principles and Practice. Philadelphia, PA: Lippincott Williams & Wilkins; 2003:1544–1551
2. Gray H. Gray's Anatomy. 20th ed. Lea & Febiger; 1918. Public domain
3. Yoganandan N, Halliday AL, Dickman CA, Benzel E. Practical anatomy and fundamental biomechanics. In: Benzel EC, ed. Spine Surgery Techniques, Complication Avoidance, and Management. 2nd ed. Philadelphia, PA: Elsevier; 2005:109–135
4. Cho SK, Skovrlj B, Lu Y, Caridi JM, Lenke LG. The effect of increasing pedicle screw size on thoracic spinal canal dimensions: an anatomic study. Spine. 2014; 39(20):E1195–E1200
5. Bogduk N, Tynan W, Wilson AS. The nerve supply to the human lumbar intervertebral discs. J Anat. 1981; 132(Pt 1):39–56
6. Bogduk N, Long DM. The anatomy of the so-called "articular nerves" and their relationship to facet denervation in the treatment of low-back pain. J Neurosurg. 1979; 51(2):172–177
7. Du Plessis AM, Greyling LM, Page BJ. Differentiation and classification of thoracolumbar transitional vertebrae. J Anat. 2018; 232(5):850–856

4 Lumbar Spine

Azeem A. Rehman and Cara Sedney

Summary
The anatomy of the lumbar spine is critical to its functions of axial forced dispersal, protection of neural elements, and allowing truncal motion. Familiarity with bony, neural, vascular, and musculoligamentous anatomy aids in safe surgery of the lumbar spine.

Keywords: anatomy, lumbar disk, alignment

4.1 Key Points

- Lumbar spine contains the largest vertebra (L1–L5).
- Function:
  - Disperses axial forces.
  - Protects spinal cord and spinal nerves.
  - Truncal motion—extension, flexion, rotation, side-bending.
    - Bipedal motion—lumbar lordosis places the body over the pelvis.

4.2 Bony Anatomy

- Components of the lumbar vertebra (**Fig. 4.1**):
  - Vertebral body.
  - Pedicle:
    - Projects posterolaterally from the posterior superior-lateral edge of the vertebral body to the lamina.
  - Lamina:
    - Projects posteromedially from the posterior medial edge of the pedicle, joining to the midline spinous process.
  - Spinous process:
    - Projects posterior from the junction of the two laminae.
    - Compared to the cervical and thoracic spine, the lumbar spinous process is short and thick relative to size of the lumbar vertebra.
  - Superior articulating process:
    - Projects superiorly from the junction of the pedicle and lamina.
    - Concave, oriented posteriorly and medially.

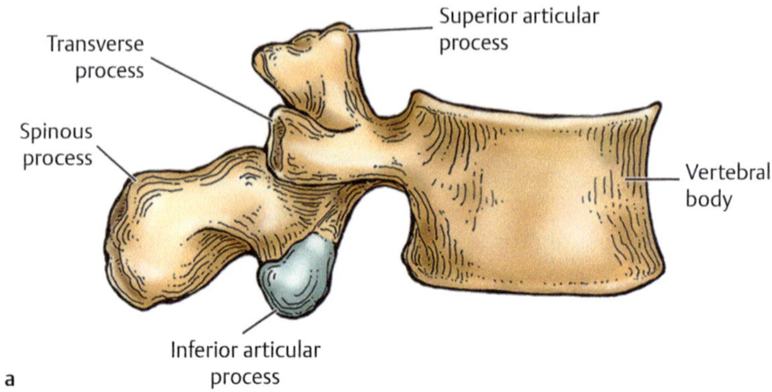

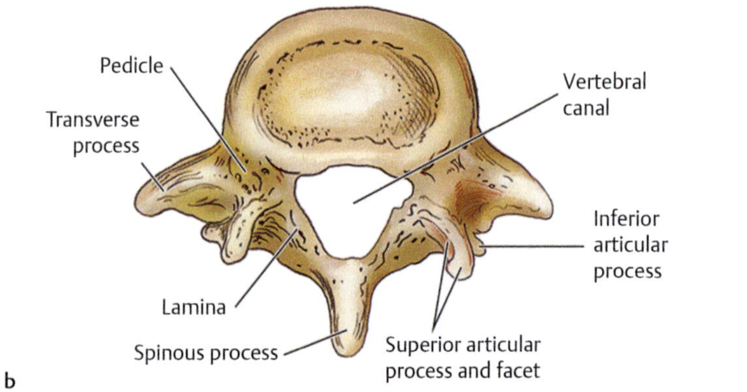

Fig. 4.1 **(a)** Lateral and **(b)** superior view of the lumbar vertebra. (Reproduced with permission from Perez-Cruet M, Fessler R, Wang M. An Anatomic Approach to Minimally Invasive Spine Surgery. 2nd ed. New York: Thieme; 2018.[1])

- Mammillary process:
  - Projects from the posterior border of the superior articulating process.
- Inferior articulating process:
  - Projects inferiorly from the junction of the pedicle and lamina.
  - Convex, oriented anteriorly and laterally.

- Zygapophyseal (facet) joint:
  - Articulation of the superior articulating process and inferior articulating process, surrounded by the articular (facet) capsule:
    - Lateral—superior articulating process of the inferior vertebra.
    - Medial—inferior articulating process of the superior vertebra.
  - Compared to the cervical and thoracic facet joints which lie in the coronal plane, the lumbar facet joint primarily lies within the sagittal plane:
    - Moving inferiorly in the lumbar spine, the orientation gradually becomes more coronal.
- Pars interarticularis:
  - Part of the lamina between the superior and inferior articulating processes.
- Transverse processes:
  - Projects laterally from the junction of the pedicle and lamina.
  - Compared to the thoracic spine, the lumbar transverse process is anterior to the articulating processes.
  - Attachment site for ligaments and muscles.
- Accessory process:
  - Projects from the posterior–inferior base of the transverse process.

- Lumbar disk:
  - Fibrocartilaginous structure between two vertebral endplates:
    - Nucleus pulposus—internal, gelatinous consistency.
    - Annulus fibrosus—external, fibrous consistency.
  - Sinuvertebral nerve:
    - Function—nociception and proprioception of disk.
    - Location—periphery of annulus fibrosis.
- Alignment:
  - Lumbar lordosis—average 33 degrees, range 20 to 45 degrees.[2]
  - Majority of lordosis due to disk spaces.

4.3 Neural Anatomy

- Spinal cord—terminates as the conus medullaris at the L1–L2 vertebral levels.
- Cauda equina—bundle of spinal nerve roots projecting from the bottom of the spinal cord.
- Five pairs of mixed (motor and sensory) spinal nerves (L1–L5):
  - Prior to exiting the neural foramen (**Fig. 4.2**), the spinal nerves branch into ventral and dorsal rami:
    - Dorsal rami:
      - Motor—erector spinae muscle.
      - Sensory—skin over back.

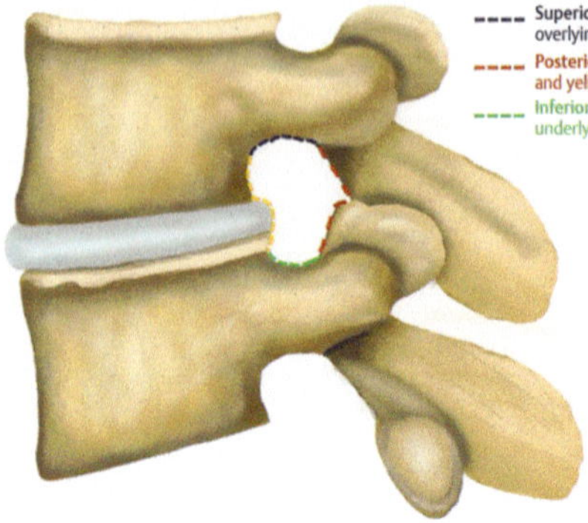

Fig. 4.2 Borders of the intervertebral foramen. (Reproduced with permission from Agarwal N. Neurosurgery Fundamentals. 1st ed. New York: Thieme; 2018.[3])

    - Ventral rami:
      - Motor—prevertebral muscles, lower extremity.
      - Sensory—prevertebral muscles, lower extremity.
  - Meningeal branches—innervate lumbar vertebra.
  - Lumbar plexus (**Table 4.1**):
    - Composition—ventral rami of spinal nerves from T12 to L5 that combine to create multiple, larger functioning nerves (**Fig. 4.3**).
      - T12—subcostal nerve.
    - Location:
      - Deep to psoas major muscle.
      - Anterior to transverse processes.
      - Nerves exit inferior to inguinal ligament:
        - Exception—obturator nerve exits via obturator foramen.

4.4 Vascular Anatomy (Fig. 4.4)

- Arterial:
  - Lumbar arteries (four paired segmental arteries):
    - Origin—abdominal aorta.
    - Pathway—project dorsolaterally around the middle of the vertebral body.
    - Supply—lumbar vertebral body.
    - Branches at the intervertebral foramen:
      - Medial—lumbar segments of spinal cord, regional sympathetic ganglia.

Table 4.1 Lumbar plexus motor and sensory innervation

Nerve	Muscle	Function	Sensory	Roots
Subcostal nerve	Pyramidalis	Tenses linea alba		T12
Iliohypogastric	Internal oblique Transversus abdominis	Compresses abdomen to increase intraabdominal pressure to force expiration	Lateral gluteal region Pubis	T12–L1
Ilioinguinal	Transversus abdominis	Expiration	Proximal and medial thigh Scrotum (male) Lateral labia majora (female) Mons pubis	L1
Genitofemoral	Cremaster	Elevates testicles	Scrotum (male) Labia majora (female)	L1, L2
Lateral femoral cutaneous			Anterolateral thigh Peritoneum	L2, L3
Femoral	Iliopsoas Pectineus Sartorius Quadriceps femoris	Hip flexion Thigh flexion, adduction, external rotation Hip flexion, abduction, lateral rotation Knee flexion Knee extension	Anterior thigh Medial thigh, knee, calf, heel	L2, L3, L4

(Continued)

Table 4.1 (*Continued*)

Nerve	Muscle	Function	Sensory	Roots
Obturator	Pectineus Adductor longus Adductor brevis Adductor magnus Adductor minimus Gracilis Obturator externus	Adducts thigh Laterally rotates thigh	Medial thigh	L2, L3, L4
Lumbosacral trunk				L4, L5

        - Middle—muscles of back, lumbar joints.
        - Lateral—abdominal muscles.
    - Artery of Adamkiewicz:
        - Largest radiculomedullary artery.
        - Origin—posterior intercostal or radicular artery.
        - Level of origin (variable)— T8–L2.
        - Pathway—left (typically) of spinal cord and ascends the spinal canal, making a hairpin loop before joining the anterior spinal artery.
  - Anterior spinal artery[2]:
    - Origin—two vertebral arteries at foramen magnum.
    - Supply—anterior two-thirds of spinal cord.
  - Posterior spinal arteries[1]:
    - Origin—posterior inferior cerebellar artery.
    - Supply—posterior one-third of spinal cord.
  - Iliolumbar artery:
    - Origin—internal iliac artery.
    - Supply—lumbar plexus.
- Venous:
  - Characteristics:
    - Valveless.
    - Pressure gradients move blood inferiorly and superiorly.
    - Drainage—segmental veins of trunk.

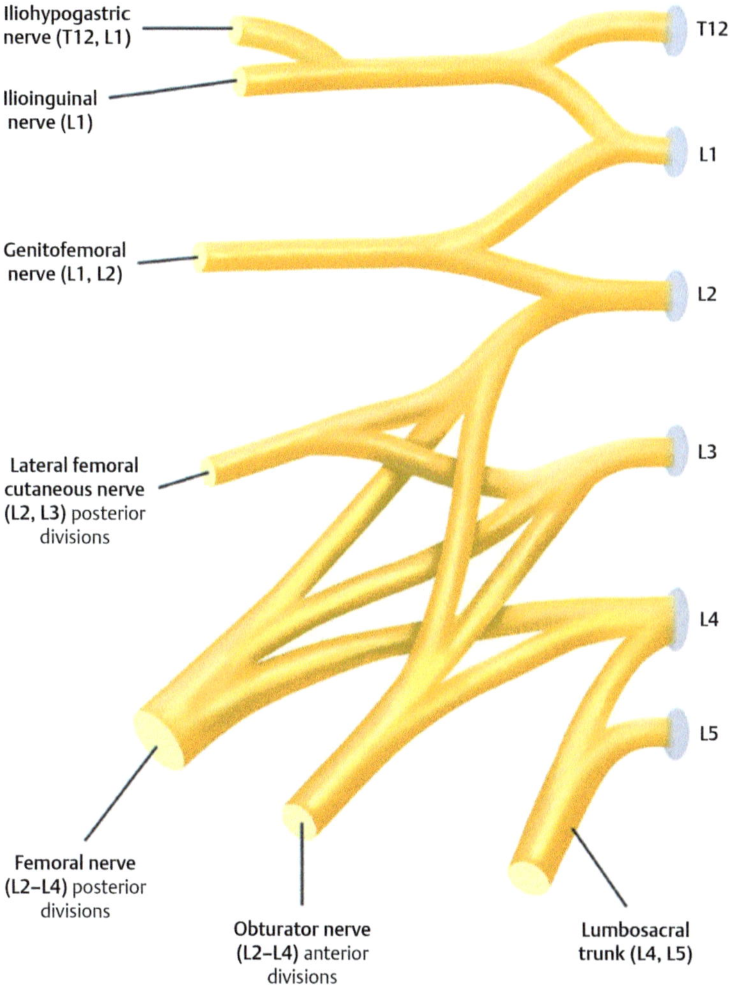

Fig. 4.3 Lumbar plexus. (Reproduced with permission from Russell S. Examination of Peripheral Nerve Injuries: An Anatomical Approach. 2nd ed. New York: Thieme; 2015.[5])

- Internal plexus:
  - Network of veins in the epidural space.
  - Communicates with the basivertebral plexus; veins tunnel through the cancellous tissue of the vertebral bodies.

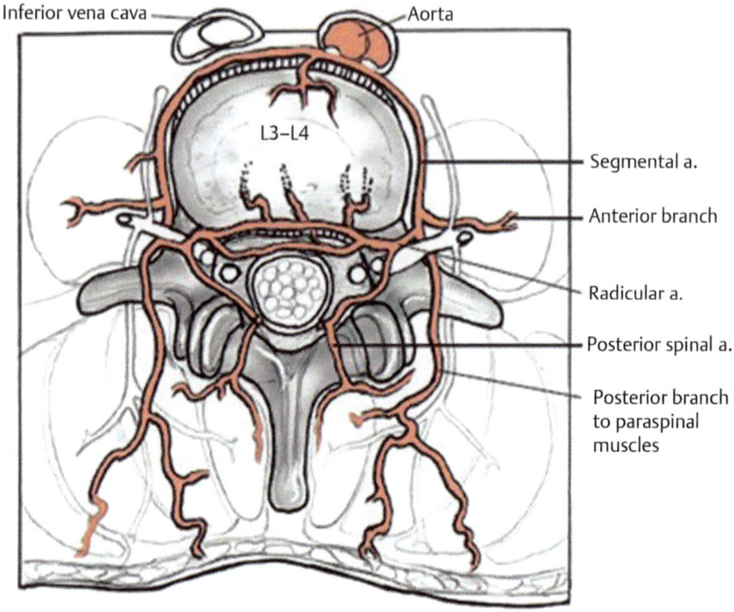

Fig. 4.4 Arterial vasculature of lumbar spine (axial section). (Reproduced with permission from Khanna A. MRI Essentials for the Spine Specialist. 1st ed. New York: Thieme; 2014.[6])

    - Intradural venous drainage of the spinal cord involves retrograde anterior and posterior central veins.
  - External plexus:
    - Anterior—anterior to vertebral bodies.
    - Posterior—posterior surface of vertebral arches.
- Lymphatic:
  - Lumbar lymph nodes:
    - Receive lymph—common iliac nodes.
    - Deliver lymph—thoracic trunk.

4.5 Ligamentous and Muscular Anatomy

- Ligaments
  - The anterior longitudinal ligament primarily resists extension while the posterior longitudinal ligament, ligamentum flavum, and supraspinous ligament resist flexion (**Table 4.2**; **Fig. 4.5**).

Table 4.2 Ligaments of the lumbar spine

Ligament	Location	Function
Anterior longitudinal ligament	Anterior margins of vertebral body and disks	Resists extension, translation, and rotation
Posterior longitudinal ligament	Posterior margins of vertebral body and disks	Resists flexion
Ligamentum flavum	Anterior margin of adjacent laminae and spinous processes	Resists flexion
Supraspinous ligament	Posterior margin of spinous processes	Resists flexion
Interspinous ligament	Inferior border of superior spinous process and superior border of inferior spinous process	Resists flexion

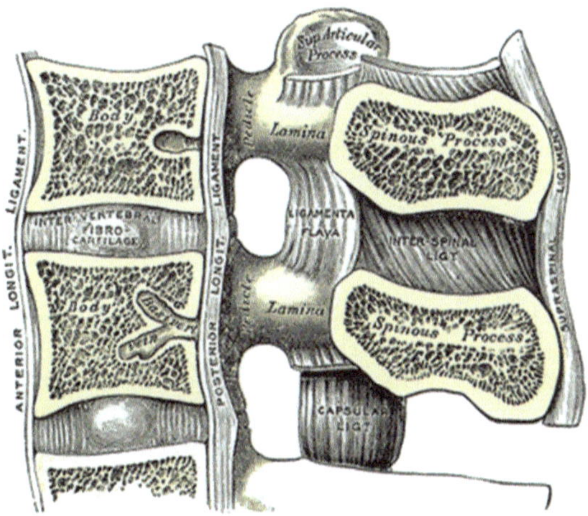

Fig. 4.5 Sagittal section of two lumbar vertebrae and their ligaments. (Reproduced from Gray H. Anatomy of the Human Body. 20th ed. Philadelphia: Lea & Febiger; 1918, in public domain.[7])

Table 4.3 Muscle groups of the lumbar spine

Muscle group	Location	Function
Erector spinae (longissimus thoracis, iliocostalis lumborum) Multifidi	Posterior to vertebra	Extension
Psoas major Abdominal muscles (internal/external oblique, rectus abdominis)	Anterior to vertebra	Truncal flexion
Quadratus lumborum Psoas major Abdominal muscles Multifidi		Rotational/ lateral flexion

- Muscle groups
  - The erector spinae muscles allow extension of the back, while the psoas major/abdominal muscles allow truncal flexion (**Table 4.3**; **Fig. 4.6**).

4.6 Surgical Pearls

- Pedicle anatomy:
  - Midpoint of transverse process correlates to midpoint of the pedicle in superior–inferior plane.
  - Lateral border of pars interarticularis correlates to midpoint of pedicle in medial–lateral plane.
  - Pedicles angulate more medial when moving inferiorly in the lumbar spine.
  - Pedicle diameter increases when moving inferiorly in the lumbar spine.
- Zygapophyseal (facet) joints:
  - Spinal synovial cysts—arise from the facet joint causing spinal stenosis.
  - Facet hypertrophy—causes foraminal stenosis compressing the exiting nerve root.
- Pars interarticularis:
  - Isthmic spondylolisthesis (spondylolysis)– fracture of the pars interarticularis leading to spondylolisthesis.
- Differences between nerve roots in cervical and lumbar spine:
  - Pedicle/nerve root mismatch:
    - Cervical nerve roots travel under the pedicle of the superior cervical vertebra. For example, C5 nerve root travels under C4 pedicle.

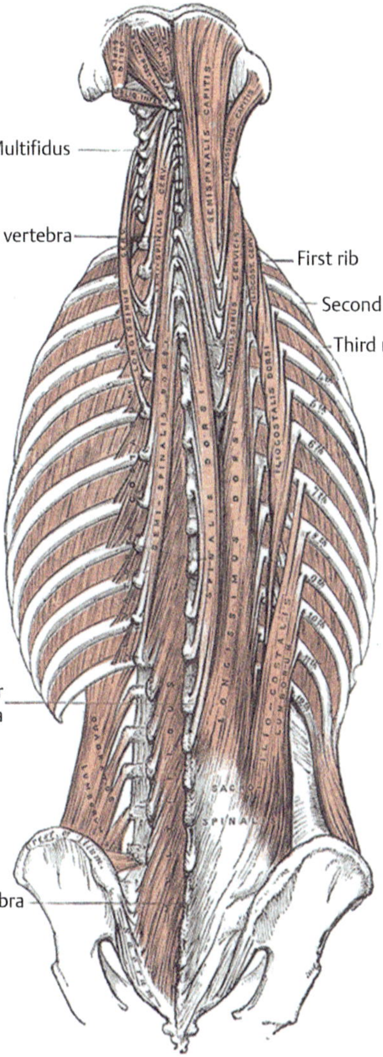

Fig. 4.6 Deep muscles of the lower back. (Reproduced from Gray H. Anatomy of the Human Body. 20th ed. Philadelphia: Lea & Febiger; 1918, in public domain.[7])

    - Lumbar nerve roots travel under the pedicle of the same lumbar vertebra. For example, L5 nerve root travels under L5 pedicle.
    - Extra C8 nerve root (no C8 vertebrae or pedicle) allows for transition.
  - Horizontal (cervical) versus vertical (lumbar) anatomy of nerve root:
    - Due to vertical orientation of the lumbar nerve root, a paracentral and foraminal disk herniation affects different nerve roots in the lumbar spine while the same nerve root is affected in the cervical spine.
- Location of disk herniation and nerve root affected:
  - For example, L4–L5 disk herniation:
    - Central—L5 nerve root, cauda equina.
    - Paracentral—L5 nerve root.
    - Far lateral (extra-foraminal)—L4 nerve root.
- The great vessels (aorta and inferior vena cava) bifurcate at the L4–L5 disk space or at the L5 vertebral body:
  - When performing an anterior approach, the L5–S1 disk space can be accessed inferior to the bifurcation while access to the L4–L5 disk space requires lateral retraction of the great vessels.
- Lateral femoral cutaneous nerve:
  - Meralgia paresthetica:
    - Pathology—entrapment of the lateral femoral cutaneous nerve.
    - Common clinical history—long-term squatting.
    - Presentation—decreased sensation over the anteromedial thigh:
      - No muscle weakness.
      - No reflex abnormalities.
    - Treatment—weight loss, loose-fitting clothes.
  - Other causes of injury—iliac crest bone graft harvest, prone positioning.
- Femoral nerve neuropathy versus L3–L4 nerve root injury.
  - Anatomy—branch to the iliopsoas muscle (hip flexion) is given off in the retroperitoneum, prior to the femoral nerve entering the leg at the level of the inguinal ligament:
    - Hip flexion weakness—L3–L4 nerve root injury.
    - Hip flexion intact—femoral neuropathy at inguinal ligament.
    - Hip flexion spared if neuropathy occurs at the level of the inguinal ligament.
  - Workup—electromyography (EMG) of lumbar paraspinal muscles:
    - Denervation—L3–L4 nerve root injury.
    - Non-denervation—peripheral nerve injury.

Common Clinical Questions

1. Which nerve root is compressed by a right L4–L5 paracentral disk herniation?
2. Which nerve root is compressed by a right L4–L5 far lateral disk herniation?
3. Compression of the exiting right L4 nerve root in the neural foramen most often results from hypertrophy of which articulating process?

Answers to Common Clinical Questions

1. The traversing right L5 nerve root.
2. The exiting right L4 nerve root.
3. The superior articulating process of L5.

References

1. Perez-Cruet M, Fessler R, Wang M. An Anatomic Approach to Minimally Invasive Spine Surgery. 2nd ed. New York: Thieme; 2018
2. Lin RM, Jou IM, Yu CY. Lumbar lordosis: normal adults. J Formos Med Assoc. 1992; 91(3):329–333
3. Agarwal N. Neurosurgery Fundamentals. 1st ed. New York: Thieme; 2018
4. Tubbs R, Loukas M, Hanna A, Oskouian R. Surgical Anatomy of the Lumbar Plexus. 1st ed. New York: Thieme; 2018
5. Russell S. Examination of Peripheral Nerve Injuries: An Anatomical Approach. 2nd ed. New York: Thieme; 2015
6. Khanna A. MRI Essentials for the Spine Specialist. 1st ed. New York: Thieme; 2014
7. Gray H. Anatomy of the Human Body. 20th ed. Philadelphia: Lea & Febiger; 1918

5 Sacral–Iliac Spine

Pedro Aguilar-Salinas and Mauricio J. Avila

Summary

The sacrum consists of five fused vertebrae (S1–S5) that form a wedge-shaped bone. It is the main structure that distributes the load from the lumbar spine to the pelvis through the sacroiliac joints. Other than the iliac joint, it also articulates with the L5 vertebral body via the disk and facet joints as well as the base of the coccyx. The sacrum has a complex neurovascular content. The main nerves originating from the lumbosacral plexus are the sciatic nerve, pudendal nerve, superior gluteal nerve, and inferior gluteal nerve. Given the pathway of the L5 nerve root, which crosses anterior and lateral to the sacral ala, pedicle screw placement at S1 could potentially injure the nerve if misplaced laterally. It is paramount to understand the general anatomy of the sacrum to perform a safer and more accurate surgery.

Keywords: sacrum, anatomy, sacroiliac joint

5.1 Key Points

- The sacrum is the structural link that distributes load from the lumbar spine to the pelvis through the sacroiliac joints (and vice versa).
- The bulbocavernosus reflex involves the S2 to S4 sacral nerves, and its absence or presence is of prognostic significance in spinal cord trauma.[1]
- Because of the location of the lumbosacral plexus in relation to the sacrum, sacral fractures have a high incidence of neurological injury (up to 25%).

5.2 Bony Anatomy

- Normal adult spine consists of five fused sacral vertebrae (S1–S5) that form the wedge-shaped sacrum. It has three surfaces: pelvic, dorsal, and lateral. The dorsal aspect includes the median (midline) sacral crest which represents the fused spinous processes.
- Three to five rudimentary fused coccygeal vertebrae form the coccyx.
- The sacrum has four paired ventral and dorsal sacral foramina, a sacral canal, a sacral promontory (anterior projection of the S1 body), and a

sacral hiatus (dorsal bony opening below the median sacral crest) (**Fig. 5.1** and **Fig. 5.2**).[2]

- The sacroiliac (SI) spine has many palpable bony landmarks. The posterior superior iliac spine may be difficult to palpate but is readily identifiable by the permanent skin dimples above the buttocks.
  - An imaginary line connecting the dimples passes through the S2 spinous process and the middle of the SI joint in the anterior–posterior plane.[3]
  - An imaginary line connecting the highest points of the iliac crest passes through the L4–L5 intervertebral disk space. This helps identify the ideal space to access cerebrospinal fluid (CSF) for sampling with a lumbar puncture.

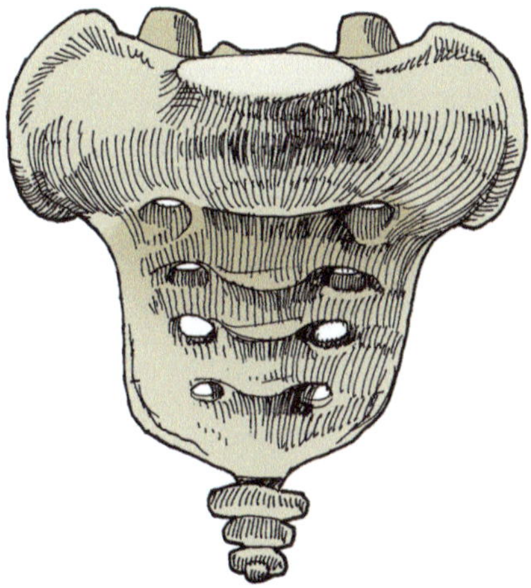

Fig. 5.1 Anterior view of bony sacrum.

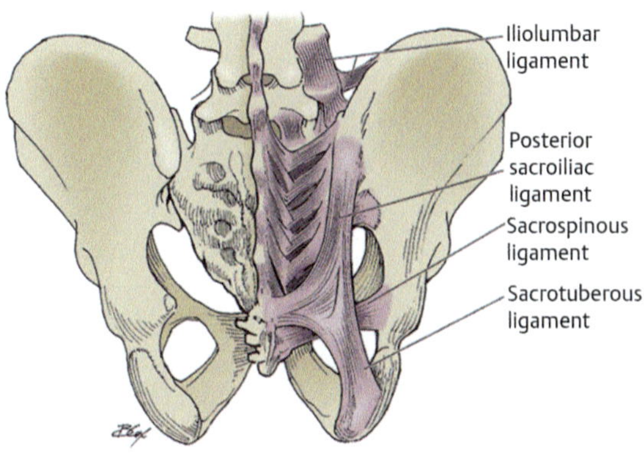

Fig. 5.2 Posterior view of bony sacrum.

- The sacrum has multiple points of articulation:
  - The S1 body articulates with the L5 body via the L5/S1 disk and facet joints. The superior articular process of S1 (part of the L5–S1 facet) faces dorsally. This orientation allows the facet joint to act as a buttress to resist anterior translation.[4]
  - The apex of the sacrum articulates with the base of the coccyx.
  - The lateral aspects of the sacrum articulate with the iliac bones to form the SI joint. The ventral part of this joint contains synovium. The posterior part is a syndesmosis and represents the interosseous sacroiliac ligament (Osborn).[3]

5.3 Neural Anatomy

- Ventral and dorsal branches of the sacral nerves exit the four pairs of anterior and posterior sacral foramina, respectively; the anterior foramina are larger in caliber than their posterior counterparts.[4]
  - These are the dermatomes supplied by sacral nerves (**Fig. 5.3**).
- The thecal sac terminates at the S2 level. The extradural component (filum terminale) attaches to the coccygeal segment (**Fig. 5.4**).[5]
- The lumbosacral trunk is composed of the ventral rami from L4 and L5 and lies posterior to the psoas muscle.[3,5]
- The following are major nerves that arise from this plexus[3]:
  - Sciatic nerve: Composed of the ventral rami from L4 to S3 and has an anterior preaxial tibial division and a postaxial peroneal division (division happens in the popliteal fossa); most commonly, it exits the pelvis via the greater sciatic foramen inferior to the piriformis muscle, and innervates the capsule of the hip joint, posterior thigh (biceps femoris, semitendinosus, semimembranosus, adductor magnus), and all leg muscles via the two distal divisions.[5]
  - Pudendal nerve: Composed of the anterior divisions of the ventral rami of S2 to S4; exits via the greater sciatic foramen between piriformis and ischiococcygeus, supplies the perineum and external genitalia.
  - Superior gluteal nerve: Composed of the posterior divisions of the ventral rami of L4 to S1 to supply the gluteus medius, gluteus minimus, and tensor fascia lata.
  - Inferior gluteal nerve: Composed of the posterior divisions of the ventral rami of L5 to S2; courses with the inferior gluteal artery to supply the gluteus maximus.
- The pelvic splanchnic nerves are composed of parasympathetic fibers derived from S2 to S4 and supply autonomic innervation to various abdominal and pelvic viscera.[1]
- The L5 nerve root crosses anterior and on the lateral edge of the sacral ala (medial to the SI joint), an important reminder when placing S1 pedicle screws.

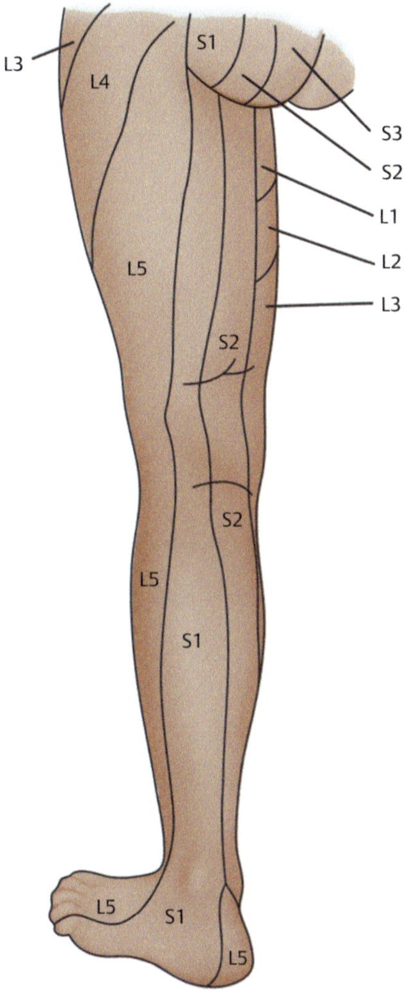

Fig. 5.3 Dermatomal map of sacral nerve roots.

5.4 Vascular Anatomy

- Common iliac artery bifurcates anterior to the SI joint to form the internal iliac artery and descends posteriorly into the greater sciatic foramen to supply the pelvis, buttocks, medial thigh, and perineum.[3]

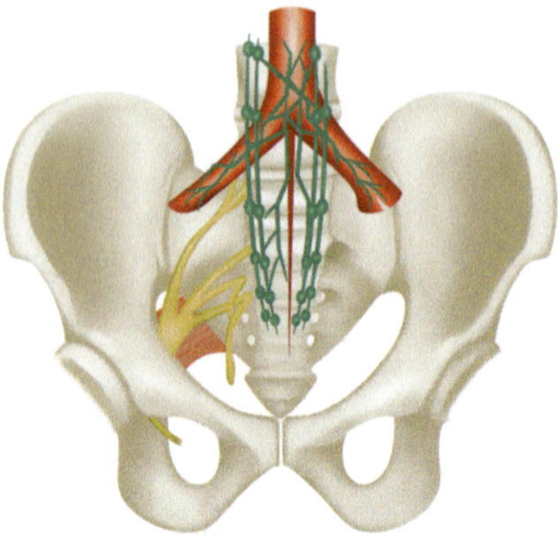

Fig. 5.4 Ventral view of the sacrum with exiting sacral nerve roots.

  - The internal iliac vein sits between the SI joint and the internal iliac artery.
- The median sacral artery is an unpaired vessel that originates from the posterior aspect of the abdominal aorta to supply the lower lumbar vertebrae, sacrum, and coccyx.[3] The median sacral vein accompanies the median sacral artery along the anterior surface of the sacrum and it drains into the left common iliac vein.
- The paired lateral sacral artery branches from the internal iliac artery and courses through the anterior sacral foramina to supply the spinal meninges.[3]

5.5 Ligamentous and Muscular Anatomy

- The anterior longitudinal ligament passes in front of sacral promontory.
- Iliolumbar ligament attaches to the transverse process of L5 with the ilium.
  - Unstable pelvic vertical shear fractures can avulse off the L5 transverse process.[1]
- The anterior SI, posterior SI, and interosseous ligaments suspend the sacrum between the ilium.[3]
  - The posterior SI and interosseous ligaments are thicker and limit motion.
- The sacrotuberous ligament attaches the lateral sacrum to the ischial tuberosity; the sacrospinous ligament attaches the lateral sacrum to the ischial spine.
  - They function to limit upward movement of the caudal portion of the sacrum and delineate the greater and lesser sciatic foramen.[3]
- See **Table 5.1** for major muscles of the sacroiliac spine.

Table 5.1 Sacroiliac muscles: anatomic relationships

Muscle	Origin	Insertion	Innervation	Comment
Gluteus maximus	Dorsal sacrum, ilium	Gluteal tuberosity	Inferior gluteal	Extends hip, externally rotates thigh
Gluteus medius	Medial ilium	Greater trochanter	Superior gluteal	Abducts thigh
Gluteus minimus	Lateral ilium	Anterior greater trochanter	Superior gluteal	Abducts thigh
Iliacus	Iliac fossa	Lesser trochanter	Femoral	Flexes hip
Psoas	T12–L5 vertebrae	Lesser trochanter	Femoral	Flexes hip, overlies lumbosacral plexus
Erector spinae	Sacrum, iliac crest, lumbar spinous process	Thoracic and cervical spinous processes, mastoid process	Dorsal rami	Composed of iliocostalis, longissimus, and spinalis
Multifidus	C2–S4 transverse process	Spinous process	Dorsal rami	Flexes, rotates spine

5.6 Surgical Pearls

- Transitional vertebra can lead to incorrect surgical localization. May be present in up to 25% of patients.[5] Requires counting down, ideally from C2.
- Sacralization: Expanded transverse processes of the L5 vertebrae articulating with top of sacrum.
- Lumbarization: Elevation of S1 vertebrae above the sacral fused mass to assume a lumbar shape.
- Low L5 to S1 disk may not be accessible via an anterior approach as a result of pubic symphysis obstruction.

- Anterior dissection of the superior hypogastric sympathetic plexus can result in retrograde ejaculation in males, a consideration when performing anterior diskectomies at L4–L5, L5–S1.

Common Clinical Question

1. Of the listed nerves, which is the most susceptible to injury during an anterior approach to the SI joint?
   A. S1 nerve root.
   B. Femoral.
   C. Ilioinguinal.
   D. L5 nerve root.
   E. Genitofemoral.

Answer to Common Clinical Question

1. D. The L5 nerve root runs just anterior to the SI joint and is susceptible to injury not only in open procedures, but also with percutaneous SI screw placement. It courses 2 to 3 mm medial to the SI joint.

References

1. Mehta S, Auerbach JD, Born CT, Chin KR. Sacral fractures. J Am Acad Orthop Surg. 2006; 14(12):656–665
2. Hollinshead WH. Anatomy for Surgeons: The Back and Limbs. 3rd ed. Philadelphia, PA: Harper & Row; 1982:88–92
3. Moore KL, Dalley AF. Clinically Oriented Anatomy. 4th ed. Philadelphia, PA: Lippincott; 1999:339–340, 347–355, 434–467
4. Herkowitz HN, Garfin SR, Eismont FJ, et al. The Spine. 5th ed. Philadelphia, PA: Saunders Elsevier; 2006:22
5. Harnsberger HR, Osborn A, MacDonald A, Ross J, eds. "Diagnostic and Surgical Imaging Anatomy: Brain, Head and Neck, Spine. Amirsys; 2006:600

II
Clinical Spine Surgery

6 Physical Examination

Mark S. Greenberg

Summary

The neurological physical examination is an essential component in the evaluation of a patient presenting with a potential neurosurgical diagnosis. It is critical to understand, assess, and differentiate radiculopathy from myelopathy. For example, lumbar spinal findings may mask cervical ones and vice versa. A thorough knowledge of upper and lower motor neuron conditions, and how to evaluate for these during an examination, is paramount.

Keywords: Spurling's maneuver, radiculopathy, Babinski sign, Hoffmann's sign, Lasègue's sign, straight-leg-raising test, femoral stretch test, muscle strength grading, sensory dermatomes, dermatomes, muscle stretch reflexes, Fortin finger test

6.1 Key Points

- There are four main components to the spinal examination: motor, sensory, reflex, and mechanical. This is in addition to the general examination, which includes observation for cutaneous and nail changes, deformity, pain behaviors, and so forth.
- Although components of a general survey nature should always be included, the physical examination is tailored to specific situations based on the history, the region of suspected involvement, and abnormal findings during the survey examination.
- No protocol can cover every contingency, and the examination must be individualized based on patient-specific factors. The order of the examination must also be tailored to the situation.

6.2 Main Components of the Spinal-Related Examination

- Motor (strength, coordination, spasticity, and muscle bulk/tone, including atrophy/fasciculations):
  - Strength evaluation is usually graded using the Royal Medical Research Council of Great Britain (MRC) scale[1] shown in **Table 6.1**.

Table 6.1 Muscle grading (modified Medical Research Council system)

Grade	Strength
0	No contraction (total paralysis)
1	Flicker or trace contraction (palpable or visible)
2	Active movement through full ROM against gravity
3	Active movement against resistance
4	Active movement against resistance (subdivisions: 4 – , slight resistance; 4, moderate resistance; 4 + , strong resistance)
5	Normal strength (against full resistance)
NT	Not testable

Abbreviation: ROM, range of motion.

    - An overview of survey muscle groups to examine is shown in **Table 6.2**.
    - Further motor testing as indicated. It may include tibialis posterior and gluteus medius (in cases of foot drop to distinguish radiculopathy from peripheral neuropathy), first lumbrical (median nerve), and abductor digiti minimi (ulnar nerve).
- Sensation (pinprick, light touch, proprioception, temperature):
  - Pinprick testing: Dermatomes and sensory distributions of peripheral nerves are shown in **Fig. 6.1**.[1]
  - Proprioception (posterior column function) is assessed by testing joint position sense in the second toe on each foot and/or vibratory sense with a low-frequency (128 Hz) tuning fork applied to bony prominences in the ankles.
  - Temperature sense may be crudely assessed by touching the cool metal of a reflex hammer handle to the skin.
- Reflexes (muscle stretch reflexes, pathologic reflexes, cutaneous reflexes, sacral reflexes, and priapism):
  - Muscle stretch reflexes are usually graded as shown in **Table 6.3**.[1] The muscle stretch reflex involved is shown in **Table 6.4**.
  - Babinski sign and Hoffmann's sign and testing for ankle clonus: Part of assessment for long tract signs should be made in all patients to detect unsuspected cervical or thoracic myelopathy or other causes of upper motor neuron deficit.

Table 6.2 Survey muscle groups

Muscle	Major root innervation	Peripheral nerve	Action to test
Upper extremity			
Deltoid	C5, C6	Axillary	Abduct shoulder over 90 degrees above horizontal
Biceps brachii	C5, C6	Musculocutaneous	Flexion at elbow with forearm supinated
Brachioradialis	C5, C6	Radial	Flex elbow with thumb pointing up
Extensor carpi radialis	C5, C6	Radial	Wrist extension
Triceps brachii	C7, C8		Extension at elbow
Flexor digitorum profundus I and II	C7, C8, T1	Anterior interosseus	Flex distal phalanges digits 2 and 3
Lower extremity			
Iliopsoas	L1, L2, L3	Femoral	Thigh flexion
Quadriceps femoris	L3, L4	Femoral	Knee extension
Biceps femoris	L5, S1, **S2**	Sciatic	Knee flexion
Tibialis anterior	L4, L5	Deep peroneal	Ankle dorsiflexion
Extensor hallucis longus	L4, L5	Deep peroneal	Great toes extension
Gastrocnemius	S1, S2	Tibial	Ankle plantarflexion

  - Further reflex testing as indicated includes abdominal cutaneous reflexes, anal wink, and bulbocavernosus. Absence of bulbocavernosus reflex in the setting of acute spinal cord injury may indicate the presence of spinal shock.
  - Priapism may indicate spinal cord injury.
- Mechanical factors: Includes observation for cutaneous changes, pain behaviors, muscle bulk/tone, and provocative maneuvers.

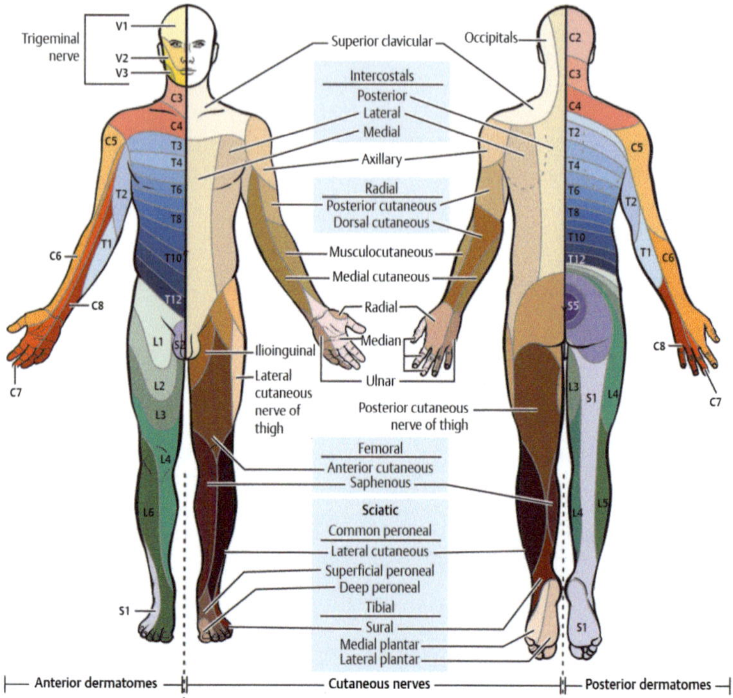

Fig. 6.1 Dermatomes and sensory distributions of peripheral nerves.

- Gait and station: Casual gait is assessed in all patients to check balance, weakness that compromises gait, and pain manifestations. Use tandem gait or Romberg's test to further assess balance and posterior column (proprioceptive) function. The ability to raise up on the toes tests gastrocnemius (S1) more reliably than does manual muscle testing.
- Cervical spine[2]:
  - Cervical range of motion and specific levels of tenderness should be documented to distinguish myofascial pain from bone pain. Specific facet pain diagram patterns can be reviewed with the patient to identify specific problem levels.
  - Spurling's maneuver (axial loading on the vertex of the head with rotation to one side, then repeating with rotation to the other side) may reproduce cervical nerve root symptoms in a patient who has herniated cervical disk or foraminal stenosis. For a positive Spurling test, the symptoms should extend beyond the shoulder girdle.

- Shoulder pathology can often mimic cervical spine pathology. Tenderness of the acromioclavicular joint to palpation or a positive empty-can test (patient extends arms in front, spread approximately 30 degrees laterally from primary position with the thumbs pointing down, and resists while the examiner pushes down on the arms; stresses supraspinatus muscle and tendon) suggests primary shoulder pathology as a cause of shoulder pain.

Table 6.3 Muscle stretch reflex (deep tendon reflex) grading scale

Grade	Definition
0	No contraction (total paralysis)
0.5 +	Elicitable only with reinforcement*
1 +	Low normal
2 +	Normal
3 +	More brisk than normal (hyperreflexic)
4 +	Hyperreflexic with clonus
5 +	Sustained clonus

Note: *In the lower extremities, reinforcement consists of having the patient hook the tips of the fingers of the left hand into the tips of the hooked fingers of the right hand and pulling (Jendrassik maneuver). Reinforcement in the upper extremities consists of having the patient clench the teeth.

Table 6.4 Muscle stretch reflexes

Nerve root involved	Corresponding muscle stretch reflex
C5	Deltoid and pectoralis*
C6	Biceps and brachioradialis
C7	Triceps
C8	Finger flexor*
L4	Patellar (knee jerk)
L5	Medial hamstrings*
S1	Achilles (ankle jerk)

Note: *This reflex is not widely used and may be difficult to elicit.

- Lumbar spine[2]:
  - Lumbar range of motion and specific levels of tenderness should be documented to distinguish myofascial pain from bone pain.
  - Nerve root tension signs: "Pull" on the nerve root that can reproduce pain in situations in which the nerve root is compressed.
  - Laségue's sign, or straight-leg-raising (SLR): With the patient supine, raise one leg at a time, keeping the knee extended. Classically positive findings: Pain or paresthesias in the distribution of the involved nerve root (not just back pain) at < 60 degrees elevation. In response, the patient may lift the hip on the involved side off the examination table. Positive in 83% of cases of nerve root compression. More sensitive for L5 or S1 compression than in upper lumbar roots.
  - Femoral stretch test or reverse straight-leg-raising: With the patient prone, flex the knee on one side at a time. More likely to be positive than SLR with upper lumbar nerve root compression (L2, L3, or L4).
- Hip and sacral pain: Important to distinguish between hip-mediated pathology and low back pathology:
  - Palpation over spinous processes, paraspinal muscles, greater trochanters (to assess for greater trochanteric bursitis), and sacroiliac (SI) joints ("Fortin finger test" suggests sacroilitis when the patient points to SI joint as the primary locus of pain). Palpation over greater trochanters: Pain suggests trochanteric bursitis.
  - FABERE, or Patrick's test (acronym: Flexion, Abduction, External Rotation), of the hip with the patient supine: Back pain suggests musculoskeletal lower back pain or sacroiliac pain; groin or hip pain suggests hip pathology.
  - The shear test can help distinguish sacral pain. With the patient prone, the examiner applies pressure to the sacrum while simultaneously applying a traction force caudal to the corresponding limb. A test is positive if it reproduces the patient's typical pain.
  - FADIR (Flexion, Adduction, Internal Rotation) can help distinguish piriformis syndrome of the hip with the patient supine. Positive response: Pain reproduction centering half the distance between the S3 foramen and the ipsilateral greater trochanter.
  - Pain and or tenderness that localizes within 3 cm of the sacroiliac joint (positive Fortin finger test) suggests possible sacroilitis.
- Vascular considerations: Palpation for pedal pulses to rule out arterial insufficiency; inspection and palpation for pedal edema suggesting venous insufficiency or congestive heart failure.

6.3 Clinical Pearls

- Babinski sign or a positive Hoffmann's sign: If there is no known etiology in a given patient, further investigation is required (to rule out cord compression or brain involvement).
- Cervical radiculopathy does not cause pain with shoulder abduction.
- Painless weakness in the LE almost never results from lumbar nerve root compression. Think of diabetic neuropathy, cervical spondylotic myelopathy, motor neuron disease, and the like.

Common Clinical Questions

1. A 55-year-old male presents to your clinic with progressive lower-extremity weakness and difficulty ambulating. He brings with him an MRI that shows grade 1 spondylolisthesis at L5–S1 with severe central canal stenosis. Flexion–extension lumbar spine X-rays show no instability. His examination shows diffuse weakness of the LEs, diffuse reduction of pinprick sensation in the LEs, reduced Achilles reflexes, and bilateral upgoing toes. Options that could be considered at this point include the following:

   I. Decompressive laminectomy of L5–S1 with attempt at reduction with bilateral pedicle screw/rod instrumentation.

   I. Lateral interbody fusion of L5–S1 with lateral vertebral body plating.

   III. Anterior lumbar interbody fusion with percutaneous L5–S1 pedicle screw/rod instrumentation.

   IV. MRI of the thoracic and cervical spine.

Which are the appropriate options to choose at this time?

A. I and III.

B. II and III.

C. I, II, and III.

D. IV.

2. A patient presents with a 2-month history of left upper extremity pain radiating to the thumb and index finger that has not responded to conservative therapy. He has a positive Spurling's sign with the head turned to the left. Strength is normal. Reflexes are normal except for a reduction in the left biceps. An MRI of the cervical spine shows disk degeneration with protrusion into the left neural foramen at both C5 to C6 and C6 to C7. Flexion–extension cervical spine X-rays are without instability. After providing informed consent, he indicates his wish to

proceed with surgical treatment. Appropriate surgical options include the following, *except* which?

A. Anterior cervical diskectomy and fusion (ACDF) of C5–C6.

B. ACDF of C5–C6 and C6–C7.

C. ACDF of C6–C7.

D. Cervical disk arthroplasty of C5–C6.

3. A 60-year-old male has diffuse weakness of the UEs with reduced reflexes and has hyperreflexia in the LEs with bilateral upgoing toes. Etiologies that could be considered include the following:

I. Cervical spinal stenosis.

II. Left C5–C6 foraminal herniated cervical disk.

III. Motor neuron disease (amyotrophic lateral sclerosis).

IV. Coincident severe lumbar and cervical spinal stenosis.

Which of the foregoing are appropriate diagnoses for this patient?

A. I and III.

B. II and IV.

C. I, II, and III.

D. IV.

Answers to Common Clinical Questions

1. D. Upgoing toes and diffuse LE weakness and hypalgesia are never caused by compromise at L5 to S1. MRI to look for cord compression above the lumbar spine is appropriate.
2. C. The sensory changes and reflex changes indicate that the C6 nerve root is involved, which implicates the disk at C5–C6. Some surgeons would also treat the disk at C6–C7 at the same time, for it may deteriorate rapidly after fusion of C5–C6; and some would perform disk arthroplasty at C5–C6 to try to shield the disk at C6–C7 from some of the forces that would occur with C5–C6 fusion. Operating on C6–C7 alone is inappropriate, for this is currently not a symptomatic level.
3. A. Both cervical spinal stenosis and amyotrophic lateral sclerosis can produce lower motor neuron findings in the UEs and lower motor neuron findings in the LEs. A unilateral foraminal herniated cervical disk will not cause this. In coincidental lumbar and spinal stenosis, the lumbar stenosis generally masks the hyperreflexia in the lower extremities.

References

1. Patton H, Sundsten J, Crill W, et al. Introduction to Basic Neurology. Philadelphia, PA: W. B. Saunders; 1976
2. Greenberg MS. Handbook of Neurosurgery. 7th ed. New York: Thieme Medical Publishers, Inc.; 2010:1352

7 Spinal Imaging

Melissa Yunting Tang, James D. Whaley, Edward L. Baldwin III, Jeremy D. Shaw, and Joon Y. Lee

Summary

Spinal imaging is a necessary tool for spine surgeons to confirm diagnosis and for surgical decision-making. There are multiple modalities of imaging available to surgeons and understanding each imaging technique is of paramount importance for clinical practice. The MRI has become the modality of choice in most cases of spinal pathology. This chapter summarizes each type of imaging modality and how they can be utilized successfully in the treatment of spinal conditions.

Keywords: spine imaging, plain radiographs, computed tomography, MRI, bone scintigraphy, spinal cord injury, spinal tumor

7.1 Key Points

- A complete history and physical examination should be undertaken first to determine the best imaging modality of choice to help with the clinical picture.
- Spinal imaging should always be interpreted in conjunction with the clinical presentation and ongoing differential diagnosis.
- Multiple different imaging modalities can help confirm the diagnosis and guide treatment recommendations.

7.2 Description

- Plain radiographs:
  - Universally available, inexpensive, and convenient.
  - Single planar imaging.
  - First modality of choice for evaluating degenerative disorders, trauma, neoplasm, infection, and deformity.
  - Unable to directly visualize nerve roots or cord compression.
  - Limited ability to determine the clinical severity of cervical and lumbar degenerative disk disease.

- Dynamic radiographs can assess instability in the setting of spondylolisthesis.[1]
- First-line evaluation in the postoperative patient to assess hardware and fusion mass for possible pseudoarthrosis.
- Use of dynamic flexion–extension X-rays is preferred over static X-rays to assess for pseudoarthrosis.

• Computed tomography (CT):
  - Optimizes bony detail visualization.
  - High sensitivity in detecting fractures, with over 99% sensitivity reported[2] (**Fig. 7.1**).
  - Reconstruction views are useful to evaluate suspected postoperative pseudoarthrosis.
  - Direct visualization of potential bony neural compression.
  - Most thin cut spinal CTs today provide submillimeter slices, allowing for optimal bony detail.[3]
  - Multirow detector technology allows for rapid 3-mm image slices with isotropic voxels and no loss in spatial resolution.[3]
  - Limited visualization of neural structures, as well as intrathecal and soft tissue pathology, in comparison to magnetic resonance imaging (MRI).

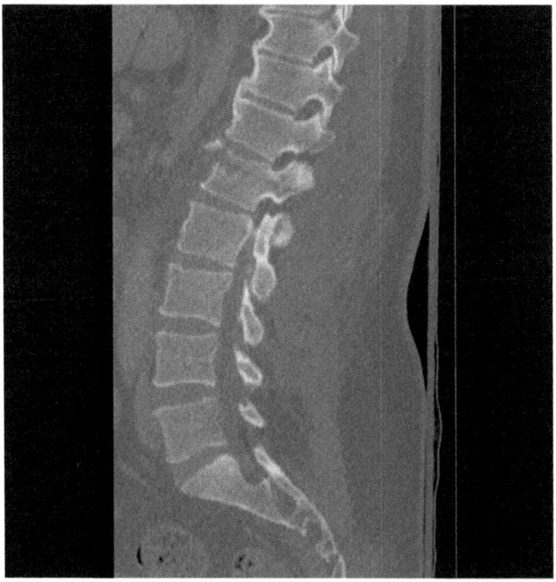

Fig. 7.1 Sagittal computed tomography (CT) image of the thoracolumbar spine demonstrating an L1 bony Chance fracture.

- Disadvantages include radiation exposure, streak artifact in cervical spine, effects of partial volume averaging, and time involved in performing multiple thin sections over multiple intervertebral disks and vertebral bodies.
- Metal artifact can lead to hollow projections causing "sunburst" or streak.
- CT myelography:
  - Can further improve visualization of foraminal and lateral recess stenosis with reconstructed images.[4]
  - Useful in patients who have implantable devices and cannot obtain MRI (e.g., pacemaker). Also useful in the setting of stainless steel implants due to significant metal artifact with MRI (e.g., Texas Scottish Rite Hospital [TSRH] spinal instrumentation).
  - Disadvantages include lack of diagnostic specificity, uncertainty of compressive lesion, and invasiveness.
- Myelography:
  - Indirect, rather than direct, assessment of extradural compression.
  - Intrathecal water-soluble contrast mixes with cerebrospinal fluid through C1 to C2 or lumbar puncture.
  - Diagnosis can be inferred based on changes in the contour of the contrast-filled thecal sac and nerve root sleeves.
  - Extradural impression on the dye column and filling defects of the nerve root sleeve demonstrate compression.
  - Water-soluble agents are available and provide excellent contrast enhancement.
  - Low rates of side effects (e.g., iohexol, iopamidol).
  - Less toxic; absorption makes removal unnecessary:
    - Newer nonionic water-soluble agents have milder side effects; severe side effects such as hallucinations, confusion, and seizures rarely occur.

- MRI[5]:
  - Modality of choice for most spinal pathology.
  - Excellent noninvasive imaging of soft tissue pathology, including hematoma, infection, spinal cord injury, and tumor, as well as identification of intramedullary, intradural, and extradural compressive lesions.
  - High sensitivity in identifying ligamentous injury (anterior and posterior longitudinal ligaments, posterior ligamentous complex [PLC]); T2 or short tau inversion recovery (STIR) sequences are particularly helpful.
  - Requires no radiation exposure, generally well tolerated, and uses pulsed radiofrequency (RF).

- Presence of facet fluid and/or interspinous fluid is associated with dynamic spondylolisthesis. Presence of these findings should lead to obtaining flexion–extension radiographs to assess presence of dynamic instability, especially for preoperative planning.[6,7]
- T1-weighted images:
  - MRI findings: Adipose, high signal; cortical bone, low signal; free water, low signal.
- T2-weighted images:
  - MRI findings: Adipose, low signal; cortical bone, low signal; free water, high signal.
- Gadolinium-based IV contrast medium can help distinguish recurrent disk herniation (avascular, no enhancement) from postoperative scar (vascular, enhancement) on T1-weighted images.
- Contrast can be useful in detecting tumor and infection:
  - Tumor: Intervertebral disk is often spared but usually involves the entire vertebral body; may show multiple noncontiguous vertebrae with metastatic disease, indicating skip lesions (highest sensitivity with STIR sequences).
  - Infection (diskitis, vertebral osteomyelitis, epidural abscess): Increased signal on T2, decreased signal on T1, enhancement with gadolinium (**Fig. 7.2**).
- Spinal cord injury:
  - MRI can quantify degree of spinal cord compression and injury.[8]
  - Can distinguish spinal cord edema from hemorrhage (T1 low, T2 high versus T1 high, T2 high, respectively).
  - STIR sequence important in identifying intramedullary cord lesions.
  - 3-Tesla magnets can image individual spinal cord tracts, providing more accurate posttraumatic neurological assessment.
- Disk degeneration:
  - MRI findings must be strictly correlated with the clinical presentation.[9]
  - In general, degenerative changes are age-related and present in both asymptomatic and symptomatic individuals.
  - Advanced imaging should be reserved for patients who have objective evidence of root irritation on examination, patients who have true radicular symptoms, and patients who have failed conservative nonoperative treatment.
  - MRI may show end plate and hypertrophic ligamentous changes, disk pathology, and evidence of instability.[10]
  - High-intensity zone (HIZ) (radial tear of the posterior annulus, fissure extending from nucleus to the periphery), dark disks with or without height loss, and Modic end plate changes have been extensively studied and have unknown clinical significance.

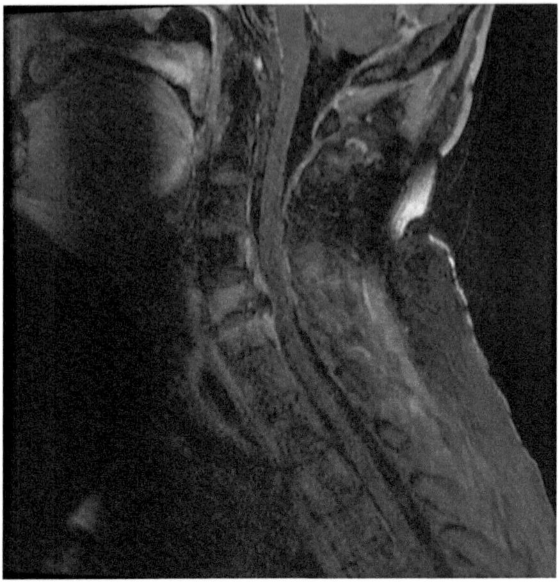

Fig. 7.2 Sagittal T1-weighted fluid-attenuated inversion recovery (FLAIR) magnetic resonance imaging (MRI) with gadolinium contrast enhancement demonstrating C5–C6 diskitis, vertebral osteomyelitis, and a large ventral epidural abscess with significant spinal cord compression.

- Modic end plate changes[11]:
  - Type 1:
    - T1 low, T2 high.
    - Associated with back pain and instability.
  - Type 2:
    - T1 high, T2 normal.
    - Presence of yellow marrow accounts for shortening of T1 signal.
    - More common than type 1.
  - Type 3:
    - T1 low, T2 low.
    - Less segmental instability secondary to advanced degeneration and sclerosis.
- Disk herniation nomenclature[12]:
  - *Protrusion:* Herniation that maintains contact with the disk of origin via a bridge as wide as or wider than the diameter of the displaced material.

- ▫ *Extrusion:* Diameter of disk material beyond interspace is greater than the width of bridge that may or may not connect to the disk of origin.
- ▫ *Sequestration:* Extrusion that is no longer contiguous with the disk of origin (**Fig. 7.3**).
- ▫ Location (axial plane): Central, subarticular or lateral recess, foraminal or pedicle zone, extraforaminal or far lateral zone, anterior zone.

- Artifact:
  - Spinal implants can result in metal artifact and poor image quality unless specific techniques are used (polymer < titanium < tantalum < stainless steel < cobalt chrome).
  - Strategies to decrease artifact include larger fields of view, smaller voxel sizes, higher readout bandwidths, and geographic orientation of the frequency-encoded direction in relation to the metal objects.

- Contraindications: Metal debris in the eye, ferrous metal implant in the brain, inner ear implant, cardiac pacemaker.
- However, 1.5-tesla MRI has been shown to be safe for most pacemakers and implantable cardioverter-defibrillators (ICDs).[13]

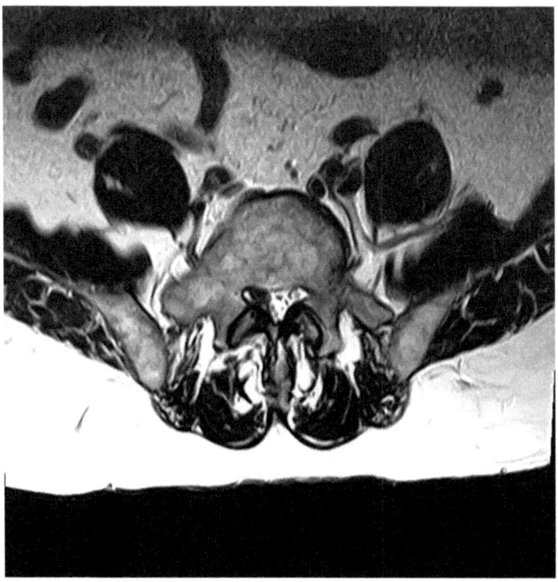

Fig. 7.3 Axial T2-weighted magnetic resonance imaging (MRI) of the lumbar spine demonstrating an L5–S1 sequestered herniated nucleus pulposus in the right subarticular recess.

- Bone scintigraphy[14]:
  - Superior sensitivity.
  - Poor specificity.
  - Can help detect lesions in symptomatic patients with negative radiographs.
  - Standard part of the workup of metastatic bone disease.
  - Can help distinguish acute versus chronic pars interarticularis fractures.

7.3 Surgical Pearls

- Before obtaining advanced imaging of the spine, a plan must be in place for how the results will be used to determine the best treatment regimen.
- A differential diagnosis should be established based on the history and physical examination and refined based on imaging findings before implementation of a nonoperative versus operative treatment plan.
- Advanced imaging can be extremely helpful in establishing a diagnosis and implementing treatment resulting in a high rate of clinical success.

Common Clinical Questions

1. Which specific combination of signal intensities and MRI sequences denote spinal cord hemorrhage?

   A. High T1, high T2.

   B. Low T1, high T2.

   C. High T1, low T2.

   D. Low T1, low T2.

2. A 35-year-old male who has previously undergone a lumbar microdiskectomy for an L4–L5 herniated nucleus pulposus presents to you with an acute onset of recurrent lower extremity radiculopathy 8 months after his previous surgery. Which MRI sequence of choice will best help distinguish a recurrent disk herniation from epidural fibrosis?

   A. Gadolinium-enhanced T1 sequence.

   B. Gadolinium-enhanced T2 sequence.

   C. STIR sequence.

   D. T1 sequence alone.

   E. T2 sequence alone.

3. Which imaging modality is most often used to assess for dynamic instability in the setting of spondylolisthesis?

A. Static radiographs.

B. Dynamic (flexion–extension) lateral radiographs.

C. CT.

D. MRI.

4. What MRI sequence is best used to differentiate myelomalacia versus spinal cord edema?[15]

A. T2.

B. T1.

C. STIR.

D. FLAIR.

Answers to Common Clinical Questions

1. A.
2. A.
3. B.
4. A.

References

1. White AP, Biswas D, Smart LR, Haims A, Grauer JN. Utility of flexion-extension radiographs in evaluating the degenerative cervical spine. Spine. 2007; 32(9):975–979
2. Brown CV, Antevil JL, Sise MJ, Sack DI. Spiral computed tomography for the diagnosis of cervical, thoracic, and lumbar spine fractures: its time has come. J Trauma. 2005; 58(5):890–895, discussion 895–896
3. Phal PM, Riccelli LP, Wang P, Nesbit GM, Anderson JC. Fracture detection in the cervical spine with multidetector CT: 1-mm versus 3-mm axial images. AJNR Am J Neuroradiol. 2008; 29(8):1446–1449
4. Patel DM, Weinberg BD, Hoch MJCT. CT myelography: clinical indications and imaging findings. Radiographics. 2020; 40(2):470–484
5. Herkowitz HN, Garfin SR, Eismont FJ, Bell GR, Balderston RA, eds. Rothman-Simeone: The Spine. 6th ed. Philadelphia, PA: Saunders Elsevier; 2011
6. Dombrowski ME, Rynearson B, LeVasseur C, et al. ISSLS PRIZE IN BIOENGINEERING SCIENCE 2018: dynamic imaging of degenerative spondylolisthesis reveals mid-range dynamic lumbar instability not evident on static clinical radiographs. Eur Spine J. 2018; 27(4):752–762

7. Even JL, Chen AF, Lee JY. Imaging characteristics of "dynamic" versus "static" spondylolisthesis: analysis using magnetic resonance imaging and flexion/extension films. Spine J. 2014; 14(9):1965–1969
8. Freund P, Seif M, Weiskopf N, et al. MRI in traumatic spinal cord injury: from clinical assessment to neuroimaging biomarkers. Lancet Neurol. 2019; 18(12):1123–1135
9. Farshad-Amacker NA, Farshad M, Winklehner A, Andreisek G. MR imaging of degenerative disc disease. Eur J Radiol. 2015; 84(9):1768–1776
10. Emch TM, Modic MT. Imaging of lumbar degenerative disk disease: history and current state. Skeletal Radiol. 2011; 40(9):1175–1189
11. Modic MT, Ross JS. Lumbar degenerative disk disease. Radiology. 2007; 245(1):43–61
12. Fardon DF, Milette PC, Combined Task Forces of the North American Spine Society, American Society of Spine Radiology, and American Society of Neuroradiology. Nomenclature and classification of lumbar disc pathology. Recommendations of the Combined Task Forces of the North American Spine Society, American Society of Spine Radiology, and American Society of Neuroradiology. Spine. 2001; 26(5):E93–E113
13. van Dijk VF, Delnoy PPHM, Smit JJJ, et al. Preliminary findings on the safety of 1.5 and 3 Tesla magnetic resonance imaging in cardiac pacemaker patients. J Cardiovasc Electrophysiol. 2017; 28(7):806–810
14. Cook GJR, Goh V. Molecular imaging of bone metastases and their response to therapy. J Nucl Med. 2020; 61(6):799–806
15. Lee MJ, Aronberg R, Manganaro MS, Ibrahim M, Parmar HA. Diagnostic approach to intrinsic abnormality of spinal cord signal intensity. Radiographics. 2019; 39(6):1824–1839

8 Radiation Exposure in Spine Surgery

Javier Quillo-Olvera, Javier Quillo-Reséndiz, and Michelle Barrera-Arreola

Summary

Fluoroscopy is a crucial tool in spine surgery, used for planning, orientation, and guidance in most spinal surgical procedures. However, it is not without risks, as it exposes both the patient and the surgical staff to radiation. Therefore, the surgeon needs to minimize radiation exposure during the procedure. It is essential for the surgeon to understand how the radiation dose emitted by the fluoroscope is measured. The direct dose is measured in mGy, while the effective dose is measured in Sieverts. This chapter outlines the health effects of direct dose exposure to ionizing radiation. Additionally, it discusses general principles of protection. For instance, the National Council on Radiation Protection and Measurements recommend an annual radiation exposure of 50 mSv or 5 rem per year. It also suggests using intraoperative image acquisition with navigation as a reasonable alternative to emitting intraoperative radiation in spine procedures. The chapter provides specific bullet points to avoid confusion and access the most relevant aspects of this topic.

Keywords: fluoroscope, intraoperative radiation, risks, spine, surgery

8.1 Key Points

- Fluoroscopy is an essential tool during many spine procedures, but its use carries a variety of radiation exposure–related risks to the patient, surgeon, and operating room (OR) staff.[1,2]
- Minimizing radiation exposure to the patient and surgical staff by optimizing the appropriate protective gear, knowledge of the position, distance from the radiation source, and using advanced image guidance navigation-assisted technology is a priority during spinal procedures.[2,3]

8.2 Description

- Ionizing radiation units of measure:
  - Gray (Gy) is an SI unit representing 1 J of radiation energy absorbed by 1 kg of mass.
  - Sievert (Sv) is an SI unit of equivalent dose or effective dose related to the biological effect of depositing a joule of radiation energy in a kilogram of human tissue.
    - It corresponds to the product of the absorbed dose of radiation and a dimensionless quality factor (Q).
  - Rem was the denomination used until January 1, 1985, for the energy created during an X-ray.
  - Gy and Sv share units (joules per kilogram), but by convention, Gy refers to dose and deterministic effects of radiation seen at high doses, whereas Sv refers to the stochastic effects of radiation seen at lower doses.
- The radiation dose emitted by the fluoroscope can be measured in two ways: the direct dose and the effective dose.
  - The direct dose of ionizing radiation is that received by the skin or the organ measured in mGy.[4]
  - The effective dose is related to the risk of cancer measured in Sieverts (Sv). A lumbar radiograph is 1.5 mSv, and a lumbar CT is 15 mSv.[4]
- For medical purposes, X-rays are produced in a vacuum tube that uses high voltage to accelerate electrons from a cathode to a metal anode releasing photons.
- A patient can then be placed between the X-ray tube and X-ray detector (image intensifier for fluoroscopy), and images are generated based on the differential X-ray absorption of tissues.
- X-rays are a type of ionizing radiation which have sufficient energy to remove electrons from atoms, so they are defined as a carcinogen by the World Health Organization.[2]
- Being directly in the X-ray beam places a patient at risk for radiation effects:
  - Radiation exposure to the patient should be minimized within the confines of appropriate medical management.[1,5]
- Radiation scatter poses a cumulative occupational risk to clinicians performing spine surgery over their careers.[2,5]
- During spine surgery, X-rays are commonly used for a variety of purposes, including the following:
  - Level confirmation.
  - Fracture–dislocation reduction.
  - Deformity correction.
  - Implant guidance for anatomic localization, orientation, or fixation.

  - Biopsy.
  - Vertebroplasty or kyphoplasty.
  - Percutaneous or minimally invasive hardware placement.
- Pathological reactions of the human body and genetic material related to the application of X-rays are called *radiological damage*.
- *Radiological risk* is the probability that a person exposed to radiation suffers a negative effect in a given time.
- *Harm risk* designates these adverse effects on a population.
- Health effects of the direct dose of ionizing radiation include the following[3]:
  - Tissue effects:
    - Testes (temporary sterility):
      - 0.1 Gy single exposure or 0.4 Gy annual exposure.
    - Testes (permanent sterility):
      - 6.0 Gy single exposure or 2.0 Gy annual exposure.
    - Ovaries (sterility):
      - 3.0 Gy single exposure or 0.2 Gy annual exposure.
    - Lens (cataract):
      - 0.5 Gy single exposure or 0.5 Gy lifetime exposure.
    - Bone marrow (depression of hematopoiesis):
      - 0.5 Gy single exposure or 0.4 Gy annual exposure.
    - Heart or brain (circulatory disease):
      - 0.1 Gy single exposure or 0.5 Gy annual exposure.
  - Stochastic effects:
    - Detriment-adjusted nominal risk coefficient after exposure to radiation at a low dose rate[3]:
      - 5.5%/Sv for cancer.
      - 0.2%/Sv for genetic effects.
    - Other factors may increase an individual's risk for cancer:
      - Younger age.
      - Female gender.
      - Autoimmune, connective tissue, or DNA repair disorders.

8.3 General Principles of Radiation Protection[1,6,7,8,9,10]

- A fundamental rule in radiation protection is to keep ionizing radiation as low as possible or "ALARA" (as low as reasonably achievable).
- Another principle is the inverse square law which states that the dose rate per surface area decreases in inverse proportion to the square of the distance.

- The National Council on Radiation Protection and Measurements recommends an annual radiation exposure limit for an occupational category of 50 mSv or 5 rem per year.
- The International Commission on Radiation Protection advises an annual exposure limit of 20 mSv or 2 rem for a 5-year average.
- The American Academy of Orthopaedic Surgeons (AAOS) recommends educating users on safe techniques to reduce exposure using protective equipment and dose-measuring methods, and regular maintenance of imaging devices and shielding.
- Certain steps can minimize radiation exposure to a spine surgeon and OR staff:
  - Equipment-based radiation protection:
    - All OR personnel should wear lead or lead equivalent shielding during fluoroscopy.
    - Eyes, thyroid, gonads, and femurs require protection.
    - Shielding should not be folded or creased and should be tested annually for defects.
    - Mobile lead glass screen can reduce the local radiation dose by 50 to 60% in the head–neck region.
    - Shielding attached to the underside of the patient table protects the surgeon in the region of the lower extremities by blocking scatter radiation emitted laterally by the patient. Local dose reduction in the lower extremities is up to 64 and 93.3% for the gonads.
    - Mobile radiation protection barriers protect the surgeon from scattered radiation depending on the size, shape, and design and can reduce the dose rate by 96.1%.
  - Personal radiation protection:
    - Best protection with one-piece lead-based aprons with an overlap in the front and a lead equivalent of 0.35 mm. A wraparound apron provides 5 times better radiation protection than a front-only apron.
    - Thyroid protection with a lead equivalent of 0.5 mm and coverage on the largest surface possible.
    - Radiation protection glasses in combination with a mobile lead glass screen can achieve a radiation dose reduction of 82.5%.
    - Wearing lead gloves during percutaneous procedures has also been reported to reduce the absorbed dose by 97.1% to the surgeon's hands.
- Other recommendations:
  - Minimize shots of fluoroscopy used per procedure.
  - Use pulsed setting rather than continuous fluoroscopy.
  - Nonessential personnel should leave the room during fluoroscopy.
  - Essential personnel should position themselves as far from the machine as the room allows (preferably behind the image intensifier) and a lead shield.

- When operating under fluoroscopic guidance, maintain a distance of 2 to 3 feet from the X-ray beam source.
- Stand opposite the source (near the image intensifier) to reduce exposure to scatter radiation during lateral fluoroscopy and position the source below the patient for anteroposterior (AP) images.
- Turn your head 90 degrees from the patient to reduce scattering to the eyes.
- Use collimation and automatic brightness control when appropriate.
- Place the image intensifier as close to the patient as possible to reduce scatter.

8.4 Evidence-Based Medicine Statements[3,9]

- Exposure to ionizing radiation is higher in minimally invasive spine procedures than in open spine surgery (level of evidence II).
- Standing contralateral to the imaging source decreases radiation exposure. Also, increasing the distance between the surgeon and the radiation source decreases radiation exposure (level of evidence IV).
- Advanced navigation-based imaging methods help reduce radiation exposure for the surgeon. Available imaging modalities include standard C-arm, mini-C-arm, and three-dimensional (3D) reconstructed C-arm. However, established workflows are required to gain that advantage (level of evidence II, III).
- O-arms can acquire more images in a shorter period than C-arms. For example, in its standard volumetric three-dimensional image mode, the O-arms can obtain about 400 images over 360 degrees in 14 seconds. However, a significant reduction in radiation exposure is exclusively for the surgeon and staff who have the advantage of leaving the OR during image acquisition, but not for the patient. Therefore, the radiation risks to the patient must be considered when choosing O-arm imaging, despite the benefit to the clinicians.

8.5 Surgical Pearls

- Always wear appropriate protection and stand as far from the X-ray beam as possible because the radiation dose to the operator decreases exponentially with distance from the source.[1,2,5]
- Use a “hands-off” technique when appropriate to minimize exposure during procedures.[1,2,5]
- Consider using intraoperative navigation guidance when many levels are involved.

Common Clinical Questions

1. Is it true or false that radiological damage refers to a breakdown in the source of ionizing radiation?
2. Is it true or false that the direct dose of ionizing radiation in the skin or an organ is measured in Sieverts?
3. Which of the following dose of ionizing radiation is associated with the risk of permanent male sterility due to testicular damage?
   A. 1.0 Gy single exposure or 2.0 Gy annual exposure.
   B. 2.0 Gy single exposure or 2.0 Gy annual exposure.
   C. 4.0 Gy single exposure or 4.0 Gy annual exposure.
   D. 6.0 Gy single exposure or 2.0 Gy annual exposure.
   E. 0.6 Gy single exposure or 0.2 Gy annual exposure.

Answers to Common Clinical Questions

1. False.
2. False.
3. D.

References

1. Rehani MM, Ciraj-Bjelac O, Vañó E, et al. ICRP Publication 117. Radiological protection in fluoroscopically guided procedures performed outside the imaging department. Ann ICRP. 2010; 40(6):1–102
2. The 2007 Recommendations of the International Commission on Radiological Protection. ICRP publication 103. Ann ICRP. 2007; 37(2–4):1–332
3. Yu E, Khan SN. Does less invasive spine surgery result in increased radiation exposure? A systematic review. Clin Orthop Relat Res. 2014; 472 (6):1738–1748
4. Giordano BD, Grauer JN, Miller CP, Morgan TL, Rechtine GR, II. Radiation exposure issues in orthopaedics. J Bone Joint Surg Am. 2011; 93(12):e69–(1–10)
5. Srinivasan D, Than KD, Wang AC, et al. Radiation safety and spine surgery: systematic review of exposure limits and methods to minimize radiation exposure. World Neurosurg. 2014; 82(6):1337–1343
6. Recommendations on Limits for Exposure to Ionizing Radiation. Bethesda, MD, USA: National Council on Radiation Protection and Measurements; 1987:91

7. Recommendations of the International Commission on Radiological Protection. New York, NY, USA: International Commission on Radiological Protection; 1990;21
8. Kaplan DJ, Patel JN, Liporace FA, Yoon RS. Intraoperative radiation safety in orthopaedics: a review of the ALARA (as low as reasonably achievable) principle. Patient Saf Surg. 2016; 10:27
9. Jenkins NW, Parrish JM, Sheha ED, Singh K. Intraoperative risks of radiation exposure for the surgeon and patient. Ann Transl Med. 2021; 9(1):84
10. König AM, Etzel R, Thomas RP, Mahnken AH. Persönliche Strahlenschutzmittel und Dosimetrie des medizinischen Personals in der interventionellen Radiologie: Aktueller Status und neue Entwicklungen [Personal radiation protection and corresponding dosimetry in interventional radiology: an overview and future developments]. Röfo Fortschr Geb Röntgenstr Neuen Bildgeb Verfahr. 2019; 191(6):512–521

9 Electrodiagnostic Testing in Spine Surgery

Kamakshi Patel and Holli A. Horak

Summary

Electrodiagnostic testing plays a crucial role in preoperative assessment and postoperative evaluation of patients undergoing spine surgery. This chapter explores the application of electrodiagnostic techniques, including electromyography (EMG) and nerve conduction studies (NCS), in the context of spine surgery. It delves into the principles, indications, and limitations of electrodiagnostic testing, emphasizing its utility in diagnosing radiculopathy, myelopathy, and peripheral nerve injuries. This chapter aims to provide spine surgeons with a deeper understanding of the role of electrodiagnostic testing in contemporary spine surgery practice.

Keywords: nerve conduction studies, electromyography, radiculopathy

9.1 Key Points

- Electromyogram/nerve conduction studies (EMG/NCSs) are performed for patients who show evidence of peripheral nervous system damage/injury.
- EMG/NCS data can be used, along with the history, physical examination, and neuroimaging, to guide the timing and localization of surgery.
- EMG/NCS cannot assess central nervous system problems such as myelopathy.
- EMG/NCS should be considered if there may be other neurologic reasons for the patient's symptoms or if the history does not match clinical examination findings. This includes evaluation for myasthenia gravis, Guillain-Barré syndrome, diabetic neuropathy, amyotrophic lateral sclerosis (ALS), and myopathies.
- EMG/NCS of the affected limb(s) can distinguish between nerve root avulsion, radiculopathy/multiple radiculopathies, plexopathy, and neuropathy.[1]
- EMG/NCS can also assist in assessing severity and time course of nerve root compression/damage.

- It is often preferable to wait 4 to 6 weeks after symptom onset before performing EMG/NCS unless the patient is critically ill or has rapid-onset paralysis. This is because of a delay in EMG manifestations owing to the time it takes for the affected axons to degenerate.

9.2 Description

9.2.1 Nerve Conduction Study

- NCS is a separate test from EMG, but the two are performed in conjunction > 90% of the time.
- NCS evaluates the integrity of the nerve itself and can assess for axonal or demyelinating damage.
- NCS parameters include the amplitude (related to the number of functional nerve fibers), latency (marker of speed of conduction from point of stimulation), and conduction velocity of individual peripheral nerves.[2,3]
- Reduced amplitude is associated with axonal loss. This is a feature of idiopathic peripheral neuropathies.
- Prolonged latency and significantly slow conduction velocity are seen in demyelinating processes. An example of this is the prolonged latency seen in carpal tunnel syndrome (CTS).
- Both motor and sensory nerve fibers can be evaluated.
- In a radiculopathy, the sensory nerve conduction study may remain normal even when the patient has clear sensory loss.
  - This is because the cell nucleus of the sensory nerve is located in the dorsal root ganglion, external to the spinal canal (and often distal to a disk herniation) (see **Fig. 9.1**).
  - Because the nucleus and distal axon are unaffected, the sensory NCS will be normal even if there are sensory symptoms (because the proximal portion of the axon is affected).

9.2.2 Electromyogram (EMG)

- EMG is the evaluation of motor unit potentials (MUPs) in the muscle.
- EMG is performed in the affected limb(s) either to evaluate the muscle fibers or to evaluate motor neuron innervation to the muscles of that specific myotome.
- EMG assesses two parameters: Spontaneous activity and MUPs[4]:
  - Spontaneous activity is the presence or absence of abnormal discharges from individual muscle fibers, the most common being fibrillations and positive waves.

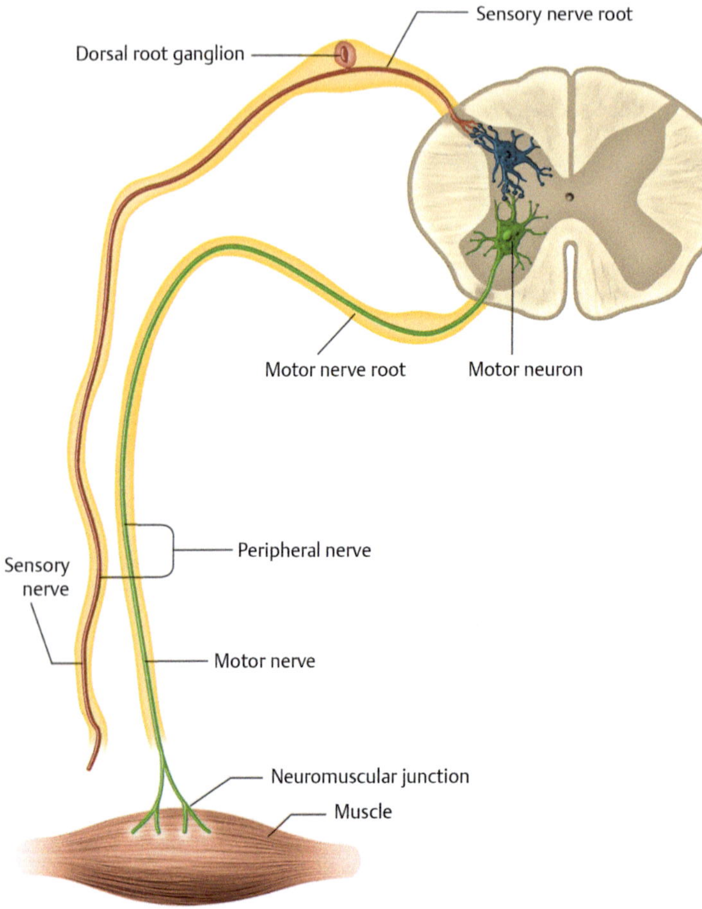

Fig. 9.1 Axial image of spinal cord showing relative location of dorsal root ganglion.

- MUPs are the electrical potentials generated by the contraction of all muscle fibers innervated by one individual motor neuron.
- EMG can potentially distinguish between hyperacute (less than 3 weeks), acute (3–12 weeks), and chronic (> 12 weeks) lesions.
- Sensitivity and specificity depend on the degree of damage/injury and presence of other coexisting peripheral nerve diseases, such as peripheral neuropathy.

9.2.3 Pathophysiology of Radiculopathy

- After 3 to 4 weeks (acute stage), fibrillations and positive waves will develop.
- Fibrillations and positive waves are strongly associated with acute axonal injury, but because they can be seen in other conditions as well, clinical correlation is needed.
- After 6 weeks or so (subacute), the surrounding remaining axons sprout new branches to the denervated muscle fibers; this is called reinnervation (see **Fig. 9.2**).[4]

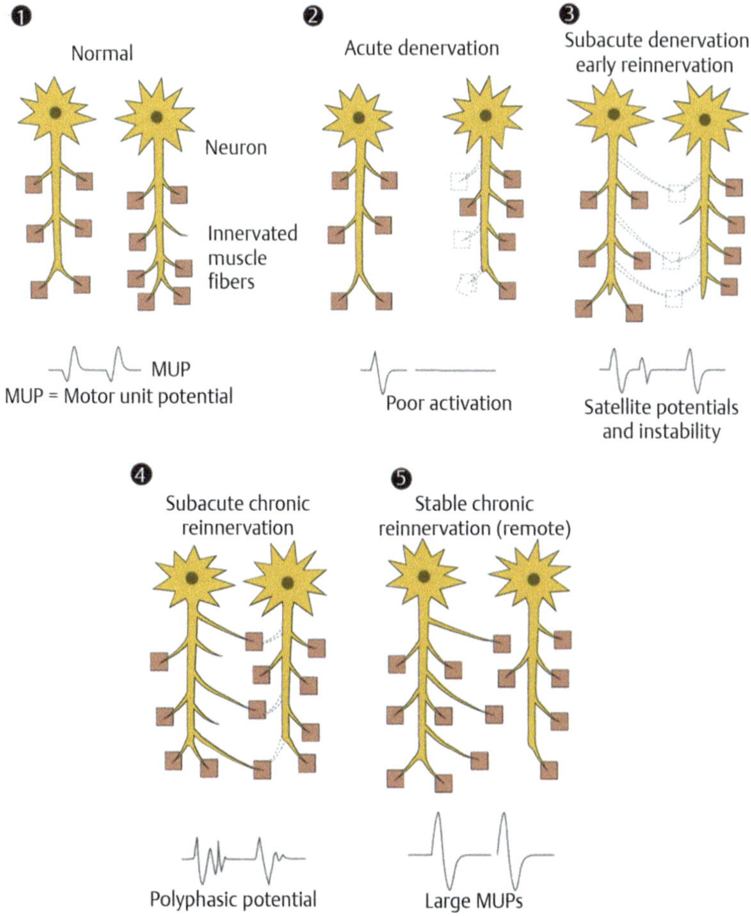

Fig. 9.2 Graphic demonstration of acute denervation and reinnervation of a motor unit.

Table 9.1 Table of radiculopathy findings

Nerve root level	Example of commonly affected muscles
C5–C6	Deltoid, biceps
C6–C7	Triceps, pronator teres
C8	First dorsal interosseous, abductor pollicis brevis
L3–L4	Vastus lateralis, vastus medialis
L4–L5	Tibialis anterior, gluteus medius
S1	Gastrocnemius, gluteus maximus, short head of biceps femoris

- With early reinnervation, the MUPs demonstrate immature potentials (satellite potentials) and irregular firing rates (also called instability).
- During reinnervation, the MUPs become polyphasic and larger as the newly reinnervated muscle fibers become integrated into the motor unit.
- After 12 weeks or so (chronic), muscle fibers are reinnervated and the potentials become more mature, giving rise to triphasic, long-duration, large-amplitude stable motor units on EMG.
- See **Table 9.1** for the more commonly affected muscles associated with specific radiculopathy levels.

9.3 EMG/NCS Pearls

- EMG does not show denervation changes initially; it may take 3 to 4 weeks for denervation (axonal injury) to be evident on EMG, in the form of abnormal insertion with fibrillations.[5]
- Accordingly, waiting 3 to 4 weeks, if possible, provides greater sensitivity.
- The earliest changes (less than 4 weeks) on EMG may simply be difficulty activating the muscles in the affected nerve root distribution.
- Sensory nerve conduction studies may remain normal in the setting of severe nerve injury (avulsion, severe radiculopathy), but motor fibers will show low or absent amplitude.

Common Clinical Questions

1. A patient who has diabetes with low amplitudes on NCS and chronic denervation changes on EMG seen only in the distal muscles of the bilateral L5 to S1 myotomes likely has what?

   A. Acute bilateral L5 and S1 radiculopathies.

   B. Acute inflammatory demyelinating polyneuropathy (Guillain-Barré syndrome).
   C. Polymyositis.
   D. Peripheral neuropathy.

2. A patient who has a suspected L5 radiculopathy has an EMG done within 1 week. What is it most likely to show?
   A. +4 fibrillations and positive waves, polyphasic, rapid-firing, large motor units.
   B. Prolonged latencies on both motor and sensory nerve conduction studies.
   C. Normal insertion but very long-duration, rapid-firing motor units.
   D. Normal insertion, but poor activation of muscles in the right L5 myotome.

3. A patient who has fibrillations, positive waves, and polyphasic motor units in the deltoids, biceps, and midcervical paraspinal muscles, but in whom all other muscles are normal, likely has what?
   A. Axillary neuropathy.
   B. Remote, inactive C5 radiculopathy.
   C. Subacute C5–C6 radiculopathies.
   D. Amyotrophic lateral sclerosis.

Answers to Common Clinical Questions

1. D.
2. D.
3. C.

References

1. Ahmad A, Barkhaus P, Levin K, Simmons Z. Basics of Lower Extremity Clinical and Electrodiagnostic Evaluation. American Association of Neuromuscular and Electrodiagnostic Medicine 2014 Course Book, 61st annual meeting
2. Preston DC, Shapiro BE. Electromyography and Neuromuscular Disorders: Clinical Electrophysiologic Correlations. Elsevier; 2020
3. Patel K, Horak HA. Electrodiagnosis of Common Mononeuropathies: Median, Ulnar, and Fibular (Peroneal) Neuropathies. Neurol Clin. 2021; 39(4):939–955
4. Dillingham TR. Evaluating the patient with suspected radiculopathy. PM R. 2013; 5(5) Suppl:S41–S49
5. Levin KH. Approach to the patient with suspected radiculopathy. Neurol Clin. 2012; 30(2):581–604

10 Intraoperative Neuromonitoring in Spine Surgery

Alexander T. Yahanda, Miguel A. Ruiz-Cardozo, and Camilo A. Molina

Summary

Intraoperative neuromonitoring in spine surgery is a valuable adjunct that assists surgeons in discerning when neural structures are at risk of being injured or have been injured. These warnings ideally provide time for interventions by surgery/anesthesia to alleviate the source of injury. This chapter discusses several intraoperative neuromonitoring methods, each of which has different utility depending on the location and type of spine surgery. Ultimately, successful neuromonitoring incorporates not just the operative site, but the long tract functions both rostral and caudal to the operative site. Since neuromonitoring may be applied to any type of spine surgery, all spine surgeons should be knowledgeable about these various techniques.

Keywords: neuromonitoring, spinal cord monitoring, somatosensory evoked potentials (SSEPs), motor evoked potentials (MEPs), transcranial electrical motor evoked potentials (TCMEPs), EMG, H reflex, mechanomyography (MMG), epidural D wave

10.1 Introduction

The purpose of intraoperative monitoring is to provide the surgeon and the anesthesiologist with immediate or close to immediate warnings that neural structures are at risk of being injured or have been injured by surgery or anesthesia. Ideally, surgeons and anesthesiologists are able to intervene when provided with a timely warning.[1,2]

10.2 Key Points

- To the extent possible, the precise nature of the operative procedure and the associated risks to structures should be known to the monitoring team in advance of the operative procedure so that the monitoring can be planned to cover the appropriate anatomical distribution and neurophysiological functions.

- The monitoring should incorporate segmental and radicular functions corresponding to the operative site, long tract functions caudal to the operative site, and long tract functions rostral to the operative site. Long tract functions rostral to the operative site should include, if possible, pathways that do not pass through the operative site. This should be done in a thoughtful way to avoid overwhelming the system and personnel with excessive data collection.
- Significant monitoring abnormalities arise from dysfunction remote to the operative site as often as they localize to the operative site. These remote monitoring abnormalities include the effects of anesthesia, hypotension, anoxia, hypothermia, neuromuscular blocking, hemorrhage, and ischemic stroke.
- Recognition of real-time or close to real-time change is critical in recognizing the offending cause and bringing about its reversal.
- Effective, reliable, comfortable communication between the monitoring team, the surgeon, and the anesthesiologist is paramount. An uneasy relationship results in delayed or incomplete communication.

10.3 Methods

- As an example, the typical setup for a patient presenting with a T12 burst fracture would include the following:
  - Median somatosensory evoked potential (SSEP) recording from EP, CII, C4′, and C3′.
  - Tibial SSEP recording from popliteal fossa, CII, Cz'.
  - Transcranial electrical motor evoked potential (TCMEP) with recordings from abductor pollicis brevis, rectus abdominis, vastus lateralis, tibialis anterior, medial gastrocnemius, abductor hallucis, flexor digiti minimi brevis pedis, and anal sphincter.
  - Free-run EMG with recordings from the same muscles.
  - Pedicle screw stimulation (triggered EMG) with recordings from the same muscles.
  - Train of four recorded at the abductor pollicis brevis.
  - EEG recorded at C4′ and C3′.

10.4 Somatosensory Evoked Potentials

Any large or small nerve in the body can be used to generate an SSEP if it is in part composed of afferent fibers. Large peripheral nerves in the extremities are typically used for intraoperative evoked potential monitoring (IOM) because they produce a larger amplitude response with a smaller number of averaged sweeps. Typically, in the upper extremities, the median and ulnar nerves are used. In the lower extremities, the tibial and fibular nerves are used. Since these nerves are composed of multiple roots, they are insensitive to single root dysfunction. If information about single root dysfunction is desired, dermatomal SSEPs would be required. If extremely caudal information is desired, pudendal SSEPs would be required.

- Technique: Upper and lower extremity SSEPs:
  - Stimulating electrodes are placed over the median or ulnar nerves at the wrists, at the tibial nerve at the ankle, or at the fibular nerve at the fibular neck.
  - For the upper extremities, the recording electrodes are placed at Erb's point (EP), over the C2 spinus process (CII), and over the contralateral cortex (C3′, C4′). For the lower extremities, the recording electrode is placed at Cz'. A variety of reference and ground electrode positions can be thoughtfully used. Typically, Fz is the common reference and FPz is the ground position.
  - The peripheral nerve can be stimulated at a frequency between 1.9 and 6.1 Hz, avoiding harmonics of 60 Hz, using a constant current stimulator. The faster the stimulating frequency, the more rapid the acquisition (up to a point, beyond which attenuated amplitude and skin blistering may result). The stimulus intensity should be sufficient to produce a muscle twitch if a mixed nerve is being stimulated (or 3 × sensory threshold if a pure sensory nerve is being stimulated). A square wave stimulus of 0.2 millisecond duration is given using a constant current stimulator.
  - Sweeps consisting of the desired waveform, EEG, EMG, EKG, and extraneous artifacts are averaged until the time-locked desired waveform is identifiable. The number of sweeps averaged is variable and depends on the signal-to-noise ratio. The sweep duration should be long enough to fully encompass the desired waveform, which could be normal or pathological. The bandwidth should be limited to the frequencies represented by the desired waveforms.
  - Typical recording and stimulating parameters for SSEPs:
    - Sensitivity: 0.5 to 2.0 uV/division.
    - Bandwidth: 30 Hz to 3000 Hz.
    - Sweep duration: 50 milliseconds for UE, 100 milliseconds for LE.
    - Pulse width: 0.2 milliseconds.
    - Stimulation rate: 1.9 to 6.1 Hz.
    - Number of sweeps: 50 to 500:
      - Alarm criteria: > 50% attenuation of amplitude or > 10% increase in latency.[3]
      - Pros: minimal disturbance to surgical procedure, can be constantly monitored, neuromuscular blocking does not impact monitoring.
      - Cons: provides information about the posterior third of the spinal cord only, N_2O impacts monitoring.

10.5 Transcranial Electrical Motor Evoked Potentials

The motor cortex is stimulated with a proprietary stimulator that provides 3 to 7 positive electrical shocks to the motor cortex. By selecting the precise location of stimulation and adjusting the stimulus intensity, TCMEPs may be set to result in focal or generalized muscle contractions, recorded from the muscles as polyphasic compound motor action potentials.

- Technique: TCMEP:
  - Stimulate the brain with the anode over appropriate motor cortex.
  - The cathode is placed over the opposite hemisphere.
  - Use a bite block.
  - Shock intensity: up to 600 V.
  - Shock duration: 50 microseconds.
  - Three to seven pulses 2 to 3 milliseconds apart:
    - Alarm criteria: Disappearance or severe attenuation of MEPs or persistent increase in the stimulation threshold by 100 V.[4]
    - Pros: Monitors motor function of the anterior two-thirds of the spinal cord.[5,6]
    - Cons: Inhalation anesthetics and neuromuscular blocking agents impact monitoring, MEPs cannot be continuously monitored, and MEPs are disturbing to the operative procedure.

10.6 Free-Run EMG

Needle electrodes are placed subcutaneously or intramuscularly in selected muscles. The purpose of this monitoring is to detect irritation or injury to peripheral nerves, which elicits solitary discharges, brief bursts, and/or prolonged trains of motor unit potential (MUP) activity.

- Technique: Free-run EMG (sEMG):
  - EMG needles are placed subcutaneously or intramuscularly above the surgical site as well as in several muscles supplied by nerve roots traversing the surgical site.
  - Sensitivity: 200 uV/div.
  - Sweep duration: 100 msec/div.
  - Bandwidth: 10 to 10,000 Hz:
    - Alarm criteria: trains of MUP activity arising from a muscle supplied by a nerve that is being physically manipulated.
    - Pros: monitors specific nerve roots within the surgical site.
    - Cons: may fail to detect acute total nerve root transection.
    - Must reverse neuromuscular blocking.

10.7 Triggered EMG

Nerve roots or peripheral nerves may be stimulated with a sterile handheld stimulator that is positioned by the surgeon in the operative field. The purpose of this technique is to identify excitable nerve tissue. The excitable nerve tissue could be hidden within tumor or a placode. The nerve could be normal but may be in closer proximity to a pedicle screw than is desirable, or there could be a breach in a pedicle with a low nerve stimulation threshold.

- Technique: Triggered EMG (tEMG):
  - The sterile stimulating electrodes are held or positioned by the surgeon to explore a tumor or placode on nerves or to explore a pedicle screw hole or to stimulate a pedicle screw to identify a breach.
  - The stimulator is triggered by the technologist.
  - The recording electrodes are the same electrodes that are used for sEMG and transcranial electrical motor evoked potentials (TCeMEP).
  - The threshold for identifying a breach is decided by the surgeon. Higher values represent a careful, conservative approach. The lumbar thresholds used would be 7.6 to 11 mA, thoracic thresholds would be 6 to 8 mA, and cervical thresholds would be 7.6 to 10 mA. A threshold in the 20 mA range would strongly suggest that a breach has not occurred. A threshold in the 3 mA range would strongly suggest that a breach has occurred.
  - Pros: Identifies viable nerve tissue in tumors or placodes. Identifies pedicle breach.
  - Cons: May fail to identify a breach if the adjacent nerve has an elevated threshold for stimulation based upon the presence of a comorbidity of nerve disease or injury.

10.8 H Reflex

- H reflexes can be recorded during surgery and under anesthesia with the same limitations as MEPs: TIVA is required, and neuromuscular block must be reversed.
- Disappearance of an H reflex unilaterally would suggest that the S1 to S2 roots have been compromised on that side.
- Disappearance of H reflexes bilaterally would suggest that the spinal cord has been severely compromised rostrally and there should simultaneously be loss of MEPs in the lower extremities.

10.9 Neuromonitoring in Spinal Deformity Surgery

The correction of spinal deformity may necessitate large fusions involving many pedicle screws, vertebral column osteotomies, and other complex techniques.

The larger the deformity correction, the higher the chance of neurological injury. Several neuromonitoring modalities have been used during spinal deformity correction.[7]

- SSEP: As SSEPs are composed of an average of signals, it is possible than an injury could be irreversible before it is identified by monitoring. In addition, many patients with deformity will have preoperative neurological deficits, which cannot be identified by SSEP. As mentioned previously, SSEPs are unable to provide information on single nerve roots. Some surgeons may elect to use SSEPs only when performing simpler posterior spinal surgeries, as SSEPs provide information from the posterior spinal cord. However, for deformity surgeries, using SSEP alone is not advised.
- TCMEP: This monitoring technique nicely complements SSEP by providing information about corticospinal/motor pathways, thus providing information about the anterior aspect of the spinal cord. Injury to the anterior spinal artery, for instance, would not be identified by SSEPs.
- EMG: Compared to SSEP and MEP, EMG provides a more "real time" monitoring modality. This may provide important information about instrumentation placement in deformity surgeries that require a large number of pedicle screws, for instance.
- Ultimately, for spinal deformity surgery, multimodal intraoperative neuromonitoring is preferred. A combination of SSEP and MEP should provide a sensitive and specific means by which to assess for impending injury. This may be supplemented by EMG.

10.10 Neuromonitoring for the Detection of Radiculopathy in Three-Column Osteotomies

- Effective neuromonitoring during three-column osteotomies would be of tremendous utility if it were able to effectively predict postoperative radiculopathy or other neurological symptoms. However, current literature on the optimal use of and outcomes for neuromonitoring during three-column osteotomies is limited.[8]
- Prior studies have determined that neuromonitoring has, at best, a modest ability to predict postoperative neurological deficits, particularly in cervical three-column surgery.[8] For lumbar three-column procedures, neuromonitoring has a low positive predictive value for postoperative deficits.[9]
- Further studies are needed to elucidate how neuromonitoring may be best incorporated into the workflow for large three-column surgeries at all levels of the spine.

10.11 Mechanomyography

- Mechanomyography (MMG) is a relatively new tool that may be used to measure the mechanical response of a muscle to a stimulus. Simplistically, it may be considered the reverse of EMG. Whereas EMG uses stimulus applied to muscles to measure potential injury to nerves, MMG involves stimulating nerves to send signals to skeletal muscles, which contract in response.[10]
- MMG measures multiple responses of muscle fibers to stimulus, including muscle fatigue, contractile force, and resonance frequency.
- MMG is not affected by the same interference or artifact as EMG. It is also less dependent on characteristics of the patient's skin (e.g., moisture). The placement of MMG sensors is not as tricky as for EMG, as the stimulus is applied via stickers rather than needles and do not need to be placed as precisely as EMG needles.[11]
- More research is required to determine the effectiveness of MMG in guiding placement of pedicle screws or other hardware during spinal surgery.

10.12 Epidural D Wave Monitoring for Intradural/Intramedullary Pathology

- D wave monitoring is similar to MEP but is recorded from the epidural space rather than in muscles of the extremities (for this reason, D wave monitoring is sometimes labeled as e-MEP).
- D waves are created by stimulation of corticospinal tract axons, which lends itself well to surgeries that extend intradural or intramedullary.
- Studies have shown that D wave monitoring for intradural/intramedullary pathology is superior to MEP and that a stable D wave may predict good motor outcomes even in instances when MEPs are lost or absent.[12] D wave monitoring may also be superior to MEP in patients who are neurologically compromised.[13,14]
- When reading epidural D wave monitoring versus MEP, it is important to note that MEPs are an "all or none" modality of monitoring. That is, the changes in amplitude of the MEP are not necessarily clinically significant compared to whether an MEP response is registered. Conversely, the amplitude of the wave matters during D wave monitoring. If the D wave amplitude is unchanged or reduced by < 50%, then a postoperative motor deficit is more likely to ultimately recover.[13] For intradural/intramedullary surgeries, this can occur in situations where the more binary MEP response has been lost.[15]

Common Clinical Questions

1. The latencies to P23 of the median SSEP are longer than the latencies to P37 of the tibial SSEP. What is the likely explanation for this problem?
   A. The patient has a cervical central cord syndrome.
   B. The technologist has inadvertently switched the electrode connections from the arms and legs.
   C. This is a normal physiological variant.
2. A patient is undergoing monitoring for a C5–C6 ACDF. TCeMEP recorded at the left deltoid shows a 55% amplitude decrease and a 12% increase in latency. These changes are sufficient to raise an alarm.
   A. True.
   B. False.
3. All of the following would represent real-time recording techniques *except* for which?
   A. sEMG.
   B. tEMG.
   C. TCeMEP.
   D. Tibial SSEP.
   E. EEG.

Answers to Common Clinical Questions

1. B.
2. B.
3. D.

Acknowledgments

Large sections of this chapter were adapted from the previous edition of this textbook. The authors are grateful to Colin R. Bamford for that prior work.

References

1. Nuwer MR, Dawson EG, Carlson LG, Kanim LE, Sherman JE. Somatosensory evoked potential spinal cord monitoring reduces neurologic deficits after scoliosis surgery: results of a large multicenter survey. Electroencephalogr Clin Neurophysiol. 1995; 96(1):6–11

2. Nuwer MR, Emerson RG, Galloway G, et al. Therapeutics and Technology Assessment Subcommittee of the American Academy of Neurology, American Clinical Neurophysiology Society. Evidence-based guideline update: intraoperative spinal monitoring with somatosensory and transcranial electrical motor evoked potentials: report of the Therapeutics and Technology Assessment Subcommittee of the American Academy of Neurology and the American Clinical Neurophysiology Society. Neurology. 2012; 78(8):585–589
3. Wagner W, Peghini-Halbig L, Mäurer JC, Perneczky A. Intraoperative SEP monitoring in neurosurgery around the brain stem and cervical spinal cord: differential recording of subcortical components. J Neurosurg. 1994; 81(2): 213–220
4. Deletis V, Sala F. Intraoperative neurophysiological monitoring of the spinal cord during spinal cord and spine surgery: a review focus on the corticospinal tracts. Clin Neurophysiol. 2008; 119(2):248–264
5. Ginsburg HH, Shetter AG, Raudzens PA. Postoperative paraplegia with preserved intraoperative somatosensory evoked potentials. Case report. J Neurosurg. 1985; 63(2):296–300
6. Chatrian GE, Berger MS, Wirch AL. Discrepancy between intraoperative SSEP's and postoperative function. Case report. J Neurosurg. 1988; 69(3):450–454
7. Laratta JL, Ha A, Shillingford JN, et al. Neuromonitoring in spinal deformity surgery: a multimodality approach. Global Spine J. 2018; 8(1):68–77
8. Lau D, Guo L, Deviren V, Ames CP. Utility of intraoperative neuromonitoring and outcomes of neurological complication in lower cervical and upper thoracic posterior-based three-column osteotomies for cervical deformity. J Neurosurg Spine. 2021; 36(3):470–478
9. Lau D, Dalle Ore CL, Reid P, et al. Utility of neuromonitoring during lumbar pedicle subtraction osteotomy for adult spinal deformity. J Neurosurg Spine. 2019; 31(3):397–407
10. Wessell N, Khalil J, Zavatsky J, Ghacham W, Bartol S. Verification of nerve decompression using mechanomyography. Spine J. 2016; 16(6):679–686
11. Zakaria HM, Tundo KM, Sandles C, et al. Mechanomyography for intraoperative assessment of cortical breach during instrumented spine surgery. World Neurosurg. 2018; 117:e252–e258
12. Ghadirpour R, Nasi D, Iaccarino C, et al. Intraoperative neurophysiological monitoring for intradural extramedullary spinal tumors: predictive value and relevance of D-wave amplitude on surgical outcome during a 10-year experience. J Neurosurg Spine. 2018; 30(2):259–267
13. Costa P, Peretta P, Faccani G. Relevance of intraoperative D wave in spine and spinal cord surgeries. Eur Spine J. 2013; 22(4):840–848
14. Bir M, Gupta U, Jaryal AK, et al. Predictive value of intraoperative D-wave and m-MEP neurophysiological monitoring in patients with preoperative motor deficits in immediate and late postoperative period. J Craniovertebr Junction Spine. 2021; 12(1):26–32
15. Avila EK, Elder JB, Singh P, Chen X, Bilsky MH. Intraoperative neurophysiologic monitoring and neurologic outcomes in patients with epidural spine tumors. Clin Neurol Neurosurg. 2013; 115(10):2147–2152

11 Bedside Procedures

Muhamed Hadzipasic, Ian David Connolly, John H. Shin, and Theresa Williamson

Summary
This chapter describes essential bedside procedures commonly utilized in spine surgery, focusing on techniques and considerations for both halo orthosis/traction and lumbar puncture or lumbar drain. It outlines key indications, proper application methods, potential complications, and postprocedure care, ensuring comprehensive guidance for clinical practice. The chapter emphasizes the critical role of bedside procedures in managing spinal conditions, particularly in acute settings, and the need for meticulous technique to optimize patient outcomes and minimize risks.

Keywords: bedside procedures, spine surgery, halo orthosis, cervical traction, lumbar puncture, lumbar drain

11.1 Key Points

- Halo orthosis and traction: Useful in reduction and stabilization in appropriately selected patients. Requires close monitoring. Skull fracture or severe skull osteoporosis is a contraindication for halo placement. Scalp abrasion or infection overlying the intended pin sites is also a contraindication for the procedure.
- Lumbar puncture (LP) or lumbar drain: Useful in diagnosis of CNS pathology and treatment of cerebrospinal fluid (CSF) leak or high-pressure phenomena. Known or suspected intracranial mass, infection, tethered cord, and coagulopathy are potential contraindications to the procedure.

11.2 Indications

- Halo orthosis: Halo orthosis is effective at controlling abnormal motion at the O-C and C1–C2 articulations resulting from fracture or ligamentous injury. The purpose of the halo is to maintain normal alignment and/or immobilize the cervical spine to prevent further spinal injury and to allow for bony fusion in cases of fractures. Halo traction is used to limit fracture–dislocations and maintain normal alignment.[1,2]

- Cervical traction: Cervical traction is useful in improving abnormal alignment caused by trauma or spinal deformity (completely flexible or partially flexible kyphotic deformities). Different vectors of traction can be employed depending on the alignment change needed to improve sagittal alignment. It is generally contraindicated in a patient without a reliable neurologic examination. Presence of a skull fracture is also a relative contraindication.
- Lumbar puncture (LP) or lumbar drain: An LP is indicated for collection and analysis of CSF for infection, subarachnoid hemorrhage, abnormal cells, or elevated intracranial pressure. Additionally, intrathecal administration of medication or contrast (for myelography) can be performed via an LP. A lumbar drain is placed if temporary CSF diversion is indicated for hydrocephalus (communicating) or wound management (pseudomeningocele, CSF leak).

11.3 Technique

11.3.1 Halo Orthosis and Traction

- Patients should be positioned either in a sitting, head-neutral position or a supine, head-neutral position at the end of the bed so that the head slightly overhangs the bed. A semirigid collar may be used to immobilize the neck during halo application.[3] It is helpful to have two providers for this procedure.
- The appropriate-sized halo ring is selected. The halo ring should accommodate the entire head circumference with clearance of approximately 1 cm to avoid pressure on the scalp.
- Halo pin sites are selected at this time, with two anterior and two posterior sites.
  - The anterior sites are centered in the groove between the supraciliary ridge and frontal prominences. Pins should be placed just superior to the lateral half of the eyebrows to avoid the supraorbital nerve and vessels. This location avoids muscular structures to diminish discomfort.
  - A posterior pin should be placed 1 cm above the apex of the pinna of each ear. A line connecting the posterior pin site with its contralateral anterior pin site should roughly bisect a line drawn between the remaining two pin sites at a right angle. This allows distribution of force for stability. The anterior and contralateral posterior pins are simultaneously tightened to ensure equal distribution of pressure.
- The planned pin sites are sterilely prepared and injected with 1% lidocaine. Patients are also often premedicated with analgesia and anxiolytics as tolerated. The two pins—one front and the diagonally opposite back pin—are then finger-tightened to just touch the skin; this is repeated for the

other pins. In children, multiple pins (> 4) are sometimes used to distribute the pressure more evenly. Positioning pins are used during this process to hold the ring in place temporarily.

- A torque screwdriver (set to 6 to 8 pounds pressure [in adults], 1 to 5 pounds in children) is then used to tighten the pins in diagonal pairs. The pins are now stabilized and locked down with appropriate locking nuts to the halo frame. The halo vest is then placed on the patient, the semirigid collar is removed, and halo and vest are stabilized with halo rods. It is important to assess alignment with lateral bedside X-ray prior to fixation to the vest and rods.
  - The halo vest should be adjusted so that the straps make contact with the patient's trapezius and shoulder area. There is a tendency for the vest to ride high and not touch the shoulders unless care is taken during vest application. Breakaway torque wrenches are used to tighten the rods to the halo ring (**Fig. 11.1**).
  - Halo care: Pin sites should be cared for with daily or every other day cleaning with hydrogen peroxide or betadine solution. Retorque each halo pin site 24 hours post-placement and then every 3 to 4 weeks. Be careful to avoid overtightening. If a pin does not torque easily, obtain cranial imaging to rule out a breach of the cranium.
- Cervical traction: Patients are commonly premedicated with muscle relaxant such as IV valium prior to traction. Care must be taken to avoid oversedation. For traction placement, a variety of devices are available. Gardner-Wells tongs or halo rings are the most common (**Fig. 11.2**). Pin sites for Gardner-Wells tongs are 2 to 3 fingerbreadths (3 to 4 cm) above

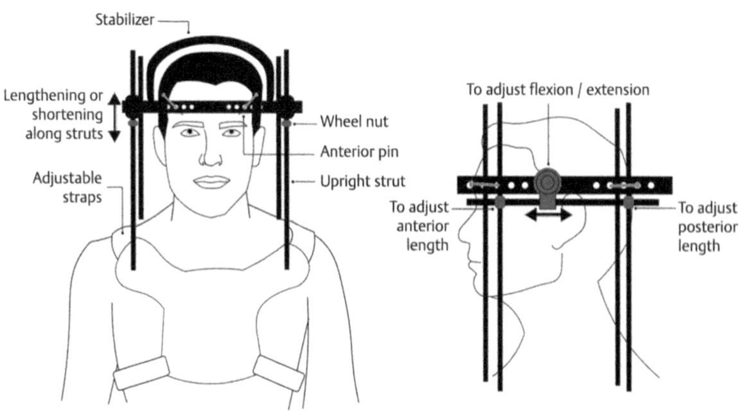

Fig. 11.1 Halo vest fixation technique.

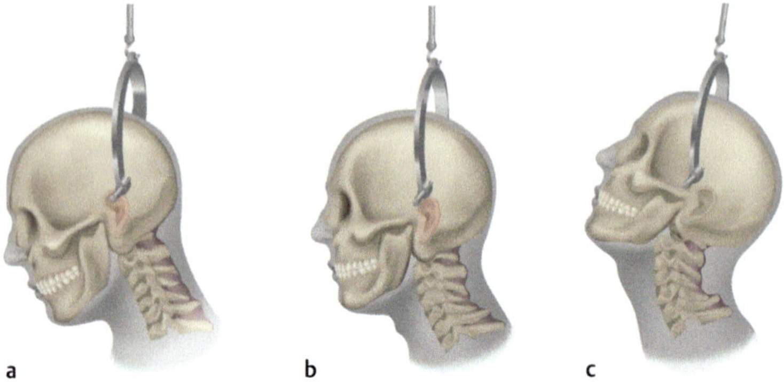

a b c

Fig. 11.2 Proper fixation points for Gardner-Wells tongs application. **(a)** Posterior placement of tongs to produce flexion of head. **(b)** Normal placement of tongs to produce straight traction. **(c)** Anterior placement of tongs to produce hyperextension of head. (Adapted from Vaccaro, AR, Albert TJ, eds. Spine Surgery: Tricks of the Trade. 2nd ed. Thieme; 2009.)

the ear pinnae. The Gardner-Wells pins are spring-loaded with a force indicator; these pins are tightened until the indicator protrudes 1 mm beyond the flat surface, which is equivalent to 31 pounds of force. Pins are retightened daily until the indicator remains at this location for 3 days. Beware of overtightening which can occur even at a fraction of a millimeter. If used, halo rings have the advantage of a compatible vest orthosis to secure the tractioned position and additionally can be secured with an adapter to intraoperative Mayfield frame.

- After tong or halo ring placement, the patient is transferred to a bed with a headboard attached to a pulley system with weights. With the pulley placed above the patient's head, flexion and traction can be accomplished. If the pulley is placed at the level of the pins, then straight traction forces can be applied. If the pulley is placed below the level of the patient's head, extension and traction are possible. True lateral X-rays should be obtained immediately after application of traction and after each weight adjustment in addition to a close neurologic examination. Typically, evaluation begins with 5 pounds of traction for upper C-spine injuries and 10 pounds for lower C-spine injuries.
- For upper cervical injuries, evaluation of the atlantooccipital joints is important to rule out atlantooccipital dislocations. Such injuries **should not** use traction. For midcervical locked facets, 5 pounds per level of traction weight should be applied to the injury (e.g., slowly work up to 25 pounds for a C5-level facet subluxation). Before applying traction for cervical facet subluxation, consider magnetic resonance imaging (MRI) to

rule out a coincidental anterior herniated disk with cord compression. If a herniated disk is present, consider anterior operative correction instead of a trial of traction.
- It is important to educate the entire care team on bedside traction and care to avoid bed height or weight changes. Additionally, any change in neurologic examination should prompt urgent decrease in weight and imaging with possible operative intervention.

11.3.2 Lumbar Puncture or Lumbar Drain

- Prior to beginning a lumbar procedure, review the patient's lumbar history and prior imaging. This bedside procedure can be performed with the patient sitting or lying down.
  - For the recumbent position, the patient is placed in a lateral decubitus posture, with neck flexed and knees brought up to the chest. This distracts the space between the spinous processes, facilitating passage of a spinal needle into the thecal sac.
  - For the sitting position, the patient should be sitting with head and arms resting on a pillow placed on a bedside stand. The back is sterilely prepared and draped.
- LP can be safely attempted at the L3 to S1 interspaces in the anatomically normal patient. The intercrestal line is identified and palpated in the midline for the L4 spinous process.
  - Initially, 1% lidocaine is infiltrated subcutaneously. Subsequently, the lumbodorsal fascia is injected.
  - The spinal needle with stylet is aimed slightly rostrally to the umbilicus to approximately parallel the spinous process, and the bevel should be turned parallel to the length of the spinal column to reduce the chance of post-LP headaches.
  - The needle is advanced in a midline trajectory, and a "pop" should be felt as the needle penetrates the ligamentum flavum and passes into the dura (**Fig. 11.3**).
  - The stylet is then withdrawn to check for CSF flow; if none is seen, reinsert the stylet and advance the needle further; if no CSF flow is present, attempt another trajectory.
  - If blood is seen, wait for the blood to drain and clear, as this may represent a traumatic tap. If it does not clear, advance the needle or attempt another trajectory as this may be epidural venous blood.
- If a lumbar drain is selected, a lumbar drain needle (14-gauge Tuohy) should be used. After entering the thecal sac with needle bevel facing laterally, the bevel is turned superiorly, and a lumbar drainage catheter with wire stylet is inserted (20–40 cm).

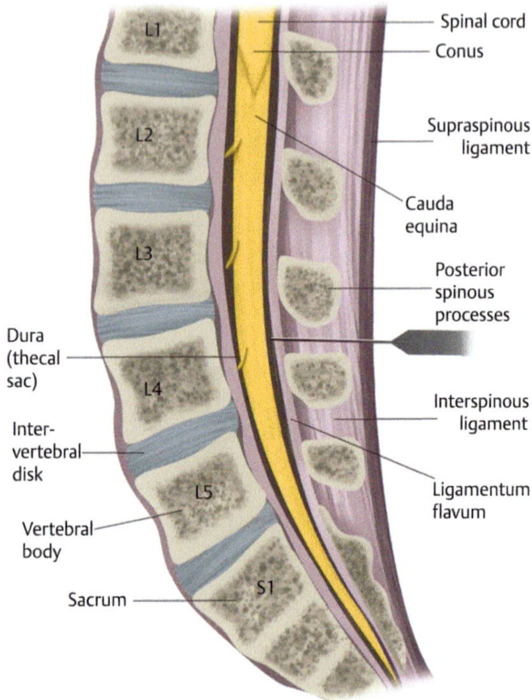

Fig. 11.3 Lumbar puncture technique, with pertinent spaces and ligaments labeled.

- The needle and stylet are sequentially removed, and CSF flow is confirmed by dropping the catheter below the patient. Do not pull the catheter back through the needle due to risk of sheering the catheter.
  - A 2 × 2 gauze section is placed around the insertion site of the catheter and a Tegaderm (3M; St. Paul, Minnesota) pad is placed on top to secure the catheter.
  - Several more Tegaderm pads are placed along the flank of the patient to secure the catheter to the patient's body.
    - Troubleshooting: If you are having difficulty accessing the intrathecal space, reassess the patient's positioning and ensure that you are on the midline and at the appropriate interspace. If the patient complains of radicular pain during the procedure, it is likely that you are lateral and need to redirect your trajectory medially. Patients with

low-pressure problems may have low flow from a lumbar drain. Avoid too many attempts at an LP or lumbar drain and consider a consult to interventional radiology if needed.

11.4 Complications

11.4.1 Halo Orthosis and Traction

- Patients who have osteoporosis may have a thin skull and suffer from skull fracture with halo pin placement or after falls while wearing their halo. Consider a head computed tomography (CT) before placing a halo in patients who have osteoporosis.
- Pin loosening occurs in 60% of patients over a 3-month period. Pins may require retightening. Overtightening can result in fracture.
- Pin site infection (10 to 20%). Treat by placing a pin at a new, adjacent site and giving the patient oral antibiotics. Recurrent or intracranial infections may require debridement.
- Neurologic deterioration after traction may occur secondary to retropulsed disk or worsened alignment. Consider obtaining a preprocedure MRI to rule out this condition before traction. Neurologic worsening following traction should be treated by reversing the previous maneuver, considering hypotension as a contributor and ensuring appropriate mean arterial pressures (typically MAP > 80), and possibly operative intervention.
- Overdistraction is another potential complication of halo/traction. This could manifest as deficits or pain and can typically be identified on the lateral X-ray.

11.4.2 Lumbar Puncture or Lumbar Drain

- Infection can occur in certain cases, especially those involving prolonged use of lumbar drains.
  - Superficial infection can be treated with drain removal and antibiotic treatment.
  - Epidural abscess (depending on size and neurologic compromise) may require surgical intervention (laminectomy and evacuation).
- Radicular pain can occur secondary to nerve root irritation. If persistent, consider repositioning of drain.
- Post-LP headache:
  - Options include bed rest (24 h), abdominal binder, desoxycorticosterone acetate, caffeine, sodium benzoate, high-dose steroids, and blood patch.
  - If related to lumbar drain, consider decreasing output.
- Spinal epidural hematoma (usually in the setting of coagulopathy or anticoagulation).

- Tonsillar herniation (in the presence of mass-occupying lesion).
- Intracranial subdural hygroma or hematoma.
- Epidermoid tumor (increased likelihood with needle introduction without stylet). This can occur in a delayed fashion, but incidence is very low.
- Abducens palsy (often delayed 5–14 days post-LP and resolving without intervention in 4–6 weeks).

11.5 Postprocedure Care

11.5.1 Halo Orthosis and Traction

- The pins should be retightened once a day for 72 hours at the same pressure and then retightened every week for 3 weeks.
  - A persistently loose pin may indicate migration into the inner table and should be removed and a new one placed at different site.
  - Postprocedure radiographs are taken to verify proper head positioning with halo orthosis and traction placement.

11.5.2 Lumbar Puncture or Lumbar Drain

- For lumbar drain care, prophylactic antibiotics may be continued while the drain is in place though there is not clear data to support their use. Maintain a clean and sterile dressing and use a barrier dressing as needed to avoid soiling. Generally, drains should be removed or changed after a week.

11.6 Outcomes

- Halo orthosis: Fusion rates are as high as 84% in nonelderly patients who have type II odontoid fracture treated with a halo; risk factors for nonunion include advanced age and displaced odontoid fractures.
- Cervical traction: Reduction of bilateral locked facets is typically easier to achieve than reduction of unilateral locked facet. Urgent reduction of fractures can result in improved neurologic outcomes for spinal cord injury patients.
- LP: Risk of persistent or disabling complication is rated at 0.1 to 0.5%.

11.7 Surgical Pearls

11.7.1 Halo Orthosis and Traction

- Pin tension should be uniform. Unequal pin tension will lead to migration of halo as pins migrate in the direction of the pin with the least tension.

- Adjustments during follow-up should not be limited to the halo pins. Inspection of alignment with the vest should be performed to ensure that shoulder straps are making contact with the trapezius and shoulder area. X-ray radiographs should accompany follow-up visits to ensure proper alignment.

11.7.2 Lumbar Puncture or Lumbar Drain

- Care must be taken when removing the Tuohy needle from the lumbar catheter to avoid shear of the catheter by the sharp bevel of the needle. The trajectory and rotation of the needle must not be altered during removal.
- Evaluation of anatomy with preoperative radiograph is essential, especially in patients who have degeneration and osteophyte formation.
- If attempts at LP or drain placement are unsuccessful, placement of lumbar drain under fluoroscopic guidance may be necessary.

Common Clinical Questions

1. Frontal halo pins may compromise which nerve?
2. During retightening of halo pins during a follow-up visit, it is found that the pins can no longer be torqued to 6 pounds after one complete turn. What has happened? What should be done?
3. A patient develops nausea, vomiting, and headaches 2 weeks after a workup for meningitis. What is the likely diagnosis? What is the treatment?

Answers to Common Clinical Questions

1. Supraciliary nerve.
2. The pin has likely breached the cortical inner table. The pin should be removed and a new pin placed at a new site. CT of head should be considered.
3. The patient has likely developed post-LP headache. Treatments include bed rest, abdominal binder, hydration, and medication. If these measures fail, a blood patch is indicated.

Acknowledgments

Thank you to the previous authors of this chapter, Daniel C. Lu and Praveen V. Mummaneni.

References

1. Chan RC, Schweigel JF, Thompson GB. Halo-thoracic brace immobilization in 188 patients with acute cervical spine injuries. J Neurosurg. 1983; 58(4): 508–515
2. Platzer P, Thalhammer G, Sarahrudi K, et al. Nonoperative management of odontoid fractures using a halothoracic vest. Neurosurgery. 2007; 61(3): 522–529, discussion 529–530
3. Greenberg MS. Handbook of Neurosurgery. 6th ed. New York: Thieme Medical Publishers; 2006:304–306

12 Orthotics in Spine Surgery

Melissa MJ Chua and Yi Lu

Summary

Orthotics in spine surgery is an important topic often overlooked. There is a wide variety of orthoses, and it is imperative to understand when and why to use each of them, particularly in cases of spinal instability or postoperative protection of spinal instrumentation. In this chapter, we detail the indications and types of orthoses by the spinal level of coverage mainly: cervical, cervicothoracic, cervicothoracolumbosacral, thoracolumbosacral, lumbosacral, and sacroiliac. We also review the technique of placing a halo fixator, an important orthosis for the most rigid cervical immobilization.

Keywords: orthotics, orthoses, spine brace, collar, halo fixator

12.1 Key Points

- There are a variety of braces, mainly classified by the area of the spine they provide support to.
- Rigidity of braces varies. It is important to select the correct brace type for the indication. For example, more rigid brace provides more immobilization in less stable spines.

12.2 Indications

- Comfort and/or pain relief.
- Stabilization and immobilization (e.g., trauma).
- Prevention of further deformity and correction of spinal deformity (e.g., scoliosis).
- Reduction of axial-loading.
- Postoperative protection of spinal instrumentation.

12.3 Biomechanics of Spinal Orthoses[1,2]

- Four biomechanical effects of spinal orthoses described by Morris[1] are: (1) motion control, (2) spinal realignment, (3) trunk support (lumbar orthoses), (4) weight transfer (cervical orthoses).

- Support types:
  - Three-point pressure system: Orthoses need at least three points of contact to create pressure equilibrium across the spine and limit movement.
  - Circumferential support: Circumferential compression of the spine to create support and restrict movement.

12.4 Classifications

- Cervical.
- Cervicothoracic.
- Cervicothroracolumbosacral.
- Thoracolumbosacral.
- Lumbosacral.
- Sacroiliac.

12.5 Cervical Orthoses (CO)

- **Halo fixator**[3]: Most rigid cervical immobilization. Consists of a rigid ring fixed around the skull by pins, an immobilizing vest around the chest, and adjustable rods and bars to affix the ring to the vest.
  - Indications: Stable Jefferson fractures (i.e., burst fractures of the atlas), type II hangman fractures (Effendi's classification), type II (if not surgical candidate) and III odontoid fractures, C2 comminuted fractures, and combinations of C1–C2 fractures. Also used for stabilization preoperatively or where surgery is contraindicated.[4]
  - Technique: Select ring with at least 1 to 2 cm distance from the skull. Select vest based on chest circumference at xiphoid process level. Sterilize skin at pin sites and infiltrate with local anesthetic. Place the ring over the head (maintained at approximately 1 cm above the pinna). Place the two anterior pins approximately 1 cm superior to orbital rim, above lateral two-thirds of orbit, and below the equator of the skull (**Fig. 12.1**). This avoids the temporalis muscle and zygomaticotemporal nerve laterally, and the frontal sinus, and supraorbital and supratrochlear nerves medially. Place the posterior pins directly opposite the anterior pins. Tighten pins to 8 in-lb (0.9 Nm) in adult patients. Place the vest and connect to the ring via the posts provided. Ensure appropriate spinal alignment with a cervical radiograph after halo fixator application. Retighten pins to 8 in-lb 48 h after initial application. Clean pin sites every other day with sterile solution (e.g., hydrogen peroxide).

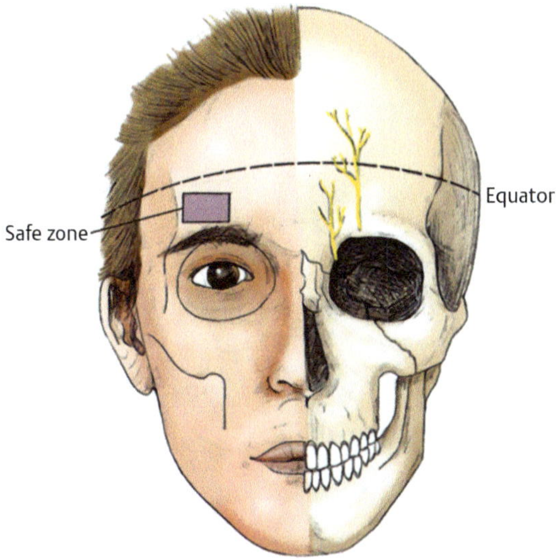

Fig. 12.1 Safe zone for anterior pin placement depicted in the shaded rectangle. Anterior pins should be placed approximately 1cm above the orbital rim and below the equator (*dotted line*). (Illustrated by Andrea Wong.)

 - Complications: Pin/ring loosening, pin-site infection, pressure-sores under the vest, frontal sinus violation, nerve injury (particularly those listed above), difficulty swallowing, dural puncture, and reduced vital capacity (**Fig. 12.1**).[5,6]
- **Soft collar:** Does not provide any significant motion restriction or support. Primarily used for patient comfort, including postoperative comfort. Contraindicated in suspected unstable cervical injury.
- **Semi-rigid collars**[7,8]: Reduce flexion/extension in middle and lower cervical spine. Less effective in reducing lateral bending and rotation motions. Limited restriction of flexion/extension from occiput to C2. Insufficient for immobilization of unstable cervical injuries. Used for emergent cervical immobilization, postoperative immobilization to protect spinal instrumentation, or stable cervical spinal injuries (e.g., stable nonoperative fractures).
  - Examples: Philadelphia collar, Miami-J collar, Aspen collar.
  - Miami-J and Aspen collars are padded and cause less contact pressure at the collar–skin interface (chin, occiput, chest) compared to the Philadelphia collar. Preferred in patients with altered mental status or elderly patients.

12.6 Cervicothoracic Orthoses (CTO)

It is more effective at restricting flexion/extension and rotation than rigid COs, particularly in middle and lower cervical spine.[9] Chin and occiput fixation are attached to trunk straps/supports.

- Examples: Aspen, Minerva, Sternal Occipital Mandibular Immobilizer (SOMI), Two-poster (one anterior and one posterior upright), Four-poster (two anterior and two posterior uprights).

12.7 Cervicothoracolumbosacral Orthoses (CTLSO)[10]

Rigid orthosis used primarily in scoliosis for frontal and sagittal correction. Main action is for elongation. Consists of a neck ring, axillary sling, thoracic and lumbar pads, and pelvic interface.

- Example: Milwaukee.

12.8 Thoracolumbosacral Orthoses (TLSO)

It consists of prefabricated braces or custom-molded casts. It restricts rotational motion (maximal restriction with custom-molded casts). Full-contact TLSO are effective in immobilizing T8–L4. Indicated for stable fractures, postoperative immobilization to protect spinal instrumentation, postural support, and scoliosis (deformity correction). Cervical extension should be added if immobilization is also needed above T8. Paradoxical increase in motion at L4–S1. Thigh cuff should be added if immobilization is also needed at L4–S1.

- Examples of limited-contact TLSO: CASH, Jewett, Knight-Taylor.
- Custom-molded TLSO are full-contact, and cervical extension or thigh cuff can be added for immobilization of additional levels as mentioned above. Custom-molded casts can be molded in hyperextension for treatment of fractures without neurologic deficit or significant instability (e.g., burst fractures, Chance fractures without ligamentous injury).

12.9 Lumbosacral Orthoses (LSO)

It immobilizes by abdominal compression and motion restriction. Mild flexion/extension restriction. Minimal side-to-side bending and rotational restriction. Not sufficient for immobilization of lumbar fractures. Indicated for patient reminder to keep good posture, supporting weak abdominal muscles (e.g., after pregnancy or abdominal surgery), and alleviating back pain by reducing motion, particularly post-surgically.

- Examples: Corset, chairback brace, custom-molded, binder.

12.10 Sacroiliac Orthoses (SIO)

For motion reduction around the SI joint to provide pelvic–sacral support and decrease pain. Includes belts or straps that wrap around the pelvis.

- Examples: Corset, trochanteric belt, sacroiliac belt.

Common Clinical Questions

1. Where is the ideal location for anterior pins when applying a halo fixator?
   A. Anywhere in the anterior skull.
   B. 1 cm superior to orbital rim, above lateral 2/3 of orbit, and below the equator of the skull.
   C. 1 cm superior to orbital rim, above medial 2/3 of orbit, and above the equator of the skull.
   D. 1 cm superior to orbital rim, above medial 2/3 of orbit, and below the equator of the skull.
2. A TLSO brace is sufficient in a stable L5 fracture.
   A. True, the brace covers all of the thoracic and lumbar spine.
   B. False, the brace causes paradoxical increase in motion at L4–S1.

Answers to Common Clinical Questions

1. B.
2. B.

References

1. Morris JM, Lucas DB. Biomechanics of spinal bracing. Ariz Med. 1964; 21: 170–176
2. Sypert GW. External spinal orthotics. Neurosurgery. 1987; 20(4):642–649
3. Botte MJ, Byrne TP, Abrams RA, Garfin SR. Halo skeletal fixation: techniques of application and prevention of complications. J Am Acad Orthop Surg. 1996; 4(1):44–53
4. Vieweg U, Schultheiss R. A review of halo vest treatment of upper cervical spine injuries. Arch Orthop Trauma Surg. 2001; 121(1–2):50–55

5. Horn EM, Theodore N, Feiz-Erfan I, Lekovic GP, Dickman CA, Sonntag VKH. Complications of halo fixation in the elderly. J Neurosurg Spine. 2006; 5(1): 46–49
6. Taitsman LA, Altman DT, Hecht AC, Pedlow FX. Complications of cervical halo-vest orthoses in elderly patients. Orthopedics. 2008; 31(5):446
7. Ivancic PC. Effects of orthoses on three-dimensional load-displacement properties of the cervical spine. Eur Spine J. 2013; 22(1):169–177
8. Horodyski M, DiPaola CP, Conrad BP, Rechtine GR, II. Cervical collars are insufficient for immobilizing an unstable cervical spine injury. J Emerg Med. 2011; 41(5):513–519
9. Holla M, Huisman JMR, Verdonschot N, Goosen J, Hosman AJF, Hannink G. The ability of external immobilizers to restrict movement of the cervical spine: a systematic review. Eur Spine J. 2016; 25(7):2023–2036
10. Negrini S, Aulisa AG, Cerny P, et al. The classification of scoliosis braces developed by SOSORT with SRS, ISPO, and POSNA and approved by ESPRM. Eur Spine J. 2022; 31(4):980–989

13 Pharmacology of Antithrombotics, Antifibrinolytics, and Osteoporosis Medications

Omar Sorour, Mohamed Macki, Alysha Jamieson, Praveen V. Mummaneni, and Leslie Robinson

Summary
Spinal surgeons need to be aware of medications that are commonly used for prevention and treatment of thromboembolism and osteoporosis. Many patients are taking these medications before and after surgery. For anticoagulant medications we review their indications and their reversal agents. For osteoporosis medications we review their indications and effects on spinal fusions.

Keywords: heparin, UFH, LMWH, pulmonary embolism, deep venous thrombosis, vitamin K, warfarin, prothrombin complex concentrate (PCC), thrombin, tranexamic acid, osteoporosis, DEXA, teriparatide, vitamin D, calcium

13.1 Key Points

- UFH and LMWH are both efficacious in preventing venous thromboembolic events.
- Treatment options for preoperative thromboembolic events include an inferior vena cava filter and a heparin bridge to oral anticoagulants.
- Various agents exist for the reversal of anticoagulation, depending on the patient history, clinical signs, laboratory values, and even thromboelastographic studies.
- Regarding treatment of osteoporosis, teriparatide has very strong evidence of augmenting bony arthrodesis after spinal fusion.

13.2 Prophylactic Anticoagulation

- Low-dose (minidose) heparin + pneumatic compression stockings.[1]
- Chemoprophylactic agents in spine surgery usually include small doses of unfractionated heparin (UFH) or low-molecular-weight heparin (LMWH) (Enoxaparin, Lovenox). According to the LMWH vs UFH in Spine Surgery

(PLUSS) Project, both are efficacious in preventing venous thromboembolic events (VTE) without an increased risk of hemorrhagic complications.[2]

- Chemoprophylactic doses:
  - UFH 5000 u subQ bid or tid (the authors' preferred protocol is 5000 u subQ bid in order to avoid postoperative hematomas).
  - LMWH 0.5 mg/kg daily or 40 mg daily. Low-weight women (< 45 kg) and low-weight men (< 57 kg) may require smaller doses.[3]
- Prophylactic doses of anticoagulation is typically started 1 to 2 days postoperatively.

13.3 Treatment of Preoperative Thromboembolic Events

- Preop: if the patient has a pulmonary embolism (PE) or deep vein thrombosis (DVT), consider
  - Inferior vena cava filter.
  - Heparin bridge to surgery.
    - High intensity heparin drip (aPTT 60–85 seconds),[4] hold 6 to 8 hours before surgery.[5]
- Preop: if the patient has an acute coronary syndrome or prosthetic cardiac valve, consider
  - Heparin bridge to surgery.
    - Low intensity heparin drip (aPTT 50–70 seconds),[4] hold 6 to 8 hours before surgery.[5]

13.4 Treatment of Postoperative Thromboembolic Events

- Postop: In the first 1 to 2 weeks after spinal surgery, because of the risk of spinal hematoma, an inferior vena cava filter is preferred for DVT/PE.
- Typically, prophylactic doses of subQ heparin 5000 u bid is started on postoperative day 1 to 2.
- Therapeutic LMWH (Enoxaparin, Lovenox) 1 mg/kg bid is started 1 to 2 weeks postoperatively, depending on risk factors.

13.5 Reversal of Anticoagulation (Table 13.1)

- Necessity of reversal agents determined by patient history of anticoagulation, clinical signs of active hemorrhage on anticoagulation, laboratory values (aPTT, INR, platelet count, fibrinogen). Thromboelastographic (TEG) studies

Table 13.1 Reversal agents of antithrombotics

Drug class	Generic drug name (Brand name)	Half-life	Holding recommendations prior to surgery	Reversal agent
Vitamin K antagonist	Warfarin (Coumadin)	20–60 hours Mean: 40 hours	5–6 days (INR ≤ 1.5)	• Vitamin K 1–10 mg IV • Prothrombin complex concentrates (PCC): 3-factor (Profilnine: II, IX, X) or 4-factor (Kcentra: II, VII, IX, X) 1. Method 1: ○ → INR 2–4: 25 IU/kg IV Push ○ → INR ≥ 4–6: 35 IU/kg IV Push ○ → INR > 6: 50 IU/kg IV Push 2. Method 2: INR < 5: 500 units; INR ≥ 5: 1000 IU 3. Method 3: Fixed dose (1500 IU)
Heparins	Unfractionated heparin	SQ: 1.5 hours IV: 30 mins	IV PPx: 4–6 hours IV Tx: 4–6 hours SQ: 24 hours	• Protamine dose per 100 units heparin: – → Immediate: 1–1.5 mg – → 30–60 mins: 0.5–0.75 mg – → > 2 h: 0.25–0.375 mg
	Low-molecular; weight heparin: Enoxaparin (Lovenox)	SQ or IV: 4 hours	24 hours	• ≤ 8 hours: 1 mg protamine for every 1 mg enoxaparin • > 8 hours: 0.5 mg protamine for every 1 mg enoxaparin • > 12–24 hours: May not need reversal

(Continued)

Table 13.1 (*Continued*)

Drug class	Generic drug name (Brand name)	Half-life	Holding recommendations prior to surgery	Reversal agent
	Low-molecular-weight heparin: Dalteparin (Fragmin)	IV: ~2 hours SQ: ~3 hours	12–24 hours	• ≤8 hours: 1 mg protamine for every 100 units dalteparin • >8 hours: 0.5 mg protamine for every 100 units dalteparin • >12–24 hours: May not need reversal
Thrombin inhibitors	Bivalirudin (Angiomax)	25–30 mins	4 hours	None (FDA approval)
	Argatroban (Acova)	40–50 mins	4 hours	None (FDA approval)
	Dabigatran (Pradaxa)	12–14 hours	1–5 + days	Idaracizumab (5 g—two separate vials each containing 2.5 g/50 mL)
Factor Xa inhibitors	Apixaban (Eliquis)	12 hours	PPx: 12–24 hours Tx: 2–3 days	• Andexanet alfa (Andexanet): – →Low dose: 400 mg IV bolus at the rate of 30 mg/min, followed by 2 h infusion 4 mg/min – →High dose: 800 mg IV bolus at the rate of 30 mg/min, followed by 2 h infusion 8 mg/min If Andexanet alfa is not available on hospital formulary, prothrombin complex concentrates may be considered

	Rivoraxaban (Xarelto)	5–13 hours	Tx: 2–3 days PPx: 12–24 hours	Andexanet alfa If Andexanet alfa is not available on hospital formulary, prothrombin complex concentrates may be considered
	Edoxaban (Savaysa)	8–14 hours	2–3 days	None (FDA approval)
	Fondaparinux (Arixtra)	17–21 hours	PPx: 24–36 hours Tx: 4–5 days	None
COX inhibitor	Aspirin	20 mins	5–7 days	Desmopressin: 0.4 mcg/kg; 1 dose
$P2Y_{12}$ inhibitors	Clopidogrel (Plavix)	6 hours	5–7 days	Platelet infusion and/or desmopressin (0.3–0.4 ug/kg)*
	Prasugrel (Effient)	7 hours	7–10 days	Platelet infusion and/or desmopressin (0.3–0.4 ug/kg)*
	Ticagrelor (Brilinta)	9 hours	5 days	None. *Note:* Breakthrough therapy designation from the FDA for a reversible inhibitor bentracimab (PB2452 monoclonal antibody). Initial IV bolus 6 g infused over 10 mins, then 6 g IV loading infusion over 4 hours, followed by 6 g IV maintenance over 12 hours
	Ticlopidine (Ticlid)	20–50 hours	10–14 days	None; platelet infusion

(Continued)

Table 13.1 *(Continued)*

Drug class	Generic drug name (Brand name)	Half-life	Holding recommendations prior to surgery	Reversal agent
GpIIb/IIIa inhibitors	Abciximab (ReoPro)	10–30 mins	48 + hours	Platelet infusion*
	Eptifibatide (Integrilin)	2.5 hours	4–8 hours	Platelet infusion*
	Tirofiban (Aggrastat)	2 hours	8–24 hours	Platelet infusion*
Phosphodiesterase inhibitors	Cilostazol (Pletal)	11–13 hours	2–3 days	Platelet infusion*
	Dipyridamole (Persantine)	10 hours	2 days	Aminophylline (50–250 mg IV push over 30–60 seconds)

Abbreviations: INR, international normalized ratio; IU, international units; IV, intravenous; PPx, prophylaxis; SQ, subcutaneous; TTx, treatment.
Note: * Efficacy not established.

are readily available at some institutions for a point-of-care evaluation of a patient's coagulation profile.

- Generalized reversal agents:
  - Fresh frozen plasma (FFP): Contains all coagulation factors (factor V, factor VII, fibrinogen, albumin, protein C, protein S, antithrombin, tissue factor pathway inhibitor) besides platelets.[6]
  - Nonactive prothrombin complex concentrates (PCC): 3-factor (factors II, IX, X), or 4-factor (Kcentra: factors II, VII, IX, X). PCC has a higher concentration of clotting factors compared to FFP. One dose equals 8 to 16 units FFP.[7]
  - Activated PCC: Anti-inhibitor coagulant complex (factor VIII inhibitor bypassing activity [FEIBA]) contains factors VIIa, X, Xa, II (Prothrombin), IIa (Thrombin), IX, and IXa.[8]
  - Recombinant activated factor VII (NovoSeven).[9,10]
  - Cryoprecipitate: High concentration of factor VIII, XIII, fibrinogen.[11]

13.6 Antifibrinolytic Agents

- May be used off-label to reduce blood loss in complex spine operations.
- These agents inhibit the conversion of plasminogen to plasmin within a clot. Plasmin promotes the breakdown of fibrin.[12]
- Thromboembolic complications have been minimal with the two drugs currently in use (aprotinin was withdrawn from the market because of these complications).
- Available agents:
  - Tranexamic acid: 10 to 30 mg/kg loading dose followed by infusion of 1 to 3 mg/kg/hr during surgery.[13]
  - Epsilon-aminocaproic acid (EACA): A common regimen is 100 mg/kg bolus, followed by 10 mg/kg/hr infusion during surgery.[13]

13.7 Osteoporosis Medications (Table 13.2)

- Treatment for documented osteoporosis is usually provided under the direction of a primary care physician and/or endocrinologist. Improvement is usually slow, and documentable changes on dual-energy X-ray absorptiometry (DEXA) scan may take up to 2 years (radiographic improvement lags behind actual reduction of fracture risk).
- Of the anabolic therapies for osteoporosis (T-score < −2.5), teriparatide (Forteo) has very strong evidence of augmenting bony arthrodesis after spinal fusion.[14]
  - Teriparatide (Forteo), a recombinant human parathyroid hormone, is the fastest-acting treatment for osteoporosis. When the risk of failure as a

result of osteoporosis is high and the downside of waiting for improvement in bone density is significant, off-label use of Forteo (teriparatide) has been described for 2 to 3 months preoperatively, as well as postoperatively in osteoporotic women, in whom it produced a slight decrease in time to fusion.[15] It is administered as a 20 mcg daily subcutaneous injection. Because of risk of osteosarcoma, Forteo should not be used in patients who are at increased risk for osteosarcoma (including patients who have Paget's disease) and should not exceed the recommended total duration of treatment of 24 months in a patient's lifetime.

Table 13.2 Medications in osteoporosis

Drug class	Mechanism of action	Generic grug name (Brand name)	Evidence in spine surgery
Parathyroid gormone (PTH) analogs	Directly stimulates bone formation by osteoblasts; indirectly increases calcium absorption in the intestines and kidney	Teriperatide (Forteo)	Randomized clinical trials have demonstrated superior efficacy in spinal fusion.
		Abaloparatide (Tymlos)	Efficacy for spinal fusion is limited to randomized controlled trial (RCT) in animals. Ongoing Phase II trial with abaloparatide vs. placebo.
Receptor activator of nuclear factor kappa-B ligand (RANK-L) inhibitors	Human monoclonal antibody that inhibits osteoclast-mediated bone destruction	Denosumab (Xgeva, Prolia)	Evidence is limited in combination with teriparatide. Ongoing Phase IV trial with denosumab vs. calcium + vitamin D.
Sclerostin inhibitors	Humanized monoclonal antibody inhibits sclerostin—a bone morphogenetic protein (BMP) osteoblast antagonist	Romosozumab (Evenity)	Although romosozumab improves lumbar bone mineral density, efficacy in lumbar fusion is limited to preclinical trials.

(Continued)

Table 13.2 (*Continued*)

Drug class	Mechanism of action	Generic grug name (Brand name)	Evidence in spine surgery
Nitrogen-containing bisphosphanates	Inhibiting farnesyl pyrophosphate synthase, thereby promoting detachment of osteoclasts from bone and halting resorption	Zoledronate (Zometa, Reclast)	Randomized clinical trials demonstrated improved fusion rate and reduced the incidence of subsequent adjacent vertebral compression fractures and pedicle screw loosening. Some studies show no difference in spinal fusion.
		Alendronate (Fosamax)	Conflicting evidence regarding efficacy on fusion rates. Animal models have demonstrated screw loosening.
		Risedronate (Actonel)	Extent of pedicle screw loosening in the risedronate group did not significantly differ from no medications.
		Ibandronate (Boniva)	Limited evidence in spinal fusion suggests that ibandronate decreases cage subsidence and increases interbody fusion.
		Pamidronate (Aredia)	Possible efficacy for spinal fusion rates is limited to RCT in rabbits.

- The authors recommend to avoid bisphosphonates 1 to 6 months preoperatively and postoperatively for patients undergoing spinal fusion surgery, as there is insufficient evidence regarding the effect of perioperative bisphonates on fusion rates.[14]
- Vitamin D and calcium may be used in conjunction with anabolic therapies in the setting of osteoporosis or alone in the setting of osteopenia (−2.5 < T-score < −1.0).

13.8 Surgical Pearls

- General agents exist for anticoagulation reversal in the setting of urgent or emergent spine surgery, including fresh frozen plasma, prothrombin complex concentrate, and cryoprecipitate.
- There exists a large variety of specific reversal agents for many anticoagulation drugs, which allows for safe spine surgery in a timely fashion (see **Table 13.1**).
- There is evidence osteoporosis medications such as teriparatide improve bony arthrodesis after spinal fusion, improving overall post-operative outcomes (see **Table 13.2**).

Common Clinical Questions

1. A 63-year-old female with a T-score of −4 is undergoing spinal fusion. Which of the following has been demonstrated to have superior efficacy in treatment of osteoporosis in this patient group in the literature?
   A. Bisphosphonates.
   B. Vitamin D.
   C. Teriperatide.
   D. High-dose vitamin D with calcium.
   E. RANK-L inhibitors.
2. A 48-year-old male with a history of atrial fibrillation treated with dabigatran (Pradaxa) presents with acute spinal cord injury. Which of the following reversal agents is appropriate prior to proceeding to the operating room for emergent decompression?
   A. Andexanet alfa (Andexanet).
   B. Prothrombin complex concentrate.
   C. Protamine.
   D. Idaracizumab.
   E. Bentracimab.

3. A 63-year-old female with a past medical history of a mechanical heart valve treated with apixaban (Eliquis) presents with acute cauda equina syndrome secondary to an L4 burst fracture. Prior to proceeding with an emergent L4 corpectomy and transpedicular fusion, which of the following reversal agents is most appropriate?
   A. Desmopressin.
   B. Andexanet alfa (Andexanet).
   C. Tranexamic acid.
   D. Protamine.
   E. Idaracizumab.

Answers to Common Clinical Questions

1. C.
2. D.
3. B.

References

1. Agnelli G, Piovella F, Buoncristiani P, et al. Enoxaparin plus compression stockings compared with compression stockings alone in the prevention of venous thromboembolism after elective neurosurgery. N Engl J Med. 1998; 339(2):80–85
2. Macki M, Haddad Y, Suryadevara R, Dabaja AL, Chedid M, Chang V, PLUSS Investigators. Prophylactic low-molecular-weight heparin versus unfractionated heparin in spine surgery (PLUSS): a pilot matched cohort study. Neurosurgery. 2021; 89(6):1097–1103
3. Sanofi. Lovenox Prescribing Information. Accessed November 4, 2022 at: https://products.sanofi.us/lovenox/lovenox.pdf
4. Alper E, Anderson F, Becker RC, et al. Guidelines for Antithrombotic Therapy. Accessed November 24, 2022 at: https://www.outcomes-umassmed.org/dvt/pdf/anticoag_guidelines.pdf
5. Yang X, Wang Q, Zhang A, et al. Strategies for sustained release of heparin: a review. Carbohydr Polym. 2022; 294:119793
6. Khawar H, Kelley W, Stevens JB, Guzman N. Fresh Frozen Plasma (FFP). StatPearls. Published online September 19, 2022. Accessed October 18, 2022 at: https://www.ncbi.nlm.nih.gov/books/NBK513347/
7. Baskaran J, Lopez RA, Cassagnol M. Prothrombin Complex Concentrate. StatPearls. Published online May 1, 2022. Accessed October 18, 2022 at: https://www.ncbi.nlm.nih.gov/books/NBK539716/

8. Awad NI, Cocchio C. Activated prothrombin complex concentrates for the reversal of anticoagulant-associated coagulopathy. P&T. 2013; 38(11): 696–701
9. Lin J, Hanigan WC, Tarantino M, Wang J. The use of recombinant activated factor VII to reverse warfarin-induced anticoagulation in patients with hemorrhages in the central nervous system: preliminary findings. J Neurosurg. 2003; 98(4):737–740
10. Jurlander B, Thim L, Klausen NK, et al. Recombinant activated factor VII (rFVIIa): characterization, manufacturing, and clinical development. Semin Thromb Hemost. 2001; 27(4):373–384
11. Blood Products. Accessed October 18, 2022 at: https://webpath.med.utah.edu/TUTORIAL/BLDBANK/BBPROD.html
12. Gill JB, Chin Y, Levin A, Feng D. The use of antifibrinolytic agents in spine surgery. A meta-analysis. J Bone Joint Surg Am. 2008; 90(11):2399–2407
13. Schulman S. Pharmacologic tools to reduce bleeding in surgery. Hematology (Am Soc Hematol Educ Program). 2012; 2012(1):517–521
14. Dimar J, Bisson EF, Dhall S, et al. Congress of neurological surgeons systematic review and evidence-based guidelines for perioperative spine: preoperative osteoporosis assessment. Neurosurgery. 2021; 89 Suppl 1:S19–S25
15. Ohtori S, Inoue G, Orita S, et al. Teriparatide accelerates lumbar posterolateral fusion in women with postmenopausal osteoporosis: prospective study. Spine. 2012; 37(23):E1464–E1468

14 Spine Biologics

Raj Swaroop Lavadi, Alexander Yahanda, Galal A. Elsayed, and Nitin Agarwal

Summary
Spine biologics are useful to achieve arthrodesis and knowledge of their utility contributes significantly to the spine surgeon's armamentarium. Optimal biologics possess osteogenic, osteoinductive, and osteoconductive properties. Each biologic has its own unique properties. This chapter summarizes the evolution, properties, and basic classification of biologics.

Keywords: spine, biologics, arthrodesis, fusion, osteobiologic, graft, autologous, allogenic, osteogenic, osteoinductive, osteoconductive

14.1 Key Points

- The ideal spine biologic should have osteogenic, osteoinductive, and osteoconductive properties.
- Autografts are the gold standard for traditional and minimally invasive spine surgery.
- Patient factors, regulatory concerns, and costs in the modern-day, value-based healthcare model should be considered before selection of a biologic.

14.2 Introduction

- Fusion/arthrodesis rates are frequently used metrics to determine satisfactory postoperative outcomes. Spine biologics are agents that function at a cellular level to facilitate arthrodesis.

14.2.1 Evolution and Market Growth

- Spine biologics have developed from bone grafts, the origin of which can be traced back to 2000 BCE, when an anthropologist discovered a skull with evidence of primitive xenograft placement. In the mid-to-late 17th century, a Dutch surgeon named Job van Meekeren continued to experiment with xenografts and observed fusion when one graft was implanted into a soldier's skull. It was not until the early 20th century when biologics were used to treat spinal pathology. Pioneers, Russell Hibbs and Fred Albee, used spinous processes and grafts from the tibia, respectively, to treat Pott's spine. By doing so, Hibbs and Albee defined the surgical utility of spine biologics and paved the way for current innovation. Fast-forward to the present day, we have the capability to manufacture biologics using a three-dimensional printer.[1,2]

- In 2019, the market value for spine biologics was approximately 1.93 billion USD. This valuation is expected to grow to approximately 2.63 billion USD by 2027.[3] The market's compound annual growth rate (CAGR) is 3.9%. The increased need for surgery to address degenerative spine disease in the geriatric population and the rising popularity of minimally invasive spine surgery (MISS) also drive this market.[3] With the need for additional spine surgery, there is a concomitant rise in the development and usage of various biologics.

14.2.2 Basic Properties

- A spinal osteobiologic has three properties:
  - Osteogenic biologics contain the necessary cells (i.e., osteoblasts and stem cells) that allow for bone formation and remodeling.
  - Osteoinductive biologics have the ability to induce differentiation of undifferentiated cells into those of a bone-forming lineage.
    - Osteoinductive property of a biologic is determined by injecting an agent into heterotopic tissue and assessing for microscopic bone formation.
  - Osteoconductive biologics facilitate the ability of bone to grow on an implant surface.
    - For a biologic to be osteoconductive, the involvement of many growth factors of dual mitogenic and angiogenic functionality is required.
    - The final fusion of the bone and implant surface is known as osseointegration.

14.3 Classification

- Autologous biologics:
  - Autograft.
  - Bone marrow aspirates.
  - Growth factors.
- Allogenic biologics:
  - Allograft.
  - Demineralized bone matrix.
  - Bone morphogenetic protein.
  - Synthetic biologics.

14.4 Autologous Biologics

14.4.1 Autografts

- Autologous bone grafts are the most commonly used spinal biologic. These grafts can be taken from various sites. The most common harvest site is the iliac crest because it contains a large quantity of graft material and may be easily accessed. Other potential sites are bony structures of the leg (e.g., the distal femur, proximal tibia, and fibula), distal radius, and ribs. Grafts may also be harvested locally from the intraoperative spinal environment, including the spinous processes, laminae, and facets.[4]
- Iliac grafts have greater osteogenic and osteoconductive potential due a higher cancellous to cortical bone ratio when compared to local autograft.[5]
- The immunologic features of autograft are favorable for arthrodesis. The quality of the graft varies according to the patient's age and the graft's metabolic activity.
- Downsides to autologous biologics include pain and bleeding at the extraction site. Complications specific to iliac crest grafts include fracture of the iliac spine, and sensory disturbances due to iatrogenic nerve injuries (i.e., cluneal and lateral femoral cutaneous nerve). Other complications such as infections, seromas, and hematomas can also occur. Due to an overall complication rate of 19% with iliac crest grafting, alternative options are preferred.[6]
- Autografts can be classified into two subtypes based on their biomechanical properties: cortical and cancellous grafts. **Table 14.1** compares these two types of grafts.
- The increased porosity of cancellous grafts allows for greater vascularization, promoting strengthening of the initially weak graft.[4] Vascularization begins 2 days after implantation with cancellous grafts. To allow for vascularization, cortical grafts need to be initially modified by

Table 14.1 Comparison of cortical and cancellous autografts[7]

Cortical grafts	Cancellous grafts
Lesser porosity	Greater porosity
Good initial strength and stability	Poor initial strength and stability
Poor vascularization	Good vascularization
Delayed osseointegration	Earlier osseointegration
Strength gradually normalizes	Strength gradually increases

osteoclasts to decrease their density. The modification stage may decrease the stability of the graft by 75%. Studies in dogs have shown that this transient instability normalizes 48 weeks after implantation.[7]

- Traditional tricortical anterior iliac crest bone graft obtained from the anterior superior iliac spine have a 6-week postoperative time for pain to subside; 4 to 10% of patients experience moderate, persistent pain at 1-year follow-up.[8]
- Automated tubular cutting bone harvest implements have anecdotally reduced pain at local graft sites.

14.4.2 Bone Marrow Aspirate

- Bone marrow aspirate (BMA) can be taken from the anterior or posterior superior iliac spine with easy access and minimal donor site complications. BMA can also be harvested through the vertebral body using an anterior or posterior approach, but the osteogenic potential of this aspirate is unclear. Since bone marrow lacks an osteoconductive ability, it requires reinforcement with allografts. BMA requires additional scaffolding to produce slightly better fusion rates when compared with standalone autograft.[9,10]

14.4.3 Growth Factors

- Extensive amounts of basic science research have been conducted on growth factors such as platelet-derived growth factor (PDGF) and transforming growth factor-beta (TGF-b), but the clinical superiority of these agents over traditional grafts has yet to be defined. The higher costs required to isolate and store the growth factors are a disadvantage.

14.5 Allogenic Biologics

14.5.1 Allografts

- Allografts are harvested from cadavers and are particularly resourceful when there is a limited supply of autograft. Allografts must undergo a thorough sterilization process, usually via gamma radiation, to eliminate microorganisms before they can be deployed. This process may intrinsically weaken the structure of certain allogenic biologics (i.e., cytokines, chemokines, growth factors). Apart from the collateral damage inflicted by the sterilization process and limited chances of acquiring hepatitis from the donor, allografts should be considered a good alternative to autografts as there is no significant difference between fusion rates and patient-reported outcome measures.[9,11,12]

14.5.2 Demineralized Bone Matrix

- Demineralized bone matrix (DBM) comes in various formulations such as putties, pastes, and gels. DBM may or may not be accompanied by a carrier. Carriers are biocompatible viscous agents that allow the DBM to set firmly within the defect sites. DBM does not have greater fusion rates compared to autografts. Ethylene glycol, a contaminant of DBM, can lead to acute tubular necrosis.[9]

14.5.3 Bone Morphogenetic Protein

- Bone morphogenetic protein (BMP) and its recombinant forms provide the most competitive outcomes to autografts. Of the many BMPs in existence, BMP-2, BMP-4, and BMP-7 have been the most thoroughly studied. The recombinant forms of BMP (rhBMP) advertise greater fusion rates when used as a graft material, with the greatest results arising when used in combination with autografts. Higher quantities of BMP do not improve fusion rates and may activate intrinsic BMP inhibitors. BMP's involvement in oncogenesis is concerning and warrants further long-term human studies.[9] Many biologics do not have standardized dosing recommendations, but lower dosing is favored for rhBMP-2. The pricing of BMP may place an added strain on the costs associated with spinal surgery, but this can be mitigated by improving surgeon's awareness of dose-associated prices.

14.5.4 Synthetic Biologics

- Synthetic biologics were designed to reduce reliance on autografts and their associated donor-site morbidity. These biologics are mainly of three types: bioactive glass, ceramics, and polymer-based compounds.

Bioactive Glass

- Bioactive glass has greater osteoblastic activity than hydroxyapatite-based ceramics and is very biocompatible. It upregulates the genes responsible for creating factors that assist bone formation (i.e., VEGF, IGF). Its antibacterial properties may limit graft invasion. Despite the microscopic advantages it carries, as a standalone biologic, it has poor fusion rates in the adult population (34%) and unknown fusion rates in the pediatric age group.[12]

Ceramics

- Commonly used ceramics include hydroxyapatite (HA) and beta-tricalcium phosphate. The advantages of ceramics include cost-effectiveness, limited chances for infections, and a long shelf-life. They are also relatively simple to manufacture and can be customized to the desired shape. Poor mechanical strength is a disadvantage of ceramics.[9]

Polymer-Based Compounds

- Two polymers used as biologics are polyetheretherketone (PEEK) and polymethyl methacrylate (PMMA). In its unadulterated form, PEEK is bio-inert, but it can be made functional by adding certain compounds such as titanium.[13] PEEK cages are biocompatible, radiolucent, have reduced implant stiffness, and, most importantly, are structurally robust. Since PEEK is MRI-compatible, the healing process can be easily tracked. PEEK can be bolstered with additional agents such as allografts and rhBMP-2. The utility of PEEK has mainly been explored for surgeries on the cervical spine. Although some studies show no significant difference in the clinical outcomes between the two, and some endorse greater clinical outcomes with the latter, bone grafts are still preferred to PEEK cages.
- PMMA, also known as bone cement, is formed by joining a sterile liquid and powder. This combination gives PMMA a solid structure and yields an exothermic reaction. It functions optimally at 73 °F, and a slight deviation from this fixed point may alter its characteristics.[14] PMMA requires additives to provide structure, stability, and added functionality. Gentamicin can be added to reduce the risk of postoperative infections and barium sulfate can be added to assist with radiological tracking. Vitamin E enhances biocompatibility and controls the heat produced from the exothermic reaction in the right concentrations. Beyond this fixed concentration range, vitamin E can prolong the cement setting time and can lead to a fragile construct.[15] Without any modifications, PMMA is associated with low fusion rates, with the upper end of the range being as low as 28%.[16] One select study found that filling a PMMA cage with a cancellous autograft could yield 90.5% and 100% fusion rates at 6- and 12-month follow-up visits, respectively, in patients who have undergone fusion for single-level cervical disk herniations with associated neurological deficits.[16] PMMA is contraindicated in patients with hypovolemia as this may potentiate hypotensive episodes.[14]

Platelet Derivatives

- Platelet concentrates/gels can be autologous or allogenic.[17] These derivatives function by directly or indirectly inducing the release of growth factors that facilitate healing. One small clinical study showed an increase in bone density following platelet gel use. The same study suggested that platelet gels can potentially overcome patient factors favoring nonfusion (i.e., smoking, diabetes).[18] Larger randomized trials must be performed before defining the appropriate indications for platelet derivatives.

- **Table 14.2** and **Table 14.3** summarize the properties and provide an overview of the advantages and disadvantages of each biologic, respectively.

Table 14.2 Properties of biologics

	Osteogenic	Osteoinductive	Osteoconductive
Autografts	✓	✓	✓
Bone marrow aspirates	✓	✓	-
Growth factors	-	✓	-
Allograft	-	✓	✓
DBM	-	✓	✓
BMP	-	✓	-
Bioactive glass	-	✓	✓
Ceramics	-	-	✓
PEEK	-	-	-
PMMA	-	-	-
Platelet Gels/Concentrates	-	✓	-

Abbreviations: BMP, bone morphogenetic protein; DBM, demineralized bone matrix; PEEK, polyetheretherketone; PMMA, polymethyl methacrylate.

Table 14.3 Biologics with their advantages and disadvantages

	Advantages	Disadvantages/ Complications
Autograft (iliac crest)	• Large amount exists • Carries all three properties of an osteobiologic	• Need for a second incision • Donor site morbidity – Pain – Fracture – Infection – Seroma – Hematoma – Nerve injury

(Continued)

Table 14.3 (*Continued*)

	Advantages	Disadvantages/ Complications
Autograft (local)[5]	• Does not require a second incision • Carries all three properties of an osteobiologic	• Lesser quantity available • Lesser osteogenic and osteoconductive properties compared to graft from the iliac crest • Potential for dural tear
Bone marrow aspirates[9,10]	• Minimal donor site morbidity	• Rare potential for procedural injury (i.e., local vessels and nerves)
Growth factors (PDGF, TGF-b)[9]	• Can be combined with allograft and used as a substitute for iliac crest graft	• High costs
Allograft[12]	• Easy to access • Unlimited quantity	• Weakened by sterilization process • Risk of communicable disease • Risk of antigenicity increases with frozen allografts
Demineralized bone matrix	• Unlimited quantity	• Poor fusion rates with open spinal surgery
Bioactive glass	• Biocompatible • Antibacterial property	• Poor fusion rates in adults • Unclear fusion potential in the pediatric population

(Continued)

Table 14.3 (*Continued*)

	Advantages	Disadvantages/ Complications
Bone morphogenetic protein (BMP)[12]	• Unlimited quantity	• Potential for oncogenesis • May activate BMP inhibitors with higher dosing • Variable/High costs
Polyetheretherketone (PEEK)[9]	• Biocompatible • MRI-compatible • Radiolucent • Robust • Reduced implant stiffness	• Potential for migration of the cage • Suboptimal fusion rates
Polymethyl methacrylate (PMMA)[14]	• Enhanced functionality with the use of additives	• Heat-sensitive • Hypotension • Infection • Heterotopic bone formation • Exothermic reaction can damage local structures including neural elements • Chances for leakage into local structures
Ceramics	• Cost-effective • Limited chance for infection • Long shelf-life • Simple to manufacture and customize	• Poor strength
Platelet gels/ Concentrates[18]	• Unlimited quantity • Low cost	• Mixed fusion results

14.6 Pediatric

- There is a general paucity of data on the usage of spine biologics in the pediatric population. This void includes lack of large sampled clinical trials, dosing recommendations, and immediate and long-term postoperative outcomes. Despite the absence of this information, autografts remain the gold standard due to their optimal fusion rates. Other biologics, such as BMP, perform close to autografts. However, its use in the clinical setting is limited due to the potential for oncogenesis and reports of many serious complications, including infection, cord compression due to osseous overgrowth, and heterotopic bone formation. All of these complications may necessitate subsequent surgery. DBM has rarely been discussed in the literature for pediatric spine surgery. A challenge in the pediatric population is the lack of adequate autograft material required for satisfactory fusion. This relative deficiency can be addressed using allografts or a local autograft and bioactive glass mixture. The lack of proper direction in this area should provide a stimulus for organizing more extensive clinical trials to identify the best biologics to be used in this vulnerable population.[12]

14.7 BOnE Classification

- A collaborative effort between several researchers and AOSpine resulted in the creation of a classification system emphasizing osteobiologic efficiency. The BOnE (Bone Osteobiologics and Evidence) classification was synthesized from a bibliometric analysis of peer-reviewed publications.[19] The evidence was presented in three levels, with each level having four subgroups. Level A data focused on human studies. The subgroups ranged from 1 to 4, with a subgroup of 1 signifying the highest level of evidence. In summation, the ultimate evidence would be categorized as A1. The creators of this classification system categorized rhBMP-2 with an A1 grade.[19] The future goals for this relatively new classification system include subjecting it to tests of reliability and validity and creating a platform to be aware of emerging biologics and literature. Such advances will help develop this classification system.[19]

14.8 MISS and Biologics

- With a growing shift toward MISS, optimal biologics need to be identified.
- MISS offers several advantages over traditional surgery, which include less trauma to the perioperative tissue, decreased postoperative pain, and shorter length of hospital stay. Despite its advantages, the superiority of MISS with added biologics has yet to be proven. In addition, the same biologics used for

a traditional open spinal surgery may yield diverse outcomes in MISS due to inherent differences in the operative environment.[4]

- The larger surface area in open operations allows for greater maneuverability and graft placement as opposed to their minimally invasive counterparts.[4]
- One such dissimilarity is the preference for local bone graft in MISS over iliac crest bone graft due to its associated complications. Awareness of the ideal biologic required for both styles of surgery can help the surgeon optimize the patient's care. The following biologics have promising fusion rates:
  - Posterior MISS approach using rhBMP-2 in combination with another bone graft (95%); iliac crest autograft (96%); autograft and allograft combination (96%).[4]
  - Anterior/Lateral MISS approach using standalone rhBMP-2 (97%); bone marrow aspirate as an extender (97%); demineralized bone matrix (98%).[4]
- Despite these high fusion rates, factors such as cost and postoperative complications must also be considered before utilizing them in practice.

14.9 Current Developments and Trends

- An optimal biologic may be considered as one that allows for the greatest rates of fusion with the least chances for complications. Peptide amphiphile (PA) based biomaterials have properties ideal for designing synthetic bone grafts. These agents are a robust, self-healing class of molecules that have the potential to contribute to regenerative medicine.[20]
- Three-dimensional printing/additive manufacturing of biologics may have the advantage of uniformity among products. The ability to combine two biologics into a single, synergistic scaffold (i.e., HA-DBM scaffold) is another advantage of this printing technique. One such promising initiative is being led by Advanced Regenerative Manufacturing Institute in Manchester, New Hampshire, USA.[20]
- Layered three-dimensional printing permits the inclusion of micro-additives into the biologic, potentially enhancing spinal fusion; thus, bringing the market closer to a biologic superior to BMP-2.[20]
- Local gene therapy is also being used to optimize fusion rates. This method promotes osteoinductive factor activity by delivering a gene or a complementary DNA sequence for the desired factor. This avoids the costs associated with isolating osteoinductive factors for later injection. In theory, by inducing DNA replication of osteoinductive factors, gene therapy may also produce a prolonged effect as opposed to the traditional injection of factors.
- As there is no emergent need to produce spine biologics, manufacturers should not rush preclinical and clinical trials prior to market testing. Adhering to preset guidelines will ensure quality, efficacy, and safety of new biologic products.

14.10 Surgical Pearls

- Autograft is the gold standard for arthrodesis in patients undergoing spinal surgery; its technical challenges, surgical site pain, and associated complications have made it a “lost art.”
- Consider the Young’s modulus versus vertebral endplate Hounsfield units on CT and static and kinetic coefficients of friction when evaluating biologics in conjunction with graft placement. These factors may play a role in determining the approach intraoperatively and evaluating future subsidence risk especially within narrow disk spaces.
- The use of combined materials such as PEEK/titanium implants can lead to fracturing intraoperatively due to the varying interfaces.
- The use of bone marrow aspirate in conjunction with a biologic can potentially offer an autologous “boost” without some of the adverse effects of a full autograft extraction.
- Off-label uses of biologics/implants are ubiquitous, but be aware of local regulatory concerns such as US FDA “blackbox” warnings for any biologic chosen before implantation.

Common Clinical Questions

1. What property of an osteobiologic is defined by its ability to grow on an implant surface?
2. What type of autograft takes longer to vascularize?

Answers to Common Clinical Questions

1. Osteoconductive.
2. Cortical.

References

1. Hampel GA, Yilmaz E, Massrey C, et al. History of bone grafts in spine surgery. Cureus. 2022; 14(5):e24655
2. Virk S, Qureshi S, Sandhu H. History of spinal fusion: where we came from and where we are going. HSS J. 2020; 16(2):137–142
3. Reports and Data. Pharma and Healthcare—Spine Biologics Market. Available from: https://www.reportsanddata.com/report-detail/spine-biologics-market
4. Chang KY, Hsu WK. Spinal biologics in minimally invasive lumbar surgery. Minim Invasive Surg. 2018; 2018:5230350

5. Tuchman A, Brodke DS, Youssef JA, et al. Iliac crest bone graft versus local autograft or allograft for lumbar spinal fusion: a systematic review. Global Spine J. 2016; 6(6):592–606
6. Dimitriou R, Mataliotakis GI, Angoules AG, Kanakaris NK, Giannoudis PV. Complications following autologous bone graft harvesting from the iliac crest and using the RIA: a systematic review. Injury. 2011; 42 Suppl 2:S3–S15
7. Pape HC, Evans A, Kobbe P. Autologous bone graft: properties and techniques. J Orthop Trauma. 2010; 24 Suppl 1:S36–S40
8. Armaghani SJ, Even JL, Zern EK, Braly BA, Kang JD, Devin CJ. The evaluation of donor site pain after harvest of tricortical anterior iliac crest bone graft for spinal surgery: a prospective study. Spine. 2016; 41(4):E191–E196
9. D'Souza M, Macdonald NA, Gendreau JL, Duddleston PJ, Feng AY, Ho AL. Graft materials and biologics for spinal interbody fusion. Biomedicines. 2019; 7(4):75
10. Kitchel SH, Wang MY, Lauryssen CL. Techniques for aspirating bone marrow for use in spinal surgery. Neurosurgery. 2005; 57(4) Suppl:286–289, discussion 286–289
11. Liao Z, Wang CH, Cui WL. Comparison of allograft and autograft in lumbar fusion for lumbar degenerative diseases: a systematic review. J Invest Surg. 2016; 29(6):373–382
12. Letchuman V, Ampie L, Choy W, DiDomenico JD, Syed HR, Buchholz AL. Bone grafting and biologics for spinal fusion in the pediatric population: current understanding and future perspective. Neurosurg Focus. 2021; 50(6):E8
13. Kumar TA, Jei JB, Muthukumar B. Comparison of osteogenic potential of poly-ether-ether-ketone with titanium-coated poly-ether-ether-ketone and titanium-blended poly-ether-ether-ketone: an *in vitro* study. J Indian Prosthodont Soc. 2017; 17(2):167–174
14. Vaishya R, Chauhan M, Vaish A. Bone cement. J Clin Orthop Trauma. 2013; 4 (4):157–163
15. Arora M, Chan EK, Gupta S, Diwan AD. Polymethylmethacrylate bone cements and additives: a review of the literature. World J Orthop. 2013; 4(2):67–74
16. Chen JF, Wu CT, Lee SC, Lee ST. Use of a polymethylmethacrylate cervical cage in the treatment of single-level cervical disc disease. J Neurosurg Spine. 2005; 3(1):24–28
17. Piccin A, Di Pierro AM, Canzian L, et al. Platelet gel: a new therapeutic tool with great potential. Blood Transfus. 2017; 15(4):333–340
18. Landi A, Tarantino R, Marotta N, et al. The use of platelet gel in postero-lateral fusion: preliminary results in a series of 14 cases. Eur Spine J. 2011; 20(Suppl 1):S61–S67
19. Wang JC, Yoon ST, Brodke DS, et al. Development of AOSpine BOnE (Bone Osteobiologics and Evidence) classification. Global Spine J. 2020; 10(7):871–874
20. Phan EN, Hsu WK. Novel approaches guiding the future of spinal biologics for bone regeneration. Curr Rev Musculoskelet Med. 2022; 15(3):205–212

III
Spinal Pathology

15 Congenital Anomalies

Mark Stephens, Jared Fridley, Eric Momin, and Andrew Jea

Summary
Congenital anomalies of the spinal cord encompass a wide variety of abnormal musculoskeletal and neural developments in utero. Developmental anomalies of the vertebrae can result in congenital scoliosis or Klippel-Feil syndrome. Abnormalities in notochord development result in split cord malformations and abnormalities in dysjunction can result in a spectrum of disorders including spinal lipomas and myelomeningoceles. In general, mild clinical presentations of congenital anomalies can be managed conservatively while surgery is reserved for more severe cases.

Keywords: MOMS trial, congenital anomalies, myelomeningocele, Klippel-Feil syndrome, congenital scoliosis, spinal lipoma, split cord malformation

15.1 Key Points

- Congenital abnormalities of the spine are a heterogenous group of disorders in which there has been compromise of one of the stages of spinal embryological development (**Fig. 15.1**).
- Other systems, including the cardiovascular, pulmonary, and genitourinary systems, may be affected.

15.2 Vertebral Developmental Abnormalities

15.2.1 Congenital Scoliosis

- Background:
  - Scoliosis that occurs secondary to abnormal vertebral development.
  - Classified based on either embryologic failure of formation (hemivertebra) or failure of segmentation (bar or block vertebra) (**Fig. 15.2**).
- Signs, symptoms, and physical examination:
  - Associated spinal abnormalities occur in approximately 20% of patients.
  - Cardiac, genitourinary, and skeletal abnormalities occur in 30 to 60% of patients.

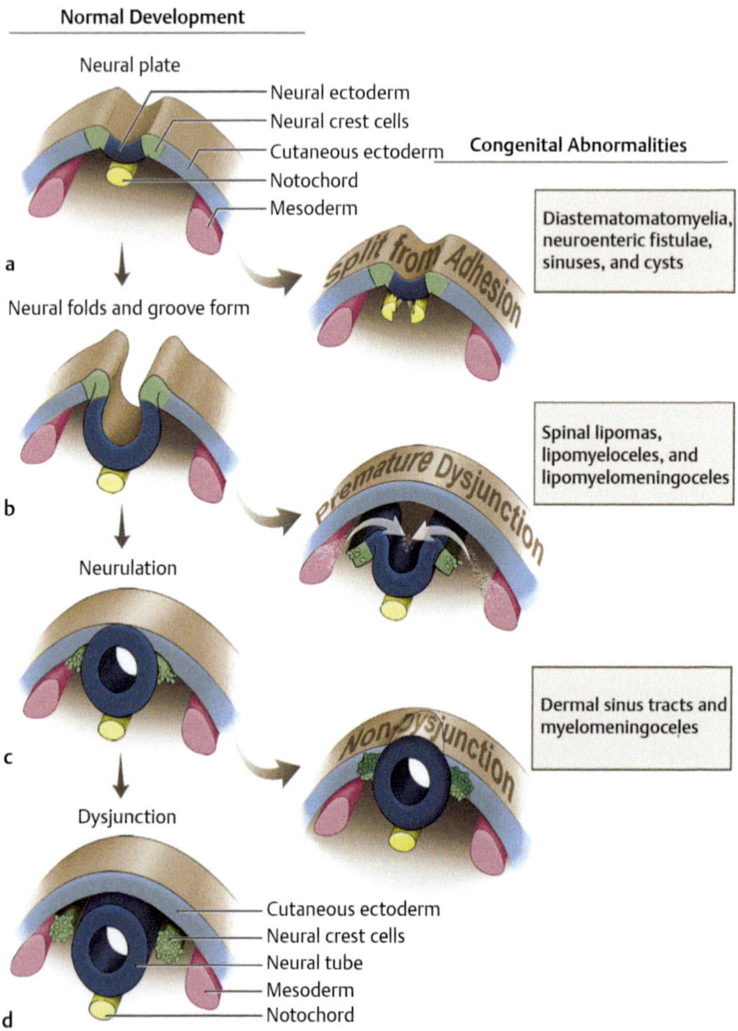

Fig. 15.1 **(a–d)** Defects during different stages of spinal cord embryology lead to congenital anomalies of the spine.

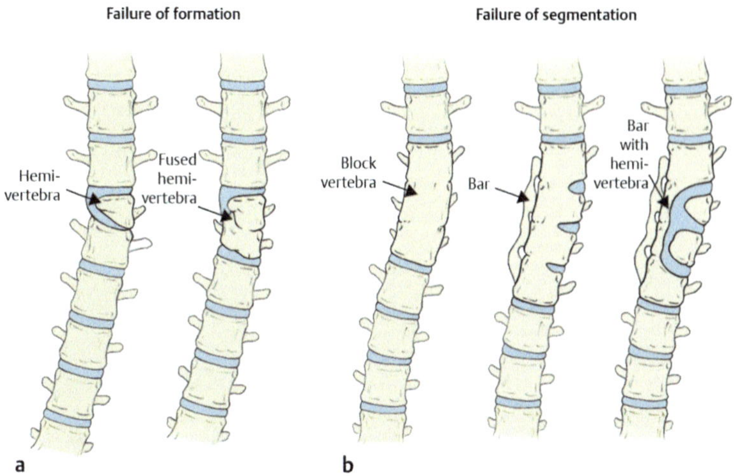

Fig. 15.2 (**a**) Formation and (**b**) segmentation anomalies in the formation of the spinal column are responsible for the development of congenital scoliosis, most evident as the child grows.

- Neuroimaging:
  - Computed tomography (CT) of the spine or spinal radiographs is used to assess bony abnormalities and to plan any surgical intervention.
  - Magnetic resonance imaging (MRI) of the spine is used to look for associated intraspinal abnormalities.
  - Echocardiogram and renal ultrasound should be performed in all patients.
- Treatment:
  - Bracing does not prevent curve progression, nor does it correct underlying pathology.
  - Surgery is considered for symptomatic curves > 45 degrees or progressing > 10 degrees per year.
  - Prophylactic surgery may be considered on a case-by-case basis (either in-situ fusion or hemiepiphysiodesis).

15.2.2 Klippel-Feil Syndrome (KFS)

- Background:
  - Characterized by multiple fused cervical vertebrae due to failure of segmentation between the 3rd and 8th weeks of gestation.
  - Three types[1]:
    - Type 1: Fusion of many cervical and upper thoracic vertebrae. High risk of scoliosis (approximately 30%).

    - Type 2: Fusion at one or two interspaces combined with other congenital spinal abnormalities.
    - Type 3: Fused cervical vertebrae with thoracic or lumbar fused vertebrae.
- Signs, symptoms, and physical examination:
  - Classic clinical triad of short neck, low posterior hairline, and decreased neck range of motion is seen in less than 50% of patients.
  - Associated with scoliosis, deafness, genitourinary abnormalities, cervical ribs, and cardiovascular abnormalities.
  - Present with neck pain or neurologic compromise.
- Neuroimaging:
  - Cervical radiographs or CT of the cervical spine reveals multiple fused cervical vertebrae.
  - MRI of the cervical spine is performed if neurologic signs/symptoms are present.
    - Echocardiogram and renal ultrasound are used to look for associated abnormalities.
- Treatment[2]:
  - Surgery is reserved for cases of spinal instability, compression of neurologic elements, or progressive spinal deformity.

15.3 Anomalies of Notochord Formation

15.3.1 Split Cord Malformations (SCMs)

- Background:
  - Classified into two types:
    - Type I: Two hemicords, each within its own dural tube, separated by a bony/cartilaginous septum.
    - Type II: Two hemicords in a single dural tube, separated by a fibrous septum.[2]
- Signs, symptoms, and physical examination:
  - Often associated with open and occult spinal dysraphism manifestations.
  - Common clinical presentations include tethered cord syndrome (TCS), pain, and/or sensorimotor disturbances, with hypertrichosis found in nearly 50% of all patients.
- Neuroimaging:
  - High-resolution thin-cut CT scans of the spine are useful for defining the type of split cord malformation.
  - MRI of the spine is useful for identifying other associated intraspinal anomalies.

- Treatment:
  - The primary goal of surgery is detethering of the spinal cord by removal of any offending bone, septa, or fibrous bands.

15.4 Anomalies of Dysjunction

15.4.1 Spinal Lipomas[3]

- Background:
  - Includes multiple pathologies: Lipomas of the filum or conus medullaris, lipomyelomeningocele, intradural spinal lipomas, epidural lipomatosis, lipomyelocele, and spinal angiolipoma.
- Signs, symptoms, and physical examination:
  - Classically associated with TCS as a result of tethering of neural tissue by the lipoma.
  - Presenting symptoms/signs can include lower extremity weakness, orthopedic abnormalities of the lower extremities, numbness, gait dysfunction, spasticity, urinary hesitancy/incontinence, back/leg pain, and cutaneous stigmata of the low back.
- Neuroimaging:
  - MRI of the lumbar spine without contrast is the modality of choice for defining the precise nature of the lipoma (T1-weighted sequence) and surrounding neural tissue (T1- and T2-weighted sequences) and is key for planning any surgical intervention.
- Treatment:
  - Natural history of these lesions is not clear, so the risk of surgical morbidity (including future retethering and neurological injury) must be weighed against any possible surgical benefit.

15.4.2 Myelomeningocele

- Background:
  - Multiple factors are involved in etiology of myelomeningocele, both maternal and fetal, including a strong association with maternal folate deficiency.
  - Nearly all patients have an associated Chiari II malformation.
- Signs, symptoms, and physical examination:
  - Neurological deficits are dependent on the location and length of the defect.
  - High risk of hydrocephalus (80–90%).
  - Associated with orthopedic and genitourinary abnormalities.
  - Risk for developing tethered cord syndrome and scoliosis.

- Neuroimaging:
  - Fetal ultrasound has nearly 100% sensitivity for detection of myelomeningocele.
  - Fetal MRI can also be useful, especially when planning surgical treatment.
- Treatment:
  - Surgical repair of the myelomeningocele should occur within the first 48 to 72 hours of life because of the risk of infection from exposure of neural elements.
  - The MOMS trial[2] has established prenatal repair as a safe alternative to postnatal repair, with a reduced incidence of hydrocephalus in prenatal repair patients.

15.5 Surgical Pearls

- The goals of surgery are to arrest progression of the deformity and to correct it, if it can be corrected safely.
- Patients who have Type I KFS should be followed closely in clinic for development of spinal deformity, particularly scoliosis.
- All Type II SCMs should be surgically explored in symptomatic patients, even if imaging does not reveal any median septae.
- Surgery carries a risk of not only neurologic injury and cerebrospinal fluid (CSF) leak, but also scar tissue formation and spinal cord tethering, all of which must be considered when deciding whether to operate on an asymptomatic patient.
- Placode is dissected from surrounding epithelium around the malformation, with care taken not to leave any attached epithelial elements because of the risk of developing dermoid tumors (**Fig. 15.3**).
- Lateral edges of the placode are reapproximated, followed by closure of the dura, the dorsal fascia/muscle layers (depending on surgeon's preference), and, finally, the skin.

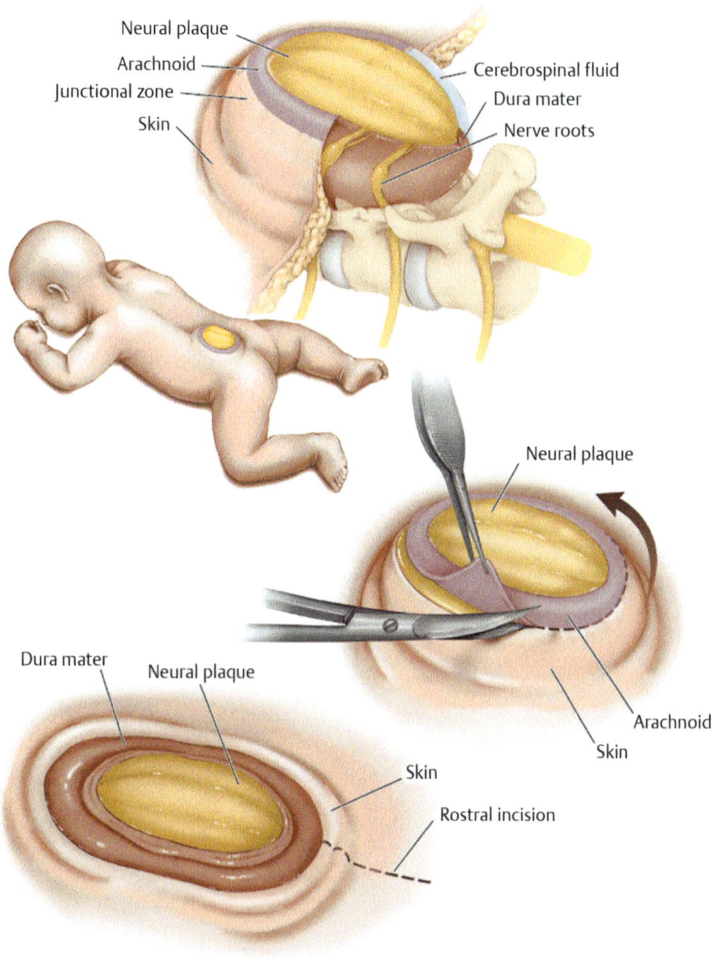

a

Fig. 15.3 **(a)** The multilayer closure begins with an initial circumferential incision following the arachnoid–skin junction to isolate the neural plaque and spinal cord. The skin incision is continued rostrally in the midline to observe the caudal-most intact lamina and the dura beneath it.

(Continued)

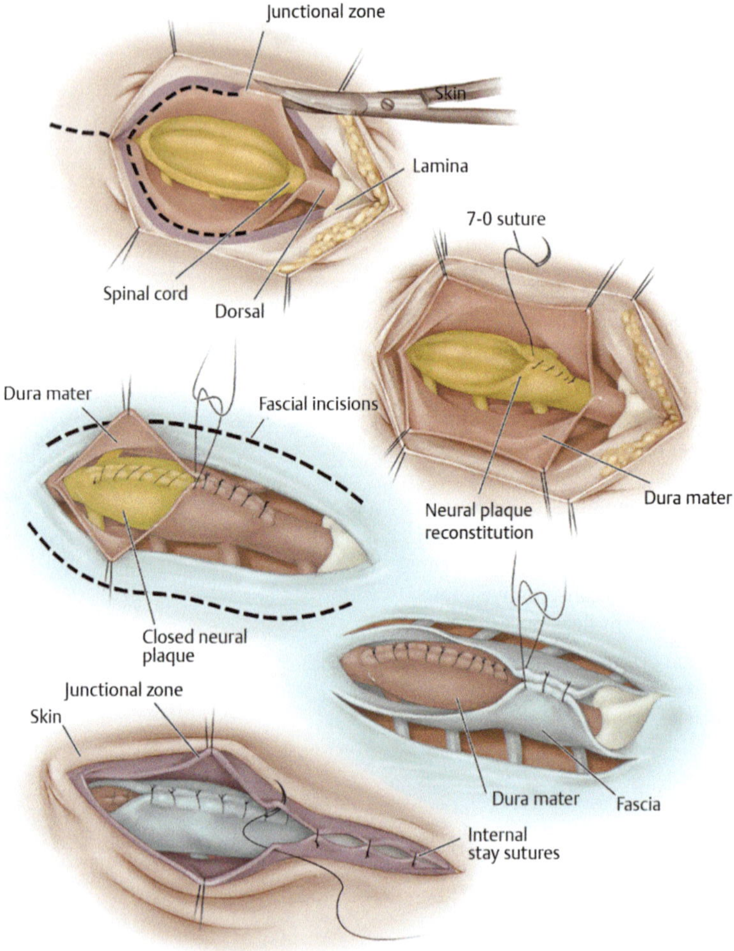

Fig. 15.3 (*Continued*) **(b)** An inferior and lateral dissection toward the caudal edge of the defect isolates the dura. The caudal defect is extended and the residual dura dissected. In the midline, the dura is then approximated following that of the lateral arachnoid. The lumbosacral fascia is identified and incised bilaterally with dissection from the posterior iliac crest and sacrospinalis muscle, with care taken to not disrupt the sacral fascial attachments. The lateral edges of the fascial flaps are then folded toward the midline and sutured in place over the dorsal surface of the dura. The subcutaneous tissue, if present, is closed. The placement of sutures in the area where the dura joins the dermis will provide for tight internal sutures that will reduce tension during later skin closure.

Common Clinical Questions

1. What other workup should be performed after diagnosing a patient with Klippel-Feil deformity?
2. Should asymptomatic patients with spinal lipoma undergo untethering?
3. What were the primary endpoints of the MOMS trial?

Answers to Common Clinical Questions

1. Klippel-Feil syndrome is not infrequently associated with midline anomalies in other organ systems such as the heart, bladder, and kidneys. Workup should include an echocardiogram and renal ultrasound[4] with possible consultation of cardiology and nephrology, respectively.
2. The utility of prophylactic untethering for spinal lipoma is widely debated. The argument for prophylactic untethering is prevention of progression of neurological deficits that may become permanent if treatment is delayed. On the other hand, many authors argue that surgery merely starts the time clock for the next tethering event, and each attempt at untethering presents with higher risks of lower chance of accomplishing the surgical goal of detethering.[5] Most contemporary pediatric neurosurgeons have adopted a conservative approach to spinal lipomas—operating only when symptoms develop.
3. The primary endpoints in the MOMS trial were need for a CSF shunt and death. The prenatal surgery group demonstrated a 50% relative risk reduction of necessitating a shunt compared to the postnatal group. When bias was removed employing a blinded adjudication committee, the risk reduction of requiring a CSF shunt was less dramatic but still showed a statistically significant decrease of about 30%. There were two deaths in both cohorts.[6]

References

1. Feil A. L'Absence et la diminution des vertèbres cervicales: Etudes clinique et pathologique. Le syndrôme de la réduction numérique cervicale. Paris, France: Librairie Littéraire et Médicale; 1919
2. Pang D, Dias MS, Ahab-Barmada M. Split cord malformation: Part I: A unified theory of embryogenesis for double spinal cord malformations. Neurosurgery. 1992; 31(3):451–480
3. Blount JP, Elton S. Spinal lipomas. Neurosurg Focus. 2001; 10(1):e3

4. Menger RP, Rayi A, Notarianni C. Klippel Feil Syndrome. [Updated 2022 Sep 26]. In: StatPearls [Internet]. Treasure Island (FL): StatPearls Publishing; January 2023. Available from: https://www.ncbi.nlm.nih.gov/books/NBK493157/
5. Kulkarni AV, Pierre-Kahn A, Zerah M. Conservative management of asymptomatic spinal lipomas of the conus. Neurosurgery. 2004; 54(4):868–873, discussion 873–875
6. Adzick NS, Thom EA, Spong CY, et al. MOMS Investigators. A randomized trial of prenatal versus postnatal repair of myelomeningocele. N Engl J Med. 2011; 364(11):993–1004

16 Cervical Trauma

Gregory D. Schroeder and Alexander R. Vaccaro

Summary
Cervical spinal trauma is common. The neuroimaging needs to be reviewed carefully so as to not miss critical injuries like atlanto-occipital dislocation. Surgical decompression surgery should be performed urgently with spinal cord injuries. Additionally, the vertebral arteries should be assessed with appropriate imaging in some cases of cervical spinal trauma, including C1/2 fractures or fractures that involve the transverse foramena.

Keywords: dens fractures, trauma, hangman fracture, ASIA

16.1 Key Points

- Early decompression increases the chance of neurologic recovery in patients who have an acute spinal cord injury.[1]
- The use of high-dose methylprednisolone in patients with an acute spinal cord injury is controversial.[2,3,4]
- C1 ring fractures rarely require surgery.
- Geriatric patients who have a type II odontoid fracture who are healthy enough to undergo general anesthesia should consider surgical stabilization—preferably a posterior C1–C2 fusion.[5,6]
- The algorithm for the treatment of subaxial cervical spine fractures is based on bone stability, injury to the diskoligamentous complex, and the neurologic injury of the patient.[7]
- Subaxial cervical facet fractures involving more than 40% of the absolute height of the intact lateral mass or more than 1 cm long from the tip of the superior articular process to the fracture line are at increased risk for failure of nonoperative treatment.[8]

16.2 General Principles

- Field management:
  - ABCs: airway, breathing, circulation.

- Spinal immobilization:
  - Rigid cervical collar, lateral bolsters, rigid backboard.
  - Pediatric patients require recessed headboard or pediatric board.
- Emergency room management:
  - ABCs plus disability and exposure.
  - Standard imaging.
  - Neurogenic shock:
    - Hypotension in the presence of bradycardia.
    - Management with vasopressors and modest fluid resuscitation.
- Classification:
  - American Spinal Injury Association (ASIA) scoring scale (**Table 16.1**):
    - Complete: No motor or sensory function below the zone of injury.
    - Incomplete: Partial motor or sensory function below the zone of injury (**Table 16.2**).
  - About 10 to 15% of patients have noncontiguous spinal fractures.
  - Orthogonal radiographs (anteroposterior [AP]/lateral cervical-thoracic, and lumbosacral spine).
  - CT:
    - Useful for visualizing occipital–cervical and cervicothoracic junctions.
    - Must include sagittal and coronal reconstructions if plain X-ray is not used.
    - Not as useful for ligamentous injury assessment.

Table 16.1 ASIA neurological scoring system

Grade	Description
A	Complete: No motor or sensory function is preserved in the sacral segments.
B	Incomplete: Sensory but not motor function is preserved below the neurologic level and includes the sacral segments.
C	Incomplete: Motor function is preserved below the neurologic level, and more than half of the key muscles below the level have a muscle grade < 3.
D	Incomplete: Motor function is preserved below the neurologic level, and at least half of the key muscle groups below the level have a muscle grade > 3.
E	Normal.

Abbreviation: ASIA, American Spinal Injury Association.
Note: The caudal-most normal level is the neurologic level.

Table 16.2 Incomplete spinal cord injury patterns

Syndrome	Prognosis	Description
Central cord	Fair	Usually due to hyperextension injury with greater upper extremity involvement and more proximal than distal muscle groups
Anterior cord	Poor	Due to injury of anterior spinal artery; loss of sense pain and temperature, and motor function
Brown-Sequard	Best	Due to hemitransection of cord or lateral injury; ipsilateral motor loss, vibration, and position sense and contralateral pain and temperature
Posterior cord	Fair	Loss of vibration and position sense

  - MRI:
    - Required in all cases with neurologic impairment or deficit.
    - Ligamentous structures visualized on T1.
    - Edema visualized on T2 with short tau inversion recovery (STIR).
- Steroid management:
  - Controversial:
    - Congress of Neurological Surgeons recommended against the use of high-dose methylprednisolone in 2013 owing to its limited efficacy and high rate of complications.[3]
    - 47.4 and 56.4% of Cervical Spine Research Society members reported using steroids in patients who had complete or incomplete spinal cord injury (SCI) in 2014.[2]
- Surgical timing:
  - Surgical decompression within 24 hours has been shown to lead to statistically significant improvements in neurologic function 6 months after injury.[1]

16.3 Upper Cervical Spine Trauma

16.3.1 Atlantooccipital Dissociation

- Background:
  - Clinical suspicion paramount.
  - Mechanism: High-energy rotational or flexion–extension force.
- Signs, symptoms, and physical examination:
  - Derangements in cardiorespiratory parameters common.

- Survivors[9]:
  - 40% quadriplegic.
  - 40% hemiplegic.
  - 20% neurologically normal.
    - Neurologic deterioration can occur in up to 35% of patients who live through the initial injury.
- Neuroimaging:
  - Radiographs:
    - Multiple radiographic measurements have been described, but none has been universally accepted as superior.
    - Powers ratio[10]: Ratio of distance from basion to C1 lamina divided by distance from opisthion to anterior ring of C1 (**Fig. 16.1**).
      - Identifies anterior subluxation if ratio is > 1.
    - Wackenheim line[11]:
      - Line from posterior surface of clivus—normally its inferior extension should barely touch posterior aspect of the odontoid tip.
      - If the line runs behind the odontoid, there is posterior dissociation.
      - If the line runs in front, there is anterior dissociation.
    - Harris's rule of 12[12]:
      - A basion–axial interval or basion–dental interval of > 12 is indicative of an atlantooccipital dissociation.

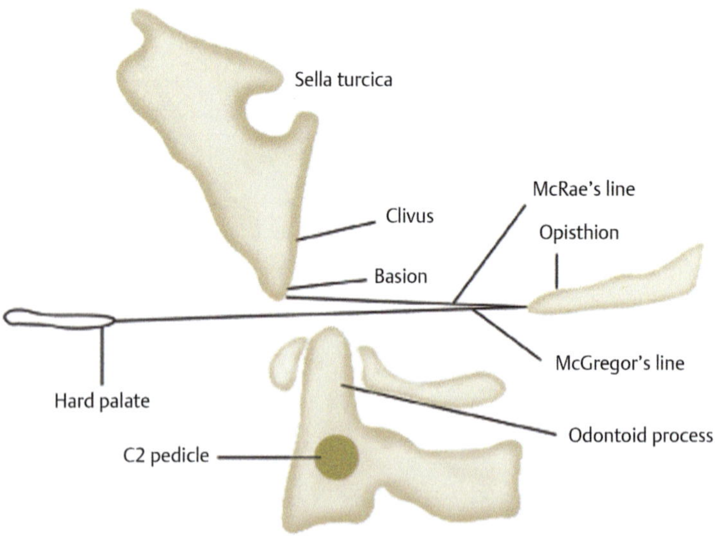

Fig. 16.1 Different lines and parameters to assess craniovertebral stability.

- CT:
  - Revised condyle–C1 interval[13]:
    - Distance between the occipital condyle and the C1 lateral mass on sagittal imaging.
    - A value of greater than 2.5 mm is consistent with a dissociation.
- Treatment:
  - Occipitocervical fusion.
- Surgical pearls:
  - Obtain a CT angiogram (CTA) or MR angiogram (MRA) to assess vertebral artery integrity as part of the preoperative planning if suspicion exists for vessel injury.
  - Use of MRI for assessing integrity of ligaments may help with decision to fuse occiput to C1, C2, or a more caudal spot.

16.3.2 Atlas (C1) Fracture

- Background:
  - Neurologic injury is rare due to large space available for the spinal cord.
  - Can occur anterior, posterior, or combined (Jefferson).
  - Mechanism is axial loading.
  - Status of transverse alar ligament (TAL) is critical to surgical decision-making.
  - Dickman classification[14] of TAL injuries:
    - Type 1—Midsubstance disruption of TAL.
      - Ligament will not heal.
    - Type 2—Avulsion of the tubercle with TAL attached.
      - Bony injury that may heal.
- Signs, symptoms, and physical examination:
  - Typically does not lead to neurologic deficits.
  - With severe fractures, complete and incomplete injuries are possible, including medullary dysfunction.
- Neuroimaging:
  - Radiographs:
    - Open-mouth odontoid view to assess the relationship of lateral mass of C1 on C2.
    - Spence rule[15]:
      - Classic rule indicating that > 7 mm composite overhang is indicative of a TAL injury.
      - Newer studies have demonstrated little correlation between bony displacement and transverse ligament integrity.[16]
  - CT scan:
    - Coronal and sagittal reconstruction can replace open-mouth radiographs.
    - Important to look for tubercle avulsion to determine the healing potential of the TAL.

    - CTA to rule out vertebral artery dissection/occlusion if suspected.
  - MRI:
    - Best method to assess the TAL.[16]
- Treatment:
  - Rigid cervical orthosis or halo:
    - TAL intact.
    - Dickman Type 2 TAL injury.
  - C1–C2 fusion:
    - Dickman Type 1 injuries.
    - Persistent instability after nonoperative treatment.
    - Clinical deformity (rotatory subluxation).
- Surgical pearls:
  - Obtain a CTA or MRA to assess vertebral artery integrity as part of the preoperative planning if vessel injury is suspected.
  - Vast majority of C1 fractures are amenable to nonoperative treatment.

16.3.3 Axis (C2) Fracture and Traumatic Spondylolisthesis of C2 (Hangman's Fracture)

- Background:
  - Associated with high-velocity trauma.
  - C2 fractures are among the most common spinal fractures in the elderly.
  - Mechanism is a combination of hyperextension, compression, and rebound flexion (**Fig. 16.2**).
- Signs, symptoms, and physical examination:
  - Patients typically present with neck pain only in nonangulated, nondisplaced fractures.
  - Complete or incomplete injuries are possible with severe fractures.
  - Cerebellar findings (nausea/vomiting, asymmetric examination, ataxia) may suggest vertebral artery injury.
- Neuroimaging:
  - CT scan with reconstructions.
  - CTA to rule out vertebral artery dissection/occlusion if suspected.
- Classification/treatment[17]:
  - Type I: Minimal displacement (< 3 mm) → hard cervical collar.
  - Type II: Significant displacement (> 3 mm) and angulation of > 11 degrees:
    - Nonoperative—reduction and halo or collar immobilization.
    - Operative:
      - Disruption of the C2/C3 disk or an inability to maintain the reduction → may consider surgery:
        - If C2 pedicle screws placement is possible, an isolated C2–C3 fusion is preferred.

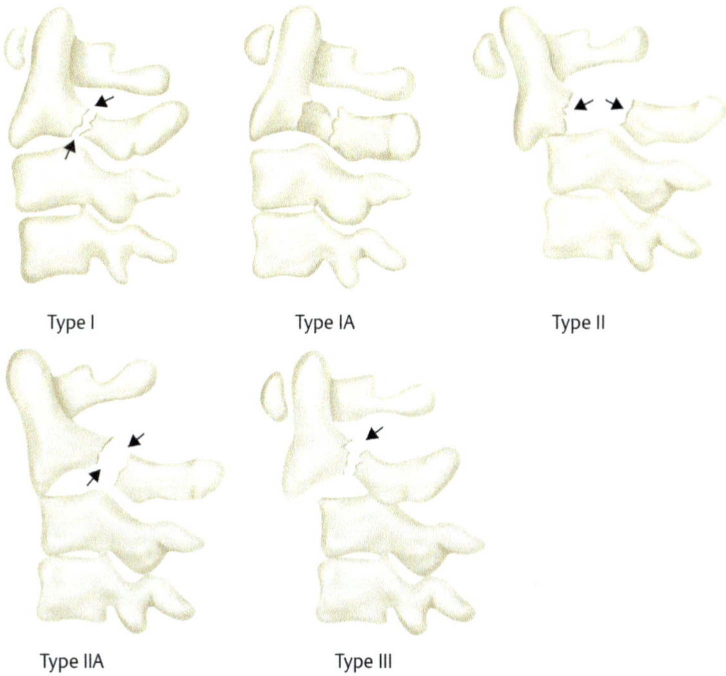

Fig. 16.2 The Effendi/Levine and Edwards classification of traumatic spondylolisthesis of the axis (hangman's fracture).

        * If C2 pedicle screw is not possible, a C1–C3 posterior fusion or C2/C3 anterior cervical diskectomy and fusion (ACDF) can be performed.
- Type IIa: Minimal displacement (< 3 mm) but angulation > 11 degrees:
    - Nonoperative—no traction:
        - Halo.
    - Operative:
        - Disruption of the C2/C3 disk or inability to maintain the reduction.
        - C2–C3 fusion preferred.
- Type III: Associated facet dislocation:
    - All require either anterior C2–C3 or posterior C1–C3 fusion.
- Atypical fracture[18]:
    - Fracture extends into the vertebral body.

    - Displacement of a portion of the posterior vertebral body attached to pedicle often significantly narrows the spinal canal.
    - Increased risk of neurologic injury, specifically Brown-Sequard injury.
- Surgical pearls:
  - Obtain a CTA or MRA to assess vertebral artery integrity as part of the preoperative planning if vessel injury is suspected.
  - Often a C2 pedicle screw can be placed, allowing for surgical treatment with only a C2–C3 fusion.

16.3.4 Dens Fracture (C2)

- Background:
  - Among the most common spinal fracture injuries in the elderly after falls.
  - Sometimes associated with simultaneous C1 fractures.
  - Mechanism: Hyperflexion or hyperextension (**Fig. 16.3**).
- Signs, symptoms, and physical examination:
  - Neck pain and tenderness on palpation are typical.
  - Usually does not cause neurologic deficits (due to the width of the canal in this region).
  - Severely angulated fractures may cause complete or incomplete injuries.
- Neuroimaging:
  - CT scan with reconstructions is recommended even if fracture is evident on plain radiograph.
  - MRI may be helpful for assessing the integrity of cruciate ligament.
- Classification:
  - Anderson and D'Alonzo[19]:
    - Type I: Avulsion fracture at tip.
    - Type II: Avulsion fracture at the waist/base.
    - Type III: Extends into the C2 vertebral body.
- Treatment:
  - Type I and type III:
    - Hard collar or halo.
    - If significant ligament disruption is associated with a type I injury, make sure there was not a spontaneously reduced atlantoaxial dissociation.
  - Type II:
    - Controversial.
    - Risk factors for nonunion[20]:
      - 5 mm of displacement, angulation > 10 degrees, age > 50, and posterior displacement.
    - A young patient having no nonunion risk factors can be treated with a halo or a hard collar.

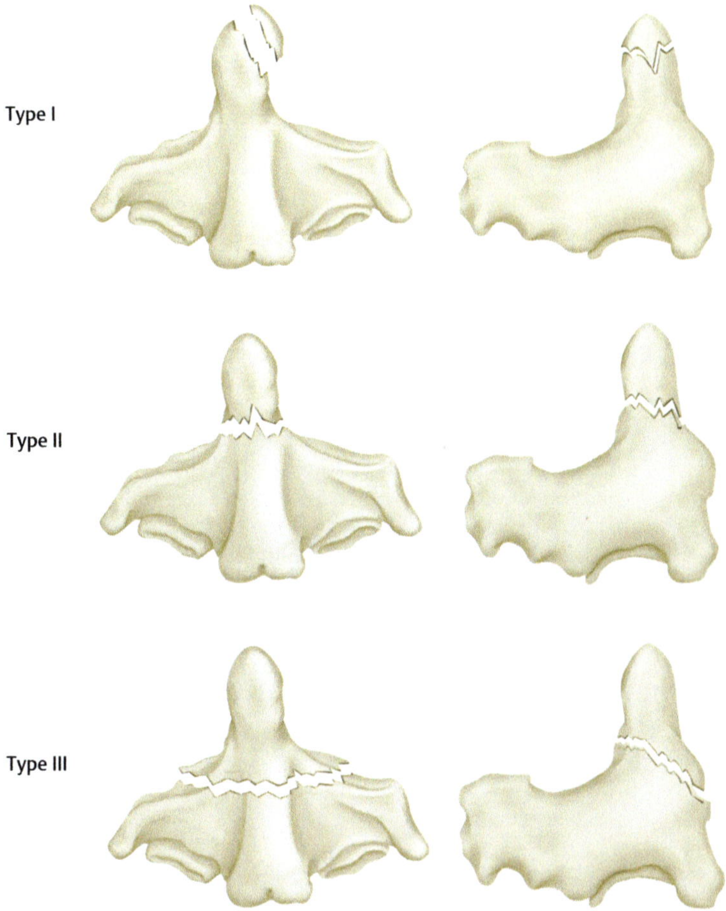

Fig. 16.3 Anderson D'Alonzo classification of dens fractures.

- Young patient with concern for nonunion:
  - Anterior odontoid screw or C1–C2 posterior fusion.
- Geriatric odontoid fracture:
  - If healthy enough to undergo general anesthesia, should undergo a C1–C2 fusion.[5,6]
  - If possible, do not treat with a halo.
- Increases the risk of dysphagia and death.

- Surgical pearls:
  - Ensure that the anterior cruciate ligament is intact before attempting an anterior odontoid screw fixation.
  - Multiple posterior fusion options for a C1–C2 fusion have been described, and the authors routinely use a C1 lateral mass and a C2 pedicle screw.

16.3.5 Subaxial Cervical Spine Trauma (C3–C7)

- Background:
  - Particularly common in high-speed motor crashes and diving accidents.
  - Wide variety of injuries that can range from benign spinous process fracture to fractures associated with complete spinal cord injuries.
- Classifications:
  - Subaxial cervical spine injury classification system[7]:
    - Assigns values based on injury morphology, integrity of the diskoligamentous complex, and neurologic status of the patient.
    - Patients with a score of > 4 should undergo surgical treatment.
    - Patients with a score of < 4 should undergo a trial of nonoperative treatment.
      - Morphology:
        - Compression = 1.
        - Burst = 2.
        - Distraction = 3.
        - Rotation = 4.
      - Diskoligamentous complex:
        - Intact = 0.
        - Indeterminate = 1.
        - Disrupted = 2.
      - Neurologic status:
        - Intact = 0.
        - Root injury = 1.
        - Complete spinal cord injury = 2.
        - Incomplete spinal cord injury = 3.
        - Persistent spinal cord compression with a neurologic deficit = + 1.
  - AOSpine Subaxial Cervical Spine Injury Classification System[21]:
    - Three types of fractures:
      - Compression (A0—Minor fractures such as an isolated lamina fracture or spinous process fracture. A1—Compression fracture involving a single end plate and not the posterior vertebral wall. A2—Coronal split of the vertebral body involving both end plates,

but not the posterior wall. A3—Burst fracture involving a single end plate and the posterior wall. A4—Burst fracture involving both end plates and the posterior wall.)
      - Tension band injury (B1—Bony injury only. B2—Posterior tension band injury including the ligamentous structures. B3—Anterior tension band injury.)
      - Translation injury (Any translation or displacement of one vertebral body in relationship to the adjacent level.)
    - Additional descriptors:
      - Facet fractures (F1—Nondisplaced fracture measuring < 40% of the height of the lateral mass and < 1 cm. F2—Displaced fracture, or a fracture measuring > 40% of the height of the lateral mass or > 1 cm. F3—Floating lateral mass. F4—Subluxed, perched, or dislocated facet. BL—Bilateral facet involvement.)
      - Neurology (N0—No neurologic injury. N1—Transient neurologic deficit. N2—Persistent radiculopathy. N3—Incomplete spinal cord injury. N4—Complete spinal cord injury. NX—Unable to evaluate neurologic status. + —Continued spinal cord compression.)
      - Patient-specific modifiers (M1—Injury to the posterior ligamentous complex. M2—Significant disk herniation. M3—Stiffening bone disease, such as ankylosing spondylitis or diffuse idiopathic skeletal hyperostosis. M4—Vertebral artery abnormality.)
    - A spine injury score will eventually be established to allow the AO classification to guide treatment.
- Signs, symptoms, and physical examination:
  - Wide variability in presentation:
    - Mild compression fractures (A1 and A2) are only associated with axial neck pain.
    - Translational injuries are often associated with significant neurologic injuries.
- Neuroimaging:
  - CT and MRI are typically necessary to determine the extent of injury.
  - CTA is recommended if any fracture involves the transverse foramen.
- Treatment:
  - Based on stability and neurologic injury.
  - Considerations:
    - Is there mechanical instability?
    - Is there neurologic compromise necessitating direct or indirect decompression?
    - Are there patient factors (e.g., multitrauma)?

- Stable: Nonoperative, rigid cervical orthosis.
- Unstable: Surgical fusion via anterior versus posterior versus combined approach.

- Surgical pearls:
  - Ongoing compression of the spinal cord is a surgical emergency.
  - Early decompression has been shown to increase the chance of neurologic recovery.[1]
  - Facet fractures measuring > 40% of the height of the lateral mass or more than 1 cm in length from the tip of the superior articular process to the fracture line have a high incidence of failing nonoperative treatment.[8]
  - C7 burst fractures have a higher likelihood of falling into significant kyphosis than do burst fractures at other levels.
  - Ensure the posterior elements are intact when an anterior cervical vertebral body fracture is present. Posterior element involvement may indicate a highly unstable injury.

Common Clinical Questions

1. List the incomplete spinal cord injuries in the order of best prognosis to worst.

   A. Brown-Sequard, anterior cord, central cord.

   B. Central cord, Brown-Sequard, anterior cord.

   C. Brown-Sequard, central cord, anterior cord.

   D. Anterior cord, central cord, Brown-Sequard.

2. A 70-year-old female presents with significant neck pain after a fall. Imaging demonstrates a type II odontoid fracture with 3 mm of displacement. What treatment will lead to the lowest mortality and highest health-related quality of life?

   A. Hard cervical collar.

   B. Halo.

   C. Posterior C1–C2 fusion.

   D. Traction and bed rest.

3. A polytrauma patient is intubated with an unknown neurologic injury. What is the best modality for assessing acute spinal cord injury?

   A. CT scan.

   B. T1-weighted MRI.

   C. T2-weighted MRI.

   D. Flexion and extension cervical radiographs.

Answers to Common Clinical Questions

1. C.
2. C.
3. C.

References

1. Fehlings MG, Vaccaro A, Wilson JR, et al. Early versus delayed decompression for traumatic cervical spinal cord injury: results of the Surgical Timing in Acute Spinal Cord Injury Study (STASCIS). PLoS One. 2012; 7(2):e32037
2. Schroeder GD, Kwon BK, Eck JC, Savage JW, Hsu WK, Patel AA. Survey of Cervical Spine Research Society members on the use of high-dose steroids for acute spinal cord injuries. Spine. 2014; 39(12):971–977
3. Hurlbert RJ, Hadley MN, Walters BC, et al. Pharmacological therapy for acute spinal cord injury. Neurosurgery. 2013; 72 Suppl 2:93–105
4. Bracken MB, Shepard MJ, Collins WF, et al. A randomized, controlled trial of methylprednisolone or naloxone in the treatment of acute spinal-cord injury. Results of the Second National Acute Spinal Cord Injury Study. N Engl J Med. 1990; 322(20):1405–1411
5. Chapman J, Smith JS, Kopjar B, et al. The AOSpine North America Geriatric Odontoid Fracture Mortality Study: a retrospective review of mortality outcomes for operative versus nonoperative treatment of 322 patients with long-term follow-up. Spine. 2013; 38(13):1098–1104
6. Vaccaro AR, Kepler CK, Kopjar B, et al. Functional and quality-of-life outcomes in geriatric patients with type-II dens fracture. J Bone Joint Surg Am. 2013; 95(8):729–735
7. Vaccaro AR, Hulbert RJ, Patel AA, et al. Spine Trauma Study Group. The subaxial cervical spine injury classification system: a novel approach to recognize the importance of morphology, neurology, and integrity of the disco-ligamentous complex. Spine. 2007; 32(21):2365–2374
8. Spector LR, Kim DH, Affonso J, Albert TJ, Hilibrand AS, Vaccaro AR. Use of computed tomography to predict failure of nonoperative treatment of unilateral facet fractures of the cervical spine. Spine. 2006; 31(24):2827–2835
9. Fisher CG, Sun JC, Dvorak M. Recognition and management of atlanto-occipital dislocation: improving survival from an often fatal condition. Can J Surg. 2001; 44(6):412–420
10. Powers B, Miller MD, Kramer RS, Martinez S, Gehweiler JA, Jr. Traumatic anterior atlanto-occipital dislocation. Neurosurgery. 1979; 4(1):12–17
11. Wackenheim A. Roentgen Diagnosis of the Craniovertebral Region. Springer; 1974

12. Harris JH, Jr, Carson GC, Wagner LK. Radiologic diagnosis of traumatic occipitovertebral dissociation: 1. Normal occipitovertebral relationships on lateral radiographs of supine subjects. AJR Am J Roentgenol. 1994; 162(4): 881–886
13. Gire JD, Roberto RF, Bobinski M, Klineberg EO, Durbin-Johnson B. The utility and accuracy of computed tomography in the diagnosis of occipitocervical dissociation. Spine J. 2013; 13(5):510–519
14. Dickman CA, Greene KA, Sonntag VK. Injuries involving the transverse atlantal ligament: classification and treatment guidelines based upon experience with 39 injuries. Neurosurgery. 1996; 38(1):44–50
15. Spence KF, Jr, Decker S, Sell KW. Bursting atlantal fracture associated with rupture of the transverse ligament. J Bone Joint Surg Am. 1970; 52(3):543–549
16. Radcliff KE, Sonagli MA, Rodrigues LM, Sidhu GS, Albert TJ, Vaccaro AR. Does C_1 fracture displacement correlate with transverse ligament integrity? Orthop Surg. 2013; 5(2):94–99
17. Levine AM, Edwards CC. The management of traumatic spondylolisthesis of the axis. J Bone Joint Surg Am. 1985; 67(2):217–226
18. Starr JK, Eismont FJ. Atypical hangman's fractures. Spine. 1993; 18(14):1954–1957
19. Anderson LD, D'Alonzo RT. Fractures of the odontoid process of the axis. J Bone Joint Surg Am. 1974; 56(8):1663–1674
20. Hsu WK, Anderson PA. Odontoid fractures: update on management. J Am Acad Orthop Surg. 2010; 18(7):383–394
21. Vaccaro AR, Koerner JD, Radcliff KE, et al. AOSpine subaxial cervical spine injury classification system. Eur Spine J. 2016; 25(7):2173–2184

17 Thoracolumbar Trauma

Anirudh Penumaka and Martina Stippler

Summary

Thoracolumbar spinal trauma is common. A thorough evaluation is critical to better understand the stability of the fracture and the potential neurological and surgical implications. There are several classification systems currently employed including the Denis, TLICS, and AO Spine, among others. Surgical intervention is reserved for those fractures demonstrating neural element compression and/or structural instability. Assessing for neurogenic or spinal shock, in addition to a complete neurological examination, is crucial.

Keywords: thoracolumbar, fracture, TLICS, AO, flexion, distraction

17.1 Key Points

- The thoracolumbar junction (T11–L2) is the most common site of traumatic spine injury in the thoracic and lumbar spine.
- Injury recognition is key in clinical decision-making and prevention of secondary neurologic injury.
- Surgery is indicated for spinal cord injury, acute or delayed mechanical instability, and intractable pain.

17.2 General Principles

- Field management:
  - ABCs: airway, breathing, circulation, and neurologic status.
  - Spinal immobilization on a rigid backboard with "log-roll" precautions.
- Emergency room management:
  - Advance trauma life support (ATLS) primary and secondary trauma assessment.
  - About 30% of patients with flexion–distraction injuries also have intra-abdominal injuries.
  - Standard trauma imaging: Noncontrast head CT; cervical, thoracic, and lumbar spine CT.
  - Treat neurogenic shock (not to be confused with spinal shock) if present.

    - Most common with cervical and high thoracic injuries.
    - Acute loss of background sympathetic tone resulting in hypotension in the presence of bradycardia.
    - Manage with vasopressors and moderate fluid resuscitation.
    - Efficacy and length of mean arterial pressure (MAP) goals is controversial. Some literature indicates MAP goals of > 85 mmHg for as long as 7 days may be beneficial. However, shorter duration (2–3 days) is commonly performed due to the risk of additional risks of vasopressor use, invasive monitoring, and longer intensive care unit (ICU) stays.[1]
- Key components of physical examination:
  - Sensorimotor examination of all dermatomes/myotomes.
  - Reflexes (deep tendon and bulbocavernosus).
  - Rectal examination: Assess tone, saddle anesthesia, and perianal sensation.
  - Assess bladder function.
- Imaging studies:
  - Plain films have limited utility in traumatic injury assessments unless CT is unavailable.[2]
  - Computed tomography (CT):
    - Primary screening tool for suspicion of thoracolumbar injury.
    - Must include axial, coronal, and sagittal reconstructions.
    - Not sensitive for assessing ligamentous injury. However, can look for splaying of spinous processes which may be indicative.
  - Magnetic resonance imaging (MRI):
    - Best for evaluation of spinal cord injury and diskoligamentous injury (such as with suspected chance injury of the disk).
    - Short tau inversion recovery (STIR) sequence should be included to assess for ligamentous injury.
- Degree of injury:
  - Determination of complete versus incomplete injury is imperative.
  - Spinal shock must be excluded if injury appears complete initially.
  - American Spinal Injury Association (ASIA) scoring scale (**Table 17.1**).[3]

17.3 Thoracolumbar Fracture

- General features:
  - The most common site of injury is at the thoracolumbar junction (T11–L2).
- Attributed to the transition from the rigid thoracic spine to the mobile lumbar spine.

Table 17.1 ASIA neurological scoring system

Grade	Description
A	Complete: No motor or sensory function is preserved in the sacral segments.
B	Incomplete: Sensory but not motor function is preserved below the neurologic level and includes the sacral segments.
C	Incomplete: Motor function is preserved below the neurologic level, and more than half of the key muscles below the level have a muscle grade < 3.
D	Incomplete: Motor function is preserved below the neurologic level, and at least half of the key muscle groups below the level have a muscle grade > 3.
E	Normal.

Abbreviation: ASIA, American Spinal Injury Association.
Note: The caudal-most normal level is the single neurologic level.

- Classification systems:
  - Thoracolumbar fractures have historically been classified as stable versus unstable based on the three-column theory[4]:
    - Anterior column: Anterior half of vertebral body and disk, as well as the anterior longitudinal ligament.
    - Middle column: Posterior half of vertebral body and disk, the posterior longitudinal ligament, and the pedicles.
    - Posterior column: Posterior bony arch as well as the posterior ligamentous complex (supraspinous and interspinous ligaments, ligamentum flavum, and facet joints).
- Thoracolumbar Injury Classification and Severity (TLICS) score is a scoring system that maintains that surgical intervention is mainly based on three factors[4,5]:
  - Morphology of the fracture.
  - Posterior ligamentous complex.
  - Neurologic status.
- Management based on the scoring system outlined in **Table 17.2**:
  - TLICS less than or equal to 3: Usually nonoperative management.
  - TLICS 4 is considered the "gray zone" in which patients may be managed surgically or conservatively.
  - TLICS ≥ 5 generally warrants surgical intervention.
- There are multiple classifications systems used to characterize fractures, including[6]:

Table 17.2 Thoracolumbar Injury Classification and Severity Scoring System

Category	Finding	Points
Radiographic findings	Compression fracture	1
	Burst component/lateral angulation > 15 degrees	1
	Distraction injury	2
	Translational/rotational injury	3
Neurologic status	Intact	0
	Nerve root injury	2
	Complete SCI	2
	Incomplete SCI (including cauda equina)	3
Posterior ligamentous complex	Intact	0
	Unknown/cannot determine	2
	Disruption	3

Abbreviation: SCI, spinal cord injury.

Criticisms of TLICS: Description of injury to the posterior ligamentous complex (PLC) is unclear and it does not account of delayed surgical treatment (Jaouim).[5]

Separated into types A (compression injuries), B (distraction injuries), and C (rotational injuries) based on pathomorphological characteristics. Literature suggests poor concordance between AO and TLICS. However, AO may be more reliable for complex injuries.

- McAfee classification system[7]:
  - Uses CT primarily to group fractures according to the type of failure seen within the middle column, which includes axial compression, axial distraction, and translation within the transverse plane.
- Load-sharing classification[8]:
  - Based on amount of comminution within the vertebral body, degree of fracture fragment displacement, and amount of kyphotic correction on later plain films.

17.3.1 Key Concepts

- The majority of isolated anterior column fractures should be considered stable, except in the following cases[9,10]:
  - Loss of > 50% vertebral body height or excessive kyphotic angulation at one segment.
  - Three or more continuous compression fractures.
  - Neurologic deficit.
  - Progressive kyphotic deformity on serial imaging studies.
- Middle column fractures are considered unstable except in the following cases:
  - Fracture above T8 with intact ribs and sternum.
  - Below L4 if posterior elements intact.
  - Neurologic deficit.
- Posterior column fractures are typically stable unless accompanied by middle column failure and/or bilateral facet fractures.
- There are six types of thoracolumbar fractures, according to the McAfee classification system, which Denis further simplifies into four categories (**Fig. 17.1**)[4]:
  - Compression fractures (AO classification A1 and A2):
    - Mechanism: Compressive flexion injury.
    - Factors of instability: > 50% loss of vertebral body height, > 30 degrees of anterior to posterior angulation, > 30 degrees of focal kyphosis.
    - If any of the foregoing factors is present, posterior fusion or percutaneous fixation at least one level above and below the affected level(s) should be performed.
  - Burst fractures (AO classification A3 and A4):
    - Mechanism: Axial compression.
    - Approximately 10 to 20% of all thoracolumbar fractures.[11]
    - Surgery is usually indicated, especially when presenting with neurologic deficit, angular deformity > 20 degrees, > 50% spinal canal compromise, anterior body height < 50% of posterior height, and/or progressive kyphosis.[12]
    - Patients presenting with a burst fracture and ***NO*** neurologic deficits: Literature has shown little or no neurologic decline with conservative measures (i.e., orthotics), with ultimately no significant difference between operative versus conservative treatment arms.[13,14,15,16] Some studies support the use of short segment instrumentation, which can be removed, especially in younger patients.
    - An anterior approach allows adequate decompression of any retropulsion, whereas a posterior approach allows reduction and restoration of sagittal balance. A combined approach could be warranted in the setting of significant instability.

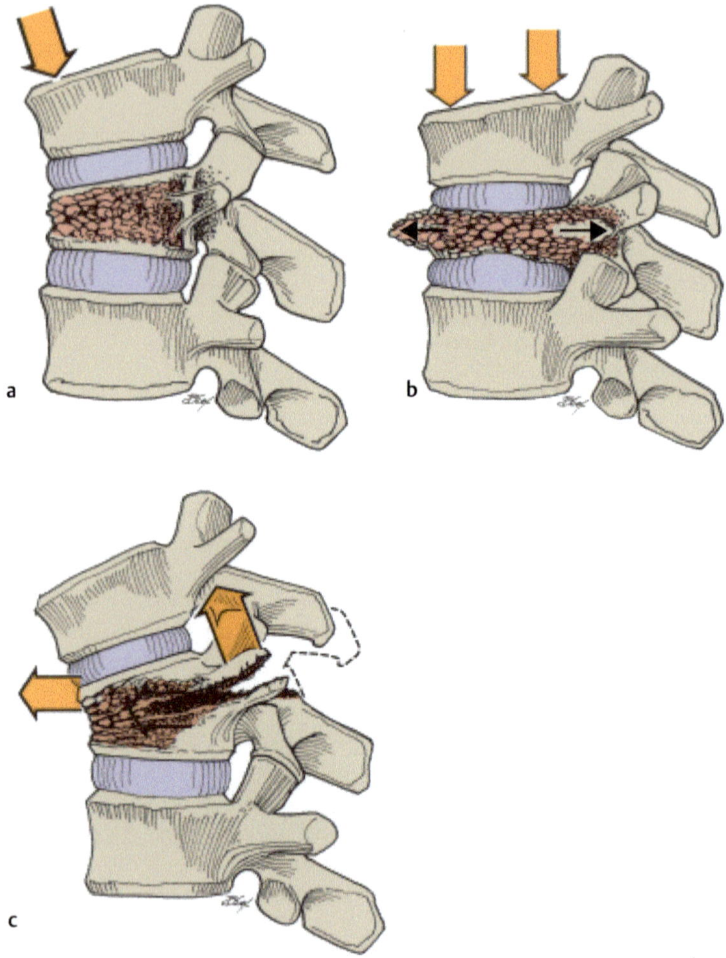

Fig. 17.1 **(a–c)** Compression: **(a)** compression fracture, **(b)** burst fracture, **(c)** chance-type fracture.

- Direct comparison of anterior/posterior approaches shows similar results regarding functional outcome and pain. Perioperatively, the anterior approach has been associated with greater intraoperative blood loss but may result in fewer long-term complications and subsequent surgeries.[17,18]

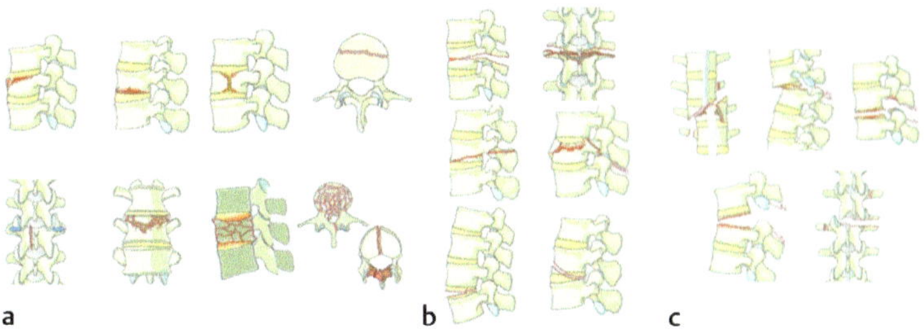

Fig. 17.2 **(a)** A-type injuries (compression injuries) in the AOSpine TL Fracture Classification. **(b)** B-typeinjuries (tension band injuries) in the AOSpine TL Classification. **(c)** C-type injuries(translation/displaced injuries) in the AO TL Classification System. (Used with permission of Springer-Verlagberlin/Heidelberg, from AO spine injury classification system: a revision proposal for the thoracic and lumbar spine. Eur Spine J. Reinhold M, Audigé L, Schnake KJ et al, 22(10), 2013)

- Chance fractures (AO classification types B1 and B2; **Fig. 17.2**):
  - Flexion–distraction injury that results in a horizontal fracture extending posteriorly through the vertebral body and into the posterior column (most often involving the pedicles).
  - A bony Chance fracture without ligamentous injury, with absence of disk injury, or with no dislocation may be treated with a hyperextension brace, such as a thoracolumbar sacral orthosis (TLSO).
  - Posterior ligamentous disruption or extension through the disk usually requires posterior fusion due to instability.
  - Rule out intra-abdominal or pelvic injury.
- Fracture–dislocation (AO classification type C):
  - Mechanism: Rotation, shear, compression, or vertebral dislocation, facet subluxation, canal compromise.
  - May result in severe subluxation or dislocation.
  - There are three main subtypes[9]:
    - Flexion rotation: Anterior compression and total rupture of the middle and posterior columns under rotational and tension forces. Imaging finding include subluxation or dislocation, increased interspinous distance, decreased canal diameter, jumped facets, and an intact posterior vertebral body.
    - Shear: All three columns, including anterior longitudinal ligament, disrupted; force directed most commonly in posteroanterior direction fracturing the posterior arch, resulting in "free-floating lamina" and the superior facet of the inferior vertebra. Often results in complete spinal cord injury (SCI).
    - Flexion distraction: Radiographically similar to a Chance-type fracture ± subluxation due to torn annulus fibrosus.

- Treatment with urgent decompression and stabilization is indicated in cases with incomplete neurologic deficit, > 50% loss of height with angulation and kyphotic angulation of > 40%.

17.4 Bracing

- High thoracic fractures (above T6):[19]
  - Stable fractures between T1 to approximately T6 may be treated with a cervicothoracic orthosis (CTO).
- Midthoracic to lumbosacral fractures (T7 – L3):
  - Stable fractures anywhere between the midthoracic spine and L5 may be treated with a hard TLSO.
  - In most cases of acute lumbosacral trauma, a soft lumbosacral orthosis (LSO) brace does not provide adequate stabilization. A TLSO remains the best option for external stabilization. In general, many thoracolumbar burst fractures are inherently stable due to the mechanical rigidity provided by the ribcage, and bracing does not appear to be necessary. There was no significant different between bracing and no bracing when kyphosis was evaluated at extended intervals after the injury.[20]
- Always assess stability of fracture in brace with upright X-rays in brace.
  - After brace is removed in 6 to 12 weeks, it is important to get flexion–extension X-rays.

17.5 Conus Medullaris and Cauda Equina Syndromes

- About 10 to 38% of thoracolumbar injuries involve the conus medullaris or cauda equina.
- Conus medullaris syndrome (ranges from lower third of T11 to L2)[21]:
  - Often presents suddenly and bilaterally.
  - Is associated more often with axial back pain than with radicular pain.
  - Features perianal numbness.
  - Features overflow incontinence.
- Cauda equina syndrome (trauma involving L3–L5)[21]:
  - Results from injury to the cauda equina below the L2 level.
  - Is associated with acute weakness either unilaterally or bilaterally, perianal or saddle anesthesia, and urinary retention.
- Both syndromes require urgent decompression.
- Often difficult to differentiate between the two conditions based on clinical examination.[21]

17.6 Spinal and Neurogenic Shock

- Speedy recognition and differentiation are crucial for acute stabilization and surgical decision-making.
- Spinal shock:
  - A temporary physiologic loss of all sensorimotor function caudal to the level of injury occurring virtually at the time of insult. Autonomic dysfunctions (i.e., loss of sympathetic tone) may occur with gradual return.
  - Mechanism is yet to be fully elucidated but may be due to displacement of K^+ into the extracellular space, thus reducing axonal transmission. As K^+ levels normalize, the manifestations of spinal shock slowly improve.
  - Separated into four clinical phases spanning from immediately postinjury up to months[22]:
    - Phase I (days 0–1): Areflexia, flaccid paralysis, anesthesia, and loss of bowel/bladder function. The bulbocavernosus reflex is typically one of the first reflexes to return and should be tested in every patient for distinguishing complete versus incomplete SCI.
    - Phase II (days 1–3): Initial reflex return; gradual recovery of deep tendon reflexes (DTRs).
    - Phase III (day 4 to 1 month): Continued return of DTRs with some early hyperreflexia.
    - Phase IV (1–12 months): Spasticity and hyperreflexia with overactivity of most cutaneous and deep tendon reflexes. Detrusor paralysis is estimated to return between 4 and 6 weeks.
      - Acute absence of the bulbocavernosus reflex after injury does not rule out incomplete SCI due to the potential presence of spinal shock.
  - Manage conservatively with observation of return of function.
- Neurogenic shock:
  - A neurological emergency resulting in loss of sympathetic tone producing unopposed vagal activity after SCI not caused by any other traumatic source.
  - Results in hypotension, bradycardia, and occasionally priapism in males.
  - Estimated to occur in up to 20% of isolated cervical injuries and 10% of isolated thoracolumbar injuries with an Abbreviated Injury Score of > 2.[23]
  - Should be treated similar to other forms of shock. IV fluids and vasopressors (e.g., phenylephrine) are warranted to achieve hemodynamic stability and prevent end-organ failure.

Common Clinical Questions

1. A 9-year-old boy was a restrained passenger in a high-speed motor vehicle accident. He presents without obvious neurological deficits, but a CT scan demonstrates a significant flexion–distraction injury at the thoracolumbar junction. Which of the following should be assessed radiographically before spinal surgical intervention is considered?
   A. The adjacent vasculature looking for potential aortic injury.
   B. The adjacent visceral organs including pancreas, spleen, and bowel.
   C. The chest cavity looking for pneumo- or hemothorax.
   D. The occipital cervical junction looking for potential atlantooccipital dislocation.
   E. All of the above.
2. A 60-year-old female with a remote history of breast cancer presents with back pain and L1 vertebral body fracture on CT. She has no neurological deficits. She denies trauma. Which of the following is an appropriate management strategy?
   A. Reassurance, discharge, and follow-up as needed.
   B. Application of TLSO brace and follow-up in 6 to 8 weeks in clinic.
   C. Scheduling an elective L1 biopsy and cement augmentation of the vertebral body.
   D. Obtaining an MRI to rule out pathologic fracture.

Answers to Common Clinical Questions

1. E.
2. D.

References

1. Saadeh YS, Smith BW, Joseph JR, et al. The impact of blood pressure management after spinal cord injury: a systematic review of the literature. Neurosurg Focus. 2017; 43(5):E20
2. Sixta S, Moore FO, Ditillo MF, et al. Eastern Association for the Surgery of Trauma. Screening for thoracolumbar spinal injuries in blunt trauma: an Eastern Association for the Surgery of Trauma practice management guideline. J Trauma Acute Care Surg. 2012; 73(5) Suppl 4:S326–S332

3. ASIA and ISCoS International Standards Committee. The 2019 revision of the International Standards for Neurological Classification of Spinal Cord Injury (ISNCSCI)—What's new? Spinal Cord. 2019; 57(10):815–817
4. Vaccaro AR, Baron EM, Sanfilippo J, et al. Reliability of a novel classification system for thoracolumbar injuries: the Thoracolumbar Injury Severity Score. Spine. 2006; 31(11) Suppl:S62–S69, discussion S104
5. Vaccaro AR, Lehman RA, Jr, Hurlbert RJ, et al. A new classification of thoracolumbar injuries: the importance of injury morphology, the integrity of the posterior ligamentous complex, and neurologic status. Spine. 2005; 30 (20):2325–2333
6. Magerl F, Aebi M, Gertzbein SD, Harms J, Nazarian S. A comprehensive classification of thoracic and lumbar injuries. Eur Spine J. 1994; 3(4):184–201
7. McAfee PC, Yuan HA, Fredrickson BE, Lubicky JP. The value of computed tomography in thoracolumbar fractures. An analysis of one hundred consecutive cases and a new classification. J Bone Joint Surg Am. 1983; 65 (4):461–473
8. McCormack T, Karaikovic E, Gaines RW. The load sharing classification of spine fractures. Spine. 1994; 19(15):1741–1744
9. Denis F. The three column spine and its significance in the classification of acute thoracolumbar spinal injuries. Spine. 1983; 8(8):817–831
10. Greenberg MS. Handbook of Neurosurgery. 8th. ed. New York: Thieme; 2016
11. Dai LY, Jiang SD, Wang XY, Jiang LS. A review of the management of thoracolumbar burst fractures. Surg Neurol. 2007; 67(3):221–231, discussion 231
12. Hitchon PW, Torner JC, Haddad SF, Follett KA. Management options in thoracolumbar burst fractures. Surg Neurol. 1998; 49(6):619–626, discussion 626–627
13. Tanasansomboon T, Kittipibul T, Limthongkul W, Yingsakmongkol W, Kotheeranurak V, Singhatanadgige W. Thoracolumbar burst fracture without neurological deficit: review of controversies and current evidence of treatment. World Neurosurg. 2022; 162:29–35
14. Wood KB, Buttermann GR, Phukan R, et al. Operative compared with nonoperative treatment of a thoracolumbar burst fracture without neurological deficit: a prospective randomized study with follow-up at sixteen to twenty-two years. J Bone Joint Surg Am. 2015; 97(1):3–9
15. Shen WJ, Liu TJ, Shen YS. Nonoperative treatment versus posterior fixation for thoracolumbar junction burst fractures without neurologic deficit. Spine. 2001; 26(9):1038–1045
16. Bakhsheshian J, Dahdaleh NS, Fakurnejad S, Scheer JK, Smith ZA. Evidence-based management of traumatic thoracolumbar burst fractures: a systematic review of nonoperative management. Neurosurg Focus. 2014; 37(1):E1
17. Esses SI, Botsford DJ, Kostuik JP. Evaluation of surgical treatment for burst fractures. Spine. 1990; 15(7):667–673

18. Wood KB, Bohn D, Mehbod A. Anterior versus posterior treatment of stable thoracolumbar burst fractures without neurologic deficit: a prospective, randomized study. J Spinal Disord Tech. 2005; 18 Suppl:S15–S23
19. Rahm MD, Brooks DM, Harris JA, Hart RA, et al. Stabilizing effect of the rib cage on adjacent segment motion following thoracolumbar posterior fixation of the human thoracic cadaveric spine: A biomechanical study. Clin Biomech (Bristol, Avon). 2019; 70:217–222
20. Chang V, Holly LT. Bracing for thoracolumbar fractures. Neurosurg Focus. 2014; 37(1):E3
21. Brouwers E, van de Meent H, Curt A, Starremans B, Hosman A, Bartels R. Definitions of traumatic conus medullaris and cauda equina syndrome: a systematic literature review. Spinal Cord. 2017; 55(10):886–890
22. Ditunno JF, Little JW, Tessler A, Burns AS. Spinal shock revisited: a four-phase model. Spinal Cord. 2004; 42(7):383–395
23. Guly HR, Bouamra O, Lecky FE, Trauma Audit and Research Network. The incidence of neurogenic shock in patients with isolated spinal cord injury in the emergency department. Resuscitation. 2008; 76(1):57–62

18 Sacropelvic Trauma

Emiliano Vialle

Summary

Sacral fractures can occur due to high-energy trauma, resulting in complex and life-threatening injuries, or due to low-energy trauma in elderly and osteoporotic patients. Several attempts have been made to classify such injuries, and the AOSpine sacral fracture classification has aggregated different types of injuries in three categories.

Identification of associated injuries is crucial for defining treatment strategies, which can vary from percutaneous fixation to open lumbopelvic stabilization.

Keywords: spinal fracture, sacral fracture, fracture fixation, pelvic fracture, polytrauma, pelvic injury, osteoporotic fracture

18.1 Key Points

- Sacral fractures are often associated with high-energy trauma and can cause pelvic ring instability.
- Highly displaced and multiplanar fractures can result in spinopelvic instability or dissociation.
- A thin-cut computed tomography (CT) scan of the sacrum with coronal and sagittal reconstructions is the imaging modality of choice for the diagnosis of high-energy traumatic sacral fractures.
- Treatment can range from observation to a variety of surgical approaches aimed at stabilizing the pelvis and sacrum.

18.2 Sacral Fractures

18.2.1 Background

- The sacrum connects the pelvis to the lumbar spine and helps dissipate the weight of the axial skeleton to the ground via the pelvis and the lower limbs.
- Sacral fractures are typically the result of high-energy trauma but can also be observed in elderly patients who have osteoporotic bone after a low-energy mechanism such as a fall.

- Fewer than 10% of sacral fractures occur in isolation, and they are often associated with other injuries to the pelvic ring.
- Denis et al[1] classified sacral fractures into three types based on the relationship of the fracture line to the sacral neuroforamen. Although commonly used, this classification does not account for all variations in sacropelvic trauma, necessitating other classifications, such as the Roy-Camille[2] and the Isler. Recently the AOSpine Classification attempted to include injury morphology in a more reliable manner, dividing sacral injuries into three types according to its importance for sacropelvic stability (**Fig. 18.1**)[3]:
  - Type A: Injuries below the sacroiliac joint without impact on pelvic stability. These injuries rarely have an impact on neurology and can be subdivided into three subtypes:
    - A1: Coccygeal or sacral compression fractures.
    - A2: Nondisplaced transverse injuries below the sacroiliac joint, usually without neurology.
    - A3: Displaced transverse injuries below the sacroiliac joint, which may be associated with neurologic deficit.
  - Type B: Unilateral longitudinal injuries, with an impact on posterior pelvic stability, and minimal or no impact on vertical stability. This is a variation of the zones of injury of Denis. Type B injuries are subdivided into:
    - B1: Central fractures involving the spinal canal with a primary longitudinal pattern. This is an uncommon fracture type that has no impact on pelvic stability and rarely has neurologic symptoms.

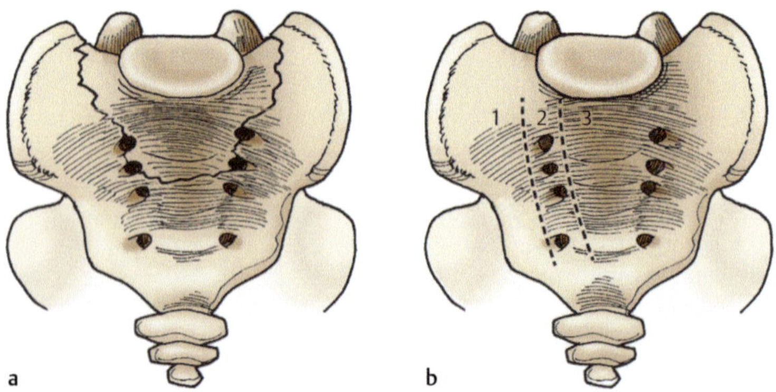

Fig. 18.1 Sacral fractures according to the Denis classification: **(a)** U-shaped fracture. **(b)** Zones 1, 2, and 3.

- B2: Transalar fracture that does not involve the spinal canal or the foramina, equivalent to Denis I injury, associated with a 5% risk of neurologic injury.
- B3: Transforaminal fracture, involving the foramina but not the canal, equivalent to Denis type II injury, associated with a 25% risk of neurologic injury.

– Type C: Bilateral injuries involving the sacroiliac joint, usually having vertical instability. These injuries have been subdivided into four groups.
  - C0: Nondisplaced U-type fractures. Usually seen as low-energy insufficiency fractures, with potential for displacement causing kyphosis.
  - C1: Any B-subtype injury where ipsilateral superior S1 facet is discontinuous with the medial part of sacrum. This may have an impact on spinopelvic instability.
  - C2: Bilateral complete B injury without transverse fracture, and potentially unstable.
  - C3: Displaced sacral U-type fracture, most likely unstable and high percentage of neurologic injury.

18.2.2 Signs, Symptoms, and Physical Examination

- Sacral injury should be suspected in any patient who has sacrococcygeal pain.
- Thorough evaluation of the pelvis should be conducted to assess stability of the pelvic ring. This can be done by applying gentle rotational pressure to the iliac wings.
- In patients who have lacerations, ecchymoses, tenderness, swelling, or crepitus around the pelvic ring, the presence of sacropelvic injury should be suspected.
- Evaluation for a sacropelvic degloving, or Morel-Lavelle lesion, should be conducted. This usually manifests as a palpable subcutaneous fluid mass.
- Digital rectal examination should be performed to evaluate for occult open fractures that might have involved the rectum. Likewise, lacerations in the perineal region should be investigated to ensure that an open fracture is not missed.
- Evaluation of the remainder of the spine should be conducted to assess for noncontiguous injuries.
- A detailed and thorough neurological examination, including motor and sensory assessments, should be performed.

18.2.3 Workup

- Standard Advanced Trauma Life Support (ATLS) protocol should be adhered to at the time of initial presentation.

- All life-threatening injuries should be addressed, and the patient adequately resuscitated.
- If provisional stabilization of the pelvic ring is necessary, placement of a pelvic binder, a pelvic sheet wrapping, or an external fixator can be performed. The principles of damage control orthopaedics—immediate and temporary stabilization with later definitive treatment—should be adhered to.

18.2.4 Neuroimaging

- The ATLS protocol for imaging a suspected sacral fracture includes obtaining an anteroposterior (AP) view of the pelvis.
- The AP view, however, is not always optimal for visualizing the fractures secondary to the inclination of the pelvis and overlying bowel gas. Approximately 30% of all sacral fractures can be identified from a single AP view of the pelvis.
- Inlet and outlet views of the pelvis are recommended to improve visualization and constitute a complete radiographic series in patients who have suspected pelvic injuries.

18.2.5 Treatment

- Nonoperative treatment is an option for patients who are neurologically intact and who have minimally displaced or angulated fractures. These are usually zone 1 or 2 injuries in conjunction with a stable pelvic fracture.[4]
- Operative techniques include sacral screws, lumbopelvic instrumentation, and a combination of the two, known as *triangular osteosynthesis.*
- Iliosacral screws can be placed by open or percutaneous techniques.
- Lumboiliac fixation offers advantages such as familiar anatomy, prevention of kyphotic deformity, and possibility of concomitant neural decompression, if necessary.
- Lumbopelvic fixation can be performed through a percutaneous or mini-open approach for fractures that do not require open reduction. These approaches have the benefit of minimal blood loss and minimal soft tissue dissection.[5]
- Sacropelvic fixation using screws placed through the S2–alar–iliac pathway has been described. The pathway is defined using intraoperative fluoroscopy and carries the benefit of a minimally invasive approach and the ease of attaching the screws to the spinal portion of the construct.[6]

18.2.6 Surgical Pearls

- Open surgical reduction and fixation continues to be recommended for sacral fractures involving the lumbosacral junction and for sacral fractures that require urgent neural decompression.

- In cases of sacral fracture involving vertical displacement, sacroiliac screws are prone to loosening and can result in loss of reduction.
- Appropriate intraoperative visualization of the necessary anatomic landmarks is crucial to performing percutaneous fixation.

18.3 Type B Injuries

18.3.1 Background

- 45% of traumatic fractures of the pelvic ring transverse the sacrum.[1]
- However, transverse sacral fractures represent only 3 to 5% of all sacral fractures.[7]
- This injury was initially termed the *suicidal jumper's fracture* because the mechanism of injury includes fall from height. Other mechanisms of injury include motor vehicle collisions, blast injuries, and rush injuries.
- As a result of potential injury to the sacral nerve roots, transverse sacral fractures often are associated with devastating complications such as bowel and bladder dysfunction, sexual dysfunction, sensory deficits, and lower motor weakness.

18.3.2 Signs, Symptoms, and Physical Examination

- The presence of root transection with a transverse sacral fracture is 35%, so a thorough neurological examination, rectal examination, and light touch and pinprick sensory examination must be performed.

18.3.3 Workup

- Adherence to standard ATLS protocols and treatment.
- Thorough and complete neurological examination, including motor testing, sensation to light touch and pinprick, rectal examination, and careful evaluation of the skin for lacerations, ecchymosis, and evidence of open factures.

18.3.4 Neuroimaging

- Radiographs, including standard pelvic views, and CT scans of pelvis and spine with reformatted coronal and sagittal view images.
- Magnetic resonance imaging (MRI) when clinically indicated.

18.3.5 Treatment

- Most stable sacral fractures can be treated nonoperatively, but those involving a pelvic ring disruption or spinopelvic instability should be stabilized.

- Historically, surgical treatment consisted of only sacral laminectomy in an effort to address and treat sacral nerve root injuries.
- New techniques have been developed to internally stabilize the fracture.
- Goal of treatment is pain relief, stabilization, and earlier mobilization. Depending on the injury, neurological recovery might not be possible, although a partial return of function often is achievable.
- The rare nature of the injury has limited published treatment strategies to case reports and case series.
- Posterior pelvic ring fixation in the form of percutaneous iliosacral screws, sacral plating, or transiliac bars is an effective treatment strategy for transverse sacral fractures. However, if associated spinopelvic instability is present, spinopelvic fixation should be applied that stabilizes the lumbar spine to the ilium.

18.3.6 Surgical Pearls

- Appropriate preoperative imaging is crucial in establishing and understanding the fracture pattern. Furthermore, adequate intraoperative radiographic visualization of the bony landmarks is essential for safe placement of iliosacral screws and spinopelvic fixation.

18.4 Type C Injuries

18.4.1 Background

- U-shaped sacral fractures can be thought of as a subdivision of transverse sacral fracture and are even rarer.[8,9]
- The injury is characterized by a transverse sacral fracture in conjunction with bilateral sacral fracture–dislocations. This results in a mechanical dissociation of the upper sacrum and spine from the pelvis.
- The injury results from a high-energy force with substantial axial load (e.g., fall or jump from height, motor vehicle collision, and crush mechanism).
- A substantial amount of associated soft tissue damage, hemorrhage, and other orthopaedic and systemic injuries are often present; 96.8% of patients who have U-shaped sacral fractures have associated injuries.
- A high mortality rate is associated with these injuries, and the injury can be missed or underdiagnosed because of the severity of the patient's other injuries.
- Sacral nerve root injuries caused by comminuted fracture fragments or displacement can present as incomplete monoradiculopathy to a complete cauda equina syndrome.

18.4.2 Signs, Symptoms, and Physical Examination

- The diagnosis might be missed or delayed because of other serious distracting injuries or difficulty visualizing the sacrum.
- Sacral injury should be suspected in any patient who has sacrococcygeal pain.
- The standard ATLS protocol should be followed at the time of initial presentation.
- Considering that the patient might be critically ill at the time of initial presentation, secondary surveys should be obtained as the patient's condition stabilizes and improves.
- The most common neurological deficit associated with U-shaped fractures is cauda equina dysfunction secondary to injury to the lower nerve roots. This will cause impaired bladder function, decreased rectal tone, and saddle anesthesia, sometimes in the absence of any lower extremity dysfunction.
- The L5 and S1 nerve roots can also be damaged, with the damage manifesting as foot drop.
- Detailed neurological examination, including rectal examination and assessment of light touch and pinprick sensation, must also be performed.

18.4.3 Workup

- Radiographic clues that suggest a U-shaped sacral fracture include bilateral transforaminal sacral fractures, irregularity of the superior sacral foraminal lines, and L5 transverse process fractures.
- Angulation of the fractured segment can also produce a pseudo inlet view on a standard AP view of pelvis.

18.4.4 Neuroimaging

- A lateral view sacral radiograph is useful when evaluating U-shaped sacral fractures, because the transverse fracture line often is difficult to appreciate.
- CT of the spine and pelvis is necessary to further define the injury and for operative planning. Coronal and sagittal reformatting are used to assess fracture angulation, translation, canal compromise, and the fracture pattern.
- MRI is obtained when patients have a known sacral fracture and neurological deficit.

18.4.5 Treatment

- Nonoperative treatment options previously included bed rest with skeletal traction or immobilization using a cast or orthoses.

- U-shaped sacral fractures typically result in spinopelvic instability and are thus not typically treated nonoperatively.
- Definitive treatment of this complex injury occurs only after all other life-threatening injuries have been addressed and the patient is adequately resuscitated.
- The principles of damage control orthopaedics should be adhered to; temporary stabilization of the pelvic ring might be necessary.
- If signs or symptoms of neurological compromise are present, decompressive maneuvers, either indirectly via fracture reduction or directly with a laminectomy or focal foraminotomy, should be performed.
- Percutaneous iliosacral screws are best used to treat a U-shaped fracture that is not comminuted and that is minimally displaced.
- Lumbopelvic fixation is best suited to treat highly unstable fractures having a substantial rotational component. The technique can be combined with iliosacral screws or a transiliac plate to form triangular osteosynthesis. This is the biomechanically superior method.

18.4.6 Surgical Pearls

- If a preoperative CT scan reveals bone fragments in the foramen, sacral nerve root decompression should be performed before fracture reduction so that the fragments do not injure the roots during a reduction maneuver.
- The sagittal relationship of the spine to the sacrum and the ilium should be reviewed preoperatively, considering that this relationship can be difficult to interpret intraoperatively because of the lack of intact bone at the sacral ala.
- A true lateral view of the pelvis, with overlap of the sciatic notches, is necessary for the safe placement of iliac screws. The obturator inlet and outlet views are used to determine the screw starting point and final position.
- A combined obturator oblique outlet view, with approximately 45 degrees caudal and 45 degrees anterolateral angulation of the radiographic beam, produces overlap of the anterior–inferior iliac spine and the posterior–superior iliac spine and is also known as the *teardrop view.*
- If adequate intraoperative visualization is not feasible, direct palpation of the sciatic notch might be necessary to ensure safe screw placement.

18.5 Traumatic Spinopelvic Dissociations (Type C3 Injuries)

18.5.1 Background

- Separate and distinct entity from lumbosacral fracture–dislocations or bilateral sacroiliac joint dislocations.

18.5.2 Signs, Symptoms, and Physical Examination

- Initial care of the patient adheres to the ATLS protocols; a pelvic compression device is sometimes necessary.
- If the patient is suffering from an active pelvic hemorrhage as a result of the injury, and if the hemorrhage cannot be adequately controlled with pelvic compression, fixation by a pelvic clamp, laparotomy, and pelvic packing should be performed, as has been described in damage control algorithms. Radiographic coiling in interventional radiology might also be necessary.

18.5.3 Workup

- Considering that spinopelvic dissociations are usually associated with other life-threatening injuries, the majority of patients are intubated and sedated. This makes a thorough and adequate neurological examination extremely difficult.
- Evaluation for ecchymosis, lacerations, and Morel-Lavelle lesions are essential components of the workup.

18.5.4 Neuroimaging

- A CT scan, often a whole-body scan, is almost universally warranted and is mandatory for these patients.

18.5.5 Treatment

- Triangular stabilization with spinopelvic fixation and iliosacral screws is the most standard method of fixation and is used for Type C3 injuries (**Fig. 18.2**).
- For C1 or C2 fractures, triangular osteosynthesis can be used, but because this fracture is not rotationally unstable, bilateral iliosacral screws or anterior tension plating might be sufficient.

18.5.6 Surgical Pearls

- The approach is based on the type of fracture and the method of stabilization.
- For direct manipulation of the sacrum to achieve reduction, a Schanz pin can be inserted into S1. Unilateral or bilateral femoral traction can also be helpful.

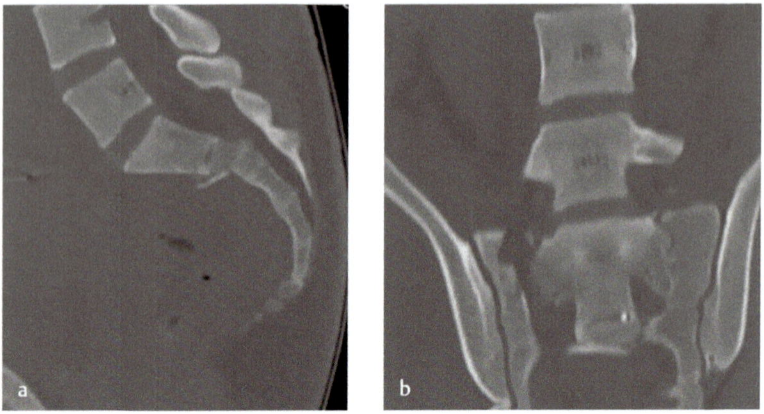

Fig. 18.2 **(a)** Computed tomographic sagittal reconstruction showing H-type sacral fracture. **(b)** Computed tomographic coronal reconstruction showing H-type sacral fracture.

Common Clinical Questions

1. According to the Denis classification of sacral fractures, which type is most likely to be associated with neural injury?
2. Indications for surgical stabilization of sacral fractures include which of the following?
   A. Zone 1 fracture with > 2 cm displacement.
   B. Minimally displaced transverse sacral fracture at S4.
   C. Lumbosacral dissociation.
   D. Nondisplaced Zone 2 fracture without neurological symptoms.
   E. A and C.

Answers to Common Clinical Questions

1. Zone 3 (central sacral canal fractures).
2. E.

References

1. Denis F, Davis S, Comfort T. Sacral fractures: an important problem. Retrospective analysis of 236 cases. Clin Orthop Relat Res. 1988; 227(227): 67–81

2. Roy-Camille R, Saillant G, Gagna G, Mazel C. Transverse fracture of the upper sacrum. Suicidal jumper's fracture. Spine. 1985; 10(9):838–845
3. Lehmann W, Hoffmann M, Briem D, et al. Management of traumatic spinopelvic dissociations: review of the literature. Eur J Trauma Emerg Surg. 2012; 38(5):517–524
4. Liu HC, Chen YZ, Sang XG, Qi L. Management of lumbosacropelvic fracture-dislocation using lumbo-iliac internal fixation. Injury. 2012; 43(4):452–457
5. Hong J, Spire WJ, Simmons NE. Mini-open stabilization of a sacral fracture: technical case report. Neurosurgery. 2013; 72(1) Suppl Operative:99–103
6. Martin CT, Witham TF, Kebaish KM. Sacropelvic fixation: two case reports of a new percutaneous technique. Spine. 2011; 36(9):E618–E621
7. Bederman SS, Hassan JM, Shah KN, Kiester PD, Bhatia NN, Zamorano DP. Fixation techniques for complex traumatic transverse sacral fractures: a systematic review. Spine. 2013; 38(16):E1028–E1040
8. Yi C, Hak DJ. Traumatic spinopelvic dissociation or U-shaped sacral fracture: a review of the literature. Injury. 2012; 43(4):402–408
9. König MA, Jehan S, Boszczyk AA, Boszczyk BM. Surgical management of U-shaped sacral fractures: a systematic review of current treatment strategies. Eur Spine J. 2012; 21(5):829–836

19 Infection

Wilson E. Vaughan, Brian Q. Hou, W. Hunter Waddell, and Byron F. Stephens

Summary
Spinal infection presents a complex challenge, encompassing a range of conditions from pyogenic vertebral osteomyelitis to epidural and intradural infections. Etiology, epidemiology, diagnostic approaches, and treatment options are discussed, with an emphasis on early detection and appropriate intervention. Multidisciplinary collaboration is highlighted for effective management, addressing key risk factors and prognostic considerations. With a focus on timely diagnosis and vigilant monitoring, this chapter serves as a practical resource for providers navigating the complexities of spinal infections.

Keywords: spinal infections, vertebral osteomyelitis, diskitis, epidural abscess, intradural abscess, postoperative infections, complications, risk factors, prophylaxis

19.1 Key Points

- A high index of suspicion is required for spinal infections, especially in at-risk patients such as the elderly, smokers, diabetics, immunosuppressed, substance abusers, and postprocedural patients (**Table 19.1**).
- Magnetic resonance imaging (MRI) of the spine with and without gadolinium contrast in conjunction with biopsy remains the most reliable means to establish a diagnosis and aid in a targeted treatment of spinal infections.
- Nonoperative treatment typically includes a 4- to 6-week course of IV antibiotics while trending the patient's inflammatory markers, namely, C-reactive protein (CRP) and erythrocyte sedimentation rate (ESR), and regularly monitoring the neurologic status.
- Nonoperative management is possible in select patients with spinal infections who have no neurologic deficit or instability of the spine.
- Surgery is typically indicated in scenarios when there is neurologic deficit, failure of medical therapy, or instability secondary to the spinal infection (**Table 19.2**).

Table 19.1 General risk factors for spinal infection

Patient-related risk factors	Procedure-related risk factors
Advanced age (65 +)	Revision procedure
Obesity	Prolonged operative time
Smoking	Instrumentation
Diabetes	Posterior approach
Immunosuppression	Tumor resection
Steroid therapy	Epidural injection
Prior surgical infection	Prolonged hospital stay
Substance abuse (drugs, EtOH)	Trauma
Poor nutritional status	Excessive blood loss

Table 19.2 Indications for surgical management of spinal infections

Failure of antibiotic/nonoperative treatment
Sepsis
Neurological degeneration
Cord compression
Severe endpoint destruction
Mechanical instability
Intractable pain

19.2 Pyogenic Vertebral Osteomyelitis and Diskitis[1,2,3]

19.2.1 Etiology, Epidemiology, and Pathogenesis

- Vertebral osteomyelitis represents 3 to 5% of all cases of osteomyelitis in patients aged > 50 years.
- Hematogenous dissemination via arterial routes occurs in 20% of cases and is the primary route of infection that involves two adjacent vertebrae in addition to the intervertebral disk (diskitis).

- The most common organism in hematogenous dissemination is *Staphylococcus aureus*, whereas *Staphylococcus epidermidis* is the second most common pathogen.
- Sites of infection: lumbar spine (50–60%), thoracic spine (30%), and cervical spine (approximately 10%).

19.2.2 Patient Presentation

- Gradually worsening axial back pain and fever (35–60%) are common presenting symptoms.
- Progression of infection may be indicated by neurologic impairment that includes sensory loss, weakness, or radiculopathy.

19.2.3 Diagnostic Workup

- If infection is suspected, immediate laboratory workup with CRP is required to shorten diagnostic delay, followed by ESR and white blood cell (WBC) count.
- Blood cultures, which are positive in approximately 30 to 70% of cases, should be obtained early in the diagnostic workup, preferably before the initiation of antibiotic therapy.
- Image-guided biopsy is warranted to guide antibiotic therapy when blood cultures are negative.
- Plain radiographs remain the basic modality of investigation.
- MRI is the preferred imaging modality for the diagnosis of vertebral osteomyelitis, which typically shows increased T2-weight signal at the endplate(s) of the affected vertebrae or soft tissue abnormalities (89%).
- The addition of gadolinium contrast to MRI increases sensitivity (96%) and specificity (94%), providing anatomic delineation of spinal abscesses.

19.2.4 Treatment

- First-line treatment includes a 4- to 6-week course of broad-spectrum IV antibiotics until culture-specific options are identified with biopsy, blood, or tissue cultures.
- Surgical treatment may be indicated in cases of significant osseous destruction resulting in instability, neurological deficits, sepsis, abscess formation, and failure of medical therapy.
- The anterior approaches allow for decompression of the neural system and removal of infected disks and vertebral bodies by way of a corpectomy and anterior column reconstruction.
- Same-day or staged posterior procedures are often performed to further stabilize the spine and decompress the neural elements.

19.2.5 Prognosis/Complications

- With aggressive medical and surgical treatment, patients with incomplete neurologic compromise may see improvement or resolution of paresis depending on the severity and chronicity of the deficit prior to initiation of treatment.
- Complications include recurrence of infection, fracture, paralysis, chronic pain, and disability.
- Mortality rate is between 5 and 20% and may be caused by the spinal–neural infection, secondary sepsis, or the original infection.

19.3 Epidural Infections[4,5]

19.3.1 Etiology, Epidemiology, and Pathogenesis

- Hematogenous spread is most common (50%) via the contamination of bacteria in the epidural space from soft tissue infections, abdominal infections, infected catheters, endocarditis, urinary tract infections, or respiratory tract infections.
- Direct spread from other infections includes vertebral osteomyelitis, diskitis, and psoas abscesses.
- Most infections are caused by *S. aureus* (63%) followed by streptococcal infections (9%).

19.3.2 Patient Presentation

- Early presentations of disease are often subtle and include back pain (70–100%), fever, and neurologic symptoms of myelopathy or paraplegia.
- Progressive neurologic deficits may include urinary retention, bowel incontinence, sensory disturbances, motor weakness, or paralysis depending on lesion size and overall cord compression.

19.3.3 Diagnostic Workup

- Standard inflammatory tests (WBC, ESR, and CRP) are recommended.
- Initial lab evaluation should also include blood cultures (× 2), electrolyte levels, and other preoperative laboratory studies such as coagulation studies, plain radiographs, or biopsy.
- MRI with gadolinium is recommended and may demonstrate fluid collection in the epidural space.

19.3.4 Treatment

- Indications for nonoperative management: neurologically intact patients, complete paralysis for more than 36 to 72 hours, poor surgical candidates, or those with multifocal epidural abscesses.
- Empiric antibiotic coverage should begin if there is a high suspicion for an epidural abscess and continue for 6 to 12 weeks with serial imaging and inflammatory lab orders.
- Indications for surgical management include failure to respond to nonoperative medical therapy, significant neurologic deficits, large paraspinal abscesses with mass effect or embolization, spinal instability, or progressive deformity.
- The treatment of the neurologically intact patient with significant stenosis from an epidural abscess requires very close monitoring and decisions are made on a case-by-case basis.
- Dorsal epidural abscesses may be surgically treated by posterior laminectomy or skip laminectomy, drainage of infected tissue, and normal saline irrigation.
- An anterior procedure may be required in the setting of a ventral epidural abscess.
- Concomitant spinal fusion may be warranted for those experiencing spinal instability due to infection and/or decompression.

19.3.5 Prognosis/Complications

- Risk factors for medical failure include a presenting motor deficit, pathologic or compression fracture in affected levels, active malignancy, diabetes mellitus, sensory changes, or dorsal abscesses due to association with cord compression.
- Failure of nonoperative management may be predicted by the SORG AI algorithm as well as in-hospital and 90-day post-discharge mortality rates.
- These algorithms are intended to serve as adjuncts for clinical care but should not substitute medical expertise and situational judgment.

19.4 Intradural Infections[6,7]

19.4.1 Etiology, Epidemiology, and Pathogenesis

- **Subdural (intradural, extramedullary)**:
  - Spinal subdural abscess is a rare infectious lesion of the spinal cord with an unknown incidence rate.
  - Hematogenous spread from an extra-spinal infection is a common cause of this condition; however, cases can result from iatrogenic

mechanisms such as lumbar puncture, epidural injection, and spinal surgery.

- **Intramedullary**:
  - An intramedullary spinal cord abscess (ISCA) is a rare clinical infection of the parenchyma of the spinal cord and is associated with high mortality and neurological morbidity.
    - Infection is typically acquired by hematological transport or close contact with infected tissue or cerebrospinal fluid (CSF).

19.4.2 Patient Presentation

- Risk factors for ISCA include diabetes, HIV, glucocorticoid use, IV drug abuse, or trauma resulting in violation of the pia mater and compromise of the blood–cord barrier.
- Patients can present with localized back pain, fever, or focal neurological deficits such as paraparesis or saddle anesthesia.

19.4.3 Diagnostic Workup

- Immediate recognition and screening with labs including leukocyte count, ESR, and CRP are necessary when clinical suspicion is high.
- Contrast-enhanced MRI with gadolinium identifies the extent of infection or cord compression.
- Fat-suppression sequence and diffusion-weighted imaging (DWI) can also differentiate intradural abscesses from tumors.

19.4.4 Treatment

- Combined medical and surgical treatment is the recommended standard of care to avoid recurrence of infection and avoid progressive neurologic deficit.
- Cultures should be obtained before wound irrigation for definitive diagnosis of the pathogen.
- Decompressive surgery with laminectomy is the first stage of a multistep process followed by antiseptic subdural irrigation and appropriate antibiotic therapy.

19.4.5 Prognosis/Complications

- Intradural infections can cause permanent disability or death and require prompt surgical treatment and antibiotics.
- Complications include bowel and bladder incontinence, paraplegia, dysesthesias, or weakness.
- Spinal cord abscesses have a mortality rate of approximately 10% and most patients experience residual neurological deficits.

19.5 Postoperative Infections[8,9,10,11]

19.5.1 Etiology, Epidemiology, and Pathogenesis

- Postoperative infections, also known as surgical site infections (SSIs), are the most common hospital-acquired infection with patients typically reporting insidious onset of pain within 4 weeks postoperatively.
- SSIs are classified as superficial or deep, with superficial infections limited to subcutaneous tissue and deep infections involving the fascia and paraspinal muscles.
- Incidence of SSI may vary from 0.6 to 18% depending on the approach, instrumentation, and indication(s) for surgery.
- *S. aureus* (73%) is the most common microorganism found in spinal SSI, a substantial portion of which is methicillin-resistant *Staphylococcus aureus* (MRSA).

19.5.2 Prophylaxis

- Cefazolin (first-generation cephalosporin) is the standard, given its activity against staphylococcal species, and should be utilized within 60 minutes of the first surgical incision.
- Most surgical patients with a history of penicillin allergy can be safely administered cefazolin prophylactically.
- Intrawound vancomycin powder is increasingly being adopted due to its high local concentration, minimal systemic absorption, and risk reduction for spinal SSI.

19.5.3 Patient Presentation

- Common risk factors include obesity, smoking, antibiotic resistance, extended hospitalization, advanced age, immunosuppression, extended operative time, and revision surgery.
- Patients typically report localized pain, wound drainage, or fever.
- Subfascial SSIs may demonstrate no external signs of infection and some patients may not exhibit constitutional symptoms with SSIs.

19.5.4 Diagnostic Workup

- Lab markers for SSI should be analyzed comprehensively, with rising ESR levels after 4th postoperative day and persistently high CRP levels (> 2 weeks postoperatively) indicating infection.

- MRI with gadolinium is recommended although be conscious of postoperative hardware producing increased signal intensity on imaging reports.

19.5.5 Treatment

- Antibiotic therapy alone can be appropriate for select superficial SSIs.
- Indications for urgent surgical management include septic presentation and neurologic deficits.
- Open irrigation and debridement of SSI is the standard treatment therapy.
- Intraoperative tissue cultures are the gold standard to identify pathogens and should occur prior to antibiotic administration if the patient is not septic.
- Patients treated with debridement and hardware removal will typically continue IV antibiotics for 24 to 72 hours postoperatively with a 7-day treatment of oral antibiotics.
- In early postoperative infections (< 3 months), hardware removal is not recommended to avoid destabilization.
- Although there is no clear consensus, if hardware is retained then long-term (lifetime) IV antibiotics should be followed by a course of suppressive oral antibiotics.

19.5.6 Prognosis/Complications

- Optimization of patient risk factors, prophylactic antibiotic use, intraoperative irrigation and debridement, and continued postoperative follow-up are necessary for positive clinical outcomes.
- In patients who develop an SSI despite efforts at prevention, timely diagnosis and treatment are critical to prevent increased morbidity or medical costs incurred due to infection.

19.6 Surgical Pearls

- Acute hematogenous osteomyelitis is primarily treated with antibiotics, with surgery typically reserved for diagnostic purposes such as open biopsy.
- Late-onset infections post spinal implant surgery often require implant removal due to an increased risk of treatment failure, with reconstruction and stabilization occasionally necessary for large defects.
- Progressive neurologic deficits, deformity, and spinal instability despite antimicrobial therapy warrant surgical intervention in patients diagnosed with vertebral osteomyelitis.

- For spinal epidural abscess, urgent surgical intervention with systemic antibiotics is indicated for evolving neurological deterioration, spinal instability, and persistent infection.

Common Clinical Questions

1. Which organism is most commonly associated with vertebral osteomyelitis and diskitis?
2. What are four indications for surgical decompression of an epidural spinal infection?
3. Which topical antibiotic utilized intraoperatively has been shown to reduce risk of spinal SSIs?

Answers to Common Clinical Questions

1. Gram-positive cocci (*Staphylococcus aureus*).
2. Neurologic deficit, evidence of spinal cord compression, persistent infection, spinal instability.
3. Vancomycin powder.

References

1. Zimmerli W. Clinical practice. Vertebral osteomyelitis. N Engl J Med. 2010; 362(11):1022–1029
2. Gupta M, Birdwell K. Spinal Infection/Osteomyelitis. Bridwell and Dewald's Textbook of Spinal Surgery. 1714; 2:2019
3. Berbari EF, Kanj SS, Kowalski TJ, et al. Infectious Diseases Society of America. 2015 Infectious Diseases Society of America (IDSA) clinical practice guidelines for the diagnosis and treatment of native vertebral osteomyelitis in adults. Clin Infect Dis. 2015; 61(6):e26–e46
4. Ameer MA, Knorr TL, Mesfin FB. Spinal Epidural Abscess. Treasure Island, FL: StatPearls Publishing; 2022
5. Shah AA, Ogink PT, Nelson SB, Harris MB, Schwab JH. Nonoperative management of spinal epidural abscess: development of a predictive algorithm for failure. J Bone Joint Surg Am. 2018; 100(7):546–555
6. Ramos AD, Rolston JD, Gauger GE, Larson PS. Spinal subdural abscess following laminectomy for symptomatic stenosis: a report of 2 cases and review of the literature. Am J Case Rep. 2016; 17:476–483
7. Keefe P, M Das J, Al-Dahir MA. Spinal Cord Abscess. Treasure Island, FL: StatPearls Publishing; 2022

8. Devin CJ, Chotai S, McGirt MJ, et al. Intrawound vancomycin decreases the risk of surgical site infection after posterior spine surgery: a multicenter analysis. Spine. 2018; 43(1):65–71
9. Dowdell J, Brochin R, Kim J, et al. Postoperative spine infection: diagnosis and management. Global Spine J. 2018; 8(4) Suppl:37S–43S
10. Hegde V, Meredith DS, Kepler CK, Huang RC. Management of postoperative spinal infections. World J Orthop. 2012; 3(11):182–189
11. Sousa-Pinto B, Blumenthal KG, Courtney L, Mancini CM, Jeffres MN. Assessment of the frequency of dual allergy to penicillins and cefazolin: a systematic review and meta-analysis. JAMA Surg. 2021; 156(4):e210021

20 Primary Bony Spinal Column Tumors

Mark A. Feger, Quante Singleton, John Clayton Clohisy Jr, and Matthew L. Goodwin

Summary
Primary bony spinal column tumors are rare. Their management, however, is crucial to optimize recovery and prognosis. The most common ones include chordomas and chondrosarcomas. A thorough evaluation is needed to rule out metastatic lesions or otherwise nonsurgical tumors that may mimic primary lesions. En bloc resection of primary bony spinal column tumors remains the gold standard treatment in the appropriate clinical context.

Keywords: chordoma, chondrosarcoma, sarcoma, tumor

20.1 Key Points

- New bony spinal column lesions require a complete workup including full spine imaging, laboratory assessment, punch biopsy, and multidisciplinary treatment plan prior to surgical intervention, except in rare cases of acute neurologic decompensation.
- History, physical examination, and complete workup of new bony spinal column lesions will differentiate between primary bony spinal column tumors, metastatic disease to the spinal column, and tumor "mimickers" such as infection and metabolic bone disease.
- En bloc resection is the preferred surgical margin for malignant and benign aggressive primary bony spinal column tumors.

20.2 Background

- Primary spine tumors are relatively rare and only represent about 10% of bony spinal column tumors.[1] Chordoma, chondrosarcoma, osteosarcoma, and Ewing sarcoma are the most frequently encountered primary bony spinal column tumors.[2,3] The vast majority of these originate in the vertebral body, although they could originate from any part of the bone.[2,3] On the other hand, aneurysmal bone cysts (ABCs), osteoid osteomas, and osteoblastomas are more commonly encountered in the posterior elements of the spine. Ewing sarcoma and Langerhans cell histiocytosis are more common in pediatric patients, whereas chordoma and chondrosarcoma are more common in adults.[1,2] Some common lesions and their characteristics are listed in **Table 20.1**.

Table 20.1 Common spinal tumors, typical characteristics and recommended surgical margins

Malignant tumors of the spine	
Chordoma	Typically, slow-growing lesions (subtypes may be more aggressive) with/without high recurrence rates. Brachyury gene duplication. MRI shows dark on T1, bright on T2. Benign notochordal cell tumors (BNCTs) may be similar but enhance less and be more sclerotic on CT. En bloc resection recommended, often with adjuvant radiation.
Chondrosarcoma	Characteristic calcifications on CT ("ring and arc"). MRI dark on T1, bright on T2 and enhances; notably may be cold on bone scan. Multiple subtypes. En bloc resection recommended; radiation classically not very effective.
Osteosarcoma	Osteoid forming tumors that may metastasize to lungs. Bimodal distribution (young and old). MRI dark on T1, bright on T2 and enhances. PET positive. En bloc resection recommended with adjuvant chemotherapy.
Ewing sarcoma	More commonly seen in the first two decades of life. EWS gene mutation. MRI dark on T1, bright on T2, and enhances. Responsive to radiation although en bloc resection recommended for primary lesions of spine when possible.
Benign/benign aggressive tumors of the spine	
Aneurysmal bone cyst (ABC)	Benign aggressive lesion, classically with "fluid-fluid" levels on MRI and in posterior elements of the spine. Very vascular. En bloc resection when possible; preoperative embolization recommended.
Osteoid osteoma (<2 cm)/ osteoblastoma (>2 cm)	Benign lesion of the spine but can cause local pain. Often in posterior elements of the spine. Classically presents with night pain and relief with NSAIDs. Nidus of bone seen on CT. Intralesional resection often effective.

(Continued)

Table 20.1 (*Continued*)

Osteochondroma	Benign lesion with cortical and intramedullary continuity of bone; cartilaginous cap can undergo malignant transformation. Intralesional resection.
Giant cell tumor (GCT)	Benign aggressive lesion. Can be vascular and expansile lytic lesion of bone. Small percentage of tumors metastasize to lungs. Denosumab useful to solidify/shrink. Gross total resection effective although en bloc resection may provide more durable response.
Hemangioma	Benign lesion that is seen in 10% of spines. Classically, MRI is bright on T1 and T2, although lipid-poor lesions may be dark on T1. Classic channels or honeycomb appearance seen on coronal/axial CT. Intralesional resection is effective although preoperative embolization is recommend.
Multiple spinal lesions	
Metastatic disease	Renal, prostate, breast, and lung diseases common. Prostate disease can be very blastic and difficult to instrument; renal disease is extremely vascular and requires preoperative embolization. Must consider prognosis, neurologic compromise, and stability of spine. Multidisciplinary treatment critical.
Lymphoma/ multiple myeloma	Typically responds dramatically to radiation. Myeloma may be more destructive to bone when compared to lymphoma. Urgent/emergent radiation may be very effective.
Tumor mimickers	Numerous tumor mimickers include infections, metabolic bone diseases (e.g., Paget's disease, brown tumors), rheumatoid arthritis, sarcoid, bone islands, epidural lipomatosis, uremic calcinosis, among others. Rarely surgical.

20.3 Signs, Symptoms, and Physical Examination

- The history, physical examination, and workup for a new spinal lesion collectively serve to differentiate primary bony spine tumors from metastatic disease to the spinal column and from tumor "mimickers" (e.g., infection, metabolic bone disease, sarcoid, bone islands, etc.) as well as to guide surgical decision-making.[2,4,5] Incidental identification of a new spinal lesion is not uncommon, and in these cases, patients are asymptomatic or minimally symptomatic. Clinical presentation for symptomatic lesions is dictated by the location of the tumor, extent of bony destruction, associated segmental instability, presence or absence of neural compression, and rate of tumor growth. Pain is the most common presenting complaint, but motor/sensory/autonomic dysfunctions are also frequently encountered.[2,4] Pain can be differentiated into localized pain related to rapid tumor expansion or pathologic fracture, radicular pain from nerve root compression/foraminal stenosis, and mechanical pain from spinal instability as a result of bony destruction and altered spinal biomechanics. History and examination should focus on: (1) risk factors and family history for metastatic disease and risk factors for tumor mimics (infections history, immunocompromised status, intravenous drug use, travel history for atypical infections), (2) prognostic factors related to the extent of neural compression (nerve root vs. cord compression, ability to ambulate, or bowel/bladder compromise), (3) presence/absence and rate of neurological decline (to help determine the need for surgical intervention and the associated surgical urgency), and (4) systemic disease burden/prognosis (to determine individual fitness and ability to tolerate a spine surgery or to determine if the patient will live long enough to recover and realize medium/long-term benefit from spine surgery).[2]

20.4 Workup and Neuroimaging

- Comprehensive evaluation for a new spinal lesion is crucial and will allow the spine surgeon to narrow the differential from primary spinal column tumors, metastatic disease, and tumor "mimickers."[2,5] A full-spine magnetic resonance imaging (MRI) with and without contrast allows for high-resolution evaluation of the neural axis (evaluate tumor burden, epidural spread, nerve root/cord compression, evaluate for skip lesions, and for surgical planning).[2] CT scan of the chest, abdomen, and pelvis assesses for other lesions or may identify an unknown primary tumor in the setting of metastatic disease to the spine. These CT scans can often be reformatted into thoracic or lumbar spine CT images for assessment of bony involvement and surgical planning. A dedicated cervical spine CT scan can be obtained if appropriate for upper thoracic or cervical lesions. Upright radiographs, if feasible, should be obtained to assess for alignment/mechanical instability and for improved understanding of intraoperative fluoroscopy/radiographs. Laboratory analysis (complete blood count, basic metabolic panel, C-reactive protein, erythrocyte sedimentation rate, serum/urine electrophoresis) is also invaluable in the comprehensive evaluation to assess for infection, multiple myeloma, and metabolic causes of a new spinal lesion. Tissue biopsy is crucial prior to surgical intervention except in very rare circumstances (i.e., emergent decompression) and this should be planned and completed at the surgical center where any subsequent spinal surgery would take place to ensure there is no unnecessary tissue contamination. Midline punch biopsies are preferred as fine-needle aspirates can often be nondiagnostic. It is preferred that each case is reviewed by a spine tumor board that consists of experts from different specialties (typically radiation oncology, interventional radiology, orthopedic spine surgery, neurosurgery).[2] This multidisciplinary approach is always preferred given the complexity of these cases. Final diagnosis is established via surgical pathology after resection, if performed.

20.5 Treatment

- Spinal tumor resections are classified based upon the surgical margin as en bloc, gross total, or intralesional.[6] En bloc refers to removing the entire tumor altogether without violating the tumor capsule whereas gross total is a complete resection of the tumor in pieces.[6] En bloc resection is the goal in most cases for malignant and benign aggressive primary spine tumors (high rate of local recurrence). Capsule breach during en bloc resection is correlated with higher rates of local recurrence and decreased survival.[2] Benign lesions such as osteochondromas, hemangiomas, and osteoid osteoma can often be treated via intralesional resection, if surgery is required. Surgery is planned/performed after a complete workup, including a biopsy in the vast majority of cases. Rarely, an acutely neurologically decompensating patient may require decompression and reconstruction prior to a tissue diagnosis. In these case, imaging/labs will be completed, and the surgeon will need to determine if the patient is a candidate for en bloc resection. If so, the patient should be taken for an urgent open biopsy with limited decompression and reconstruction to restore/preserve neurologic function. If the patient is not a candidate for en bloc resection, then a more definitive urgent decompression and reconstruction should be performed. Some patients will present with a subacute neurologic decline (weeks to a couple months) and in these cases, steroids can be beneficial while completing an expedited workup, including biopsy, often on an inpatient basis. If lymphoma is suspected, biopsy should be obtained prior to steroid administration so as to not decrease the diagnostic yield.[2]

If biopsy confirms lymphoma or myeloma, treatment is often nonsurgical with radiation and chemotherapy.[2] In most cases of neurologically intact patient with a new bony spinal lesion, a complete workup can be performed on an outpatient basis and a multidisciplinary treatment approach should be established prior to surgical intervention.

20.6 Surgical Pearls

- Preoperative preparation is key. Preoperative central line placement, bilateral lower extremity duplex ultrasound for identification of unknown venous thrombosis, and spinal angiography can all be beneficial. Angiography can guide preoperative embolization to minimize intraoperative blood loss and help ensure there will be preservation of adequate spinal cord/brain perfusion if the en bloc resection requires any arterial sacrifice.[2]
- T1-weighted MRI provides the highest resolution to determine the extent/location of tumor within the bony spinal column, and the Weinstein-Boriani-Biagini classification system is useful to characterize the radial location and depth of the tumor within the spinal column, which can aid in formulating a plan for any required bony cuts.[7] The number of bony cuts should be minimized, should be outside of the tumor margin when possible, and those that are utilized should be quickly cauterized/waxed to prevent inadvertent tumor spread.[2] Bleeding should be minimized with attention to careful hemostasis and use of hemostatic agents and tranexamic acid when appropriate.[2] Sterile water irrigation can also be utilized to lyse free tumor cells after removal of the tumor.
- During reconstruction, general deformity principles should be applied to maximize long-term clinical outcomes. In particular, positive sagittal balance and mismatch between pelvic incidence and lumbar lordosis are not well tolerated.[8]
- When a spinal column tumor is susceptible to chemotherapy and/or radiosensitive (e.g., Ewing sarcoma, multiple myeloma, plasmacytomas, lymphoma, etc.), surgery is typically reserved only for cases with marked spinal instability or rapid neurologic decline.[2]

Common Clinical Question

1. A patient presents with a large sacral lesion suspicious for tumor. He has no history of cancer and demonstrates mild urinary retention. What is the next best step in management?
   A. Urgent decompression.
   B. Full workup, including CT-guided biopsy.
   C. Follow-up MRI in 6 months.
   D. Urgent preoperative embolization followed by surgical decompression.

Answer to Common Clinical Question

1. B.

References

1. Groves ML, Zadnik PL, Kaloostian P, et al. Epidemiologic, functional, and oncologic outcome analysis of spinal sarcomas treated surgically at a single institution over 10 years. Spine J. 2015; 15(1):110–114
2. Goodwin ML, Buchowski JM, Schwab JH, Sciubba DM. Spinal tumors: diagnosis and treatment. J Am Acad Orthop Surg. 2022; 30(17):e1106–e1121
3. Sundaresan N, Rosen G, Boriani S. Primary malignant tumors of the spine. Orthop Clin North Am. 2009; 40(1):21–36, v
4. Sciubba DM, Gokaslan ZL. Diagnosis and management of metastatic spine disease. Surg Oncol. 2006; 15(3):141–151
5. Knoeller SM, Uhl M, Gahr N, Adler CP, Herget GW. Differential diagnosis of primary malignant bone tumors in the spine and sacrum. The radiological and clinical spectrum: minireview. Neoplasma. 2008; 55(1):16–22
6. Enneking WF, Spanier SS, Goodman MA. A system for the surgical staging of musculoskeletal sarcoma. Clin Orthop Relat Res. 1980(153):106–120
7. Hart RA, Boriani S, Biagini R, Currier B, Weinstein JN. A system for surgical staging and management of spine tumors. A clinical outcome study of giant cell tumors of the spine. Spine. 1997; 22(15):1773–1782, discussion 1783
8. Le Huec JC, Faundez A, Dominguez D, Hoffmeyer P, Aunoble S. Evidence showing the relationship between sagittal balance and clinical outcomes in surgical treatment of degenerative spinal diseases: a literature review. Int Orthop. 2015; 39(1):87–95

21 Surgical Management of Spinal Metastases

Esteban Quiceno, Amna Hussein, Michael Galgano, and Ali A. Baaj

Summary

The effective surgical management of spinal metastases is crucial for spinal surgeons, given the rising incidence of this pathology due to advancements in cancer treatment and increased longevity among oncology patients. Although en bloc resections remain an option for highly specific cases, the NOMS framework should guide management decisions. Separation surgery combined with radiosurgery is considered the standard of care for surgical cases, and spine surgeons should be well versed in this technique and judiciously select appropriate patients for it.

Keywords: oncologic disease, spinal metastases, epidural compression, NOMS framework, radiosurgery, radiotherapy, separation surgery

21.1 Key Points

- Surgical decompression, in addition to adjuvant therapy, is considered the standard in the setting of symptomatic spinal cord compression from epidural tumor disease in most cases.[1]
- The main indications for surgery in metastatic spinal disease are mechanical instability and neural element compression.[2]
- Intralesional gross total or en bloc excisions are usually no longer required and have been replaced by separation surgery to create a safe target for stereotactic radiosurgery through the epidural compression.[3]
- The treatment goals for patients with spinal metastasis are palliative, including preservation of ambulatory status, neurological function, and maintenance of spinal stability.[4]

21.2 Background

- Spinal metastasis is a common entity in oncologic patients. In observation cohort studies of oncologic population with solid tumors, the mean cumulative incidence of spinal metastasis is approximately 15.6%.[5]

- The most common causes of spinal metastasis arise from lung (24.6%), prostate (20.7%), and breast carcinoma (16.5%).[5]
- Spinal metastasis will develop metastatic epidural cord compression in 1 out of 10 patients.[5]
- Metastasis most commonly affects the thoracic spine (70%), followed by the lumbar spine (20%) and cervical spine (10%).[4]
- The NOMS decision framework is an assessment tool to determine the optimal management of patients with metastatic spinal cord compression, which takes into account the neurological, oncological, mechanical, and systemic status of the patient.[4]
- Radiosurgery offers a significantly higher biologic effective dose and more precise dose when compared with external beam radiotherapy.[4]

21.3 Signs, Symptoms, and Physical Examination

- Pain is the initial symptom in 90 to 95% of the patients.[6]
- Classic findings that make malignancy the most likely cause of back pain are: history of malignancy, age more than 50 years, weight loss of more than 10 pounds, lymphadenopathy, and multiple medical visits.[7]
- Pain associated with metastatic spinal tumors can be divided into two: biologic pain and spinal instability associated pain.[8]
- The biologic pain is typically constant, is worse when lying down, and at night. These characteristics are explained as due to the venous compression by the epidural component of the tumor and by the physiological secretion variation of endogenous steroids.[8]
- Pain associated with spinal instability presents with severe movement-related pain that is characteristic to the specific spinal level involved.[8]

21.4 Workup and Neuroimaging

- Every patient with spinal metastasis should undergo a spine computed tomography (CT) of the compromised segment to determine the presence of instability.
- A whole-spine magnetic resonance imaging (MRI) is mandatory to determine the presence of epidural compression and rule out polymetastatic disease.
- Staging with a CT of the chest, abdomen, and pelvis or if available a position emission tomography (PET-CT) is required.[8]
- Before determining the appropriate treatment, the histology of the tumor should be known. This doesn't apply in acute neurological deterioration scenarios where decompression and stabilization are the rule.[8]

- In cases of solitary masses of the spine, the biopsy is the initial approach. Metastatic disease should be differentiated from primary bone tumors; the treatment is radically different.
- Tumors are considered radiosensitive or radioresistant according to their response to conventional external beam radiation.
- Lymphoma, seminoma, and myeloma are considered highly radiosensitive.
- Some solid tumors such as seminomas, breast, prostate, and neuroendocrine carcinomas, and ovarian carcinomas are considered radiosensitive.[4,8]
- Sarcoma, melanoma, and renal cell, thyroid, hepatocellular, colorectal, and non-small cell lung carcinomas are considered radioresistant.[4]
- A six-point grading system[9] describes the degree of epidural spinal cord compression. This system uses an axial T2 MRI sequence at the anatomical point with the most important compression.
- Grade 0 indicates bone-only disease; 1a, epidural impingement without deformation of the thecal sac; 1b, deformation of the thecal sac; 1c, deformation of the thecal sac with spinal cord abutment but without compression; 2, spinal cord compression but cerebrospinal fluid (CSF) visible around the cord; and 3, spinal cord compression and no visible CSF around the cord.
- The assessment of spinal stability depends on clinical and radiological criteria.
- The SINS score (Spinal Instability in Neoplastic Disease) is used to determine the presence of instability. Several factors are analyzed, including: global spine location of the tumor, pain, bone lesion quality, spinal alignment, vertebral body collapse, and posterior involvement.[10]
- In general, palliative surgery is considered in patients with a survival of at least 3 months after the procedure.
- Historically multiple scores have been used; among them is the Tomita and Tokuhashi score, which has yielded results that are difficult to be generalized and tended to be inaccurate.[11]
- The Skeletal Oncology Research Group (SORG) nomogram uses hemoglobin levels, white cell count, age, previous systemic therapy, presence of visceral and brain metastasis, and number of spine metastasis.
- The SORG nomogram also divides the types of cancer into good prognosis (lymphoma, multiple myeloma, breast, kidney, prostate, or thyroid) and poor prognosis (all other types of cancer) and takes into account the ECOG performance status.
- The SORG nomogram has demonstrated the best survival estimation at 1 month, 3 months, and 1 year in approximately 90, 71, and 78% of the cases.[11,12]

21.5 Treatment

- Patients with radiosensitive tumors and no myelopathy can be treated with external beam radiation therapy.[4]
- Radiosurgery has redefined radiosensitivity. It yields a clinical benefit regardless of histology, providing a more durable and symptomatic response and higher local control rates than historical controls using conventional radiotherapy.[4]
- Spinal metastatic diseases with an epidural spinal cord compression of grades 0, 1a, and 1b in the absence of mechanical instability are considered for radiation as initial treatment.
- Tumor grades 2 and 3 require surgical decompression prior to radiation unless the tumor is highly radiosensitive.[8]
- Patients with radioresistant tumors and epidural spinal cord compression of grades 0, 1a, and 1b can be treated with image-guided radiation therapy (stereotactic radiosurgery) which can deliver high doses of radiation in close proximity to the spinal cord.[8]
- Radiosurgery related complications are: esophagitis, mucositis, dysphagia, diarrhea, paresthesia, transient laryngitis, transient radiculitis, and radiation-induced spinal cord injury.[7]
- An important complication associated with radiosurgery is the delayed vertebral body fracture,[13] which is more common in the presence of lytic disease, spinal location at T10 or lower, and high percentage of the vertebral body involved with the disease.
- Lesions with a low SINS score are generally stable and do not require stabilization.
- Lesions with a high SINS score[13,14,15,16,17] require fixation to restore spinal stability.
- Intermediate SINS score tumors require further assessment and are considered a gray zone regarding stabilization.
- Some authors recommend elective stabilization with minimally invasive surgery (MIS) or vertebroplasty in patients with intermediate SINS score who will undergo radiosurgery due to the reported risk of associated vertebral fractures.[14]

21.6 Surgical Pearls

- The main objective of separation surgery is to create a minimum amount of space, 2 to 3 mm margin, between the tumor and spinal cord to allow for safe postoperative radiosurgery.[15]
- Cement augmentation through fenestrated pedicle screws is a safe and effective option in patients with oncologic disease.[16]

- The percutaneous instrumentation should be performed first, usually two levels above and two levels below the affected segment.
- Longer constructs may be required depending on the bone quality and presence of multiple lytic lesions.
- A focal laminectomy or transpedicular approach can be performed at the affected level.
- To access the ventral dura, unilateral or bilateral facetectomies should be performed.
- The transpedicular approach allows a good exposure of the posterior longitudinal ligament and the ventral portion of the tumor.
- Following coagulation and proper hemostasis, the posterior longitudinal ligament should be removed from the superior free tumor edge to the inferior free tumor edge.
- If needed the roots can be sacrificed in the thoracic spine below T2, always proximal to the dorsal root ganglion.[16]
- If an important amount of vertebral body is resected, it can be reconstructed with polymethylmethacrylate or a cage.[16,17]

Common Clinical Questions

1. What is the initial approach for newly diagnosed solitary masses of the spine?
2. What is the current ideal management for radioresistant metastasis of the spine with an epidural component?

Answers to Common Clinical Questions

1. Percutaneous biopsy.
2. Separation surgery + radiosurgery.

References

1. Patchell RA, Tibbs PA, Regine WF, et al. Direct decompressive surgical resection in the treatment of spinal cord compression caused by metastatic cancer: a randomised trial. Lancet. 2005; 366(9486):643–648
2. Sciubba DM, Pennington Z, Colman MW, et al. NASS Spine Oncology Committee. Spinal metastases 2021: a review of the current state of the art and future directions. Spine J. 2021; 21(9):1414–1429
3. Newman WC, Bilsky MH. Fifty-year history of the evolution of spinal metastatic disease management. J Surg Oncol. 2022; 126(5):913–920

4. Barzilai O, Laufer I, Yamada Y, et al. Integrating evidence-based medicine for treatment of spinal metastases into a decision framework: neurologic, oncologic, mechanicals stability, and systemic disease. J Clin Oncol. 2017; 35 (21):2419–2427
5. Van den Brande R, Cornips EM, Peeters M, Ost P, Billiet C, Van de Kelft E. Epidemiology of spinal metastases, metastatic epidural spinal cord compression and pathologic vertebral compression fractures in patients with solid tumors: a systematic review. J Bone Oncol. 2022; 35:100446
6. Jacobs WB, Perrin RG. Evaluation and treatment of spinal metastases: an overview. Neurosurg Focus. 2001; 11(6):e10
7. Bates DW, Reuler JB. Back pain and epidural spinal cord compression. J Gen Intern Med. 1988; 3(2):191–197
8. Laufer I, Rubin DG, Lis E, et al. The NOMS framework: approach to the treatment of spinal metastatic tumors. Oncologist. 2013; 18(6):744–751
9. Bilsky MH, Laufer I, Fourney DR, et al. Reliability analysis of the epidural spinal cord compression scale. J Neurosurg Spine. 2010; 13(3):324–328
10. Fisher CG, DiPaola CP, Ryken TC, et al. A novel classification system for spinal instability in neoplastic disease: an evidence-based approach and expert consensus from the Spine Oncology Study Group. Spine. 2010; 35(22): E1221–E1229
11. Smeijers S, Depreitere B. Prognostic scores for survival as decisional support for surgery in spinal metastases: a performance assessment systematic review. Eur Spine J. 2021; 30(10):2800–2824
12. Paulino Pereira NR, Mclaughlin L, Janssen SJ, et al. The SORG nomogram accurately predicts 3- and 12-months survival for operable spine metastatic disease: external validation. J Surg Oncol. 2017; 115(8):1019–1027
13. Mehta N, Zavitsanos PJ, Moldovan K, et al. Local failure and vertebral body fracture risk using multifraction stereotactic body radiation therapy for spine metastases. Adv Radiat Oncol. 2018; 3(3):245–251
14. Sullivan PZ, Albayar A, Ramayya AG, et al. Association of spinal instability due to metastatic disease with increased mortality and a proposed clinical pathway for treatment. J Neurosurg Spine. 2020:1–8Epub ahead of print
15. Echt M, Stock A, De la Garza Ramos R, et al. Separation surgery for metastatic epidural spinal cord compression: comparison of a minimally invasive versus open approach. Neurosurg Focus. 2021; 50(5):E10
16. Massaad E, Rolle M, Hadzipasic M, Kiapour A, Shankar GM, Shin JH. Safety and efficacy of cement augmentation with fenestrated pedicle screws for tumor-related spinal instability. Neurosurg Focus. 2021; 50(5):E12
17. Moussazadeh N, Laufer I, Yamada Y, Bilsky MH. Separation surgery for spinal metastases: effect of spinal radiosurgery on surgical treatment goals. Cancer Contr. 2014; 21(2):168–174

22 Intradural Extramedullary and Intramedullary Spinal Tumors

Esteban Quiceno, Amna Hussein, Jose Manuel Orenday-Barraza, and Ali A. Baaj

Summary
Intradural extramedullary and intradural intramedullary spine tumors can significantly impact patient's function and quality of life. Their resection should prioritize safety, utilizing adjuncts such as neuromonitoring, ultrasound, and an ultrasonic aspirator, alongside a clean surgical technique. Paramount importance must be placed on arachnoid dissection, and in cases of intramedullary tumors, employing relatively safe entry zones to the spinal cord. This chapter focuses on the surgical technique for the safe resection of intradural spine tumors.

Keywords: intradural, intramedullary, spine tumor, neuromonitoring

22.1 Key Points

- Intradural spinal tumors are divided into intradural extramedullary and intradural intramedullary according to their anatomical location.
- The most common types of intradural extramedullary tumors are: schwannomas, meningiomas, and neurofibromas.[1]
- The most common types of intradural intramedullary tumors are: ependymomas, astrocytomas, and hemangioblastomas.
- Metastatic disease and lymphoma should always be on the differential.
- Diffuse intramedullary enhancing lesions should be differentiated from demyelinating disease.
- The main surgical goal is to achieve gross total resection if clinically indicated.
- The keys are adequate tumor exposure and proper arachnoid dissection.

22.2 Indications

- In general, intradural spinal tumors are considered surgical entities if the patient is symptomatic. In rare cases they can be found incidentally in patients with other spinal complaints.

22.3 Technique

22.3.1 Surgical Technique for Intradural Extramedullary Tumors

- Proper preoperative planning with correct localization of the tumor according to the magnetic resonance imaging (MRI).
- Positioning of the patient in prone position without compression of the abdomen to avoid bleeding due to high venous pressure.
- Neuromonitoring is used during the procedure including somatosensory-evoked potentials (SSEPs), motor-evoked potentials (MEPs), and electromyography (EMG).
- In most cases intradural extramedullary tumors are approached through a midline incision; some exceptions are when a unilateral minimally invasive approach is selected, and a para-median or lateral approach and incision are used. This could be the case with schwannomas that have an important foraminal component without central canal involvement.
- Subperiosteal dissection is performed in a standard fashion.
- Laminectomy without fusion is often feasible. Occasionally, instrumented fusion is indicated if significant facetectomy is anticipated.
- In the thoracic spine, transpedicular or costotransversectomy approach may be needed for ventrally located lesions.
- Intraoperative ultrasound should be used to determine the margins and correct localization of the tumor to have a good surgical exposure. Further bony decompression should be avoided after dural opening.
- The dura is opened longitudinally except in cases of dumbbell schwannomas in which a "T-shaped" incision could be beneficial.
- The dura is tacked up with Nurolon sutures.
- During the dural opening the arachnoid should be preserved.
- Bleeding from the surgical field should be minimized to reduce the rate of chemical meningitis. It is recommended to keep patties at the superior and inferior edges of the exposure.
- After proper arachnoid dissection, a monitoring probe or stimulator should be used in case the tumor has originated from a rootlet or the filum terminale, which is the case with schwannomas and ependymomas, respectively. The stimulation should start at low voltage, 0.1 to 0.3 mV, and should be increased progressively. Sometimes it is difficult to isolate responses from a single rootlet, especially at the lumbar spine (**Fig. 22.1**).
- There is debate regarding the sacrifice of the root in cases of schwannomas that originate in the cervical and lumbar spine due to the fact that these roots are usually considered eloquent.[2] All efforts should be made to preserve motor rootlets.

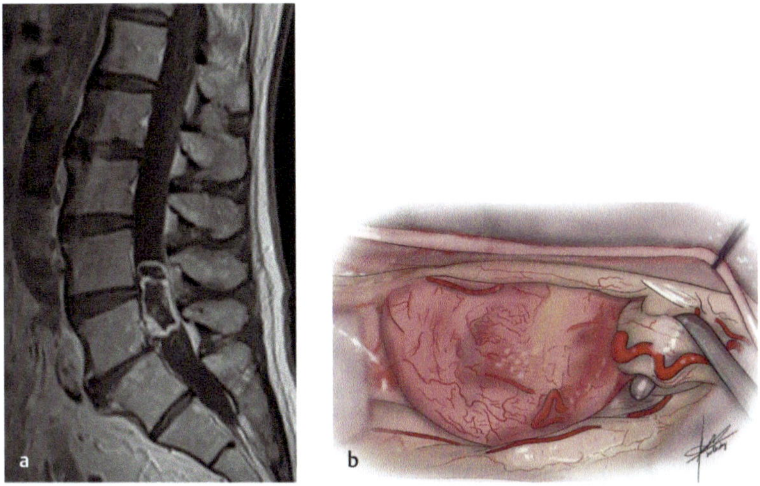

Fig. 22.1 (a) Gadolinium-enhanced sagittal magnetic resonance imaging (MRI) sequence demonstrating cystic lesion in the lumbar intradural extradural space. Final pathology confirmed schwannoma. (b) Schematic illustration demonstrating afferent/efferent rootlet identification that needs to be stimulated prior to sectioning.

- After stimulating, the nerve root attachment or filum terminale should be coagulated and sharply cut.
- In case of meningiomas, the arachnoid from the spinal cord or nerve roots and the tumor should be dissected. In the thoracic and cervical spine, the spinal cord can be safely rolled with gentle traction on the dentate ligament after it is incised (**Fig. 22.2**).
- Usually, intradural extramedullary tumors can be resected en bloc after precise detachment and arachnoid exposure of the upper and lower poles of the tumor.
- In cases of thoracic or cervical tumors, especially in meningiomas, initial debulking with ultrasonic aspirator is helpful to reduce the traction on the spinal cord.
- In cases of meningiomas with Simpson grade I resection, the recurrence rate has been reported to be as low as 0% compared with rates of recurrence as high as 40% in series with higher Simpson resections.[3] Resection of the ventral dura should be avoided due to the risks of cerebrospinal fluid (CSF) leak and spinal cord herniation through the defect. Achieving complete resection of the affected ventral dura and suturing a patch from a posterolateral approach can be technically demanding.[4]

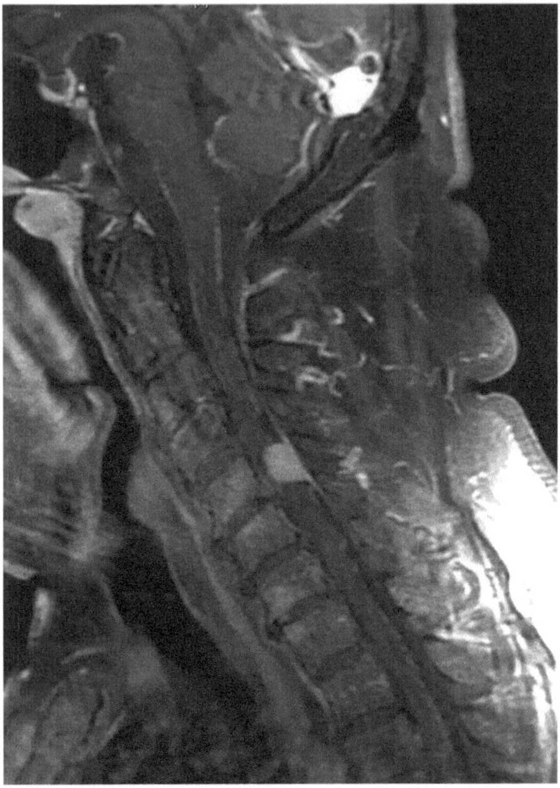

Fig. 22.2 Gadolinium-enhanced sagittal magnetic resonance imaging (MRI) sequence demonstrating avidly enhancing dural-based lesion in the cervical spine. Final pathology confirmed meningioma.

- For meningiomas we don't recommend peeling off the inner and external dural layers because histopathological studies have showed residual tumor cell infiltrates between the inner and outer dural layers. Instead if dural resection is not completed, we recommend coagulating the dural attachment of the tumor.[4]
- Watertight dural closure is of paramount importance to avoid complications such as CSF leak and meningocele.
- Leaving a subfascial drain without negative pressure is optional but it is our preference.
- Instrumentation after an intradural extramedullary tumor is typically not required except in cases of preoperative instability or deformity, significant facetectomy, or destabilizing laminectomy.

22.3.2 Surgical Technique for Intradural Intramedullary Tumors

- As in extramedullary tumors, preoperative planning according to the extension of the tumor and levels involved on the MRI is a must.
- During surgery for intramedullary tumors SSEPs will almost always be affected due to the posterior midline myelotomy approach.
- In addition to MEPs, D wave monitoring (direct waves of the spinal cord) is an important adjunct and may allow continued safe surgical resection of intramedullary lesions even with a significant drop of the MEPs.[5]
- Most of the tumors will be approached with a midline incision in prone position. There are authors who suggest a lateral approach through a lateral or lateral oblique position for high cervical tumors with a predominant intramedullary lateral location to be approached through the dorsal root entry zone (**Fig. 22.3**).
- The disadvantage of the dorsal root entry zone approach is the greater chance of neurological deficit related to its proximity with the lateral columns.
- Prior to the myelotomy, the midline should be identified, which is difficult in intramedullary tumors due to the deformation and change of shape of the spinal cord.
- Intraoperative mapping of the anatomic trajectory of the posterior tracts[6] is one option to find the median sulcus. Another option is identifying the area where multiple small vessels are diving into the midline.[7]
- Coagulation of the multiple veins that come from the posterior median sulcus can be done if needed. It should be done with the bipolar in a low mode (8–10 power intensity).
- The myelotomy can be performed with a number 11 blade, with continuous dissection with gentle opening and closure of bipolar forceps.
- 10/0 sutures can be used to tack up the pial borders of the myelotomy.
- A biopsy as the initial step is mandatory. In the case of ependymomas gross total resection should be pursued.
- In cases of low-grade or high-grade astrocytoma, resection should be pursued only if there are clear planes and if intraoperative monitoring (IOM) continues to be favorable during attempted resection (**Fig. 22.4**).
- Hemangioblastomas are usually superficial and make an appearance into the pial surface, which makes an extensive myelotomy unnecessary.
- When resecting a hemangioblastoma the main draining veins should be preserved until the feeding arteries are well controlled.
- We avoid leaving any hemostatic material inside the tumoral cavity. Usually with proper surgical technique and patience good hemostasis is achieved.
- Laminoplasty is an option in patients with intramedullary cervical tumors, especially in the growing spine.[8]

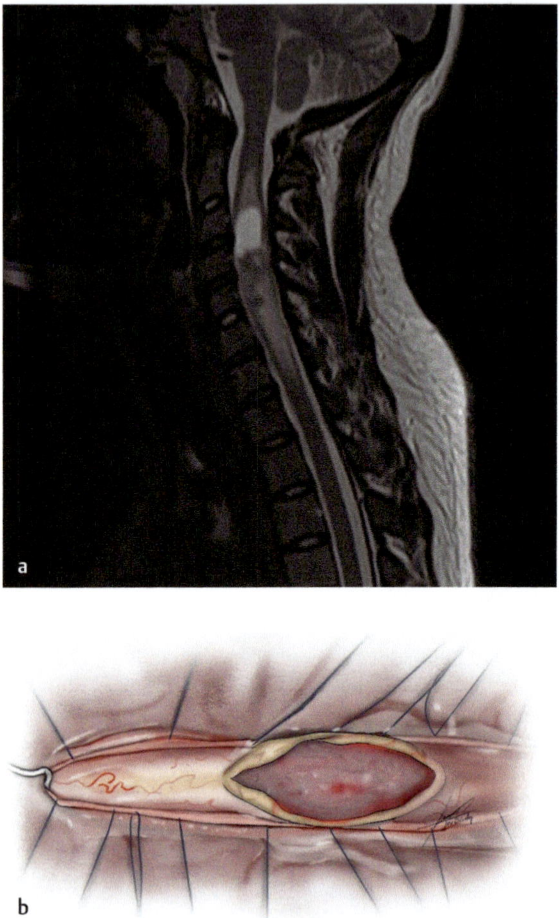

Fig. 22.3 (a) T2-weighted sagittal magnetic resonance imaging (MRI) sequence demonstrating cystic, mixed-signal intramedullary lesion proven to be ependymoma. (b) Schematic illustration demonstrating dural opening and midline myelotomy for access to intramedullary lesions.

22.4 Complications

- The main complications after the resection of intradural extramedullary tumors and intramedullary tumors are CSF leak and neurological deterioration respectively.

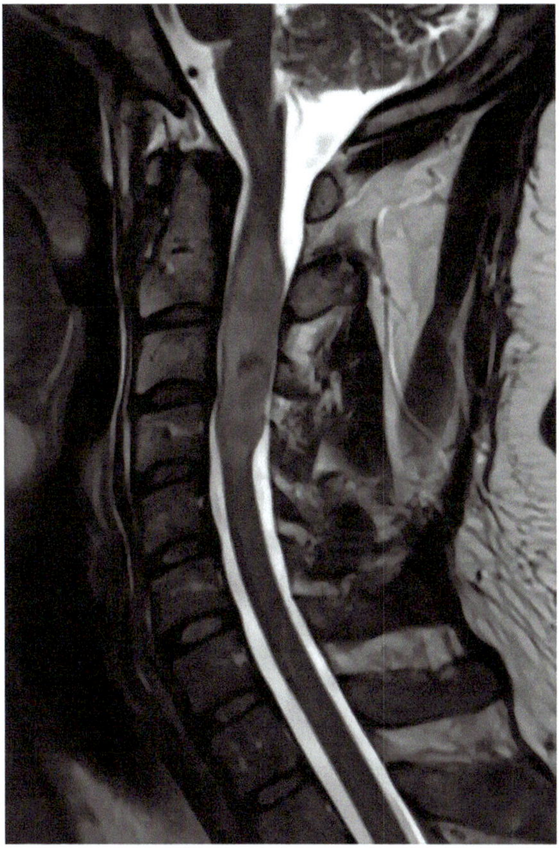

Fig. 22.4 T2-weighted sagittal magnetic resonance imaging (MRI) sequence demonstrating expansile intramedullary lesion with pathology consistent with high-grade astrocytoma.

- CSF leak in intradural extramedullary tumors is approximately 5%.[9]
- Immediate postoperative neurological deficit in intramedullary tumors can be as high as 50%, with various degrees of improvement in the months to follow.[10]

22.5 Postoperative Care

- Intramedullary tumors require postoperative observation in intensive care unit (ICU) during the first 24 to 48 hours to maintain the spinal cord perfusion.

- Steroids are weaned progressively.
- Postoperative MRI within 2 to 4 weeks is recommended to serve as a baseline for the annual surveillance imaging (especially for intramedullary tumors).

22.6 Surgical Pearls

- Accurate and precise localization of the levels involved and lesion using fluoroscopy and ultrasound is critical.
- Understanding IOM and how it can change, as well as how to address signal changes, is an important aspect of spinal intradural tumor surgery.
- Rarely is instrumented fusion necessary during middle approaches for intradural tumors.

22.7 Outcomes

- The neurological outcome will depend on the preoperative neurological status.
- Resection of intradural extramedullary tumors is usually associated with improved disability, pain, and health status.[11]
- The best predictor of a good outcome in intramedullary tumors is the preoperative ability to walk,[12] and high-grade tumors have poor neurological outcomes.

Common Clinical Questions

1. What are the common IOM modalities in spinal intradural tumor surgery?
2. When should angiography be considered preoperatively?
3. How is a drop in MEPs addressed during spinal tumor surgery resection?

Answers to Common Clinical Questions

1. EMG/SSEP/MEP for extramedullary lesions; additionally D wave monitoring should be considered for intramedullary lesions.
2. When hemangioblastoma or other vascular lesions are suspected.
3. Check the IOM wire leads; check with anesthesia if relaxants were administered or if blood pressure has dropped. Administer additional steroid dose if needed. If signals do not respond and return to previous baseline, discontinuing further resection of intramedullary lesion may be considered.

References

1. Koeller KK, Shih RY. Intradural extramedullary spinal neoplasms: radiologic-pathologic correlation. Radiographics. 2019; 39(2):468–490
2. Kim P, Ebersold MJ, Onofrio BM, Quast LM. Surgery of spinal nerve schwannoma. Risk of neurological deficit after resection of involved root. J Neurosurg. 1989; 71(6):810–814
3. Klekamp J, Samii M. Surgical results for spinal meningiomas. Surg Neurol. 1999; 52(6):552–562
4. Nakamura M, Tsuji O, Fujiyoshi K, et al. Long-term surgical outcomes of spinal meningiomas. Spine. 2012; 37(10):E617–E623
5. Olmsted ZT, Ryu B, Phayal G, et al. Direct wave intraoperative neuromonitoring for spinal tumor resection: a focused review. World Neurosurg X. 2022; 17: 100139
6. Yanni DS, Ulkatan S, Deletis V, Barrenechea IJ, Sen C, Perin NI. Utility of neurophysiological monitoring using dorsal column mapping in intramedullary spinal cord surgery. J Neurosurg Spine. 2010; 12(6):623–628
7. Takami T, Naito K, Yamagata T, Ohata K. Surgical management of spinal intramedullary tumors: radical and safe strategy for benign tumors. Neurol Med Chir (Tokyo). 2015; 55(4):317–327
8. Sun S, Li Y, Wang X, et al. Safety and efficacy of laminoplasty versus laminectomy in the treatment of spinal cord tumors: a systematic review and meta-analysis. World Neurosurg. 2019; 125:136–145
9. Cofano F, Giambra C, Costa P, et al. Management of extramedullary intradural spinal tumors: the impact of clinical status, intraoperative neurophysiological monitoring and surgical approach on outcomes in a 12-year double-center experience. Front Neurol. 2020; 11:598619
10. Jecko V, Roblot P, Mongardi L, et al. Intramedullary spinal cord lesions: a single-center experience. Neurospine. 2022; 19(1):108–117
11. Newman WC, Berry-Candelario J, Villavieja J, et al. Improvement in quality of life following surgical resection of benign intradural extramedullary tumors: a prospective evaluation of patient-reported outcomes. Neurosurgery. 2021; 88(5):989–995
12. Lee SM, Cho YE, Kwon YM. Neurological outcome after surgical treatment of intramedullary spinal cord tumors. Korean J Spine. 2014; 11(3):121–126

23 Cervical and Thoracic Spine Degenerative Disease

Jean-Valery Coumans

Summary

Cervical degenerative disease can be associated with disk herniations and stenosis. A subset of patients requires surgical intervention for persistent symptoms. A neurological examination combined with imaging is used to confirm the diagnosis. The choice of surgical approach is dictated by the location of the compression relative to the spinal cord, the extent of the stenosis, and the overall sagittal alignment.

Keywords: cervical stenosis, cervical myelopathy, cervical laminectomy, ACDF, laminoplasty

23.1 Key Points

- There is a continuum between the normal aging of the spine and symptomatic degeneration.[1,2]
- Cervical and thoracic degenerative disease is a chronic condition but can present acutely.
- Magnetic resonance imaging (MRI) is usually the imaging modality of choice for diagnosis.
- Weight-bearing X-rays provide information on sagittal and coronal balance.
- Radicular and axial pain may be treated conservatively, but myelopathy and/or worsening neurologic function generally requires surgical intervention.

23.2 Cervical Disk Herniation

23.2.1 Background

- Dehydration, fissuring, and fragmentation of the nucleus pulposus of cervical disks with age are natural processes.[1,2]
- The annulus and the posterior longitudinal ligament may tear, allowing the nucleus to herniate into the spinal canal, where it may compress the cord and/or the adjacent root at its foramen.[2]

- Acute disk rupture occurs more often laterally in the spinal canal due to the relative weakness of the posterior longitudinal ligament in that area; as a result, root compression occurs more often than cord compression.
- Most herniations resolve spontaneously as the fragment involutes.

23.2.2 Signs, Symptoms, and Physical Examination

- The pain correlates most closely with the affected myotome, whereas numbness and paresthesia correlate with the affected dermatome.[3]
- Lateral disk herniations cause pain that radiates from the neck to the shoulder/arm and into the hand; disk usually impinges on nerve exiting from the neural foramen at the level of the herniation (e.g., a C6/C7 disk causes C7 radiculopathy).
- C5 symptoms: Shoulder abduction (deltoid and supraspinatus) weakness; lateral upper arm paresthesias; deltoid and pectoralis reflexes diminished.[3] Can resemble rotator cuff tear; be sure to test shoulder.[3]
- C6 symptoms: Forearm flexion (biceps) weakness; upper arm, thumb, and radial forearm sensory alteration; biceps and brachioradialis reflexes diminished.[3]
- C7 symptoms: Latissimus dorsi (shoulder adduction), elbow extension (triceps), and finger extension weakness; second- and third-digit sensory alteration; triceps reflex diminished. Pain often occurs over latissimus dorsi, mimicking posterior chest wall pain and not to be confused with thoracic radiculopathy. Symptoms are often alleviated with shoulder abduction or shrug (to decrease nerve tension).[3]
- C8 symptoms: Intrinsic hand muscle weakness; fourth- and fifth-digit sensory alteration; finger-jerk reflex diminished (rarely used).[3]
- Central disk herniation can cause myelopathy and central cord syndrome.

23.2.3 Workup

- Complete history and physical.
- Neuroimaging studies based on localization of signs and symptoms (**Fig. 23.1**)[4]:
  - MRI is the imaging modality of choice for visualizing soft tissue and the spinal cord/nerve roots.[4]
  - Use CT or CT myelogram when MRI cannot be done.[4]
  - Plain CT is good for bone detail and evaluation of the foraminal size.
  - Plain X-rays are good for bone imaging, anteroposterior/lateral views are useful for visualizing alignment, and flexion–extension views are useful for assessing subluxation/dynamic instability (instability with movement).

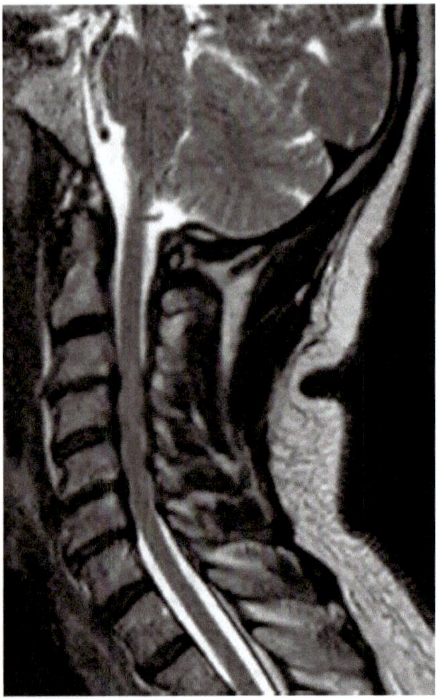

Fig. 23.1 Magnetic resonance imaging (MRI) is the imaging modality of choice for visualizing soft tissue and the spinal cord/nerve roots but cannot distinguish between disk and bone.

23.2.4 Treatment

- More than 80% of patients who have acute cervical radiculopathy as a result of cervical disk herniation can improve without surgery.
- Surgery is indicated for those who fail to improve or those who have progressive neurologic deficit while undergoing nonsurgical management.
- Anterior surgical options: Anterior cervical diskectomy with bone graft/ cage insertion and plating (ACDF), or artificial disk (arthroplasty), anterior cervical foraminotomy (done less commonly).
- Posterior surgical options: Posterior cervical laminectomy/foraminotomy with or without fusion, keyhole laminectomy (for lateral "soft disk" herniation).[5]

23.2.5 Surgical Pearls

- Posterior approaches are not well suited when the compressive pathology is anterior to the spinal cord.[5]

- Partial or complete corpectomy may be required if herniated disk is sequestered posterior to vertebral body and is not accessible by diskectomy.

23.3 Cervical Spondylotic Myelopathy

23.3.1 Background

- Caused by the reduction of the sagittal diameter of the cervical spinal canal as a result of congenital and degenerative changes.[2]
- Often caused by degeneration of the intervertebral disk producing a focal stenosis as a result of a “cervical bar” that is usually a combination of osteophytic spurs and/or protrusion of disk material.
- Most common type of spinal cord dysfunction in patients older than 55 years.
- Cord injury likely occurs as the result of several interrelated factors: Direct compression of the cord, microtrauma associated with neck flexion and extension, and vascular injury.[2]
- Signs and symptoms may overlap with those of amyotrophic lateral sclerosis (ALS; also known as motor neuron disease). Both conditions may present with upper motor neuron findings in the lower extremities (hyperreflexia, spasticity) and lower motor neuron findings in the upper extremities (weakness, hyporeflexia). However, sensory disturbance is only present in cervical myelopathy. Dysarthria and tongue fasciculations may occur in ALS.

23.3.2 Signs, Symptoms, and Physical Examination

- Cervical pain can occur and is related to the degenerative disease that often accompanies myelopathy.
- Earliest motor findings are typically weakness in the triceps, finger extensors, and hand intrinsic muscles (lower cervical myotomes are affected at all levels involved).
- Gait disturbance, often with lower extremity weakness or stiffness, is a common finding.
- Clumsiness with fine motor skills (writing, texting, buttoning).
- Glove-distribution sensory loss in the hands or sensory level below the area of cord compression.
- Hyperactive reflexes below the level of stenosis, pathologic reflexes (Hoffmann’s, Babinski, clonus, etc.).
- Hypertonia may be observed on passive movement of the extremities.
- Central cord syndrome, characterized by motor and sensory deficits affecting the upper extremities more than the lower extremities, may occur acutely after trauma with hyperextension in those who have cervical stenosis.

23.3.3 Workup

- Complete history and physical.
- Neuroimaging studies based on localization of signs and symptoms.
  - Plain X-ray: Good for bone imaging. May demonstrate narrow canal (posterior vertebral line to spinolaminar line < 12 mm). Flexion–extension view may demonstrate dynamic instability.
  - MRI is the imaging modality of choice for visualizing soft tissue and the spinal cord and nerve roots. Acute disks are hyperintense on T2 images to normal disks; osteophytes are hypointense to disks on T2 images. T2 hyperintensity in the spinal cord is generally an indicator of cord edema or ischemia and affects the recommendation for surgery (**Fig. 23.2**).[4]
  - Plain CT: Good for bone imaging. May demonstrate a narrow canal but does not provide adequate information regarding soft tissues.
  - CT myelogram: Used when MRI cannot be done. Can still visualize spinal cord/nerve roots but does not provide information about changes within the spinal cord parenchyma.

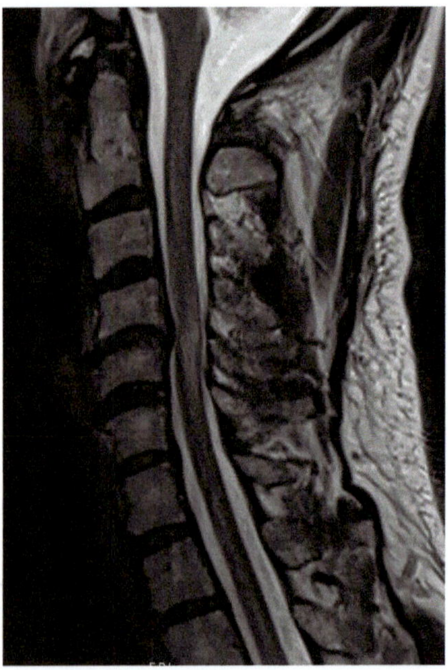

Fig. 23.2 T2 sagittal magnetic resonance imaging (MRI) scan showing disk/osteophyte with cord compression at C4–C5 and myelomalacia (T2 signal hyperintensity in the spinal cord).

23.3.4 Treatment

- Nonoperative management (eliminating "high-risk" activities, monitoring symptoms) may be considered for mild myelopathy.
- There is a 20 to 40% chance of needing surgery at 5 years after initial diagnosis of minimally symptomatic cervical stenosis.
- More severe myelopathy should be treated with surgical decompression.
- Surgical approaches:
  - Posterior: Not ideal for correction of kyphotic deformity. Preferred for most cases of myelopathy due to ossification of the posterior longitudinal ligament (OPLL).[5]
    - Laminectomy alone (higher incidence of late kyphotic deformity, ideal for rapid and simple decompression in elderly patients).[5]
    - Laminectomy + instrumentation/fusion (affords stabilization and some correction of kyphosis).
    - Laminoplasty (preserves movement, ideal if patient is younger and has a congenitally narrow canal).
  - Anterior: Ideal for correction of kyphotic deformities.[6]
    - Anterior cervical diskectomy and fusion (ACDF).
    - Arthroplasty.
    - Corpectomy and fusion: When compression extends beyond region of disk space.

23.3.5 Surgical Pearls

- Choice of approach is largely affected by the location of the compression.
- In general, older patients with multilevel compression and preserved lordosis can undergo a laminectomy.[5]
- In general, young patients with a congenitally narrow canal in whom it is desirable to preserve movement are good candidates for a laminoplasty.[6]
- Patients with loss of lordosis and one to three levels of anterior cord compression are treated with anterior approaches.
- MRI scan is done in the supine position and does not provide reliable information on cervical lordosis which is best assessed with a weight-bearing lateral X-ray.[2]

Common Clinical Questions

1. Physical therapy and pain management should be the treatment of choice initially for patients with severe cervical stenosis and myelopathy. True or false?
2. A laminectomy without fusion is a good treatment option for patients with multilevel cervical stenosis, neck pain and radiculopathy, and cervical kyphosis. True or false?

Answers to Common Clinical Questions

1. False.
2. False.

References

1. Matsumoto M, Okada E, Ichihara D, et al. Age-related changes of thoracic and cervical intervertebral discs in asymptomatic subjects. Spine. 2010; 35(14): 1359–1364
2. Nouri A, Tetreault L, Singh A, Karadimas SK, Fehlings MG. Degenerative cervical myelopathy: epidemiology, genetics, and pathogenesis. Spine. 2015; 40(12):E675–E693
3. Abbed KM, Coumans JV. Cervical radiculopathy: pathophysiology, presentation, and clinical evaluation. Neurosurgery. 2007; 60(1) Supp1 1: S28–S34
4. McDonald MA, Kirsch CFE, Amin BY, et al. Expert Panel on Neurological Imaging. ACR Appropriateness Criteria® cervical neck pain or cervical radiculopathy. J Am Coll Radiol. 2019; 16 5S:S57–S76
5. Rissanen A, Hämäläinen M, Marjamaa J, et al. Long-term follow-up after cervical laminectomy without fusion for cervical spondylotic myelopathy. World Neurosurg. 2022; 167:e222–e235
6. Ghogawala Z, Terrin N, Dunbar MR, et al. Effect of ventral vs dorsal spinal surgery on patient-reported physical functioning in patients with cervical spondylotic myelopathy: a randomized clinical trial. JAMA. 2021; 325(10): 942–951

24 Degenerative Lumbar Spine Disease

Juan Emmerich

Summary

This chapter discusses degenerative lumbar spine disease, emphasizing its prevalence due to natural aging, environmental factors, and genetic predisposition. Key conditions include the following:

Radicular pain is diagnosed by correlating pain distribution with nerve root compression seen on imaging. Conservative treatment is preferred initially, with surgery considered if conservative methods fail, focusing on nerve decompression techniques like laminoforaminotomy or microdiskectomy.

Neurogenic claudication presents with leg symptoms induced by walking, often managed conservatively but may require surgical decompression like laminectomy with foraminotomies.

Axial back pain from disk disease may require surgical intervention if conservative measures fail, typically involving disk removal or fusion procedures.

Facet joint disease manifests with pain worsened by back extension and is diagnosed using MRI and injections for confirmation. Treatment involves injections or rhizolysis, alongside physical therapy.

Spondylolisthesis may necessitate decompression and fusion, with options like laminectomy and instrumented fusion considered.

Degenerative scoliosis/kyphosis requires comprehensive preoperative planning due to its complexity. Treatment options vary based on symptoms, degree of deformity, and patient factors, aiming to restore spinal balance.

Surgical pearls emphasize careful surgical approaches to preserve spinal stability and nerve function. Overall, treatment decisions are guided by symptom severity, imaging findings, and patient-specific factors, with a range of surgical and conservative options available.

Keywords: lumbar spine, degenerative pathology, radicular pain, neurogenic claudication, spondylolisthesis, back pain

24.1 Key Points

- Degenerative disease of the spine is a ubiquitous problem and a part of the natural aging process. It includes a group of different pathologies that have

a big impact in the quality of life of the patients. Treatment, surgical or otherwise, is directed at specific symptoms, pathologies, and syndromes.
- Skeletoligamentous disorders are typically the result of intervertebral disk disease or facet disease or both. Sacroiliac and hip joint pain can also be contributors to back pain.
- Determining the "pain generator" is not always straightforward, because different modalities of degenerative disease could be present in the same patient, and determination of the main cause usually requires a synthesis of data from the medical history, physical examination, provocative testing, and imaging.

24.2 Background

- Degeneration of the lumbar spine is the result of natural aging, environmental insults, and genetic predisposition.
- Comorbidities, such as smoking, diabetes, and especially obesity, could play a big role in the development of the disease.
- Degenerative changes may be asymptomatic.[1]
- Specific disease states, such as rheumatoid arthritis and ankylosing spondylitis, can accelerate or alter the pathology and clinical presentations.
- Changes that develop over time include loss of water volume within the nucleus pulposus with loss of disk height, disk bulging, facet joint degeneration, and osteophyte formation across the joints (both the intervertebral disks and facet joints). Eventual loss of motion occurs.

24.3 Specific Conditions

24.3.1 Radicular Pain

- Signs, symptoms, and physical examination:
  - Diagnosis requires a correlation between the pain distribution and the compressed nerve root identified on imaging. The correlation with the clinical presentation is particularly important because the patient could have small–medium compression in the MRI without symptoms.
  - Sharp, shooting pain in a given dermatome, but it sometimes may be dull or aching.
  - Pain, the most frequent symptom, followed by paresthesias, weakness, and diminished reflexes can be found on examination.
- Workup and neuroimaging:
  - Diagnostic testing includes MRI, the current gold standard, CT scan (if the offending pathology is suspected to be osseous), and X-rays to assess the general alignment and the stability of the spine.

  - If there is doubt about the level or location of the pathology, a test nerve root injection with anesthetic may be diagnostically helpful. Electromyography (EMG) is also frequently used to confirm the radiculopathy or to distinguish it from a peripheral nerve problem.
  - Classic pathology is a paracentral disk herniation. Other possibilities include compression as a result of foraminal collapse, facet joint overgrowth, or a far lateral disk herniation.
- Treatment:
  - Conservative treatment is usually the first option, with a combination of pain medicine, and anti-inflammatory drugs, opioids, and injections, with good results, especially in medium paracentral disk herniation.
  - When the conservative treatment (following the correct guidelines) fails to control the symptoms, surgical treatment is the recommended option.
  - Treatment of radiculopathy is directed at nerve decompression. This can be done with a laminoforaminotomy or microdiskectomy. Different techniques from traditional approach to minimal invasive techniques such as tubular decompression or endoscopy decompression are accepted options, each one with pros and cons.
  - In cases in which compression is caused by foraminal collapse resulting from loss of spinal alignment (e.g., spondylolisthesis or degenerative scoliosis), a fusion with intervertebral height restoration may be indicated.
- Surgical pearls:
  - During a laminoforaminotomy, or microdiskectomy, care must be taken to avoid excessive facet joint removal. These joints are critical to the stability of the spine, and no more than half of a joint should be removed in a unilateral approach.
  - After surgical decompression, scar formation can result in radiculitis or, rarely, arachnoiditis. Minimizing manipulation and nerve root retraction may be helpful.

24.3.2 Neurogenic Claudication

- Signs, symptoms, and physical examination:
  - Diagnosis is highly dependent on the history. Patients typically complain of unilateral or bilateral leg pain, numbness, and weakness that can be precipitated by walking or standing.
  - The physical examination is frequently completely normal.
  - The ability to walk farther when bending forward (such as when pushing a shopping cart) is classic.
  - Vascular claudication is suggested when relief occurs with rest without the need to flex at the waist and must be ruled out by evaluating peripheral pulses (for suspected cases, an ankle–brachial index [ABI] may be useful).

- Workup and neuroimaging:
  - Diagnostic testing includes an MRI, the current gold standard, or CT myelogram to evaluate the size of the lumbar spinal canal and neuroforamina.
  - Compression may result from congenital stenosis, disk bulging, ligamentum flavum hypertrophy, facet joint overgrowth, or spondylolisthesis or any combination of these.
- Treatment:
  - Conservative treatment is not as effective as in acute irradiation pain, but helps to reduce symptoms, which could be important in elderly patients or patients with comorbidities to delay or even avoid the surgical treatment.
  - Surgical intervention is directed at patients who have failed conservative measures, such as epidural injections, and includes decompression with the possibility of an adjunct fusion.
  - Standard treatment involves the use of a midline laminectomy with foraminotomies.
  - Unilateral hemilaminotomy for bilateral decompression is another less invasive option that preserves more of the skeletoligamentous structures.
- Surgical pearls:
  - Curved Kerrison rongeurs can be useful to reach out to the distal foramina and should be placed on the caudal and dorsal aspect of the foramen; this being the least likely location for the exiting nerve root.
  - In performing a hemilaminotomy for bilateral decompression, care should be taken to preserve the ipsilateral ligamentum flavum, which will displace the dura ventrally. This reduces the risk of dural injury while work is being performed on the contralateral nerve roots. Ipsilateral decompression can be performed after the opposite side has been decompressed.
  - It is important to perform a lateral decompression of the canal, not just a central decompression, because the symptoms rarely improve unless a correct release of all the nervous structures is achieved.
  - MISS procedure, especially tubular surgery, could be a good option in patients with comorbidities, particular in the elderly.

24.3.3 Axial Back Pain from Intervertebral Disk Disease (without Deformity)

- Signs, symptoms, and physical examination:
  - The most classic disk-related mechanical pain syndromes present as pain that worsens with activity and lessens with rest.
  - Anterior thigh pain can also be associated with low back pain, as the symptoms may follow a somatotopic pattern.

 - Physical examination may reveal pain relief with extension maneuvers and provocation with flexion, although these findings are not universal.
 - It is important to eliminate other insidious causes of axial pain, such as infection or malignancies.
- Workup
 - MRI to examine the disk and neighboring structures.
 - CT myelogram when MRI is contraindicated.
 - Flexion–extension films to rule out spondylolisthesis.
- Neuroimaging:
 - The disk nucleus progressively loses the high signal on T2 (so-called black disk), and loss of disk height will also occur.
 - Adjacent bony end plates may exhibit high T2 signal, classified as Modic changes, that shows a compromise of the end plate.
 - Plain X-rays may also reveal degeneration, but dynamic flexion and extension views may be more effective in revealing any instability.
 - CT scans may demonstrate osteophytes and are less useful. In marginal cases, a provocative diskogram can be used to assess the disk's internal morphology and ability to tolerate the injectate's pressure, as well as any symptoms associated with injection.[2]
- Treatment:
 - Treatment of disk-related pain remains controversial and requires that patients must have failed conservative treatment measures.
 - For patients who have intractable symptoms and demonstrable pathology, treatment may be directed at disk removal or the elimination of motion, but there is some controversy about the ideal indication and the best timing for performing the surgical treatment.
 - This can be performed with a posterolateral instrumented fusion; anterior (ALIF), posterior (PLIF), or transforaminal lumbar interbody fusion (TLIF); lateral interbody fusion; extreme lateral interbody fusion (XLIF); or total disk arthroplasty.[3]
- Surgical pearls:
 - It is generally believed that if surgical treatment of disk-related pain is warranted, then an interbody fusion is preferable to posterolateral fusion.
 - For patients who will undergo disk arthroplasty, care must be taken to exclude those who have facet disease, as the posterior joints must continue to function after the operation.

24.3.4 Axial Back Pain from Facet Joint Disease

- Signs, symptoms, and physical examination:
 - The zygapophyseal joint (facet joint) is a synovial joint that is prone to arthritic changes and is a possible pain generator (**Fig. 24.1**).
 - Pain that worsens with provocative maneuvers such as back extension may be a simple diagnostic clue.

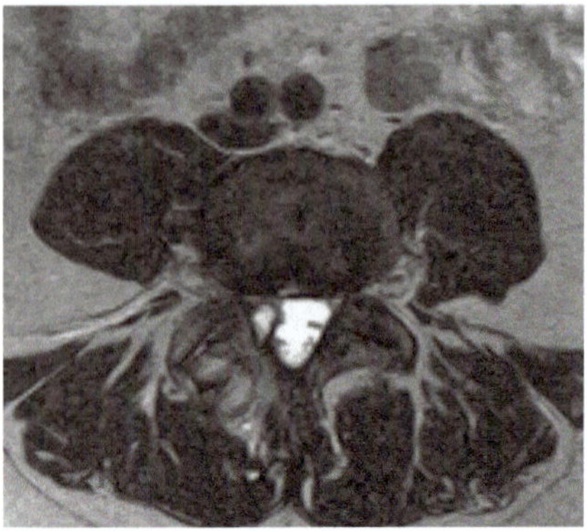

Fig. 24.1 Right synovial cyst causing radiculopathy at the L5/S1 level.

- Facet pain can radiate into the lower extremity, mimicking a painful radiculopathy.

- Workup:
  - MRI, flexion–extension X-ray, and single-photon emission computed tomography (SPECT) bone scan are helpful.
  - The definitive diagnostic test is an anesthetic or steroid injection (controversy surrounds the relative efficacy of intra-articular versus periarticular joint injections).
  - Hip or sacroiliac joint pathology must also be considered as a possible source of "back pain," and requires a good examination of this joints to avoid an incorrect diagnosis.
- Neuroimaging:
  - High T2 signal in the joint as well as increased focal uptake on SPECT bone scans can be valuable predictors.[4]
- Treatment:
  - Interventional treatment of isolated facet joint disease is with anesthetic/steroid injections or dorsal ramus rhizolysis.
  - In addition, physical therapy and anti-inflammatory medications are often helpful.
- Surgical pearls:
  - Obtain dynamic films to rule out spondylolisthesis.
  - Fusion/fixation of the facet joint remains controversial.

24.3.5 Spondylolisthesis

- Signs, symptoms, and physical examination:
  - Spondylolisthesis may be the result of congenital, traumatic, degenerative, or iatrogenic etiologies.

- A degenerative spondylolisthesis typically affects the L4–L5 level, although any level may become involved.
- A fatigue fracture of the pars followed by progression of slippage may also be classified as a form of degeneration caused by chronic mechanical load.
- The clinical syndrome may cause leg pain, back pain, or both.

• Workup:
  - MRI and flexion–extension films are mandatory.
• Neuroimaging:
  - Diagnostic testing can include MRI to evaluate neural entrapment. Flexion–extension X-rays are mandatory to assess the gross stability of the level, which affects treatment decisions (**Fig. 24.2**).
• Treatment:
  - Typically involves decompression and fusion. A common approach is laminectomy for decompression followed by instrumented fusion.
  - Controversy exists over the utility of correcting the slippage.
  - The use of interbody fusion increases the rate of arthrodesis but poses the threat of higher complication rates.

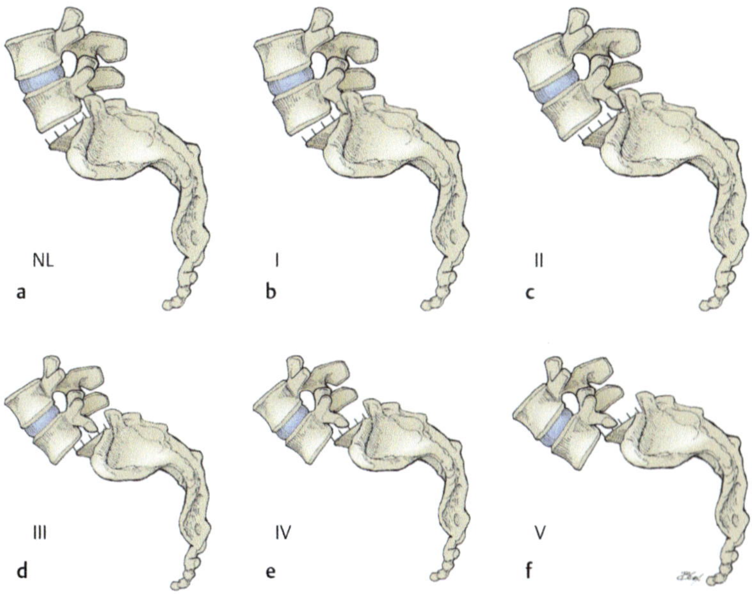

Fig. 24.2 **(a–f)** Meyerding classification of spondylolisthesis: **(a)** Normal; **(b)** Grade I: 0 to 25%; **(c)** Grade II: 26 to 50%; **(d)** Grade III: 51 to 75%; **(e)** Grade IV: 76 to 100%; **(f)** Grade V: > 100% (spondyloptosis).

- Surgical pearls:
  - High-grade slips where realignment is desired can often be treated more effectively by instrumenting the level above (L4–S1 in a L5/S1 slip) to bring the middle intermediary screw up to a rod connecting the two end screws.
  - The exiting nerve root at the slip level is displaced ventrally. Aggressive correction of a high-grade slip can result in foot drop. Close EMG monitoring for nerve root irritation may allow assessment of the stretch/ tension on this structure.

24.3.6 Degenerative Scoliosis and Kyphosis

- Signs, symptoms, and physical examination:
  - Evaluation of patients with spinal deformity requires not only a standard physical examination, but also an assessment of the patient's standing and lying postures.
  - Any progression of deformity should also be evaluated with serial imaging. The frequent coincidence of hip and sacroiliac joint arthritis and leg length discrepancies needs to be assessed.
  - Because this disease entity typically affects older females, an evaluation of bone density may be warranted and appropriate measures to augment bone density must be undertaken.
  - In addition, assessment of any contributing hip flexion contractures may be necessary.
- Workup:
  - Diagnostic imaging requires an assessment of neural element integrity (MRI or myelography) and disk and facet joint disease, as well as local and global spinal alignment.
- Neuroimaging:
  - MRI, dynamic X-rays, and CT scanning are essential for preoperative planning.
  - To determine coronal alignment (Cobb angle) and loss of sagittal balance, 36-inch standing X-rays are mandatory.
- Treatment:
  - The treatment of this patient population is complicated, requiring significant investment in preoperative planning, surgical intervention, and postoperative care. Critical decision-making factors include the following:
    - Source and nature of complaints (pain, reduced activities of daily living [ADLs], neurologic symptoms, abnormal postures, cosmetic concerns).
    - The degree of deformity and its relative contribution to the patient's symptoms.

    - The extent (levels and amount of correction) of the deformity that needs treating.
    - The amount (quality and number of levels) of fixation needed.
    - The surgical technique necessary to achieve correction.
    - Need for fusion adjuncts (osteobiologics, bracing, and bone stimulation).
    - Anesthetic considerations and risks.
    - Nutrition and metabolic concerns.
    - The extent to which rehabilitation will be necessary after surgery.
- Surgical pearls:
  - Careful preoperative planning, including measurements of preoperative sagittal/coronal imbalance, is essential to achieve good clinical and surgical outcomes.
  - There is no clear consensus on which is the best surgical treatment in these cases. While some surgeons prefer the global correction of the balance, others prefer to perform a punctual treatment of the most affected levels without seeking global correction.

Common Clinical Questions

1. Lumbar facet joint pain is best treated with what?
   A. Massage therapy.
   B. Electrostimulation.
   C. Joint injections.
   D. Surgical fusion.
2. Causes of spondylolisthesis include all of the following *except* what?
   A. Neoplastic.
   B. Degenerative.
   C. Traumatic.
   D. Iatrogenic.
3. Studies critical to the evaluation of a spinal deformity include what?
   A. Blood tests for rheumatoid arthritis.
   B. Genetic assessment of predilections for deformity.
   C. SPECT nuclear medicine bone scan.
   D. 36-inch standing X-rays.

Answers to Common Clinical Questions

1. C.
2. A.
3. D.

References

1. Jensen MC, Brant-Zawadzki MN, Obuchowski N, Modic MT, Malkasian D, Ross JS. Magnetic resonance imaging of the lumbar spine in people without back pain. N Engl J Med. 1994; 331(2):69–73
2. Carragee EJ, Chen Y, Tanner CM, Truong T, Lau E, Brito JL. Provocative discography in patients after limited lumbar discectomy: a controlled, randomized study of pain response in symptomatic and asymptomatic subjects. Spine. 2000; 25(23):3065–3071
3. Fujiwara A, Tamai K, Yamato M, et al. The relationship between facet joint osteoarthritis and disc degeneration of the lumbar spine: an MRI study. Eur Spine J. 1999; 8(5):396–401
4. Kim KY, Wang MY. Magnetic resonance image-based morphological predictors of single photon emission computed tomography-positive facet arthropathy in patients with axial back pain. Neurosurgery. 2006; 59(1): 147–156, discussion 147–156

25 Congenital and Neuromuscular Scoliosis

Michael J. Yang, Steven W. Hwang, and Amer F. Samdani

Summary

This chapter summarizes key concepts underlying the etiology, classification, and management of congenital and neuromuscular scoliosis. The chapter will highlight key principles permeating the care of neuromuscular scoliosis in pediatrics such as growth, progression of curvature, the relationship of functional status and curve progression, and risk stratification. Even though the diagnoses are heterogeneous, similar themes are common across all patients, and similar approaches can be used to optimize care and minimize complications. The chapter will touch on proper evaluation of patients with congenital and neuromuscular scoliosis as well as surgical indications and optimization. The chapter will also highlight tricks and tips in the management of these complex patients.

Keywords: congenital, neuromuscular, scoliosis, pediatric, deformity, spine, surgery, outcomes

25.1 Key Points

- Congenital and neuromuscular scoliosis differ from idiopathic scoliosis by the presence of vertebral anomalies and an underlying neurologic disorder, respectively.
- Both conditions may be accompanied by significant medical comorbidities and decreased pulmonary function, necessitating thorough preoperative evaluation.
- Initial treatment is often conservative and may involve bracing. Surgical correction is indicated in cases of severe or progressive scoliosis, particularly in cases of increasing curve magnitude in skeletally immature patients.

25.2 Congenital Scoliosis

- Background:
  - Scoliosis is defined by abnormal coronal curvature of the spine.

- Congenital scoliosis is distinguished from other etiologies of scoliosis by the presence of vertebral anomalies at birth.
- Congenital vertebral anomalies are classified according to the underlying error in embryologic development: (1) failure of formation, (2) failure of segmentation, or (3) failure of both formation and segmentation[1] (**Table 25.1**).
- Incomplete and complete failure of formation result in wedged or completely absent vertebrae, respectively. Asymmetric failure of formation results in a hemivertebra consisting of a single pedicle and hemilamina, which is the most common cause of congenital scoliosis.[2]

Table 25.1 Etiologies of congenital and neuromuscular scoliosis

Congenital scoliosis	Neuromuscular scoliosis[7]
Failure of formation Fully segmented hemivertebra Semi-segmented hemivertebra Incarcerated hemivertebra Nonsegmented hemivertebra Failure of segmentation Unilateral bar Block vertebra Mixed anomalies Dysplastic spondylolisthesis	• Primary neuropathies – Upper motor neuron pathology ▪ Cerebral palsy ▪ Spinocerebellar degeneration ▪ Charcot-Marie-Tooth disease ▪ Syringomyelia ▪ Spinal cord tumor ▪ Spinal cord trauma – Lower motor neuron pathology ▪ Poliomyelitis ▪ Other viral myelitides ▪ Traumatic ▪ Spinal muscular atrophy ▪ Myelomeningocele • Primary myopathies – Muscular dystrophy – Duchenne's muscular dystrophy – Limb-girdle dystrophy – Facioscapulohumeral dystrophy – Arthrogryposis – Congenital hypotonia – Myotonic dystrophy

Note: Congenital scoliosis is classified by the underlying error in development. In contrast, the Scoliosis Research Society classifies neuromuscular scoliosis according to whether the underlying cause is a primary neuropathy or myopathy.

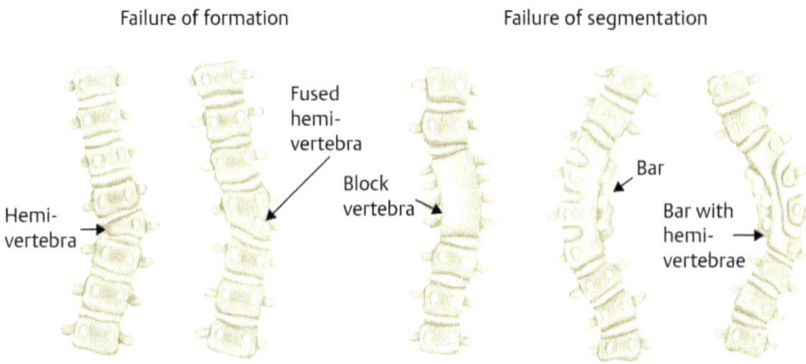

Fig. 25.1 The failures of formation and segmentation.

- Failure of segmentation can occur unilaterally or bilaterally, resulting in a fused unsegmented bar of bone or a block vertebra, respectively (**Fig. 25.1**).
- Although the vertebral anomaly is present at birth, scoliosis typically does not develop until the growth phases of childhood or adolescence. Congenital scoliosis develops when spine growth is not balanced bilaterally. For example, the lack of growth plate in a unilateral unsegmented bar coupled with normal growth in the contralateral side from a hemivertebra has the highest risk of progressive deformity.
- Other types of congenital deformity include congenital kyphosis, congenital lordosis, congenital stenosis, and dysplastic spondylolisthesis.

• Signs, symptoms, and physical examination:
  - Pelvic and truncal imbalance can be identified on physical examination based on head tilt, shoulder height asymmetry, leg length discrepancy, and pelvic tilt.
  - Adam's forward bend test assesses thoracic rotation and is quantified through a scoliometer.[3]
  - Thorough neurologic examination including strength, sensation, and reflex testing evaluates neurologic spinal cord and/or nerve root impingement.
  - Neurocutaneous stigmata of spinal dysraphism including skin tags, hair tufts, dermal sinus tracts, or abnormal pigmentation as well as musculoskeletal abnormalities such as asymmetric calves or club feet may be found on dermatologic and orthopaedic examination.

• Workup:
  - A complete patient history includes prenatal and birth history in addition to developmental motor and cognitive milestones.
  - Medical comorbidities are common; renal, respiratory, and cardiac anomalies are frequently present with congenital spine disorders.[4]

- Pulmonary function testing should be included in the thorough preoperative workup as associated congenital rib fusions may lead to restrictive lung disease and thoracic insufficiency.
- Entire spine upright posteroanterior (PA) and lateral X-rays are often initially acquired to evaluate clinically suspected scoliosis and serially performed to monitor curve progression over time.
- Computed tomography (CT) enables imaging of bony anatomy including pedicle and vertebral size for preoperative surgical planning, and three-dimensional CT reconstruction may improve visualization of complex deformity (**Fig. 25.2**).
- Magnetic resonance imaging (MRI) is warranted to evaluate potential coexisting abnormalities, such as syringomyelia or diastematomyelia, as well as to image the relationship of neural structures to abnormal bony structures.

• Treatment:
  - Initial management is typically conservative and may involve bracing. Unfortunately, nearly 75% of patients treated conservatively for congenital scoliosis will progress significantly.[5] Early surgery is warranted for severe or progressive congenital scoliosis. Surgical options include spinal fusion, growing systems, hemivertebrectomy, and/or hemiepiphysiodesis.

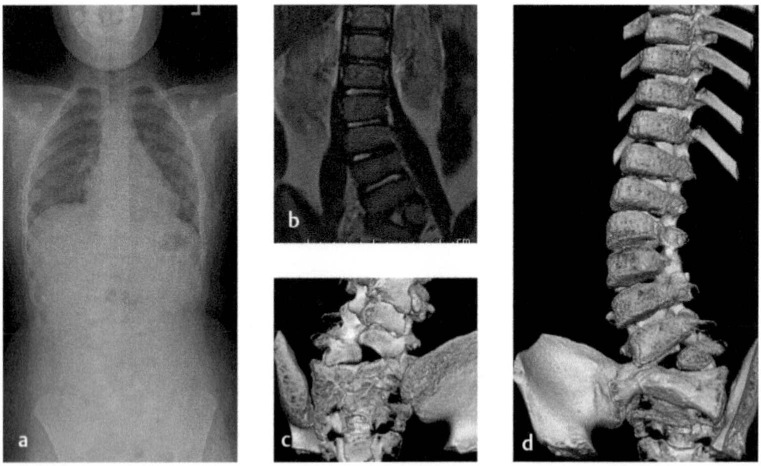

Fig. 25.2 **(a)** Posteroanterior (PA) X-ray depicting a scoliotic deformity involving seven lumbar vertebrae and an L7 hemivertebra in a patient. **(b)** A coronal MRI image demonstrating the L7 hemivertebra. **(c)** A three-dimensional CT image demonstrating the lamina of the L7 hemivertebra and the absent contralateral posterior elements. **(d)** An anterior view of the CT reconstruction image depicting the vertebral anomaly.

- Surgery carries significant morbidity and mortality. Reames et al reported a morbidity of more than 10% and mortality of 0.3% in a series of 2,000 patients who underwent surgical treatment for congenital scoliosis.[6]
- Surgical pearls:
  - Perioperative evaluation for associated renal, cardiac, respiratory, and congenital anomalies is imperative.
  - Surgical treatment is indicated for severe or progressive congenital scoliosis.

25.3 Neuromuscular Scoliosis

- Background:
  - Scoliosis commonly occurs in patients with neuromuscular disease, and it is often more severe and progressive than in patients without an underlying neuromuscular disorder.
  - The Scoliosis Research Society classifies neuromuscular scoliosis by etiology: upper motor neuron disease, lower motor neuron disease, mixed pathology, and primary muscle disease[7] (**Table 25.1**).
  - Asymmetric paraplegia and muscle tone, mechanical force imbalance across the spine, related congenital spine and/or neural anomalies, altered sensory feedback, and abnormal posture contribute to the development of scoliosis in patients with neuromuscular disease.
  - The severity of underlying neuromuscular disease often determines whether spine deformity will develop. Scoliosis develops in up to 74% of patients with cerebral palsy,[8] up to 90% of males with Duchenne's muscular dystrophy not treated with corticosteroids,[9] and in nearly 100% of patients with onset of traumatic tetraplegia prior to skeletal maturity.[10]
- Signs, symptoms, and physical examination:
  - Signs and symptoms of neuromuscular scoliosis are similar to those found in congenital scoliosis. In addition, joint contractures and spasticity are common, and scoliosis is more likely to involve the pelvis with an associated "windswept" deformity; both may result in significant postural difficulty and functional impairment.
  - Patients with neuromuscular disorders are often nonambulatory at presentation and may have significant medical comorbidities. Pulmonary and nutritional status should be considered, and pressure sores may be present at scoliotic apices and other pressure-bearing sites.
- Workup:
  - Thorough evaluation includes a complete history, physical examination, and neurological examination.

- Static conditions such as cerebral palsy or myelomeningocele should be distinguished from progressive conditions such as Duchenne's muscular dystrophy.
- The purpose and utility of radiographs, CT, and MRI are similar in the evaluation of neuromuscular scoliosis as in congenital scoliosis, as previously discussed.

• Treatment:
  - Initial conservative treatment is frequently the first-line treatment, including bracing and customized wheelchair seating systems to provide balanced support for the head, back, and pelvic girdle. Although the role of bracing in the prevention of curve progression is controversial, it may delay surgery in very young children with neuromuscular scoliosis.[12]
  - The goals of surgical treatment are often augmented quality of life via pain relief, improved seating posture and pulmonary mechanics, prevention of deformity progression, and alleviation of caregiver burden.
  - An exact curve severity threshold as an indication for surgery has not been established, and evaluation of surgical candidacy is made on a case-by-case basis. However, surgery is often recommended for coronal curves > 50 degrees. Surgery may include growing systems in skeletally immature patients or long fusion constructs.
  - As with congenital scoliosis, surgical intervention for neuromuscular scoliosis is associated with high morbidity and mortality. Reames et al found the morbidity to be greater than 18% and mortality 0.3% in a series of nearly 5,000 patients undergoing surgical correction of neuromuscular scoliosis.[6]
• Surgical pearls:
  - The severity of underlying disease determines the development and progression of scoliosis in patients with neuromuscular conditions.
  - Surgical correction is indicated for severe or progressive scoliosis, although the high surgical morbidity must be considered.

Common Clinical Questions

1. What developmental event leads to the formation of a hemivertebra?

   A. Bilateral failure of formation.

   B. Unilateral failure of formation.

   C. Failure of segmentation.

   D. Both failure of formation and segmentation.

2. Which of the following pathologic entities carries the highest risk of developing scoliosis?

   A. Cerebral palsy.

   B. Duchenne's muscular dystrophy.

   C. Skeletally immature tetraplegic spinal cord injury.
   D. Rett syndrome.
3. Which of the following is associated with the highest risk of scoliotic progression?
   A. Growth spurts.
   B. Skeletal maturity.
   C. Ambulatory status.
   D. Vitamin deficiency.

Answers to Common Clinical Questions

1. B. A hemivertebra results from unilateral failure of formation.
2. C. Skeletally immature cervical spine injuries carry a nearly 100% risk of scoliosis.
3. A. Growth spurts are associated with the highest risk of scoliotic progression.

References

1. Hedequist D, Emans J. Congenital scoliosis: a review and update. J Pediatr Orthop. 2007; 27(1):106–116
2. Mackel CE, Jada A, Samdani AF, et al. A comprehensive review of the diagnosis and management of congenital scoliosis. Childs Nerv Syst. 2018; 34 (11):2155–2171
3. Chan G, Dormans JP. Update on congenital spinal deformities: preoperative evaluation. Spine. 2009; 34(17):1766–1774
4. Ferguson RL. Medical and congenital comorbidities associated with spinal deformities in the immature spine. J Bone Joint Surg Am. 2007; 89 Suppl 1: 34–41
5. McMaster MJ, Ohtsuka K. The natural history of congenital scoliosis. A study of two hundred and fifty-one patients. J Bone Joint Surg Am. 1982; 64(8): 1128–1147
6. Reames DL, Smith JS, Fu K-MG, et al. Scoliosis Research Society Morbidity and Mortality Committee. Complications in the surgical treatment of 19,360 cases of pediatric scoliosis: a review of the Scoliosis Research Society Morbidity and Mortality database. Spine. 2011; 36(18):1484–1491
7. Berven S, Bradford DS. Neuromuscular scoliosis: causes of deformity and principles for evaluation and management. Semin Neurol. 2002; 22(2):167–178

8. Miyanji F, Nasto LA, Sponseller PD, et al. Assessing the risk-benefit ratio of scoliosis surgery in cerebral palsy: surgery is worth it. J Bone Joint Surg Am. 2018; 100(7):556–563
9. Lebel DE, Corston JA, McAdam LC, Biggar WD, Alman BA. Glucocorticoid treatment for the prevention of scoliosis in children with Duchenne muscular dystrophy: long-term follow-up. J Bone Joint Surg Am. 2013; 95 (12):1057–1061
10. Dearolf WW, III, Betz RR, Vogel LC, Levin J, Clancy M, Steel HH. Scoliosis in pediatric spinal cord-injured patients. J Pediatr Orthop. 1990; 10(2):214–218
11. Li Y, Swallow J, Gagnier J, et al. Pediatric Spine Study Group. A report of two conservative approaches to early onset scoliosis: serial casting and bracing. Spine Deform. 2021; 9(2):595–602
12. Fletcher ND, McClung A, Rathjen KE, Denning JR, Browne R, Johnston CE, III. Serial casting as a delay tactic in the treatment of moderate-to-severe early-onset scoliosis. J Pediatr Orthop. 2012; 32(7):664–671

26 Scheuermann's Kyphosis

Venkat Boddapati and Han Jo Kim

Summary

Scheuermann's kyphosis is a common pathology found in the adolescent population, and is defined as anterior wedging >5 degrees at three or more adjacent segments. The pathology most commonly occurs in the thoracic spine, followed by the thoracolumbar junction. Patients may present with pain, postural concerns, self-esteem issues, and if larger deformities with compressive pathology (disk, cysts, etc.) may have symptoms of spinal cord compression. Imaging should include long-cassette films, flexibility films, and MRI. Although the mainstay of treatment is nonoperative, with physical therapy and bracing, a subset of patients may require surgery. Indications include larger deformities, restrictive pulmonary disease, and neurological deficits, among others. LIV level selection may include fusing to the first lordotic disk, to the neutral vertebra, or to the stable sagittal vertebra.

Keywords: Scheuermann's kyphosis, spine deformity, level selection

26.1 Key Points

- The etiology of Scheuermann's disease remains unknown. Prevailing theories related to its etiology include avascular necrosis of the vertebral ring apophyses, collagen fibril dysfunction, and postural factors, among others. Genetics may play a role as familial studies have shown an autosomal dominant inheritance pattern (incomplete penetrance).
- Adolescents with significant deformity may have self-esteem issues, postural concerns, and pain located about the apex of the kyphosis. Neurological symptoms in Scheuermann's disease are rare.
- Patients should be examined carefully to exclude spastic paraparesis manifested by ataxia and hyperreflexia, which may rarely be present and is secondary to cord compression by the angular deformity, herniated thoracic disk, or a spinal epidural cyst. Magnetic resonance imaging (MRI) is warranted in these situations.
- Successful surgical management of Scheuermann's disease requires addressing sagittal imbalance and choosing the correct upper (UIV) and

lower (LIV) instrumented levels in order to sufficiently correct the sagittal plane deformity as well as to prevent postoperative junctional pathology.

26.2 Background

- Scheuermann's disease (kyphosis dorsalis juvenilis) is a structural kyphosis of the thoracic spine initially described by Scheuermann in 1921 in a series of 105 adolescent patients.[2] It occurs commonly in adolescents (0.4–8.3% of the general population), with roughly equal male and female prevalence, and is often asymptomatic but can present with self-esteem issues, postural concerns, and pain around the apex of the deformity.[4] Scheuermann's disease is rarely associated with neurological complications.
- Sorensen defined the radiographic criteria of Scheuermann's disease as anterior vertebral wedging of > 5 degrees at ≥ 3 adjacent segments or > 15 degrees in over 3 adjacent levels.[5]
- The two types of Scheuermann's disease are: (1) thoracic variant, apex at T6–T8 (most common variant); and (2) thoracolumbar variant, apex at thoracolumbar junction, T10–L1 (less common variant).
- The natural history of Scheuermann's disease is poorly understood. The treatment is based on the age of the patient, the severity of the deformity, the curve pattern, the progression and presence or absence of pain, and neurological deficits. Operative intervention for Scheuermann's disease is indicated for patients who have progressive deformity, painful curves, unacceptable cosmetic appearances, restrictive pulmonary disease, and neurological deficits.

26.3 Signs, Symptoms, and Physical Examination

- Adolescents who have deformity greater than 75 degrees often have self-esteem or postural concerns. Curves greater than 100 degrees may present with neurological symptoms or cardiopulmonary issues; however, this is rare.
- The deformity may be associated with pain typically centered at the apex of the kyphosis and fatigue. Prior studies have shown pain in only 20% of their patients, whereas prior studies have reported an incidence greater than 60%. Speck and Chopin note higher rates of pain with larger deformities.[6] Pain is more commonly the chief complaint of adults. The pain of Scheuermann's disease is usually intermittent, aching, and nonradiating in nature, localized over the kyphotic region.

- Spondylolysis or spondylolisthesis has been identified in up to 50% of adolescents with Scheuermann's disease[7] and must be excluded in any Scheuermann's patient who presents with back pain. Concomitant scoliosis, while uncommon, may impact fusion level selection.[8]
- On physical examination, the patient who has Scheuermann's kyphosis typically has a well-demarcated angular deformity that is accentuated in Adam's forward bend test. Often there is compensatory hyperlordosis of the cervical or lumbar spine, characterized by a prominent head and neck thrust. The kyphosis is normally rigid and not fully correctible when the patient attempts extension of the thoracic spine in the prone position.
- The thoracic deformity may be increased with forward bending, when viewed from the side. Thoracolumbar or lumbar kyphosis is not easily visible but may be detected by prominent spinous processes of the thoracolumbar or lumbar spine. A mild scoliosis of 10 to 20 degrees may be noted on forward bending in 20 to 30% of patients.
- Muscle tightness and apparent contractures, particularly of the hamstrings, are common findings.
- Patients should be examined carefully to exclude spastic paraparesis manifested by ataxia and hyperreflexia, which may rarely be present and be secondary to cord compression by the angular deformity, herniated thoracic disk, or a spinal epidural cyst.

26.4 Workup

- The criteria for the diagnosis of Scheuermann's disease is > 5 degrees of wedging of at least three adjacent vertebrae at the apex of the kyphosis or > 15 degrees at three adjacent vertebrae.[5]
- Associated findings may include end plate abnormalities and disk wedging.
- Radiographic evaluation of Scheuermann's disease involves acquiring orthogonal standing (posteroanterior and lateral) views of the spine. Full-length films (36-inch cassette) of the spine and/or full-length standing films are recommended to identify concomitant pathology and compensatory changes.
- EOS imaging is preferred as this unique digital imaging system enables long-length PA and lateral images to be acquired simultaneously and at a 9.2 times lower radiation dose, with a quality that is 97.2% equivalent to or better than conventional radiology.
- Standing PA radiographs are required to exclude an associated scoliosis and may also be used to determine interpedicular distance, which is increased in patients who have spastic paraparesis secondary to a spinal epidural cyst.

- Successful surgical management of Scheuermann's disease requires addressing this sagittal imbalance and choosing the correct upper (UIV) and lower (LIV) instrumented levels.
- Any Scheuermann's patient who has a neurological deficit or significant back pain requires further evaluation with an MRI scan of the whole spine.
- A hyperextension lateral radiograph is an important part of the workup and may aid in surgical management of Scheuermann's kyphosis by providing valuable information on the flexibility of the deformity. There is some evidence that simple supine imaging or scout images from advanced imaging may also provide information on deformity flexibility.[9]
- Important radiographic parameters to measure in all patients include the end vertebra, first lordotic disk, last touched proximal vertebra by the posterior sacral vertical line (PSVL), the stable sagittal vertebra (SSV), global sagittal balance (sagittal vertebral axis), magnitude of thoracic kyphosis, compensatory cervical and lumbar lordosis, and pelvic parameters (pelvic incidence, pelvic tilt, sacral slope).

26.5 Neuroimaging

- MRI may reflect changes seen on plain films more clearly and earlier.
- Indications for MRI include patients with neurological symptoms, evidence of congenital anomalies on plain films, and rapidly progressive kyphosis.
- Schmorl's nodes may be easily seen on MRI, where disk material herniates through the end plate defect beneath the nonfused ring apophysis.
- Sometimes prolapse of large foci of intervertebral disk tissue may be observed anteriorly and appear submarginally behind the anterior longitudinal ligament; subsequently, a portion of the apophyseal ossification center may be separated from the vertebral body and produce a limbus vertebra.
- Some authors recommend MRI in all patients undergoing deformity surgery as disk herniations may cause neurological symptoms intraoperatively or postoperatively after cantilever correction of the kyphotic deformity.[10]

26.6 Treatment

26.6.1 Nonoperative Treatment

- The treatment is based on the age of the patient and skeletal maturity, the severity of the deformity, the curve pattern, and the progression and presence or absence of pain and neurological deficits. Nonoperative treatment using an extension-type brace with corrective sternal pad is usually the mainstay of initial treatment if the curve measures between 60 and 75 degrees, is passively correctible, and the patient has mild symptoms.

- Riddle et al, however, have found that patients who have curves greater than 75 degrees will respond less favorably to bracing, and surgical intervention should be considered in these patients.[11]
- If nonoperative treatment is pursued, then the brace should be worn for more than 18 hours per day and should be accompanied by an exercise program. Brace noncompliance will hinder the effectiveness of this treatment modality so proper patient and family motivation is vital.
- In addition to bracing, physical therapy is an important mainstay of nonoperative management as it may help improve muscle tone, trunk stabilization, and posture.

26.6.2 Operative Treatment

- Operative intervention for Scheuermann's disease is indicated for patients who have progressive deformity with high kyphosis (e.g., > 75 degrees), painful curves, unacceptable cosmetic appearances, restrictive pulmonary disease, and neurological deficits.
- The main goals of surgery are to relieve pain, improve cosmesis and quality of life, and improve sagittal balance.
- Surgical management can be through an anterior-only, combined anterior–posterior, or posterior-only techniques. With the maturation of pedicle screw technology, a majority of current surgical management is being performed through a posterior-only approach with posterior column osteotomies.[6] Riouallon et al compared 64 patients with Scheuermann's disease who had anterior–posterior surgery and 67 patients who had posterior-only surgery and found similar functional improvements and kyphosis correction between both the cohorts. They advocate for posterior-only fusion in a majority of cases, reserving combined approaches for the most severe deformities.[11] An example of a posterior-only construct is shown in **Fig. 26.1**.
- Appropriate level selection is important to minimize risk of adjacent segment deformity (e.g., proximal and distal junctional kyphosis).[6] The UIV is typically selected as the proximal end vertebra.
- Current concepts and literature support symmetry, with the number of levels above the apex being equal to the number of levels fused distally.
- A number of methods have been described to identify the LIV. These include: (1) fusing to the first lordotic disk beyond the end vertebra, (2) fusing to distal neutral vertebra, and (3) fusing to the SSV.[12] Kim et al

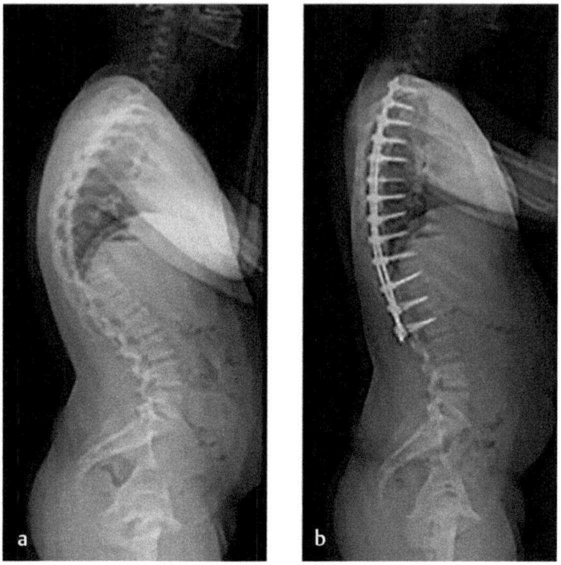

Fig. 26.1 **(a, b)** A 17-year-old adolescent male with 85 degrees kyphosis who underwent posterior spinal fusion and Ponte-type posterior column osteotomies from T2 to L2 with 45 degrees residual thoracic kyphosis.

compared LIV selection between the first lordotic disk and the SSV in patients with Scheuermann's disease and found that fusing to the SSV leads to a lower rate of distal junctional pathology at the expense of fusing more motion segments.[13]

- Correction is usually obtained by a cantilever reduction technique followed by sequential rounds of rod compression. The rods are placed in the proximal screws, and the reduction is achieved by using a cantilever maneuver with the rod while inserting it into the distal anchors, thus engaging and reducing the rods in a sequential and bilateral manner. This is facilitated by the use of reduction screws below the apex of the deformity.
- Posterior column osteotomies around the apex of the deformity aids in increasing curve flexibility and reducing the deformity. There is no consensus on the number of posterior column osteotomies that need to be performed, but it is influenced by the magnitude of the kyphosis (as each posterior column osteotomy imparts approximately 10 degrees of correction) and rigidity of the kyphosis. Three-column osteotomies may be required in cases of significant rigid deformity.

26.7 Surgical Pearls

- Generous posterior column osteotomies about the apex improve curve flexibility and ease of reduction.
- Use of reduction screws to facilitate correction and rod reduction.
- Maintain appropriate thoracic kyphosis after deformity correction. Overcorrecting the deformity may lead to neurological compromise, sagittal imbalance postoperatively, and increase in the rates of junctional pathology. Some authors recommend correcting to 50% of the preoperative kyphosis and avoiding less than 40 degrees of thoracic kyphosis postoperatively.[13]
- Intraoperative flat plate radiographs may aid in visualizing the magnitude of deformity correction achieved.
- Given the high rates of junctional pathology noted after Scheuermann's disease, close follow up with serial radiographs is warranted. Meticulous handling of soft tissues at the proximal and distal ends of the constructs is paramount, and using a modified Wiltse approach at cephalad end of construct to potentially protect the posterior soft tissue sleeve and lessen the risk of proximal junctional kyphosis may be warranted. Additional mitigative techniques include but are not limited to ensuring a "smooth landing" between fused and unfused segments with the utilization of transition rods, transverse process hooks at the cephalad segments, or spinous process tethering. Ultimately the best way to prevent junctional pathology is appropriate level selection.

Common Clinical Questions

1. A 13-year-old skeletally immature boy is brought to your office because his mother is concerned about his poor posture. A lateral radiograph shows thoracic kyphosis of 68 degrees. It is partially correctable on hyperextension. What is the initial course of management?
2. What are the radiographic criteria for the diagnosis of Scheuermann's kyphosis?
3. Based on the current literature, what is the best way to prevent distal junctional kyphosis in a patient who undergoes fusion for Scheuermann's kyphosis?

Answers to Common Clinical Questions

1. A corrective extension-type brace worn for 18 + hours to prevent progression of kyphosis.

2. The radiographic criteria for the diagnosis of Scheuermann's disease are more than 5 degrees of wedging of at least three adjacent vertebrae at the apex of the kyphosis; additional findings that may be noted are end plate irregularities.
3. LIV is typically the vertebra that is most closely bisected by the PSVL, and this vertebra should be positioned distal to the first lordotic disk and rostral to a lordotic disk. When fused short of the PSVL, the rate of distal junctional kyphosis has been found to be dramatically higher.

References

1. Scheuermann HW. Kyphosis dorsalis juvenilis. Orthop Chir. 1921; 41:305–317
2. Scheuermann HW. The classic: kyphosis dorsalis juvenilis. Clin Orthop Relat Res. 1977(128):5–7
3. Wenger DR, Frick SL. Scheuermann kyphosis. Spine. 1999; 24(24):2630–2639
4. Tribus CB. Scheuermann's kyphosis in adolescents and adults: diagnosis and management. J Am Acad Orthop Surg. 1998; 6(1):36–43
5. Sorensen K. Scheuermann's juvenile kyphosis: clinical appearances, radiography, aetiology, and prognosis. Enjar Munksgaard Forlag Copenhagen; Munksgaard; 1964
6. Speck GR, Chopin DC. The surgical treatment of Scheuermann's kyphosis. J Bone Joint Surg Br. 1986; 68(2):189–193
7. Ogilvie JW, Sherman J. Spondylolysis in Scheuermann's disease. Spine. 1987; 12(3):251–253
8. Dai Y, Li Y, Li P, Li L, Tu Z, Wang B. Familial lumbar Scheuermann disease with idiopathic scoliosis in China: first case report. Medicine (Baltimore). 2017; 96(25):e7100
9. Kaiser R, Behrbalk E, Walsh M, Waldauf P, Perez Romera AB, Mehdian H. Can MRI predict flexibility in Scheuermann kyphosis patients? Clin Spine Surg. 2017; 30(7):E938–E941
10. Lee SS, Lenke LG, Kuklo TR, et al. Comparison of Scheuermann kyphosis correction by posterior-only thoracic pedicle screw fixation versus combined anterior/posterior fusion. Spine. 2006; 31(20):2316–2321
11. Riouallon G, Morin C, Charles YP, et al. French Scoliosis Study Group. Posterior-only versus combined anterior/posterior fusion in Scheuermann disease: a large retrospective study. Eur Spine J. 2018; 27(9):2322–2330
12. Cho KJ, Lenke LG, Bridwell KH, Kamiya M, Sides B. Selection of the optimal distal fusion level in posterior instrumentation and fusion for thoracic hyperkyphosis: the sagittal stable vertebra concept. Spine. 2009; 34(8):765–770
13. Lowe TG, Kasten MD. An analysis of sagittal curves and balance after Cotrel-Dubousset instrumentation for kyphosis secondary to Scheuermann's disease. A review of 32 patients. Spine. 1994; 19(15):1680–1685

27 Adolescent Idiopathic Scoliosis

Kevin Kwan, Josephine Coury, Yong Shen, and Lawrence G. Lenke

Summary
Adolescent idiopathic scoliosis (AIS) is classified according to the Lenke system, guiding treatment options such as bracing, physical therapy, and selective spinal fusion. Prediction of AIS progression relies on the scoliotic curve's magnitude in relation to skeletal maturity. Curves under 25 degrees should be monitored every 4 to 6 months until maturity, while bracing is recommended for curves over 25 degrees or if there is a 5-degree progression in two visits, or a 10-degree progression in one visit, occurs. Surgical intervention is indicated for skeletally immature patients with over 40-degree curve or skeletally mature patients with over 50-degree curve. The objectives of surgery are to achieve optimal three-dimensional alignment and balance while minimizing fused levels and preserving pulmonary function. Selective fusion should be considered based on specific radiographic criteria.

Keywords: adolescent idiopathic scoliosis, bracing, Lenke classification, selective fusion, physical therapy, level selection

27.1 Key Points

- The progression of adolescent idiopathic scoliosis (AIS) can be predicted based on the degree of a patient's existing scoliosis in relation to skeletal maturity.
- Patients with a scoliotic curve under 25 degrees should be observed radiographically and clinically every 4 to 6 months until skeletal maturity.
- Brace treatment should be initiated for scoliotic curves greater than 25 degrees or if greater than a 5 degrees progression in two consecutive visits, or 10 degrees progression in one follow-up visit, occurs.
- AIS patients who are either skeletally immature with over a 40 degrees major curve or skeletally mature with greater than a 50 degrees major curve are indicated for surgical management.
- The goals of spinal instrumentation and fusion include creating an optimal three-dimensional alignment and balanced spine while minimizing vertebral levels fused and optimizing pulmonary function.
- Selective thoracic or thoracolumbar/lumbar fusion should be performed in patients who meet specific radiographic criteria.

27.2 Definition

- AIS is defined as a coronal Cobb angle of at least 10 degrees as measured by an anteroposterior radiograph in children 10 to 18 years of age.
- AIS patients have three-dimensional deformities with abnormalities in the coronal, sagittal, and axial planes.
- AIS has no clear etiology, but a strong genetic component. About 30 to 40% of AIS patients have a family history of scoliosis.[2]

27.3 Prevalence

- AIS has a prevalence of 0.47 to 5.2%.[3] The incidence of AIS in the general population is 1 to 3%, but only 0.15 to 0.30% of AIS patients develop curves in the surgical range.[4]
- In patients from 10 to 18 years of age, the incidence of a coronal Cobb angle of 10, 20, and > 40 degrees is 1 to 3%, 0.3 to 0.5%, and 0.1%, respectively.[4]
- The female-to-male ratio ranges from 1.5:1 to 3:1, increasing with Cobb angle measurements. The female-to-male ratio ranges from 1.4:1 in curves between 10 and 20 degrees to up to 7.2:1 in curves > 40 degrees.[4]

27.4 Clinical Evaluation

- A thorough history and physical examination should be performed for AIS patients.
- History should include growth history, age of menarche, and voice changes to determine peak growth velocity.
- Physical examination should include a full upper and lower extremity neurologic evaluation.
- Trunk shift, shoulder balance, rib prominence, and waist crease or pelvic obliquity should be noted both statically and dynamically while the patient ambulates (**Fig. 27.1**).
- Curve rotation should be assessed by performing an Adam's forward bend test and quantified with a scoliometer. A 7-degree scoliometer measurement of the thoracic and thoracolumbar curve on Adam's forward bend test correlates to a 20-degree trunk rotation.

27.5 Radiographic Evaluation

- Radiographic assessment involves standing anteroposterior and lateral 36-inch scoliosis radiographs. Standing full-length EOS head-to-toe

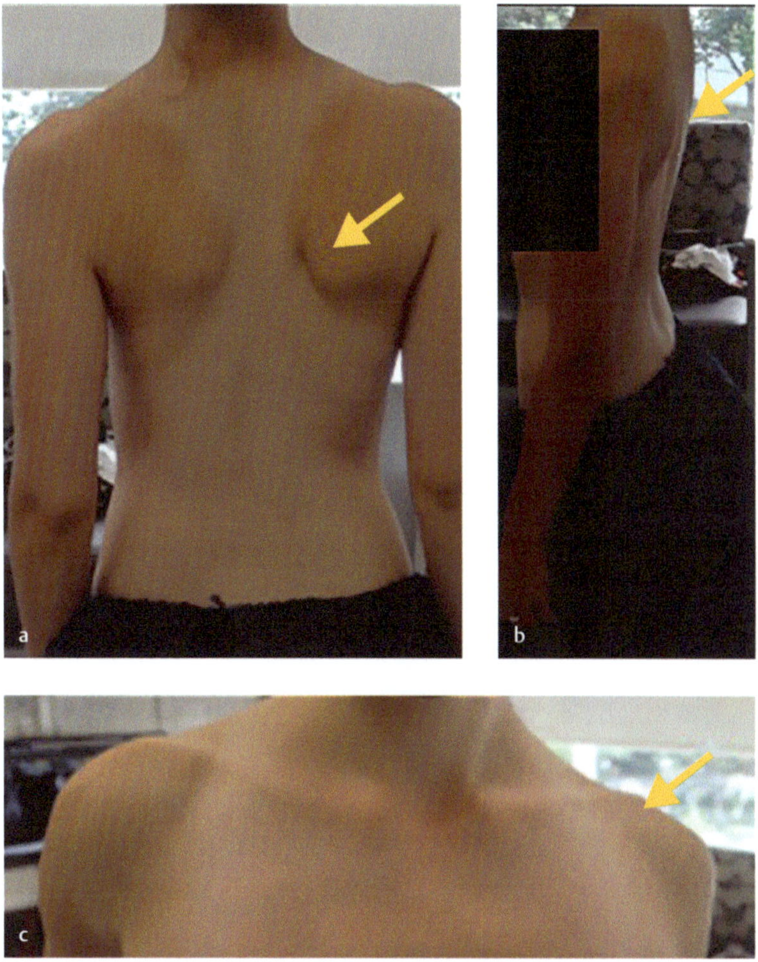

Fig. 27.1 Adolescent idiopathic scoliosis (AIS) patient with a scapular hump **(a)**, thoracic hypokyphosis **(b)**, and shoulder asymmetry **(c)**.

imaging is ideal as it allows for visualization of the sagittal and coronal harmony between the skull, shoulder, hips, knees, and ankles (**Fig. 27.2**).

- In patients being prepared for surgical correction, side-bending radiographs and/or supine radiographs, both anterior–posterior and lateral, should be performed to assess the flexibility of the scoliosis.[5]

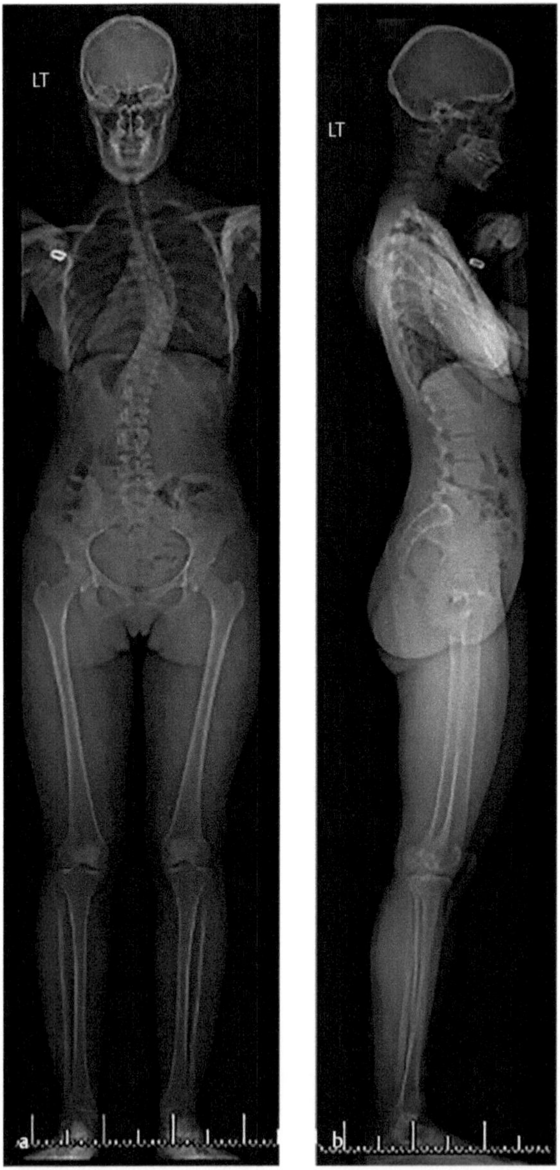

Fig. 27.2 Full-length anteroposterior (AP) **(a)** and lateral **(b)** EOS films of an adolescent idiopathic scoliosis (AIS) patient.

- A total spine MRI should be performed in patients with significant back pain, neurologic deficits, atypical curve pattern, sagittal plane hyperkyphosis, or rapid curve progression.[6]
- The preoperative total spine MRI will evaluate for syrinx, Chiari malformation, or tethered cord. MRI is also used to evaluate the spinal cord shape at the apex of the major scoliotic curve.
- A spinal cord shape classification system (SCSCS) designated three spinal cord types at the apex of a major scoliotic curve.[7] In type 1, the spinal cord is surrounded by cerebrospinal fluid (CSF). In type 2, the spinal cord is draped across the pedicle or vertebral body with no CSF in between. In a type 3 cord, the spinal cord is both draped and deformed at the apex.[7]
- Patients with a type 3 cord have a 28 × greater chance of neuromonitoring changes during surgery.[7]
- Routine CT scan of the spine is avoided to minimize radiation in AIS patients. Pedicle morphology can also be evaluated on MRI.

27.6 Skeletal Maturity

- Skeletal maturity can be evaluated using bone age radiographs, pubertal phase, and chronologic age.
- In terms of radiographs, ossification of the iliac apophysis (Risser score), triradiate cartilage, and hands (Sanders hand score) are utilized to assess skeletal maturity.
- Skeletal maturity is achieved when there is less than 1 cm of height difference over a 6-month interval or approximately 2 years post-menarche in females.

27.7 Management Overview

- AIS treatment includes observation, physical therapy, and bracing or surgical intervention depending on scoliotic curve size, progression, and skeletal maturity.
- AIS in adolescents who are skeletally immature and at peak growth velocity is most likely to progress.[4]
- Curvatures greater than 50 degrees at skeletal maturity have an annual progression of 1 to 3 degrees per year. Curve magnitude is the greatest risk factor for curve progression. Curves most likely to progress are thoracic, followed by lumbar, thoracolumbar, and double major.[8]
- Progression of moderate-sized idiopathic curves into adulthood without intervention has no dissimilarity concerning mortality to age-matched

controls, but may have increased aesthetic deformity, discomfort, or functional disability.[9]

- Surgical management of AIS curvatures in adulthood is associated with greater surgical time, blood loss, construct length, and overall morbidity.[10]

27.8 Observation

- Observation is appropriate for skeletally immature patients with a scoliotic curve under 25 degrees. These patients should be evaluated radiographically and clinically every 4 to 6 months until skeletal maturity.
- The typical AIS curve progresses 1 degree per month, accelerating during the growth phase of puberty.

27.9 Bracing

- Bracing should be initiated for skeletally immature patients with curves between 25 and 40 degrees. The goal of bracing is to halt or slow the progression of a patient's scoliosis.
- The appropriate brace should be selected depending on the apex of the curve and physician's preference. Patients should be monitored every 4 to 6 months for curve progression during bracing.
- The BRAIST study, a multicenter trial investigating the role of bracing in AIS, showed that bracing significantly reduced the rate of high-risk curves progressing to surgery.[11] Surgery was not required in 72% of patients in the bracing group versus 48% in the observational group.[1]
- Although longer treatment time with the brace was beneficial in preventing curve progression, patient compliance in wearing the brace significantly affects outcomes.[11]
- It is essential to understand that bracing can negatively affect a patient's overall quality of life regarding psychological and social aspects.[12]

27.10 Physical Therapy

- Physiotherapeutic scoliosis-specific exercises (PSSE), including the Schroth method, may be used with brace treatment to prevent curve progression in low-medium degree curvatures.[13]
- However, uncertainty remains over the effectiveness of PSSE as there is a lack of high-quality research supporting its efficaciousness.[14] There is also a lack of research on the interaction between factors such as skeletal maturity, curve characteristics, therapy compliance, and PSSE in treating AIS.[15]

27.11 Surgical Intervention

- Skeletally immature AIS patients with over 40 degrees of major curve and skeletally mature patients with greater than 50 degrees of major curve are indicated for surgical management.
- Surgery involves posterior spinal instrumentation and fusion (PSIF) to keep or improve spine balance while minimizing the levels fused and maximizing the surgical three-dimensional correction.
- Inferior facetectomies are used for visualization of pedicle screw start point, flexibility, bone graft, and fusion. Osteotomies may be performed to improve mobilization of the spine.
- Posterior column osteotomies are typically performed peri-apically for at least three to five vertebral levels to allow for derotation and optimal three-dimensional deformity correction.
- Rarely, three-column osteotomies, such as pedicle subtraction and/or vertebral column resection, are used in severe and rigid deformities.

27.12 Lenke Classification

- The Lenke AIS classification is used to guide surgical management including which curves should be fused while also providing advice on the upper instrumented vertebra (UIV) and lower instrumented vertebra (LIV) selection.[17]
- The classification separates curve patterns into six types based on the location of the major curve (largest Cobb measurement) and whether the minor curves (other two curves) are nonstructural or structural.[7] The three regions of the spine are the proximal thoracic (PT) region (T2 to T5), the main thoracic (MT) region (T6 to T11–T12 disk space), and the thoracolumbar/lumbar (TL/L) region (T12 vertebra to L4). (**Table 27.1**).
- The most tilted vertebrae above and below the curve's apex are termed the end vertebrae. The Cobb angle is measured from the cephalad endplate of the superior end vertebra to the caudal endplate of the inferior end vertebra.
- Minor curves are designated as structural or nonstructural based on side-bending flexibility and/or hyperkyphosis in the sagittal plane. Minor structural curves have ≥ 25 degrees residual side bending Cobb measurements and/or ≥ 20 degrees of PT kyphosis or TL kyphosis in the standing sagittal X-ray.
- The second component of the Lenke classification is the lumbar spine modifier. The central sacral vertical line (CSVL) is drawn on the coronal radiograph. In lumbar modifier A, the CSVL lies between the pedicles at the curve apex. In modifier B, the CSVL contacts the pedicle at the apex.

Table 27.1 Curve type 1 through 6 based on curve location and major, structural minor, and nonstructural curves

		Curve location		
Type	**Name**	**Proximal thoracic**	**Major thoracic**	**Thoracolumbar/ Lumbar**
Type 1	Main thoracic (MT)	Nonstructural	Major	Nonstructural
Type 2	Double thoracic (DT)	Structural minor	Major	Nonstructural
Type 3	Double major (DM)	Nonstructural	Major	Structural minor
Type 4	Triple major (TM)	Structural minor	Major	Major
Type 5	Thoracolumbar (TL/L)	Nonstructural	Nonstructural	Major
Type 6	Thoracolumbar, main thoracic (TL/L-MT)	Nonstructural	Structural minor	Major

In modifier C, the CSVL does not touch the pedicles/vertebral body at the apex (**Fig. 27.3**).

- The sagittal thoracic modifier is the third component to the AIS classification system. T5 to T12 kyphosis is measured on the lateral upright X-ray. For hypokyphosis under 10 degrees, the designated modifier is a "–." Kyphosis of between 10 and 40 degrees is considered normal kyphosis or "N." Above 40 degrees is considered hyperkyphosis and is designated as a "+."
- Thus, the complete Lenke AIS classification system is a triad system that combines the curve type (1–6), the lumbar modifier (A, B, or C), and the sagittal thoracic modifier (–, N, or +). A representative example is a 1AN classification, which is the most common.

27.13 Instrumented Level Selection

- The selection of the appropriate fusion levels for operative AIS patients remains controversial but should typically include all major curves and structural minor curves.

THE LENKE CLASSIFICATION SYSTEM FOR AIS

Curve type	Proximal thoracic	Main thoracic	Thoracolumbar/Lumbar	Description
1	Nonstructural	Structural*	Nonstructural	Main thoracic (MT)
2	Structural†	Structural*	Nonstructural	Double thoracic (DT)
3	Nonstructural	Structural*	Structural†	Double major (DM)
4	Structural†	Structural§	Structural§	Triple major (TM)
5	Nonstructural	Nonstructural	Structural*	Thoracolumbar/Lumbar (TL/L)
6	Nonstructural	Structural†	Structural*	Thoracolumbar/Lumbar-Main thoracic (TL/L-MT)

*Major curve: largest Cobb measurement, always structural; †Minor curve: remaining structural curves; §Type 4 - MT or TL/L can be the major curve

STRUCTURAL CRITERIA
(Minor curves)

Proximal thoracic - Side bending cobb ≥25°
- T2–T5 Kyphosis ≥+20°

Main thoracic - Side bending cobb ≥25°
- T10–L2 Kyphosis ≥+20°

Thoracolumbar/Lumbar - Side bending cobb ≥25°
- T10–L2 Kyphosis ≥+20°

LOCATION OF APEX
(SRS definition)

CURVE	APEX
Thoracic	T2 to T11–12 Disc
Thoracolumbar	T12–L1
Lumbar	L1–2 Disc to L4

MODIFIERS

Lumbar spine modifier	Center sacral vertical line to lumbar apex
A	Between pedicles
B	Touches apical body(ies)
C	Completely medial

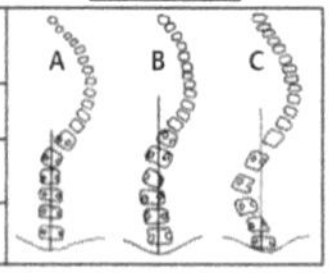

Thoracic sagital profile T5–T12	
Modifier	Cobb angle
- (Hypo)	<10°
N (Normal)	10° – 40°
+ (Hyper)	>40°

Curve type (1–6) + Lumbar spine modifier (A, B, C) + Thoracic sagital modifier (-, N, +) =
Curve classification (e.g. 1B+):

Fig. 27.3 Summary of the Lenke classification. (Reproduced with permission from Dr. Lenke. Lenke LG, Betz RR, Harms J, et al. Adolescent idiopathic scoliosis: a new classification to determine the extent of spinal arthrodesis. J Bone Joint Surg Am 2001;83–A(8):1172.)

- The standard selection of the UIV is often based on the clinical shoulder balance as follows (for a typical right thoracic MT curve): T2 if the left shoulder is high, T3 if the shoulders are neutral, and T4 if the right shoulder is elevated. If the PT curve is structural, T2 is typically selected as the UIV.
- The LIV can be determined based on the location of the last touched vertebra (LTV) by the CSVL. The LTV is typically the LIV. LIV selection aims to preserve as many mobile lumbar segments as possible while allowing for adequate correction of the thoraco/lumbar curvature. This can vary based on the degree of vertebral tilt, rotation, and flexibility.
- The LTV can also be designated as the third modifier of the classification system. Thus, for a 1AN curve where L2 is the LTV, the complete classification will be 1AN/L2.
- A selective fusion is performed by instrumenting only the major curve and allowing the other minor curves to compensate and spontaneously correct. Selective thoracic fusion (STF) can typically be performed not only in Lenke type 1 and 2 curves but also in select type 3 and 4 curves. Selective thoracolumbar fusion can be completed in Lenke type 5 and some type 6 curves.[17]

- STF can typically be performed if the apical vertebral rotation (AVR), apical vertebral translation (AVT), and Cobb ratio are above 1.2. The AVT is the ratio of the distance from the C7 plumb line to the center of the apex of the T curve as compared to the CSVL to the apex of the TL/L curve. The AVR is a ratio of the T to TL/L rotation based on Nash-Moe grading of the radiographic appearance of the pedicles.[18] The Cobb angle ratio compares the T to TL/L coronal curve magnitude.
- Correction of the three-dimensional deformity utilizes many different techniques including differential rod contouring, translation, cantilever, compression on the convexity, distraction on the concavity, in-situ coronal contouring, and derotational maneuvers.[19] In the thoracic region optimal production of thoracic kyphosis is important to improve postoperative pulmonary function outcomes.[20]
- Alternative surgical techniques with anterior vertebral body tethering (VBT) using bony anchors supplemented by elastic cords allow compression on the convexity of the curvature while preserving spinal motion.[21] These methods are still somewhat controversial and have much higher reoperation rates than PSIF procedures in AIS patients. Patient selection is crucial for VBT techniques: VBT is contraindicated for patients with curvatures > 60 degrees, thoracic kyphosis > 40 degrees, or rotational deformity > 20 degrees.[21]

Common Clinical Questions

1. An 11-year-old premenarchal female presents to your office for follow-up with a 21 degrees increase in her thoracic curve over the last 6 months. What is the appropriate next step for management?
   A. Total spine MRI.
   B. Observation with repeat imaging in 4 to 6 months.
   C. Physical therapy with repeat imaging in 4 to 6 months.
   D. Bracing with repeat imaging in 4 to 6 months.
   E. Surgical intervention given the rapid progression.
2. A 12-year-old premenarchal female presents to your office as she was noted to have scoliosis on a routine school examination. Her mother asks: What is the most predictive factor of AIS curve progression?
   A. Chronologic age.
   B. Sanders score.
   C. Peak height velocity.
   D. Tanner stage of development.
   E. Curve magnitude.

3. A 14-year-old skeletally immature male presents to your office for an initial scoliosis evaluation. On radiographs, he has a 30 degrees thoracic curve with no previous imaging. What is the most appropriate next step in management?
   A. Observation with repeat imaging in 4 to 6 months.
   B. Physical therapy only with repeat imaging in 4 to 6 months.
   C. Initial bracing with repeat imaging in 4 to 6 months.
   D. Surgical management including a selective thoracic fusion.
   E. Further workup is needed including MRI and CT.

Answers to Common Clinical Questions

1. A. MRI is appropriate due to the rapid degree of curve progression of >1 degree per month.
2. E. Curve magnitude is the greatest risk factor for curve progression in a skeletally immature female.
3. C. The patient meets criteria for bracing with close follow-up. Given his age and that he has likely not reached skeletal maturity, his curvature will likely progress.

References

1. Edery P, Margaritte-Jeannin P, Biot B, et al. New disease gene location and high genetic heterogeneity in idiopathic scoliosis. Eur J Hum Genet. 2011; 19(8):865–869
2. Mathieu H, Patten SA, Aragon-Martin JA, et al. Genetic variant of TTLL11 gene and subsequent ciliary defects are associated with idiopathic scoliosis in a 5-generation UK family. Sci Rep. 2021; 11(1):11026
3. Weinstein SL, Dolan LA, Cheng JC, Danielsson A, Morcuende JA. Adolescent idiopathic scoliosis. Lancet. 2008; 371(9623):1527–1537
4. Konieczny MR, Senyurt H, Krauspe R. Epidemiology of adolescent idiopathic scoliosis. J Child Orthop. 2013; 7(1):3–9
5. Cheh G, Lenke LG, Lehman RA, Jr, Kim YJ, Nunley R, Bridwell KH. The reliability of preoperative supine radiographs to predict the amount of curve flexibility in adolescent idiopathic scoliosis. Spine. 2007; 32(24): 2668–2672
6. Ozturk C, Karadereler S, Ornek I, Enercan M, Ganiyusufoglu K, Hamzaoglu A. The role of routine magnetic resonance imaging in the preoperative evaluation of adolescent idiopathic scoliosis. Int Orthop. 2010; 34(4):543–546

7. Sielatycki JA, Cerpa M, Baum G, et al. A novel MRI-based classification of spinal cord shape and CSF presence at the curve apex to assess risk of intraoperative neuromonitoring data loss with thoracic spinal deformity correction. Spine Deform. 2020; 8(4):655–661
8. Westrick ER, Ward WT. Adolescent idiopathic scoliosis: 5-year to 20-year evidence-based surgical results. J Pediatr Orthop. 2011; 31(1) Suppl:S61–S68
9. Danielsson AJ. Natural history of adolescent idiopathic scoliosis: a tool for guidance in decision of surgery of curves above 50°. J Child Orthop. 2013; 7(1):37–41
10. Lonner BS, Ren Y, Bess S, et al. Surgery for the adolescent idiopathic scoliosis patients after skeletal maturity: early versus late surgery. Spine Deform. 2019; 7(1):84–92
11. Weinstein SL, Dolan LA, Wright JG, Dobbs MB. Effects of bracing in adolescents with idiopathic scoliosis. N Engl J Med. 2013; 369(16):1512–1521
12. Piantoni L, Tello CA, Remondino RG, et al. Quality of life and patient satisfaction in bracing treatment of adolescent idiopathic scoliosis. Scoliosis Spinal Disord. 2018; 13:26
13. Zhou Z, Liu F, Li R, Chen X. The effects of exercise therapy on adolescent idiopathic scoliosis: an overview of systematic reviews and meta-analyses. Complement Ther Med. 2021; 58:102697
14. Romano M, Minozzi S, Bettany-Saltikov J, et al. Exercises for adolescent idiopathic scoliosis. Cochrane Database Syst Rev. 2012; 2012(8):CD007837
15. Fan Y, Ren Q, To MKT, Cheung JPY. Effectiveness of scoliosis-specific exercises for alleviating adolescent idiopathic scoliosis: a systematic review. BMC Musculoskelet Disord. 2020; 21(1):495
16. Lenke LG, Betz RR, Harms J, et al. Adolescent idiopathic scoliosis: a new classification to determine extent of spinal arthrodesis. J Bone Joint Surg Am. 2001; 83(8):1169–1181
17. Lenke LG, Edwards CC, II, Bridwell KH. The Lenke classification of adolescent idiopathic scoliosis: how it organizes curve patterns as a template to perform selective fusions of the spine. Spine. 2003; 28(20):S199–S207
18. Nash CL, Jr, Moe JH. A study of vertebral rotation. J Bone Joint Surg Am. 1969; 51(2):223–229
19. Seki S, Newton PO, Yahara Y, et al. Differential rod contouring is essential for improving vertebral rotation in patients with adolescent idiopathic scoliosis: thoracic curves assessed with intraoperative CT. Spine. 2018; 43(10):E585–E591
20. Kim YJ, Lenke LG, Bridwell KH, Kim KL, Steger-May K. Pulmonary function in adolescent idiopathic scoliosis relative to the surgical procedure. J Bone Joint Surg Am. 2005; 87(7):1534–1541
21. Samdani AF, Ames RJ, Kimball JS, et al. Anterior vertebral body tethering for idiopathic scoliosis: two-year results. Spine. 2014; 39(20):1688–1693

28 Adult Degenerative Deformity

Hai Le, Wyatt D. Vander Voort, Joseph Wick, and Eric Klineberg

Summary

Adult degenerative deformity is a common condition that can result in back pain, neurogenic claudication, and radiculopathy. Assessing the global deformity parameters on standing full-length scoliosis X-rays is critical. Optimizing the patient medically, including the bone health, is equally paramount before any surgery is undertaken.

Keywords: adult degenerative deformity, scoliosis, kyphosis

28.1 Key Points

- Adult degenerative deformity is characterized by abnormal coronal and sagittal spinal curvature in the adult spine.
- Asymmetric disk and facet joint degeneration are thought to be the most common causes of degenerative deformity.
- The most commonly presenting symptom is intractable back pain, but other symptoms such as radiculopathy and neurogenic claudication may also be present.
- The primary goals of surgery are to restore sagittal balance, decompress the neural elements, and achieve stabilization and arthrodesis.
- The absolute degree of coronal curve correction in an adult degenerative deformity patient is less important than maintaining or restoring sagittal balance.
- Despite the high risk of complications in patients undergoing reconstructive surgery for adult degenerative deformity, most studies suggest a significant improvement in quality of life and high rate of patient satisfaction if the surgical objectives are achieved.
- In general, the goal of surgery is to correct Pelvic Incidence-Lumbar Lordosis (PI-LL) mismatch to within ±10 degrees for patients with sagittal spinal deformity.

28.2 Background

- Spinal deformity is a dynamic process involving coronal, sagittal, and rotational elements. Any coronal plane deformity > 10 degrees is called scoliosis, whereas sagittal plane deformity can result in kyphosis or hyperlordosis.
- Adult spinal deformity refers to abnormal curvatures of the spine in patients who have completed their growth.
- There are several terms used to describe the adult degenerative deformity: adult degenerative scoliosis, degenerative lumbar scoliosis, de novo scoliosis, collapsing scoliosis, senescent lumbar scoliosis, and primary degenerative scoliosis.
- The pathophysiology of adult degenerative deformity is associated with degenerative changes.
- The asymmetrical degeneration of disk and facet joints puts an asymmetric load on the spine that leads to degenerative deformity.
- Degenerative changes in the vertebral body and disks are more obvious in adult degenerative deformity, commonly resulting in spinal stenosis.
- Degenerative deformity is characterized by a curve in the lumbar area and no compensatory curve in the thoracic vertebra, while adult idiopathic scoliosis has a major curve as well as compensatory curve similar in size to the major curve.
- Rotatory deformity is limited to the apex of the curve in adult degenerative deformity accompanied by lateral subluxation, while it is observed in the entire lumbar spine in adult idiopathic scoliosis.
- Sagittal imbalance is more common in adult degenerative deformity than adult idiopathic scoliosis.
- The risk factors of curve progression may be a curve with Cobb angles over 30 degrees, an asymmetric disk above and below the apical vertebra, a lateral listhesis of over 6 mm, an apical rotation greater than Grade II, osteopenia, and L5 vertebra being located above rather than below the intercrest line.
- Patient's age or sex is not associated with curve progression in adult degenerative deformity.
- Adult degenerative deformity curves tend to progress 1 to 6 degrees per year (average 3 degrees per year).[4]

28.3 Signs, Symptoms, and Physical Examination

- The most common symptom of adult degenerative deformity is back pain.
- Back pain results from degenerative changes in the lumbar disk and facet joint, as well as from muscle fatigue.

- Spinal stenosis is present in only 31% of adult idiopathic scoliosis, whereas it is observed in 90% of adult degenerative deformity.[4]
- Leg pain presents as intermittent claudication or radiating pain caused by spinal stenosis.
- Spinal stenosis more frequently presents as foraminal stenosis than central stenosis, and more commonly on the concave side than on the convex side.
- In addition to scoliosis, sagittal and coronal imbalance is frequently observed in adult degenerative deformity, which causes improper posture leading to low back pain.
- Pain at the convexity is caused by fatigue of the paraspinal muscles or arises from the facet joints.
- Pain at the concavity of the curve is thought to be caused by destruction of the facet joints and degenerative changes in disk spaces.
- Radicular pain at the concavity can arise from narrowed foramina or ruptured disks causing radiculopathy.
- Hip extension and knee flexion may be observed in patients who are compensating to maintain sagittal spinal alignment.

28.4 Evaluation of Adult Degenerative Deformity

- A detailed neurologic examination, including muscle power, reflexes, sensory testing, and gait testing, is necessary for patients with spinal deformity.
- Any degree of shoulder or pelvic asymmetry as well as pelvic obliquity and leg length discrepancy should be evaluated.
- The range of motion in hip and knee joints is evaluated to identify any contracture.
- Full-length (36-inch) standing posterior–anterior and lateral X-ray images should be obtained to assess sagittal and coronal balance. Full-body X-rays, if available, may allow for evaluation of global alignment.
- All images should be compared with any previous films to assess curve progression.
- Lateral flexion and extension views may suggest curve flexibility and can reveal dynamic instability. However, adult degenerative lumbar deformity is typically a fixed deformity.
- If neurological symptoms are present, magnetic resonance imaging (MRI) is recommended to evaluate compression of the neural elements.
- In patients with significant risk factors for osteoporosis (e.g., female, age ≥ 65 years, prior fragility fracture), dual-energy X-ray absorptiometry (DEXA) is recommended.

- Assessment of previous treatments is essential. A trial of conservative treatment is mandatory before surgical intervention is considered.
- In surgical candidates, workup may include cardiac echo and pulmonary function tests (PFTs) to ensure patients are fit for extensive spinal surgical reconstruction surgery.

28.5 Spinopelvic Parameters

- Sagittal vertical axis (SVA) > 5 cm is associated with worse clinical symptoms and quality of life measures.[5]
- Pelvic incidence (PI) = pelvic tilt (PT) + sacral slope.
- In general, PI-LL mismatch should be within ±10 degrees for adult spinal deformity.[6]

28.6 Treatment

- Initial intervention might include weight loss, physical therapy, exercise, oral nonsteroidal anti-inflammatory drugs (NSAIDs), and epidural steroid injections (ESIs).
- Given the high complication risks associated with surgery, careful patient selection, preoperative medical optimization, and expectation management are important when indicating patients for surgery.
- Surgical intervention is considered if there is neurologic deterioration or high risk for curve progression, or if back pain becomes refractory to nonsurgical treatment.
- The goal of surgery is to relieve back pain, improve radiating pain and claudication, and correct deformity.
- Surgical options include decompression alone, decompression and limited short fusion, and decompression and long fusion with correction of deformity.
- Decompression alone may induce curve progression and worsening of subluxation.
- In large scoliosis curve and severe subluxation of the apical vertebra, correction of deformity with decompression and long segment fusion is required.
- Restoration of sagittal imbalance is achieved by anterior column release or additional posterior techniques such as osteotomies.
- Posterior-based osteotomy techniques include Smith-Petersen osteotomy, pedicle subtraction osteotomy (PSO), and vertebral column resection (VCR).

- Typical surgical constructs include thoracic to sacral or to iliac stabilization with pedicle screw and rod systems, coupled with osteotomy techniques to provide decompression and correction.
- Spinopelvic fixation is typically recommended for long fusion constructs with the upper instrumented vertebra (UIV) at or above L2.
- Anterior interbody techniques can provide additional corrective and enhanced arthrodesis capabilities.
- Surgery should be selected with a full understanding of the cause of symptoms while considering the advantages, disadvantages, indications, and complications of each surgical option.

28.7 Complications

- There are substantial surgical risks for patients with adult degenerative deformity because of their increased age and frequently associated medical comorbidities.
- The reported complication rates of adult degenerative deformity surgery are as high as 40%, and the rates are even higher in the population older than 75 years and in the revision setting.[4]
- The most common complications are excessive blood loss, deep wound infection, and pulmonary embolism.
- Increase in fusion level and longer operation time are associated with more blood loss. This is particularly the case where osteotomy techniques such as PSO or VCR techniques are employed.
- Late complications include adjacent segment disease, pseudarthrosis, proximal junctional kyphosis (PJK), and proximal junctional failure (PJF).

Common Clinical Questions

1. What are the indications for surgery in adult degenerative deformity?
2. What are the most common complications of surgical intervention in adult degenerative deformity?

Answers to Common Clinical Questions

1. Surgical intervention is considered if there is neurologic deterioration or curve progression, or if back pain becomes refractory to nonsurgical treatment.
2. The most common complications are excessive blood loss, deep wound infection, and pulmonary embolus.

References

1. Silva FE, Lenke LG. Adult degenerative scoliosis: evaluation and management. Neurosurg Focus. 2010; 28(3):E1
2. Heary RF, Kumar S, Bono CM. Decision making in adult deformity. Neurosurgery. 2008; 63(3) Suppl:69–77
3. Cho KJ, Kim YT, Shin SH, Suk SI. Surgical treatment of adult degenerative scoliosis. Asian Spine J. 2014; 8(3):371–381
4. Ledonio CGT, Polly DW, Jr, Crawford CH, III, et al. Adult degenerative scoliosis surgical outcomes: a systematic review and meta-analysis. Spine Deform. 2013; 1(4):248–258
5. Glassman SD, Berven S, Bridwell K, Horton W, Dimar JR. Correlation of radiographic parameters and clinical symptoms in adult scoliosis. Spine. 2005; 30(6):682–688
6. Schwab F, Patel A, Ungar B, Farcy JP, Lafage V. Adult spinal deformity-postoperative standing imbalance: how much can you tolerate? An overview of key parameters in assessing alignment and planning corrective surgery. Spine. 2010; 35(25):2224–2231

29 Radiographic Parameters of Spinal Deformity

Alexander Aabedi, Vijay Letchuman, Andrew K. Chan, and Praveen V. Mummaneni

Summary

Radiographic parameters of spinal deformity are evidence-based metrics that help surgeons analyze a patient's spinal alignment, identify sources of sagittal and coronal (scoliotic) deformity, and guide correction to improve pain, disability, and quality of life. Studies ranging from bioenergetic analyses to cross-sectional population studies have refined the goals of adult spinal deformity correction. All patients evaluated for spinal deformity should undergo full-length anteroposterior and lateral standing X-rays. The sagittal vertical axis (SVA) is a reliable metric for global sagittal alignment (ideally less than 5 or 6 cm). Abnormal curvatures in the cervical, thoracic, and lumbar spine relative to the pelvis can increase the SVA, leading to pain, fatigue, and accelerated degenerative disk/joint disease. In the lumbar spine, sagittal deformity often results from a mismatch between pelvic incidence (PI) and lumbar lordosis (LL, ideally within 10 degrees). As the mismatch severity increases, compensatory mechanisms such as pelvic retroversion and knee flexion emerge, causing fatigue and disability. Deformity correction involves strategic placement of osteotomies and/or interbodies, the latter of which can be achieved through a minimally invasive (MIS) approach for faster recovery and better postoperative pain control.

Keywords: adult spinal deformity, osteotomy, minimally invasive deformity surgery, scoliosis

29.1 Key Points

- Sagittal vertical axis (SVA) less than 5 to 6 cm is the most utilized postoperative radiographic goal following surgery for adult spinal deformity.
- The ideal lumbar lordosis is within 10 degrees of the pelvic incidence (LL-PI), though there is an increasing awareness that age adjustment is important for both LL-PI and the SVA.

29.2 Background

- Normal or near-normal sagittal alignment has been directly correlated with clinical outcomes regarding pain and functional status.
- The sagittal profile is a harmonious relationship between the cervical, thoracic, and lumbar curvatures but is also influenced by the association between the pelvis and the spine. This relationship is better known as "spinopelvic balance."[1]
- Assuming a normal distribution and negative values for kyphosis and positive values for lordosis, there is a wide variation of neutral upright curvatures among normal, asymptomatic adults.
  - The C2–C7 angle (the greatest variation in regional curves) ranges from −11 degrees of kyphosis to + 45 degrees of lordosis.
  - The thoracic kyphosis (T1–T12) ranges from 25 to 65 degrees of kyphosis.
  - The lumbosacral lordosis (T12–S1) ranges from + 40 to + 84 degrees. Of note, approximately 70% of the total lumbosacral lordosis occurs between the superior end plate of L4 to the superior end plate of S1.
  - Various radiographic parameters have been associated with spinal deformities. For example, higher pelvic incidence has been correlated with isthmic spondylolisthesis.[1,2,3,4,5,6,7,8,9,10]

29.3 Signs, Symptoms, and Physical Examination

- Initial clinical evaluation of patients includes assessment of their main complaints and comorbidities.
- Physical examination includes assessment of neurological deficits, rigidity of their clinical deformity (i.e., lie down test, etc.), body habitus, posture, muscle contractures (hip flexion, knee flexion, etc.), pelvic obliquity, shoulder imbalance, and limb deformities.

29.3.1 Neuroimaging

- Radiographic assessment includes standing, global, full-length X-rays with anteroposterior and lateral views of the whole skeleton, including the spine, to evaluate sagittal and coronal alignment, and measure the sagittal, coronal, and lumbo-sacral–pelvic parameters. Pelvic obliquity, leg length discrepancy, and lower extremity compensation, such as asymmetric knee bending, should be assessed.

- Additional radiographic evaluation may include a lumbar magnetic resonance imaging (MRI) or computed tomography (CT) myelogram (for patients with previous lumbar instrumentation), dynamic lumbar radiographs to help identify mobile listhesis, and side-bending or supine X-rays in scoliosis cases to evaluate curve flexibility. Assessment of bone density is also of importance in patients who will undergo surgical treatment.[6,9,11,12,13,14,15,16]
- Several forms of measurements have been proposed to assess a patient's global sagittal balance (**Fig. 29.1**).
  - One important parameter is a vertical line drawn from the center of the C7 vertebral body with respect to the posterior superior corner of the S1 end plate (the "sacral reference point"). This "C7 plumb line" should be less than 6 cm from the sacral reference point in normally aligned, asymptomatic individuals. The C7–SVA has a positive value when the vertical plumb line is anterior to the sacral reference point and a negative value when posterior to it.[8,17,18]

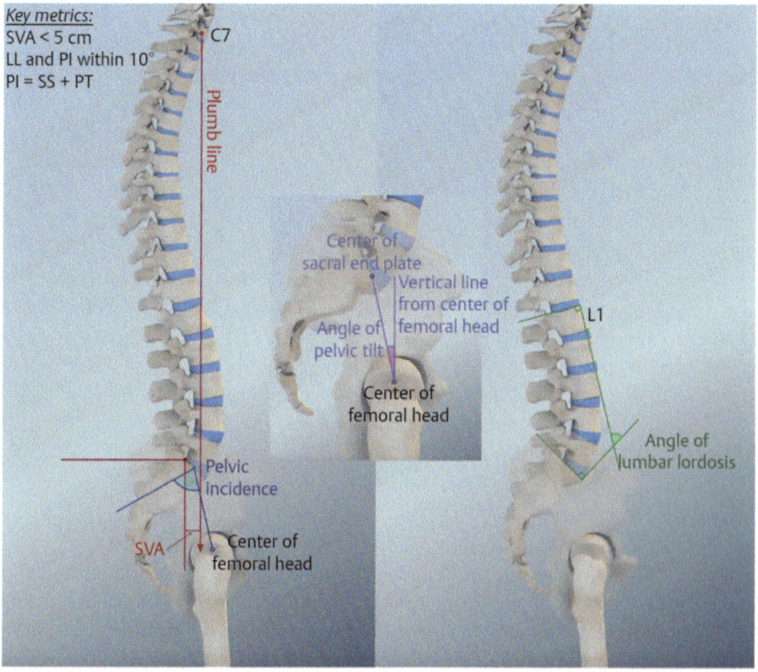

Fig. 29.1 Calculation of sagittal vertical axis (SVA), pelvic incidence (PI), pelvic tilt (PT), and lumbar lordosis (LL). SS, sacral slope.

- Pelvic incidence (PI) is defined as the angle formed by a line drawn from the midpoint of the approximated center of the femoral heads to a line perpendicular to the center of the sacral end plate. The PI is established at the end of adolescence and is a constant value unaffected by body posture. Typical values range from 48 to 55 degrees.[3,4,8,10]
- Pelvic tilt (PT) is defined as an angle formed between a vertical reference line at the midpoint of the approximated center of the femoral heads and a line drawn from the femoral head center point to the midpoint of the sacral end plate. Normal values are under 20 degrees.[4] Pelvic retroversion occurs at higher values of PT.
- Sacral slope (SS) is defined as an angle formed between a horizontal reference line and the sacral end plate. Normal values range from 36 to 42 degrees.

- From a geometrical point of view, PI = SS + PT. Spinopelvic alignment is normal when there is a direct relationship between the PI, SS, and lumbar lordosis (LL). An elevated PT is a sign of compensated sagittal imbalance.
- Considering that PI cannot be changed, surgeons must pursue an adequate LL when planning surgeries to achieve a normal sagittal balance and improve patients' final outcome. To determine the ideal LL, we can use the equation LL = PI ± 10 degrees. However, there are age-adjusted alignment goals.[19]
- A more recently described radiographic parameter known as the T1 pelvic angle is another measure of sagittal alignment that is independent of compensatory mechanisms such as pelvic retroversion.[20] It is measured by taking the angle between a line from the center of the femoral heads to the center of the T1 vertebral body and from the center of the femoral heads to the center of the superior end plate of S1. An angle greater than 20 degrees indicates malalignment.
- The central sagittal vertical line (CSVL) provides a measurement of global coronal balance, which can be perturbed in both adolescent and adult degenerative scoliosis. It is acquired by measuring the distance from the C7 plumb line to the midline of the sacrum. Values greater than 2 cm (a rightward deviation of the plumb line being defined as positive) or less than −2 cm indicate coronal imbalance. Coronal imbalance is typically generated by scoliosis, a lateral curvature of the spine. Cobb angles > 10 degrees are considered abnormal, though, depending on the presence of compensatory curves, they are not always associated with coronal imbalance.

29.4 Treatment

- Operative treatment is recommended in patients who have moderate to severe symptoms, patients who fail conservative measures for pain control, and patients with neurological deficits. Surgical planning is highly dependent on the radiographic parameters discussed above. Additional factors that may influence surgical planning are revision status (e.g., pseudarthrosis or instrumentation failure), patients' comorbidities, previous surgeries, bone quality, and body habitus.[6,9,10,11,16,21,22,23,24,25,26,27,28,29,30]

- Decompression without fusion can be considered in patients without evident instability, in patients without severe sagittal imbalance (mild curves), and when symptoms are secondary to nerve root compression (i.e., in patients with minimal axial low back pain). Minimally invasive decompressive techniques can be used to decrease blood loss and hospital stay. The main limitations of decompressive techniques are the inabilities to restore sagittal balance and improve axial back pain. There is also a small risk of later instability secondary to decompression. The MISDEF2 algorithm was created for this reason to provide a framework to assist surgeons in the decision-making when considering minimally invasive spinal (MIS) surgery techniques for deformity corrections (**Fig. 29.2**).[22,26]

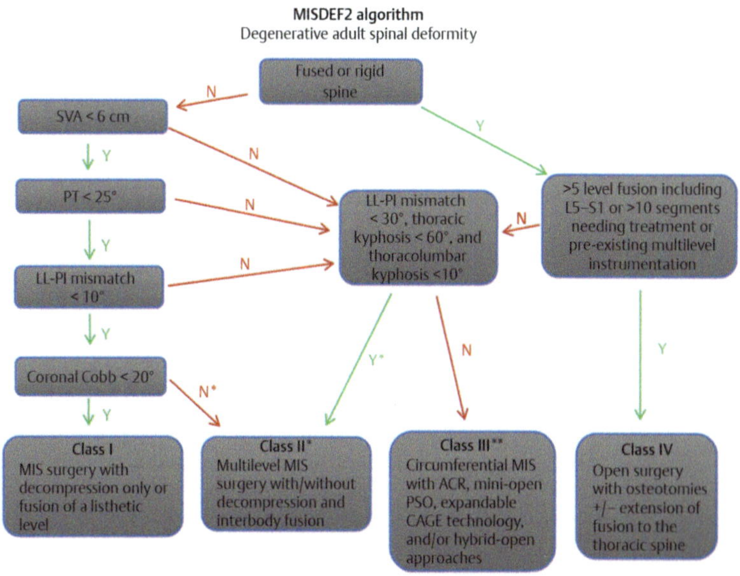

Fig. 29.2 MISDEF2 algorithm for decision-making in minimally invasive spinal (MIS) deformity surgery. ACR, anterior column realignment; LL-PI, lumbar lordosis–pelvic incidence; PSO, pedicle subtraction osteotomy; PT, pelvic tilt; SVA, sagittal vertical axis. (This figure was published in *Neurosurgery Clinics of North America*, vol 29, issue 3, Choy W, Miller CA, Chan AK, Fu KM, Park P, Mummaneni PV, Evolution of the Minimally Invasive Spinal Deformity Surgery Algorithm: An Evidence-Based Approach to Surgical Strategies for Deformity Correction, pp 399–406, copyright Elsevier (2018). Reprinted with permission from Elsevier.)

- Anterior and lateral approaches include the anterior lumbar interbody fusion (ALIF) and lateral lumbar interbody fusion (LLIF) techniques, respectively. Potential advantages of these approaches include indirect decompression via expanded foraminal height, as well as avoidance of posterior lumbar muscle trauma. ALIF can provide 5 to 10 degrees of additional lumbar lordosis while LLIF can provide 2 to 5 degrees of correction. The LLIF technique can also improve coronal spine alignment, especially from L1 to L4 levels (the L5–S1 level is limited by the iliac crest unless an oblique approach is selected). ALIF may have approach-related complications, such as retrograde ejaculation or vascular injuries. LLIF has some risk of lumbar plexus injuries as the psoas muscle is traversed and may rarely result in vascular injury to the iliac vein. In general, anterior spine techniques are useful to restore lumbar lordosis and to provide interbody fusion with indirect nerve root decompression but most of the time will require a combined posterior approach to achieve normal or near-normal restoration of the spinopelvic measurements. The additional benefit of the anterior or lateral approach is a larger cage footprint which enhances biomechanical stability, increases fusion surface area, and reduces subsidence given that the cages may span the ring apophyses.
- The majority of spinal deformities are treated by a posterior approach with instrumentation and fusion, with or without an anterior approach. Posterior approaches allow direct decompression of a stenotic spinal canal or foramina. Advantages of the posterior approach include direct decompression, the possibility to perform interbody fusion using posterior or transforaminal techniques (posterior lumbar interbody fusion or transforaminal lumbar interbody fusion, respectively), and access to perform spinal osteotomies that can correct coronal and sagittal imbalance. Banana-shaped and expandable-type cages are increasingly leveraged to optimize restoration of segmental lordosis and disk height.
- Osteotomies are used to attain coronal and sagittal deformity correction, especially in rigid deformities. In general, the goal of spinal osteotomies is to restore the SVA to under 6 cm and to attain LL within 10 degrees of the PI. However, age-adjusted thresholds may be followed (**Table 29.1**).[19] The chosen osteotomy technique may vary according to the degree of correction required to restore sagittal balance. Smith-Petersen osteotomy (SPO) includes resection of the adjacent facet joints, narrow resection of the lamina, and ligaments of the involved level and may correct 5 to 10 degrees of lordosis per level and is used for patients with ankylosing spondylitis.[8,31,32] The Ponte osteotomy is similar with up to 10 degrees of lordosis per level and is performed in patients without ankylosing spondylitis.[33]

Table 29.1 Age-adjusted ideal alignment goals

	Age group (years)				
	<45	45–54	55–64	65–74	≥74
PT (°)	11.0	18.8	22.0	25.1	28.8
PI-LL (°)	−10.5	0.5	5.8	10.5	17.0
SVA (cm)	−3	1–2	3–4	5–6	8

Abbreviations: PI-LL, pelvic incidence–lumbar lordosis; PT, pelvic tilt; SVA, sagittal vertical axis.

- The pedicle subtraction osteotomy (PSO) consists of resection of the facet joints, lamina, pedicles, and wedge-shaped portion of the vertebral body. Closure of osteomy gap in PSO can result in 20 to 35 degrees of lordosis correction and significant improvement of the SVA. The complication potential of PSO compared with SPO is higher, including blood loss and neurological deficits.[8] However, a PSO is often needed when there is a rigid deformity without open disk spaces (a situation where an SPO may not suffice).
- A less invasive approach known as anterior column realignment (ACR), which involves removal of the disk via a lateral approach with division of the anterior longitudinal ligament/annulus and placement of a hyperlordotic cage, has emerged as a potentially less morbid alternative to three-column osteotomy with ≥ 15 degrees correction per level when an open, unfused disk space is present at the apex of the desired lordosis.[32]
- An additional less invasive approach, when the single-level lordotic restoration of an ACR is not required, is multilevel ALIF/LLIF along with fully percutaneous posterior instrumentation (i.e., circumferential minimally invasive surgery). This multilevel interbody approach is sometimes combined with an open posterior approach with or without osteotomies (i.e., hybrid surgery).
- In cases in which there is a rigid coronal and sagittal deformity, surgeons can perform a vertebral column resection, which consists of resection of the vertebral body, the adjacent disks, and all the posterior elements of the affected level, resulting in the most significant correction rate of all osteotomies (≥ 40 degrees) but having a significant risk of new neurological deficits and blood loss.
- New techniques including patient-specific rods and kickstand rods can help achieve coronal alignment goals in appropriate patients by pushing the thoracolumbar junction toward midline.

Common Clinical Questions

1. Above what value is the sagittal vertical axis considered abnormal?
2. How does one measure pelvic incidence?
3. What is the ideal relationship between lumbar lordosis and pelvic incidence?

Answers to Common Clinical Questions

1. Above 5 to 6 cm.
2. Pelvic incidence (PI) is defined as the angle formed by a line drawn from the midpoint of the approximated center of the femoral heads to a line perpendicular to the center of the sacral end plate.
3. They should be within 10 degrees of one another.

References

1. Kuntz C, IV, Levin LS, Ondra SL, Shaffrey CI, Morgan CJ. Neutral upright sagittal spinal alignment from the occiput to the pelvis in asymptomatic adults: a review and resynthesis of the literature. J Neurosurg Spine. 2007; 6(2):104–112
2. Kanter AS, Shaffrey CI, Mummaneni P, Wang MY, Uribe JS. Introduction: Adult spinal deformity: pathophysiology and corrective measures. Neurosurg Focus. 2014; 36(5):Introduction
3. Legaye J, Duval-Beaupère G, Hecquet J, Marty C. Pelvic incidence: a fundamental pelvic parameter for three-dimensional regulation of spinal sagittal curves. Eur Spine J. 1998; 7(2):99–103
4. Lafage V, Schwab F, Patel A, Hawkinson N, Farcy JP. Pelvic tilt and truncal inclination: two key radiographic parameters in the setting of adults with spinal deformity. Spine. 2009; 34(17):E599–E606
5. Lau D, DiGiorgio AM, Chan AK, et al. Applicability of cervical sagittal vertical axis, cervical lordosis, and T1 slope on pain and disability outcomes after anterior cervical discectomy and fusion in patients without deformity. J Neurosurg Spine. 2019:1–8. Online ahead of print.
6. Moal B, Schwab F, Ames CP, et al. International Spine Study Group. Radiographic outcomes of adult spinal deformity correction: a critical analysis of variability and failures across deformity patterns. Spine Deform. 2014; 2(3):219–225
7. Okonkwo DO, Mummaneni PV. Introduction: Adult spinal deformity. Neurosurg Focus. 2010; 28(3):E1
8. Rose PS, Bridwell KH, Lenke LG, et al. Role of pelvic incidence, thoracic kyphosis, and patient factors on sagittal plane correction following pedicle subtraction osteotomy. Spine. 2009; 34(8):785–791

9. Than KD, Park P, Fu KM, et al. International Spine Study Group. Clinical and radiographic parameters associated with best versus worst clinical outcomes in minimally invasive spinal deformity surgery. J Neurosurg Spine. 2016; 25 (1):21–25
10. Uribe JS, Januszewski J, Wang M, et al. Minimally Invasive Surgery Section of the International Spine Study Group. Patients with high pelvic tilt achieve the same clinical success as those with low pelvic tilt after minimally invasive adult deformity surgery. Neurosurgery. 2018; 83(2):270–276
11. Bae J, Theologis AA, Strom R, et al. Comparative analysis of 3 surgical strategies for adult spinal deformity with mild to moderate sagittal imbalance. J Neurosurg Spine. 2018; 28(1):40–49
12. Blondel B, Schwab F, Bess S, et al. Posterior global malalignment after osteotomy for sagittal plane deformity: it happens and here is why. Spine. 2013; 38(7):E394–E401
13. Horn SR, Passias PG, Oh C, et al. International Spine Study Group. Predicting the combined occurrence of poor clinical and radiographic outcomes following cervical deformity corrective surgery. J Neurosurg Spine. 2019; 32 (2):182–190
14. Park P, Wang MY, Nguyen S, et al. International Spine Study Group. Comparison of complications and clinical and radiographic outcomes between nonobese and obese patients with adult spinal deformity undergoing minimally invasive surgery. World Neurosurg. 2016; 87:55–60
15. Than KD, Mehta VA, Le V, et al. Role of obesity in less radiographic correction and worse health-related quality-of-life outcomes following minimally invasive deformity surgery. J Neurosurg Spine. 2022:1–10. Online ahead of print.
16. Wang MY, Park P, Tran S, et al. MIS-ISSG Group. Intermediate-term clinical and radiographic outcomes with less invasive adult spinal deformity surgery: patients with a minimum follow-up of 4 years. Acta Neurochir (Wien). 2020; 162(6):1393–1400
17. Glassman SD, Bridwell K, Dimar JR, Horton W, Berven S, Schwab F. The impact of positive sagittal balance in adult spinal deformity. Spine. 2005; 30 (18):2024–2029
18. Xi Z, Duan PG, Mummaneni PV, et al. Posterior displacement of L1 may be a risk factor for proximal junctional kyphosis after adult spinal deformity correction. Global Spine J. 2023; 13(4):1042–1048
19. Lafage R, Schwab F, Glassman S, et al. International Spine Study Group. Age-adjusted alignment goals have the potential to reduce PJK. Spine. 2017; 42 (17):1275–1282
20. Protopsaltis T, Schwab F, Bronsard N, et al. International Spine Study Group. The T1 pelvic angle, a novel radiographic measure of global sagittal deformity, accounts for both spinal inclination and pelvic tilt and correlates with health-related quality of life. J Bone Joint Surg Am. 2014; 96(19):1631–1640

21. Berven S, Jain D, O'Neill C, Selinger A, Mummaneni P. Team approach: degenerative spinal deformity. JBJS Rev. 2017; 5(4):e1
22. Choy W, Miller CA, Chan AK, Fu KM, Park P, Mummaneni PV. Evolution of the minimally invasive spinal deformity surgery algorithm: an evidence-based approach to surgical strategies for deformity correction. Neurosurg Clin N Am. 2018; 29(3):399–406
23. Mummaneni PV, Dhall SS, Rodts GE, Haid RW. Circumferential fusion for cervical kyphotic deformity. J Neurosurg Spine. 2008; 9(6):515–521
24. Mummaneni PV, Hussain I, Shaffrey CI, et al. International Spine Study Group. The minimally invasive interbody selection algorithm for spinal deformity. J Neurosurg Spine. 2021; 34(5):741–748
25. Mummaneni PV, Park P, Fu KM, et al. International Spine Study Group. Does minimally invasive percutaneous posterior instrumentation reduce risk of proximal junctional kyphosis in adult spinal deformity surgery? A propensity-matched cohort analysis. Neurosurgery. 2016; 78(1):101–108
26. Mummaneni PV, Park P, Shaffrey CI, et al. International Spine Study Group (ISSG). The MISDEF2 algorithm: an updated algorithm for patient selection in minimally invasive deformity surgery. J Neurosurg Spine. 2019; 32(2):221–228
27. Mummaneni PV, Shaffrey CI, Lenke LG, et al. Minimally Invasive Surgery Section of the International, Spine Study Group. The minimally invasive spinal deformity surgery algorithm: a reproducible rational framework for decision making in minimally invasive spinal deformity surgery. Neurosurg Focus. 2014; 36(5):E6
28. Mummaneni PV, Tu TH, Ziewacz JE, Akinbo OC, Deviren V, Mundis GM. The role of minimally invasive techniques in the treatment of adult spinal deformity. Neurosurg Clin N Am. 2013; 24(2):231–248
29. Park P, Than KD, Mummaneni PV, et al. International Spine Study Group. Factors affecting approach selection for minimally invasive versus open surgery in the treatment of adult spinal deformity: analysis of a prospective, nonrandomized multicenter study. J Neurosurg Spine. 2020:1–6. Online ahead of print.
30. Wang MY, Mummaneni PV. Minimally invasive surgery for thoracolumbar spinal deformity: initial clinical experience with clinical and radiographic outcomes. Neurosurg Focus. 2010; 28(3):E9
31. Chan AK, Lau D, Osorio JA, et al. Asymmetric pedicle subtraction osteotomy for adult spinal deformity with coronal imbalance: complications, radiographic and surgical outcomes. Oper Neurosurg (Hagerstown). 2020; 18(2):209–216
32. Saigal R, Mundis GM, Jr, Eastlack R, Uribe JS, Phillips FM, Akbarnia BA. Anterior column realignment (ACR) in adult sagittal deformity correction: technique and review of the literature. Spine. 2016; 41 Suppl 8:S66–S73
33. Ponte A, Orlando G, Siccardi GL. The true Ponte osteotomy: by the one who developed it. Spine Deform. 2018; 6(1):2–11

30 Vascular Pathology of the Spine

Michael D. White, Timothy D. Uschold, and Steve W. Chang

Summary
This chapter offers readers a detailed exploration of the classification, diagnosis, and management of complex vascular lesions in the spine. It begins with a discussion of spinal cavernous malformations, with a focus on epidemiology, symptomatology, diagnostic workup, and treatment. Readers will also find an extensive overview of arteriovenous malformations and arteriovenous fistulas. This chapter discusses the classification of these lesions based on anatomical location using the Spetzler et al nomenclature, which can provide insight into the most appropriate management. The text also navigates the current treatment paradigms for arteriovenous malformations and fistulas, highlighting key challenges and strategies for both endovascular and surgical interventions. With clear and concise descriptions and practical insights, this chapter serves as an invaluable resource for readers seeking to further their understanding of complex vascular lesions in the spine and improve their clinical practice.

Keywords: spinal vascular lesions, arteriovenous malformation, arteriovenous fistula, spinal cavernous malformation, spinal AVM, spinal AVF, spinal fistula

30.1 Key Points

- The Spetzler et al nomenclature for spinal vascular lesions classifies arteriovenous malformations (AVMs) and arteriovenous fistulas (AVFs) according to their anatomic locations. Lesion classification does not rigidly dictate optimal treatment strategy but can provide a useful decision-making framework.[1]
- Spinal angiography is the gold standard and is warranted for all arteriovenous lesions.
- Thorough understanding of spinal angiographic anatomy, surgical vascular anatomy, and segmental variability is essential for decision-making.
- A high index of suspicion should be maintained in the presence of spinal vascular lesions. Protean clinical findings, imaging appearance, and low incidence often result in diagnostic delays.

30.2 Cavernous Malformations

- Background:
  - Cavernous malformations are benign vascular neoplasms that may occur in sporadic or familial forms. Spinal cavernomas favor thoracic over cervical locations, followed by lumbar locations.
  - Spinal cavernous malformations constitute about 5% of all spinal vascular lesions. There is a slight female preponderance, with a ratio of 2:1.[2]
  - Intramedullary is the most common location, although intramedullary exophytic, intradural extramedullary, and extradural locations have been reported.
  - Peak incidence of symptomatic hemorrhage is reported in the fourth decade.
- Signs, symptoms, and physical examination:
  - Acute: Large hemorrhages can result in long-tract dysfunction or radicular symptoms (including pain) depending on location. Acute meningeal signs are rare.
  - Progressive decline or stepwise deterioration due to repeated hemorrhages or hemosiderin toxicity. Improvement between events is usually incomplete.
  - Estimated bleed rates of 1.4 to 4.5% per patient-year have been reported. The rate of subsequent hemorrhage may approach 66% per patient-year.
- Workup:
  - Magnetic resonance imaging (MRI) with gradient-recalled echo (GRE) sequences.
  - Detailed family history, MRI of the brain, and possible familial screening should be considered. As many as 50% of patients may harbor intracranial cavernomas as well.[3]
- Neuroimaging:
  - MRI is the modality of choice. Cavernomas are angiographically occult.
  - MRI appearance: T1 and T2 "popcorn" heterogeneity reflects vascular sinusoids containing blood products of different ages. Surrounding T1 and T2 hypointensity reflects the rim of hemosiderin-stained parenchyma. Hypointense "blooming" is notable with GRE sequences, with the absence of flow voids.[4]
  - Although a hypointense peripheral T2 signal can indicate a cavernous malformation on MRI, this can also be observed in roughly 22 to 33% of spinal cord ependymomas, also known as the "cap sign."[5] Small size, eccentric axial location, minimal enhancement, and absence of or minimal cord edema are often seen in cavernous malformations and can aid in diagnosis.[6]

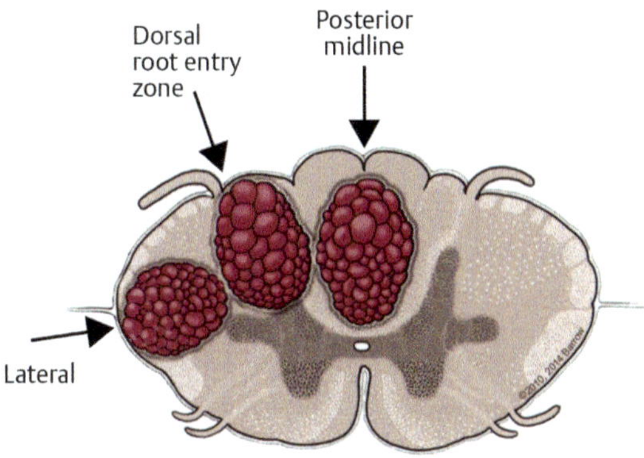

Fig. 30.1 Safe entry zones for intramedullary lesions. (Reproduced with permission from Barrow Neurological Institute, Phoenix, Arizona.)

- Treatment:
  - Gross total excision is the treatment goal and is protective against future hemorrhage.
  - Conservative management is a consideration for small asymptomatic lesions, especially deep-seated lesions that fail to reach the pial surface on axial images.[3,7]
  - Lesions that demonstrate growth on interval imaging, repeat hemorrhages, or those that become symptomatic should be considered for surgical resection.
- Surgical pearls:
  - Appropriate entry zones from a posterior or posterolateral approach include midline myelotomy, dorsal lateral sulcus at the dorsal root entry zone, or laterally between the dentate ligaments (**Fig. 30.1**).
  - Whenever possible, sharp dissection is preferred. However, some coagulation of the cavernoma may be necessary to debulk the lesion internally. Piecemeal excision is common.
  - Care is necessary to preserve hemosiderin-stained parenchyma surrounding the cavernoma. The developmental venous anomaly should be preserved whenever possible.[3,7]

30.3 Arteriovenous Lesions

- Background:
  - Intradural–dorsal AVF:
    - Considered an acquired lesion attributed to venous outflow dysfunction.

   - Low-flow fistulas involve a radiculomedullary artery as it pierces the dural root sleeve resulting in an arterialized coronal venous plexus. Type B lesions recruit feeders from adjacent levels, but a single fistulous point is always present.
   - Accounts for 60 to 80% of spinal vascular lesions. Typically affects males more than females, 40 to 60 years of age, and has a predilection for the thoracolumbar spine.
  - Intradural–ventral AVF:
    - High-flow anastomosis between the anterior spinal artery (ASA) and ventral venous plexus. Varix formation, flow rate, complexity, and a multiplicity of feeding pedicles increase with types A to C.
    - Occurs in younger patients (20–60 years of age) and favors the thoracolumbar spine.
  - Extradural AVM:
    - High-flow direct anastomosis between the epidural artery and vein may receive multisegmental arterial contributions.[1]
    - Sporadic de novo formation, congenital, syndromic associations (e.g., neurofibromatosis [NF]-1), and traumatic etiologies have all been reported (**Table 30.1**).
  - Extradural–intradural AVM:
    - High-flow AVM, irrespective of tissue boundaries, commonly involving multiple or entire spinal segments. May interdigitate with functional cord tissue. Commonly fed by ASA and posterior spinal artery (PSA). Rare.
  - Intramedullary AVM:
    - High-flow AVM with diffuse and compact forms. High-risk features, including varix formation and associated aneurysms, are common.
    - Typically symptomatic early in life (10–30 years of age), with a predilection for the cervical spine. These AVMs represent 15 to 20% of all spinal vascular lesions.
  - Conus AVM: High-flow, complex shunting pattern found at conus. Multiple shunts and nidi may be pial or intramedullary. Rare (**Table 30.2**).[1]
- Signs, symptoms, and physical examination:
  - Intradural–dorsal AVF: Protean history of progressive myelopathy, dominated by gait and sphincter dysfunction. Patients most commonly become symptomatic due to vascular congestion rather than hemorrhage, although hemorrhage can occur in rare instances.
  - Intradural ventral: Similarly protean, progressive, and variable history dominated by myelopathic findings. Symptomatic progression resulting from steal, compression, and hemorrhage increases with grade and flow rate.
  - Extradural: Myeloradiculopathy is common, with symptoms due to compression, steal, and hemorrhage. Venous congestion is typically rare.

Table 30.1 Spetzler et al's arteriovenous fistula classification[1]

Type	Shunt location	Pathophysiology	Symptoms	Imaging	Treatment
Intradural dorsal—type A (single-level feeder), type B (multiple feeders)	Intradural entry of radiculomedullary artery at root sleeve	Vascular congestion as a result of venous outflow obstruction	Progressive myelopathy	MRI shows dorsal flow voids and T2 cord change; DSA is gold standard	Surgery versus endovascular
Intradural ventral*: type A, type B, and type C	Direct fistula to anterior spinal artery	Mass effect, steal, or hemorrhage progresses with higher grades	Progressive myelopathy	MRI shows ventral flow voids; DSA is gold standard	Surgery; endovascular treatment may be a more appropriate alternative with higher grades
Extradural	Epidural artery and vein	Primarily compression and steal rather than congestion; may hemorrhage	Progressive myelopathy or radiculopathy or both	MRI shows epidural engorgement; DSA is gold standard	Primarily endovascular, except when the decline is a result of hemorrhage

Abbreviation: DSA, digital subtraction angiogram; MRI, magnetic resonance imaging.
Note: * Intradural ventral type A fistulas are small shunts in which blood flow is slow and venous hypertension is moderate. Types B and C have progressively larger shunts; the latter are characterized by a giant fistula and a markedly distended venous network. As the size and flow of the fistula increases, the signs and symptoms attributable to progressive vascular steal and spinal cord compression become more pronounced.

Table 30.2 Spetzler et al's arteriovenous malformation classification[1]

Type	Distinguishing features	Pathophysiology	Symptoms	Treatment
Extradural–intradural	Irrespective of normal tissue planes; may involve the entire metamere	Steal, compression, hemorrhage	Progressive myelopathy, often with radicular-type pain	Multimodality, typically palliative
Intramedullary: Compact nidus Diffuse nidus	Typically with at least one ASA feeder; PSA feeders are also common High-flow aneurysms and varices	Hemorrhage, steal, compression	Acute or stepwise progression of radicular pain and long-tract signs (e.g., myelopathy)	Primarily surgical; preoperative embolization is typically useful
Conus	Complex shunting and nidal patterns typically involve ASA and PSA	Steal, hemorrhage, venous congestion	Progressive myelopathy or radiculopathy, or both; symptoms are referable to conus location	Multimodality (endovascular + surgery)

Abbreviations: ASA, anterior spinal artery; PSA, posterior spinal artery.

- Extradural–intradural AVM: Malignant natural history characterized by progressive myelopathy. Radicular pain referable to the involved segment is typical. The pathophysiology involves mass effect, steal, hemorrhage, and compression.
- Intramedullary AVM: Malignant natural history characterized by progressive myeloradiculopathy. Stepwise deterioration or acute decline attributable to repeated hemorrhage, steal, and compression.
- Conus AVM: Progressive myeloradiculopathy, symptoms referable to conus.[1]

• Workup:
  - Spinal MRI/magnetic resonance angiography (MRA) has proven especially useful for intradural dorsal lesions. MRA may be sufficiently sensitive to identify the fistula type, pinpoint the level(s) of the shunt, and to confirm treatment at follow-up.
  - Spinal angiography, however, remains the gold standard imaging modality (for all spinal AVFs and AVMs) and may be directed more precisely after careful inspection of prior MRA.

• Neuroimaging:
  - AVMs:
    ▪ MRI is most useful to delineate the size and configuration of the nidus (compact versus diffuse), to evaluate for hemorrhage, and to assess the angioarchitecture.
  - Intradural dorsal AVF:
    ▪ MRI: In the appropriate clinical setting, extensive intramedullary T2 hyperintensity and intradural flow voids along the dorsal pial surface are nearly pathognomonic. Enhancement can be variable.
    ▪ Angiography: Venous outflow is sluggish, and a long venous phase may be necessary. Suspected but occult intradural–dorsal fistulas require surgical exploration.
  - Intradural ventral:
    ▪ MRI: Reveals variable T2 hyperintensity and enhancement with dilated flow voids along the ventral surface of the spinal cord, including varix formation.
    ▪ Angiography: Reveals a direct fistula between the radiculomedullary artery and ASA. The ASA is identified by the classic hairpin loop and could be displaced from the midline. The ventral arterialized vein often harbors a prominent venous varix.
  - Extradural:
    ▪ MRI/MRA: Prominent epidural flow voids and enhancement, typically with significant mass effect. Variable T2 intramedullary signal change.[4]

• Treatment:
  - Intradural–dorsal AVF: Microsurgical clip occlusion at intradural fistulous point remains the gold standard. Embolization with a liquid

  agent is now an acceptable first-line treatment but is associated with a greater risk of recurrence.[8]
  - Intradural–ventral AVF: Microsurgical fistula obliteration remains the treatment of choice, but embolic strategies are also often used. Vessel caliber (particularly types A and B) and proximity to ASA present challenges to endovascular management. However, relatively high rates of complete obliteration have been reported for both open surgical and endovascularly treated lesions, around 88 and 74%, respectively.[9]
  - Extradural AVF: Endovascular treatment is favored, especially for lesions with large-caliber feeding vessels. For large venous pouches, embolization may be difficult due to the large quantity of embolic material needed for obliteration.[10]
  - Extradural–intradural AVM: Curative resection is atypical. Multimodal palliation strategies alleviate symptoms of steal, compression, and hemorrhage.
  - Intramedullary AVM: Surgical resection, typically via a posterior or posterolateral approach, remains the gold standard and is typically preceded by attempts at embolization in appropriately selected patients.[11]
  - Conus AVM: Multimodal strategies include aggressive embolization and resection.[1]
- Surgical pearls:
  - Indocyanine green angiography (ICG) is ideal for intraoperative confirmation of location and is essential for identifying angiographically occult lesions.
  - Intramedullary AVMs are commonly fed by at least one branch of the ASA. Steal phenomena may obscure ASA involvement on preoperative angiography, but serial runs mid-resection may reveal the ASA as shunting is progressively eliminated.
  - Arterial supply is circumferentially addressed first for intramedullary AVMs. Venous outflow is spared until the lesion is sufficiently devascularized.

Common Clinical Questions

1. The Spetzler et al nomenclature divides arteriovenous lesions solely on the basis of what characteristic?
2. What imaging modality is the gold standard and is mandatory for all spinal arteriovenous lesions?
3. Describe the typical imaging findings of an intradural–dorsal fistula on MRI.

Answers to Common Clinical Questions

1. Anatomic location; all other characteristics follow suit.
2. Angiography.
3. Dorsal flow voids, extensive T2 signal change, variable and patchy enhancement.

References

1. Spetzler RF, Detwiler PW, Riina HA, Porter RW. Modified classification of spinal cord vascular lesions. J Neurosurg. 2002; 96(2) Suppl:145–156
2. Saliou G, Krings T. Vascular diseases of the spine. Handb Clin Neurol. 2016; 136:707–716
3. Perrini P, Uygur E, Spetzler RF, Lanzino G. Cavernous malformations of the spinal cord. In: Lanzino G, Spetzler RF, eds. Cavernous Malformations of the Brain and Spinal Cord. Thieme Medical Publishers; 2008:88–93
4. Jackson J, Partovi S. Imaging of spinal cord vascular malformations. Operative Techniques in Neurosurgery. 2003; 6(3):125–140
5. Fine MJ, Kricheff II, Freed D, Epstein FJ. Spinal cord ependymomas: MR imaging features. Radiology. 1995; 197(3):655–658
6. Jeon I, Jung WS, Suh SH, Chung TS, Cho YE, Ahn SJ. MR imaging features that distinguish spinal cavernous angioma from hemorrhagic ependymoma and serial MRI changes in cavernous angioma. J Neurooncol. 2016; 130(1):229–236
7. Vishteh AG, Sankhla S, Anson JA, Zabramski JM, Spetzler RF. Surgical resection of intramedullary spinal cord cavernous malformations: delayed complications, long-term outcomes, and association with cryptic venous malformations. Neurosurgery. 1997; 41(5):1094–1100, discussion 1100–1101
8. Steinmetz MP, Chow MM, Krishnaney AA, et al. Outcome after the treatment of spinal dural arteriovenous fistulae: a contemporary single-institution series and meta-analysis. Neurosurgery. 2004; 55(1):77–87, discussion 87–88
9. Ozpinar A, Weiner GM, Ducruet AF. Epidemiology, clinical presentation, diagnostic evaluation, and prognosis of spinal arteriovenous malformations. Handb Clin Neurol. 2017; 143:145–152
10. Brinjikji W, Lanzino G. Endovascular treatment of spinal arteriovenous malformations. Handb Clin Neurol. 2017; 143:161–174
11. Connolly ES, Jr, Zubay GP, McCormick PC, Stein BM. The posterior approach to a series of glomus (Type II) intramedullary spinal cord arteriovenous malformations. Neurosurgery. 1998; 42(4):774–785, discussion 785–786

31 Spondyloarthropathies

Joshua Vignolles-Jeong, Alexander Keister, Samuel Ammerman, and Andrew J. Grossbach

Summary

Spondyloarthropathies are a group of inflammatory rheumatic diseases associated with the HLA-B27 gene which affect the sacroiliac joints, spine, and peripheral joints. Articular manifestations include enthesitis, dactylitis, and inflammatory pain and stiffness in the sacroiliac joints and spine. Extraarticular manifestations include uveitis, inflammatory bowel disease, and psoriasis. Neuroimaging combined with a thorough history and physical examination is key to determine the extent of disease progression and to inform treatment. Medical management options include nonsteroidal anti-inflammatory drugs, methotrexate, sulfasalazine, and tumor necrosis factor-alpha inhibitors. Surgical intervention is indicated in the setting of unstable fractures, atlantoaxial instability, or progressive disease that is refractory to medical treatments. In this chapter, the authors outline treatment options and surgical pearls in the management of ankylosing spondylitis, rheumatoid arthritis, diffuse idiopathic skeletal hyperostosis, and ossification of posterior longitudinal ligament.

Keywords: spondyloarthropathies, ankylosing spondylitis, rheumatoid arthritis, diffuse idiopathic skeletal hyperostosis, ossification of posterior longitudinal ligament

31.1 Key Points

- Spondyloarthropathies are stratified into seronegative and seropositive arthropathies according to antinuclear antibody (ANA) and rheumatoid factor (RF) status.
- Comprised of a variety of disorders/syndromes with overlapping symptomology with varying human leukocyte antigen (HLA) associations including ankylosing spondylitis (AS), psoriatic arthritis, enteropathic arthritis, Reiter syndrome, ossification of the posterior longitudinal ligament (OPLL), and rheumatoid arthritis (RA).
- Cervical spine involvent is present in up to 80% of RA cases.[1]

- In RA, atlantoaxial subluxation (AAS) classified by anterior atlantodental interval (ADI) of ≤ 3 mm (stable) and posterior atlantodental interval (PADI) of ≤ 14 mm (increased risk of injury).
- OPLL: Highest incidence is in Asian population and is mostly asymptomatic. Computed tomography (CT) preferred over X-ray for evaluation of posterior longitudinal ligament (PLL) calcification/ossification when OPLL is suspected.
- Diffuse idiopathic skeletal hyperostosis (DISH): Not associated with SI joint involvement/pathology. Associated with osteophytic changes, spine stiffness, difficulty breathing, and dysphagia.

31.2 Ankylosing Spondylitis Seronegative Arthropathy

31.2.1 Background

- Also known as Marie-Strümpell disease.[2] Ankylosing spondylitis (AS) is a rare chronic systemic inflammatory disease most strongly correlated with HLA-B27. Mediated by tumor necrosis factor (TNF)-alpha, TNF-beta, CD-4, and CD-8.[3,4]
- Peak incidence is in the teen years to the fourth decade of life with males more commonly affected than females at a ratio of 3:1.[5] Prevalence rates range from 0.9 to 1.4%.[6]
- An estimated 90% of the risk of developing AS is heritable.[7]
- Characterized by chronic back pain and progressive stiffness involving the sacroiliac joints, shoulders, peripheral joints, and digits.
- In cases of advanced disease progression, fibrosis and calcification of the spine result in loss of flexibility and a rigid "bamboo" appearance (**Fig. 31.1**).
- Extra-articular manifestations include anterior uveitis, inflammatory bowel disease, psoriasis, and cardiovascular disease.[8]

31.2.2 Signs, Symptoms, and Physical Examination

- Sacroiliac stiffness progresses to the entirety of the spinal column resulting in decreased range of motion.[1]
- Initially presents with nonradiating back pain and morning stiffness lasting longer than 45 minutes that improves with activity.
- Structural deformities are primarily a result of osteoproliferation as opposed to osteodestruction.[9]
- Atlantoaxial subluxation may occur in up to 21% of patients and can cause compression of the spinal cord.

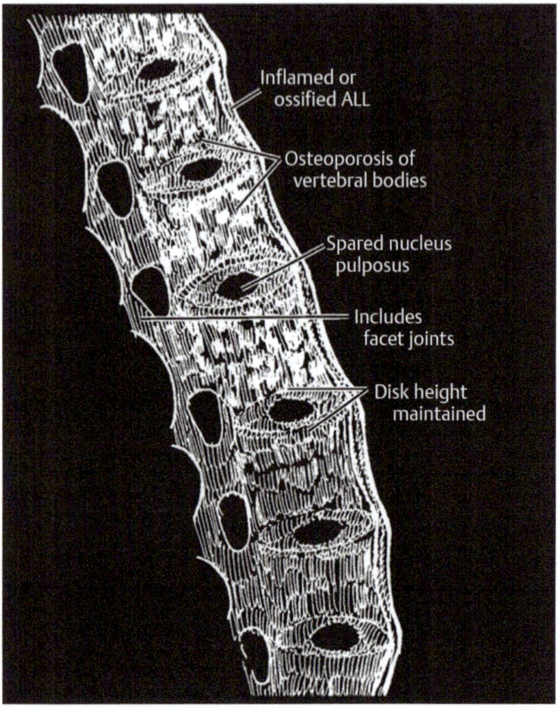

Fig. 31.1 Features of "bamboo spine" in ankylosing spondylitis. ALL, anterior longitudinal ligament.

- Involvement of tendons/ligaments may present as plantar fasciitis or Achilles tendonitis.
- Cauda equina syndrome may arise in long-standing cases of AS.[10]
- Vertebral fractures can occur with minimal or no trauma, most commonly in the C5–C6 interspace.[11]
- Certain diseases can mimic AS and must be ruled out. These include mechanical low back pain, rheumatoid arthritis, lumbar spinal stenosis, and diffuse idiopathic skeletal hyperostosis (DISH).

31.2.3 Workup

- Diagnosis is made using the Modified New York Criteria which includes: (1) low back pain/stiffness for over 3 months which improves with physical activity, but not with rest; (2) limited mobility in the lumbar spine in both the sagittal and frontal planes; and (3) limited chest wall expansion corrected for sex and age.[12]

31.2.4 Neuroimaging

- Plain X-ray series are the gold standard for assessing structural damage in the spine (e.g., bamboo spine) and SI joint.
- Magnetic resonance imaging (MRI) to evaluate soft tissue pathology in the disk space and ligamentous structures.[13]

31.2.5 Treatment

- Medical management includes nonsteroidal anti-inflammatory drugs (NSAIDs), TNF-a antagonists, methotrexate, sulfasalazine, and corticosteroids.
- Stable fractures are managed with rigid bracing and unstable fractures are managed surgically with decompression and fusion.
- Advanced hip arthritis and severe hip pain are managed with arthroplasty.[8]

31.2.6 Surgical Pearls

- AS patients tend to have their neck fixed in a flexed position. Following trauma and immobilization, intraoperative forced inline fixation may have deleterious results. Therefore, the neck should be fixed in natural position.
- If traction is utilized, it should be in line with the patient's natural degree of kyphosis and not strictly horizontal.
- There is no universal consensus for management of spinal cord injury in patients with AS (e.g., internal fixation vs. halo) without obvious compression.
- Laminectomy and fusion are the recommended interventions for root/cord compression.
- In cases of severe kyphotic deformity, consider posterior osteotomy and fusion for correction.[14,15]

31.3 Rheumatoid Arthritis

31.3.1 Background

- Rheumatoid arthritis (RA) affects 1 to 2% of the world population. Cervical involvement is observed in up to 80% of RA cases.
- Cervical spine involvement manifests as atlantoaxial subluxation (anterior > posterior), basilar impression, and pannus granulation of odontoid process.[16]
- Up to 36% of patients with preexisting cervical spine instability will develop neurologic deficits.[17]

31.3.2 Signs, Symptoms, and Physical Examination

- Morning stiffness, symmetric arthritis especially of the proximal interphalangeal, metacarpophalangeal, and metatarsophalangeal joints, rheumatoid nodules on extensor surfaces.
- Neck pain with possible C2 radiculopathy.
- Signs of vertebrobasilar insufficiency including tinnitus, visual disturbance, vertigo, and dysphagia.[16]
- Occipital headache.[17]

31.3.3 Workup

- Anterior atlanto-odontoid interval (ADI): ≤ 3 mm used for evaluation of the integrity of the transverse ligament; this was not found to correlate with risk of injury.
- Posterior atlanto-odontoid interval (PADI): evaluation of the amount of space for the spinal cord at the level of C1–C2; found to correlate with risk of injury if ≤ 14 mm.[18]
- Evaluate degree of cervicomedullary junction compression and basilar impression.

31.3.4 Neuroimaging

- Lateral cervical spine X-ray: Evaluate (1) anterior atlantodental interval (AADI)—posterior margin of the anterior arch of C1 to the anterior margin of the dens; and (2) posterior atlantodental interval (PADI)—posterior aspect of vertebral body to spinolaminar line.[17]
- Contrast-enhanced MRI: Evaluate degree of soft tissue compression and pannus.

31.3.5 Treatment

- In cases of asymptomatic atlantoaxial subluxation (AAS), prophylactic surgical treatment may be considered in instances of 6 to 10 mm of mobile atlantoaxial instability.[19]
- AAS will progress over time in patients with RA; therefore, intervention is recommended, particularly in cases of existing myelopathy.
- Immobilization of the C1–C2 joint via posterior fusion or halo may reduce pannus size over time.
- Halo traction may be utilized to align the odontoid and restore its natural positioning.
- A rigid collar does not support the C1–C2 joint and is not recommended.

31.3.6 Surgical Pearls

- In most cases of anterior, posterior, or vertical subluxation, 360 degrees of fusion will be required.
- A posterior-only approach is sufficient in cases of rotational or lateral subluxation.
- Posterior fusion with or without laminectomy (C1): C1–C2 fusion, occiput–C2.
- It is important to consider the course of the vertebral arteries prior to C1–C2 fusion.[20]
- Anterior approach: Odontoidectomy. In the transoral approach, the patient's mouth must be able to open at least 25 mm. The patient should remain in halo traction until fusion.
- The transoral approach is associated with higher rates of morbidity and should be considered as a second option to posterior fusion.
- In cases of combined RA with basilar impression, reduction should occur prior to fusion.

31.4 Diffuse Idiopathic Skeletal Hyperostosis

31.4.1 Background

- Noninflammatory condition characterized by aberrant ossification of the spine, peripheral joints, and peripheral entheses.
- Vertebral ossification independent of degenerative changes at respective levels and not associated with SI joint pathology (**Fig. 31.2**).[21]
- Increased risk of spinal fracture.[22]
- Risk factors: age, male sex, metabolic syndrome.[23,24]

31.4.2 Signs, Symptoms, and Physical Examination

- Often asymptomatic, but may present with spine stiffness.[25]
- Cervical spine: dysphagia and difficulty in breathing.[26]
- Extraspinal joint stiffness and decreased range of motion.[27]

31.4.3 Workup/Neuroimaging

- Spine radiograph demonstrating ossification connecting four or more contiguous vertebrae in the absence of significant degenerative changes.[28]

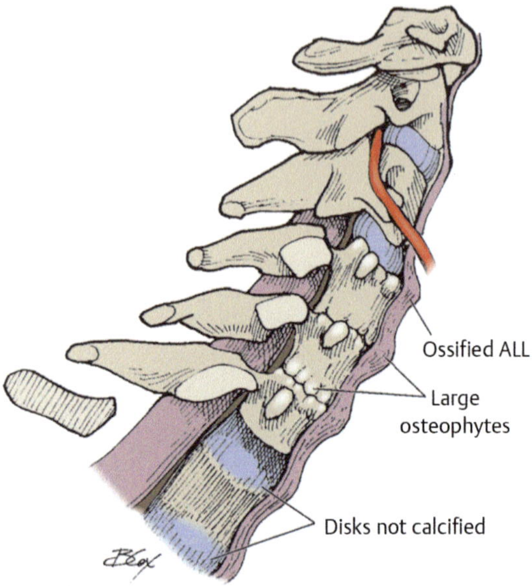

Fig. 31.2 Diffuse idiopathic skeletal hyperostosis in the cervical spine. Note the continuous osteophyte formation along the anterior border of the cervical spine. ALL, anterior longitudinal ligament.

31.4.4 Treatment

- Physical therapy and NSAIDs for symptomatic pain relief.[29]
- Glucocorticoid injections at enthesopathic sites.
- Surgical intervention (e.g., cervical osteophytectomy) indicated upon failure of conservative management of dysphagia and airway compromise.[30]

31.4.5 Surgical Pearls

- Debulking of anterior cervical osteophytes.
- Avoid disrupting adhesions between osteophytes and esophagus due to high risk of esophageal tear.
- Evaluation with fluoroscopic imaging to ensure complete osteophyte excision.[31]

31.5 Ossification of the Posterior Longitudinal Ligament

31.5.1 Background

- Calcification with subsequent endochondral ossification of PLL. Can occur in any part of the spine and may extend into dura. Most common in the subaxial cervical region, although dural ossification is most common in the thoracic region.[32]
- Classified as localized (confined to disk space), segmental (confined to vertebral body), continuous, and mixed (combination of segmental and continuous) (**Fig. 31.3**).
- Incidence highest in Asian population (between 2 and 3%), twice as common in men than in women, and prevalence increases with age (presents most commonly in 40- to 59-year-old individuals).[33]

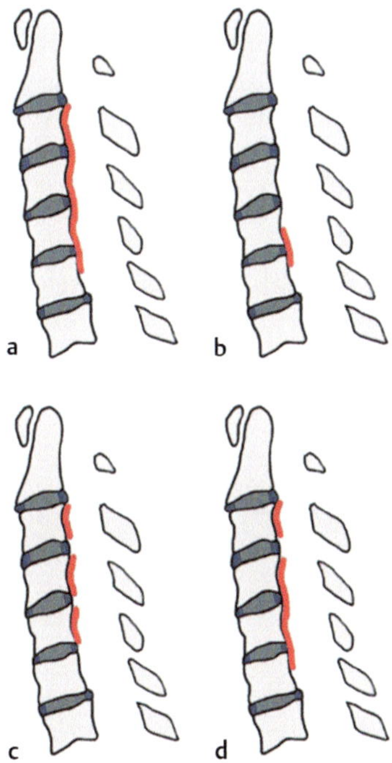

Fig. 31.3 Different classes of ossification of the posterior longitudinal ligament. **(a)** Continuous. **(b)** Localized. **(c)** Segmental. **(d)** Mixed.

31.5.2 Signs, Symptoms, and Physical Examination

- Many affected individuals are asymptomatic with approximately 30% rate of progression to myelopathy over a 30-year period.[33]
- Neck pain that may progress to severe myelopathic symptoms (e.g., loss of balance and weakness).

31.5.3 Workup/Neuroimaging

- Although visible on plain X-ray, ossification is commonly missed and underdiagnosed, so evaluation with CT is suggested when OPLL is suspected.
- Axial MRI (dark on T1 and T2) and CT for evaluation of degree of stenosis.
- Consider serum glucose when clinical suspicion is high, given diabetes mellitus is a distinct risk factor for OPLL development.[33]

31.5.4 Treatment

- Mild and/or asymptomatic cases are treated conservatively, given relatively low rate of progression to myelopathy.[34]
- Surgical intervention aims to decompress the spinal cord and is indicated for refractory and/or severe cases, especially in the setting of myelopathic symptoms.

31.5.5 Surgical Pearls

- To prevent intraoperative hyperextension, fiberoptic intubation is recommended.
- If there is dural extension, it is generally inextricable without sacrificing the dura, making it the surgeon's decision whether to leave this ossification. Preservation of arachnoid is essential if electing to remove dural ossification.
- Anterior (e.g., corpectomy) as opposed to posterior (e.g., laminoplasty) approaches for decompression is a long-standing debate. Perioperative complications are higher in the anterior approach, especially in the setting of complete removal of the OPLL, including dural portion, but clinical outcomes tend to be better at 1- and 2-year follow-up.[35]

Common Clinical Questions

1. A 42-year-old male presents to your clinic complaining of recent leg pain in the setting of a long-standing history of back pain and gluteal stiffness that improves after his morning run. Scoliosis X-rays demonstrate a "bamboo

spine" with pathologic thoracic kyphosis. It is decided he needs an L2–L4 TLIF. What is a consideration during surgery that might make operating much more difficult on this patient?

A. Maintaining patient's natural kyphosis.
B. Using a lateral approach.
C. Using an anterior approach.
D. Using a posterior approach.

2. After obtaining cervical imaging for a 17-year-old girl with a past medical history significant for Down syndrome, you determine she has atlantoaxial subluxation in the setting of early-onset rheumatoid arthritis. Her father mentioned he noticed her neck stiffness last month at her brother's basketball game. She currently denies any inflammatory neck pain, loss of balance, and weakness. What is the best next step in her management?

   A. Rigid neck collar.
   B. Halo collar with NSAIDs.
   C. Posterior C1–C2 fusion.
   D. Transoral odontoidectomy.

3. In rheumatoid arthritis, an ADI of > 3 mm indicates a need for surgery. True or false?

4. A 53-year-old male visits you in clinic complaining of "morning neck pain" for the last 2 years. His primary care provider prescribed him naproxen for pain relief when he initially presented 2 years ago. When questioned further, he reports being involved in a motor vehicle accident 10 years ago. He also describes a "lump" in his throat and difficulty swallowing solid food for the last 3 months and recent neck stiffness without crepitus. He tells you that this made him concerned for his health and he started rigorous exercise therapy for his neck. Further workup reveals a normal pelvic X-ray and a cervical X-ray showing contiguous osteophytic bridging of C3–C7. What is the best next step in his management?

   A. Analgesics.
   B. Continue PT and NSAIDs until respiratory complications develop.
   C. Glucocorticoid injections and close follow-up.
   D. Offer surgery.

5. X-ray is the imaging method of choice to visualize OPLL. True of false?

Answers to Common Clinical Questions

1. A. Keeping an AS patient in the natural kyphosis is essential, and a posterior approach for most spine surgeries is recommended. A lateral approach is not necessarily going to make operating harder, like an anterior approach would, considering how common anterior osteophytic bridging is in AS patients.
2. C. Fixation of the atlantoaxial joint with or without odontoidectomy is not particularly indicated over conservative therapy like a halo collar and NSAIDs in a younger patient with very early disease and no myelopathic symptoms. It should be noted a rigid collar does *not* support the atlantoaxial joint, so it is not indicated.
3. False. Although ADI > 3 mm may indicate instability, it does not warrant operating, while ADI > 10 mm does. Moreover, a PADI > 14 mm indicates risk for neurologic injury, which would indicate surgery.
4. D. This patient's presentation is most consistent with DISH, given a globus sensation and neck stiffness in the absence of SI joint pathology otherwise characteristic of seronegative spondyloarthropathies. Given the development of dysphagia, this will likely progress to compress the trachea, leading to respiratory difficulty. Although the patient has not received glucocorticoid injections, he has certainly failed conservative management. Surgery to decompress his esophagus and mitigate the threat of tracheal compression is the best option in this case.
5. False. Although surgeons can sometimes see OPLL on plain X-ray, it is often missed and underdiagnosed, so CT is the method of choice.

References

1. Nguyen HV, Ludwig SC, Silber J, et al. Rheumatoid arthritis of the cervical spine. Spine J. 2004; 4(3):329–334
2. Ausman JI. Handbook of Neurosurgery. 7th ed. Book Reviews. Surg Neurol Int. May 31, 2010;1:19. eCollection 2010
3. Reveille JD, Ball EJ, Khan MA. HLA-B27 and genetic predisposing factors in spondyloarthropathies. Curr Opin Rheumatol. 2001; 13(4):265–272
4. Reveille JD, Arnett FC. Spondyloarthritis: update on pathogenesis and management. Am J Med. 2005; 118(6):592–603
5. Braun J, Sieper J. Ankylosing spondylitis. Lancet. 2007; 369(9570):1379–1390
6. Reveille JD, Witter JP, Weisman MH. Prevalence of axial spondylarthritis in the United States: estimates from a cross-sectional survey. Arthritis Care Res (Hoboken). 2012; 64(6):905–910

7. Dakwar E, Reddy J, Vale FL, Uribe JS. A review of the pathogenesis of ankylosing spondylitis. Neurosurg Focus. 2008; 24(1):E2
8. Zhu W, He X, Cheng K, et al. Ankylosing spondylitis: etiology, pathogenesis, and treatments. Bone Res. 2019; 7:22
9. Ramos-Remus C, Gomez-Vargas A, Guzman-Guzman JL, et al. Frequency of atlantoaxial subluxation and neurologic involvement in patients with ankylosing spondylitis. J Rheumatol. 1995; 22(11):2120–2125
10. Tang C, Moser FG, Reveille J, Bruckel J, Weisman MH. Cauda equina syndrome in ankylosing spondylitis: challenges in diagnosis, management, and pathogenesis. J Rheumatol. 2019; 46(12):1582–1588
11. Vosse D, Feldtkeller E, Erlendsson J, Geusens P, van der Linden S. Clinical vertebral fractures in patients with ankylosing spondylitis. J Rheumatol. 2004; 31(10):1981–1985
12. van der Linden S, Valkenburg HA, Cats A. Evaluation of diagnostic criteria for ankylosing spondylitis. A proposal for modification of the New York criteria. Arthritis Rheum. 1984; 27(4):361–368
13. Ostergaard M, Lambert RG. Imaging in ankylosing spondylitis. Ther Adv Musculoskelet Dis. 2012; 4(4):301–311
14. Quiñones-Hinojosa A. Schmidek and Sweet Operative Neurosurgical Techniques: Indications, Methods, and Results. 6th ed. Elsevier; 2012
15. Burkus JK. Esophageal obstruction secondary to diffuse idiopathic skeletal hyperostosis. Orthopedics. 1988; 11(5):717–720
16. Krauss WE, Bledsoe JM, Clarke MJ, Nottmeier EW, Pichelmann MA. Rheumatoid arthritis of the craniovertebral junction. Neurosurgery. 2010; 66 (3) Suppl:83–95
17. Gillick JL, Wainwright J, Das K. Rheumatoid arthritis and the cervical spine: a review on the role of surgery. Int J Rheumatol. 2015; 2015:252456
18. Boden SD, Dodge LD, Bohlman HH, Rechtine GR. Rheumatoid arthritis of the cervical spine. A long-term analysis with predictors of paralysis and recovery. J Bone Joint Surg Am. 1993; 75(9):1282–1297
19. Papadopoulos SM, Dickman CA, Sonntag VK. Atlantoaxial stabilization in rheumatoid arthritis. J Neurosurg. 1991; 74(1):1–7
20. Ebraheim N, Rollins JR, Jr, Xu R, Jackson WT. Anatomic consideration of C2 pedicle screw placement. Spine. 1996; 21(6):691–695
21. Le HV, Wick JB, Van BW, Klineberg EO. Diffuse idiopathic skeletal hyperostosis of the spine: pathophysiology, diagnosis, and management. J Am Acad Orthop Surg. 2021; 29(24):1044–1051
22. Westerveld LA, Verlaan JJ, Oner FC. Spinal fractures in patients with ankylosing spinal disorders: a systematic review of the literature on treatment, neurological status and complications. Eur Spine J. 2009; 18(2): 145–156
23. Weinfeld RM, Olson PN, Maki DD, Griffiths HJ. The prevalence of diffuse idiopathic skeletal hyperostosis (DISH) in two large American Midwest metropolitan hospital populations. Skeletal Radiol. 1997; 26(4):222–225

24. Okada E, Ishihara S, Azuma K, et al. Metabolic syndrome is a predisposing factor for diffuse idiopathic skeletal hyperostosis. Neurospine. 2021; 18(1): 109–116
25. Forestier J, Rotes-Querol J. Senile ankylosing hyperostosis of the spine. Ann Rheum Dis. 1950; 9(4):321–330
26. Verlaan JJ, Boswijk PF, de Ru JA, Dhert WJ, Oner FC. Diffuse idiopathic skeletal hyperostosis of the cervical spine: an underestimated cause of dysphagia and airway obstruction. Spine J. 2011; 11(11):1058–1067
27. Belanger TA, Rowe DE. Diffuse idiopathic skeletal hyperostosis: musculoskeletal manifestations. J Am Acad Orthop Surg. 2001; 9(4):258–267
28. Resnick D, Niwayama G. Radiographic and pathologic features of spinal involvement in diffuse idiopathic skeletal hyperostosis (DISH). Radiology. 1976; 119(3):559–568
29. Mader R, Verlaan JJ, Eshed I, et al. Diffuse idiopathic skeletal hyperostosis (DISH): where we are now and where to go next. RMD Open. 2017; 3(1): e000472. Erratum in: RMD Open. 2017 Nov 14;3(2):e000472
30. Lofrese G, Scerrati A, Balsano M, et al. Surgical treatment of diffuse idiopathic skeletal hyperostosis (DISH) involving the cervical spine: technical nuances and outcome of a multicenter experience. Global Spine J. 2022; 12(8):1751–1760
31. Hamouda WO. Timing for surgical intervention in DISHphagia. J Craniovertebr Junction Spine. 2018; 9(4):227–231
32. Saetia K, Cho D, Lee S, Kim DH, Kim SD. Ossification of the posterior longitudinal ligament: a review. Neurosurg Focus. 2011; 30(3):E1
33. Inamasu J, Guiot BH, Sachs DC. Ossification of the posterior longitudinal ligament: an update on its biology, epidemiology, and natural history. Neurosurgery. 2006; 58(6):1027–1039, discussion 1027–1039
34. Pham MH, Attenello FJ, Lucas J, He S, Stapleton CJ, Hsieh PC. Conservative management of ossification of the posterior longitudinal ligament. A review. Neurosurg Focus. 2011; 30(3):E2
35. Inoue T, Maki S, Yoshii T, et al. Japanese Multicenter Research Organization for Ossification of the Spinal Ligament. Is anterior decompression and fusion more beneficial than laminoplasty for K-line (+) cervical ossification of the posterior longitudinal ligament? An analysis using propensity score matching. J Neurosurg Spine. 2022:1–8. Online ahead of print.

32 Spinal Emergencies

Mohammad Hassan A. Noureldine and Puya Alikhani

Summary
This chapter focuses on spinal emergencies, highlighting the importance of prompt diagnosis and intervention for optimal outcomes. Spinal hematomas present with initial intense pain and progressive neurologic symptoms. MRI is the preferred imaging for diagnosis, and treatment often involves surgical decompression and correction of coagulopathy. Cauda equina syndrome and conus medullaris syndrome result from conus medullaris and lumbar/sacral nerve root pathology, often due to disk herniation. They manifest with severe back pain, sciatica, and urinary dysfunction. Prompt surgical decompression within 24 hours is crucial for better outcomes. Spinal epidural abscess may present challenges in diagnosis due to vague symptoms, with characteristic features on MRI. Treatment involves surgical decompression and prolonged antibiotic therapy, with early surgery associated with better outcomes. Overall, the chapter emphasizes the significance of early diagnosis and intervention in spinal emergencies to prevent permanent neurological damage and improve patient outcomes.

Keywords: spinal hematoma, cauda equina syndrome, conus medullaris syndrome, spinal epidural abscess, spinal emergency, early diagnosis, surgical decompression

32.1 Key Points

- Prompt and accurate diagnosis of spinal emergencies is critical because return of function is highly dependent on early intervention.
- Magnetic resonance imaging (MRI) is the imaging modality of choice in diagnosing ligamentous injury, spinal hematomas, acute herniated nucleus pulposus, spinal epidural abscesses, and neoplastic conditions.
- Computed tomography (CT) myelogram is the preferred alternative when MRI is contraindicated (e.g., incompatible pacemaker) or not available.
- Most spinal instrumentation is safe, effective, and at times necessary in the treatment of epidural abscess or diskitis/osteomyelitis of the spine.
- Trauma and tumors may also present as "spinal emergencies," as discussed elsewhere in this book.

32.2 Spinal Hematomas

- Background:
  - Spinal hematomas may occur in the subdural, epidural, and subarachnoid spaces—similar to their cranial counterparts, as well as within the spinal cord tissue, i.e., intramedullary hematomas.
  - No etiologic factor is identified in about one-third of cases (29.8%), followed by anticoagulant therapy (17%), vascular malformations (9.2%), and spontaneous hemorrhage (8.5%) as most common causes.[1]
  - In the sagittal plane, spinal hematomas typically localize dorsal (44.3%) and dorsolateral (31%) to the spinal cord,[1] most frequently at the cervicothoracic and thoracolumbar regions in young adults and adults older than 50 years, respectively.[1,2,3,4,5]
  - The epidural type is diagnosed in up to 76% of spinal hematoma cases, followed by subarachnoid (15.9%), subdural (4.1%), combined subdural/subarachnoid (1.5%), and intramedullary (0.8%), among other rare combinations.[1]
  - The incidence of the epidural type is estimated at 0.1 per 100,000 per year[6]; rarity of other spinal hematoma types precludes calculating their incidence rates.
  - Spinal subarachnoid hemorrhages most commonly occur via redistribution of cerebrospinal fluid (CSF) containing blood products from intracranial bleeds, potentially extending along the entire length of the spinal subarachnoid space, and less frequently from coagulopathy, spinal arteriovenous malformations (AVMs), aneurysms or cavernous angiomas, or following diagnostic/interventional spinal procedures.
  - Intramedullary hemorrhages are most frequently associated with traumatic spinal cord injury leading to cord contusions with subsequent hematoma formation. Tumors, vascular pathologies, and coagulopathy are other potential etiologies.
- Signs, symptoms, and physical examination:
  - Epidural and subdural spinal hematomas present with intense, knifelike pain at the hemorrhage site, which may be followed by a pain-free interval of minutes to days. Progression of symptoms may be quicker in subdural than in epidural spinal hematomas.[7]
  - Subarachnoid hematomas are associated with nuchal rigidity, headaches, nausea and vomiting, disturbances of consciousness, and epileptic seizures in up to 35.4% of patients.[1]
  - Symptoms depend on the location and extent of hemorrhage and may include motor weakness, sensory and reflex deficits, and acute bowel/bladder dysfunction.[2]
  - Signs and symptoms may be related to radiculopathy, i.e., sensory and/or motor deficits along specific nerve root dermatomes; myelopathy, which

may present as bilateral sensory and/or motor deficits, dexterity and gait abnormalities, urinary difficulties, upper motor neuron signs, e.g., hyperreflexia, clonus, spasticity, Hoffmann's or Babinski's; or myeloradiculopathy, a mixture of radiculopathic and myelopathic signs/ symptoms.[8]
 - Acute traumatic central cord syndrome (ATCCS) is a very common acute incomplete cervical cord injury presenting with severe weakness in upper extremities more than lower extremities.[9]
- Workup:
  - Basic workup is comprised of complete blood count (CBC) with differential (including platelets), electrolytes, and partial thromboplastin time (PTT)/prothrombin time (PT)/international normalized ratio (INR).
  - Disseminated intravascular coagulation (DIC) panel and specific hematology factors may need to be assessed.
- Neuroimaging:
  - The imaging modality of choice is MRI with or without gadolinium,[10] and the appearance is highly dependent on the age of the clot (**Fig. 32.1**)[11]:
    - Hyperacute bleeding (< 24 h): T1 isointense, T2 slightly hyperintense.
    - Acute bleeding (1–3 d): T1 slightly hyperintense, T2 hypointense.
    - Early subacute bleeding (3–7 d): T1 hyperintense, T2 hypointense.
    - Late subacute bleeding (7–14 d): T1 hyperintense, T2 hyperintense.
    - Chronic bleeding (> 14 d): T1 slightly hypointense, T2 hypointense.
  - Sagittal cuts will demonstrate the rostrocaudal levels of a spinal hematoma, whereas axial cuts help in elucidating the hematoma type.

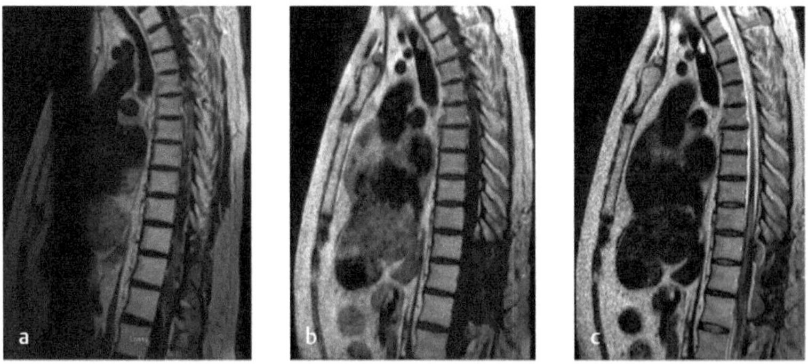

Fig. 32.1 A 33-year-old patient with intradural extramedullary metastatic lesion to the lower thoracic spine with a subacute neurological decline, necessitating urgent surgical decompression. After 4 days, he developed acute lower extremities weakness, and an emergent magnetic resonance imaging (MRI) was performed revealing a hyperacute spinal epidural hematoma. **(a)** Immediate postoperative, contrast-enhanced T1 image showing adequate decompression. **(b)** T1 image with isointense signal and **(c)** T2 image with hyperintense signal, consistent with hyperacute bleeding.

- Epidural spinal hematomas lead to epidural fat effacement and dural compression (focal or diffuse) dorsally in most cases, potentially with thecal sac and nerve roots displacement ventrally.[11]
- Subdural spinal hematomas are limited by dural reflections of the midline dorsal septum and bilateral denticulate ligaments, localizing to one anterior and two posterolateral subdural spaces, the configuration of which is referred to as "inverted Mercedes-Benz" sign.[12,13]
- Subarachnoid spinal hematomas typically appear as an intrathecal layer of blood in the dependent areas of the lower lumbar spine, i.e., the pathognomonic "sedimentation sign," or much less frequently as an intradural-extramedullary clot with possible mass effect on the spinal cord/nerves.[11,14] Arachnoiditis is a potential complication of the spinal subarachnoid hemorrhage and appears as a deformity in spinal cord shape, intradural adhesions, and clumping/peripheral displacement of nerve roots, leading to the classic "empty thecal sac" sign in advanced stages.
- Intramedullary hematomas are associated with cord edema that progresses at a rate of about one vertebral level every 24 to 36 hours in the acute phase following trauma, despite the static volume of the hematoma compared to baseline imaging.[15]

• Treatment:
  - The treatment of choice is correction of coagulopathy, if present, and surgical decompression as soon as possible.
  - Optimal timing of surgery is not known and will vary on a case-by-case basis, but the general rule is to decompress the cord within 6 to 12 hours of symptom onset to prevent permanent neurologic consequences.[16]
  - Benefit of surgical intervention is debatable if the only symptom is pain. Conservative management with serial imaging is a valid option in patients with small hematomas and mild/improving deficits.
  - Surgery typically involves laminectomy without the need for fusion.
  - For cervicothoracic and thoracolumbar junction multilevel laminectomies, instrumentation and fusion should be considered.
  - Laminoplasty is a potential alternative in the cervical region to avoid fusion.
  - Traumatic subarachnoid spinal hemorrhages may be treated conservatively, whereas those associated with large clots/adhesions and those related to vascular pathologies will likely require endovascular treatment versus open surgery.
  - Intramedullary hemorrhages caused by cavernous angiomas or AVMs typically present with devastating neurologic symptoms but are often not managed via emergent surgical decompression.

- For the ATCCS, early surgical decompression was contraindicated in the past. Newer studies advocate early decompression; however, the timing of surgery remains controversial.[9]
- Surgical pearls:
  - Subfascial drains may diminish the incidence of symptomatic epidural blood collections after multilevel laminectomy procedures.

32.3 Cauda Equina and Conus Medullaris Syndromes

- Background:
  - Cauda equina syndrome (CES) refers to a clinical condition that results from compressive, ischemic, and/or inflammatory neuropathy of multiple lumbar and sacral nerve roots in the lumbar spinal canal.[17,18]
  - Conus medullaris syndrome (CMS) has features similar to those of CES but involves compression at the level of the conus medullaris—typically at the T12–L1 level but may extend to mid-L2 vertebral body level.
  - The most common cause of CES is disk herniation in the lumbar region—L4–L5 being the most common level, although CES occurs in only 2% of disk herniations.[19,20,21]
  - It may also be caused by traumatic injury, lumbar spinal stenosis, primary or metastatic tumors, epidural abscess, ankylosing spondylitis, spinal subdural or epidural hematoma, spinal manipulation, or vascular malformation.[17,18]
- Signs, symptoms, and physical examination:
  - Severe low back pain (83–100%) and sciatica (90–100%) are the most common presenting symptoms of CES, although up to 71% of patients report prior history of back pain.[19,22,23]
  - Urinary dysfunction is the most consistent finding, occurring in 90% of patients presenting with CES.
  - Complete CES entails painless urinary retention and overflow incontinence. Poor urinary stream/micturition only with straining, loss of desire to void, and altered urinary sensation indicate incomplete CES, which is associated with more favorable outcomes.[24]
  - Diagnosis may be challenging in patients presenting with radiculopathy due to acute disk herniation along with pain- or narcotic intake-related urinary retention in the absence of true neurogenic bladder dysfunction; however, the presence of saddle anesthesia and decreased rectal tone are diagnostic of CES.
  - Saddle anesthesia is the most common sensory deficit (75% of patients), and anal sphincter tone is diminished in 80% of patients.

  - If sensory deficits progress to total perineal anesthesia, the patient will likely develop permanent bladder dysfunction.
  - Classic symptoms of CMS include symmetric saddle anesthesia, early atonic bladder/rectal sphincter, and symmetric mild lower extremity weakness.[25]
  - Depending on the injury level, other CMS features may include loss of bulbocavernosus and anal reflexes and mixed picture of upper and lower motor neuron injury.[26,27]
- Workup:
  - Basic laboratory studies and appropriate neuroimaging.
  - If imaging demonstrates pathology other than herniated nucleus pulposus (HNP), further workup is indicated (e.g., tumor or infection workup).
- Neuroimaging:
  - MRI is the best initial study if CES or CMS is suspected, both of which are among the few neurosurgical emergencies that require emergent MRI.
  - MRI assesses soft tissue compression as well as signal changes within the spinal cord, especially with T2-weighted images.
  - Unenhanced CT scan demonstrates bony anatomy, which may be helpful when the structural integrity of the spine is compromised and for surgical planning. CT scan with intrathecal contrast (CT myelogram) is the test of choice when MRI is contraindicated or spinal structures are obscured by artifact from extensive prior instrumentation (**Fig. 32.2**).
- Treatment:
  - Prompt surgical decompression is key. Timing is controversial but should ideally be < 24 hours.[28] In cases of spinal cord compression, the literature suggests better outcomes with significant improvement in sensory/motor deficits and urinary/rectal function if surgery is performed within 48 hours.[17,29]
  - Surgical strategy is usually focused on the underlying causes and typically involves laminectomy and diskectomy (for HNP). More extensive surgery (e.g., vertebrectomy, tumor removal) may be necessary for other pathologies.
  - Return of function is dependent on the extent and duration of preoperative deficits, and it may be a slow process taking several months to years.[30,31]
  - Methylprednisolone therapy remains controversial, with recent re-evaluation of the literature arguing against steroid therapy in patients with acute spinal cord injury.[25,32]
- Surgical pearls:
  - Complete hemilaminotomy or laminectomy may be required for removal of a large central disk fragment causing CMS or CES.

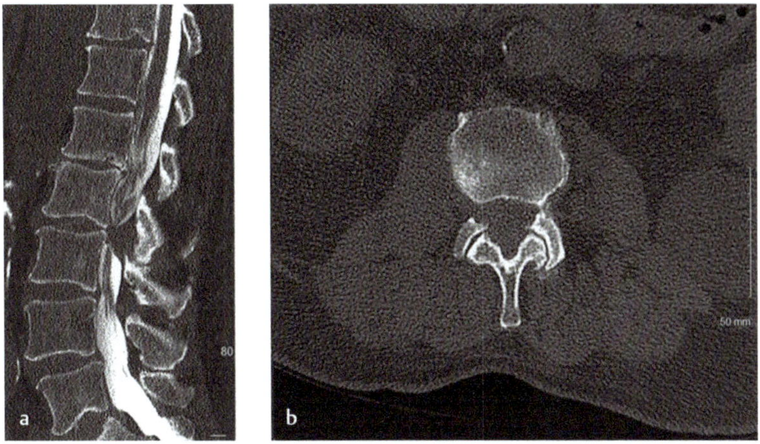

Fig. 32.2 A 61-year-old male with a cardiac pacemaker that is not magnetic resonance imaging (MRI) compatible who presented with numbness and weakness in different dermatomes of both the legs, saddle anesthesia, and overflow urinary incontinence. Sagittal **(a)** and axial **(b)** computed tomography (CT) myelogram showed severe stenosis at L2–L3, with absence of contrast signal/flow at that level.

32.4 Spinal Epidural Abscess

- Background:
  - The incidence of spinal epidural abscesses (SEA) has been shifting over the past two decades and reportedly increased from 2.5 to 8 per 10,000 admissions in a large case-control study.[33]
  - The most common site is lumbar (51%), followed by thoracic (26%) and cervical (23%).[34] The majority of cases involve a single anatomic level (one to two adjacent levels in up to 92%), whereas "skip lesions" are reported in 9.8%.[33]
  - SEA is often associated with vertebral osteomyelitis/diskitis.
  - Risk factors include known focus of infection, intravenous drug abuse, diabetes mellitus, hepatitis, cardiac/renal/liver disease, trauma, and epidural anesthesia/analgesia, although risk factors may be absent in up to 22%.[35]
  - Factors associated with better neurologic outcomes include age less than 60, absence of comorbidities, and smaller abscess size compressing less than 50% of thecal sac.[36]
  - Gram-positive *Staphylococcus aureus* is the most common causative agent.[34]

- Signs, symptoms, and physical examination:
  - Diagnosis in the emergency department may be challenging and is often achieved in a delayed fashion due to the vagueness of presenting signs and symptoms.[37]
  - Initial misdiagnosis rates may be up to 89%,[38] and the classic triad of axial back pain, neurologic deficits, and fever occurs in less than 10% of patients upon presentation.[34,37]
  - The severity of neurologic deficits upon definitive diagnosis and prior to surgery is the greatest predictor of overall outcome.[37,39]
  - The most common presenting symptoms include excruciating axial back pain, paralysis, radicular pain, weakness, and sensory deficits.
  - Average time from back pain to root symptoms is 3 days, and from root pain to weakness is 4.5 days.
  - Leukocytosis and fever may be absent.
- Workup:
  - CBC with differential will show leukocytosis in two-thirds of the patients.[40]
  - Acute phase reactants (erythrocyte sedimentation rate [ESR], C-reactive protein [CRP]) are elevated in almost all cases.
  - Blood cultures are positive in up to 70% of cases.[38]
  - Cardiac echo to rule out endocarditis may be indicated.
- Neuroimaging:
  - MRI with gadolinium is the modality of choice for diagnosing SEA.
  - Whole-spine MRI should be obtained upon initial diagnosis to look for secondary infection foci.
  - Typical findings include an epidural mass with T1 hypointense/isointense and T2/short tau inversion recovery (STIR) hyperintense signals, as well as epidural thickening with peripheral enhancement on T1-contrasted images (**Fig. 32.3**).[41,42]
  - CT myelogram is the preferred alternative when MRI is contraindicated (e.g., incompatible pacemaker) or not available.
  - Plain radiographs are often helpful for suspected diskitis and will show chronic, erosive changes in the end plates. Standing scoliosis X-ray images help in detecting sagittal/coronal alignment changes in cases of advanced osteomyelitis, although these changes may happen after several weeks.
  - CT scan is helpful in diagnosing osteomyelitis.
- Treatment:
  - For SEAs that show clear involvement of the spinal canal and cause dural compression, the treatment of choice is surgical decompression and intravenous antibiotic therapy for 6 weeks (range 2–24 weeks), followed by switching to oral antibiotics.[34]
  - Surgical therapy is associated with improved motor function in comparison to delayed surgery after failure of medical management.

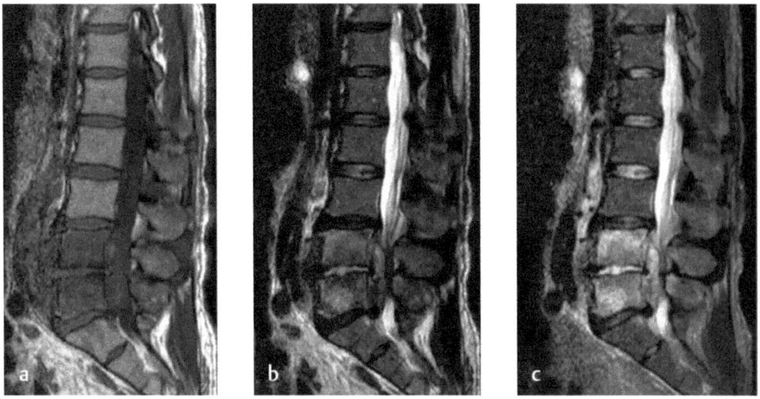

Fig. 32.3 A 54-year-old male with history of intravenous (IV) drug use who presented with progressive weakness in lower extremities as well as urinary/stool incontinence. Magnetic resonance imaging (MRI) without contrast revealed a large anterior epidural mass highly suspicious for an abscess, which was emergently evacuated in the operating room. **(a)** The anterior epidural mass appears isointense and infected vertebral bodies appear hypointense on nonenhanced T1 image. Both the epidural abscess and infected vertebral bodies appear hyperintense on **(b)** T2 and **(c)** short tau inversion recovery (STIR) images.

Diabetes mellitus, leukocytosis > 12.5 k, CRP > 115, and positive blood cultures have been identified as predictors of failure of medical management alone.[35]
- Another consideration in favor of early surgery is to obtain samples for culture so that antibiotic treatment is not delayed and is pathogen-specific.
- SEA is often seen in association with diskitis/osteomyelitis. In these cases, typically only a thin film of epidural enhancement is seen. Surgical intervention is not necessarily indicated in these situations.
- SEA is fatal in up to one-third of elderly patients, and mortality is usually due to the original focus of infection or as a complication of neurologic compromise.
- Severe neurologic complications (e.g., paralysis) and delay in diagnosis and treatment may have medicolegal implications, often associated with alleged negligence-based lawsuits.[43]

- Surgical pearls:
  - Most spinal instrumentation is safe, effective, and at times necessary in the treatment of epidural abscess or diskitis/osteomyelitis of the spine.[44,45]
  - Instrumentation in patients who have spinal infection after decompressive surgery does not increase the recurrent rates of infection.[46]

Common Clinical Questions

1. Cauda equina syndrome describes the clinical condition that results from what neuropathy type involving multiple lumbar and sacral nerve roots?
   A. Compressive.
   B. Ischemic.
   C. Inflammatory.
   D. All of the above.
2. Which of the following factors has been shown to correlate with worse neurologic outcomes in patients with spinal epidural abscesses?
   A. Absence of risk factors/comorbidities.
   B. Age > 60.
   C. Thecal sac involvement, regardless of epidural abscess size.
   D. Rostorcaudal extension of abscess, i.e., number of vertebral levels.

Answers to Common Clinical Questions

1. D.
2. B.

References

1. Kreppel D, Antoniadis G, Seeling W. Spinal hematoma: a literature survey with meta-analysis of 613 patients. Neurosurg Rev. 2003; 26(1):1–49
2. Groen RJ. Non-operative treatment of spontaneous spinal epidural hematomas: a review of the literature and a comparison with operative cases. Acta Neurochir (Wien). 2004; 146(2):103–110
3. Liu W-H, Hsieh C-T, Chiang Y-H, Chen G-J. Spontaneous spinal epidural hematoma of thoracic spine: a rare case report and review of literature. Am J Emerg Med. 2008; 26(3):384.e1–384.e2
4. Franscini L, Ballmer PE, Sturzenegger M, Beer JH, Tuncdogan E, Straub PW. Evaluation of back pain secondary to spinal epidural hematoma associated with aspirin intake and a partial platelet glycoprotein Ia/IIa deficiency. Arch Intern Med. 1994; 154(23):2769–2771
5. Arseni C, Chimion D, Georgian M. Hématome épidural spinal spontané conditionné par une dysimmunoglobulinémie maligne. Rev Roum Neurol. 1968; 5:145–152
6. Holtås S, Heiling M, Lönntoft M. Spontaneous spinal epidural hematoma: findings at MR imaging and clinical correlation. Radiology. 1996; 199(2): 409–413

7. Braun P, Kazmi K, Nogués-Meléndez P, Mas-Estellés F, Aparici-Robles F. MRI findings in spinal subdural and epidural hematomas. Eur J Radiol. 2007; 64 (1):119–125
8. Babu JM, Patel SA, Palumbo MA, Daniels AH. Spinal emergencies in primary care practice. Am J Med. 2019; 132(3):300–306
9. Molliqaj G, Payer M, Schaller K, Tessitore E. Acute traumatic central cord syndrome: a comprehensive review. Neurochirurgie. 2014; 60(1–2):5–11
10. Bozzo A, Marcoux J, Radhakrishna M, Pelletier J, Goulet B. The role of magnetic resonance imaging in the management of acute spinal cord injury. J Neurotrauma. 2011; 28(8):1401–1411
11. Pierce JL, Donahue JH, Nacey NC, et al. Spinal hematomas: what a radiologist needs to know. Radiographics. 2018; 38(5):1516–1535
12. Grassner L, Grillhösl A, Griessenauer CJ, et al. Spinal meninges and their role in spinal cord injury: a neuroanatomical review. J Neurotrauma. 2018; 35(3): 403–410
13. Kasliwal MK, Shannon LR, O'Toole JE, Byrne RW. Inverted Mercedes Benz sign in lumbar spinal subdural hematoma. J Emerg Med. 2014; 47(6):692–693
14. Crossley RA, Raza A, Adams WM. The lumbar sedimentation sign: spinal MRI findings in patients with subarachnoid haemorrhage with no demonstrable intracranial aneurysm. Br J Radiol. 2011; 84(999):279–281
15. Leypold BG, Flanders AE, Burns AS. The early evolution of spinal cord lesions on MR imaging following traumatic spinal cord injury. AJNR Am J Neuroradiol. 2008; 29(5):1012–1016
16. Al-Mutair A, Bednar DA. Spinal epidural hematoma. J Am Acad Orthop Surg. 2010; 18(8):494–502
17. Ahn UM, Ahn NU, Buchowski JM, Garrett ES, Sieber AN, Kostuik JP. Cauda equina syndrome secondary to lumbar disc herniation: a meta-analysis of surgical outcomes. Spine. 2000; 25(12):1515–1522
18. Hussain SA, Gullan RW, Chitnavis BP. Cauda equina syndrome: outcome and implications for management. Br J Neurosurg. 2003; 17(2):164–167
19. Gitelman A, Hishmeh S, Morelli BN, et al. Cauda equina syndrome: a comprehensive review. Am J Orthop. 2008; 37(11):556–562
20. Podnar S. Epidemiology of cauda equina and conus medullaris lesions. Muscle Nerve. 2007; 35(4):529–531
21. Bagley CA, Gokaslan ZL. Cauda equina syndrome caused by primary and metastatic neoplasms. Neurosurg Focus. 2004; 16(6):1–18
22. Shapiro S. Medical realities of cauda equina syndrome secondary to lumbar disc herniation. Spine. 2000; 25(3):348–351, discussion 352
23. Shapiro S. Cauda equina syndrome secondary to lumbar disc herniation. Neurosurgery. 1993; 32(5):743–746, discussion 746–747
24. Gleave JR, Macfarlane R. Cauda equina syndrome: what is the relationship between timing of surgery and outcome? Br J Neurosurg. 2002; 16(4):325–328
25. Radcliff KE, Kepler CK, Delasotta LA, et al. Current management review of thoracolumbar cord syndromes. Spine J. 2011; 11(9):884–892

26. Pavlakis AJ, Siroky MB, Goldstein I, Krane RJ. Neurourologic findings in conus medullaris and cauda equina injury. Arch Neurol. 1983; 40(9):570–573
27. Brouwers E, van de Meent H, Curt A, Starremans B, Hosman A, Bartels R. Definitions of traumatic conus medullaris and cauda equina syndrome: a systematic literature review. Spinal Cord. 2017; 55(10):886–890
28. Nater A, Fehlings MG. The timing of decompressive spinal surgery in cauda equina syndrome. World Neurosurg. 2015; 83(1):19–22
29. Quraishi NA, Rajagopal TS, Manoharan SR, Elsayed S, Edwards KL, Boszczyk BM. Effect of timing of surgery on neurological outcome and survival in metastatic spinal cord compression. Eur Spine J. 2013; 22(6):1383–1388
30. Chang HS, Nakagawa H, Mizuno J. Lumbar herniated disc presenting with cauda equina syndrome. Long-term follow-up of four cases. Surg Neurol. 2000; 53(2):100–104, discussion 105
31. Hellström P, Kortelainen P, Kontturi M. Late urodynamic findings after surgery for cauda equina syndrome caused by a prolapsed lumbar intervertebral disk. J Urol. 1986; 135(2):308–312
32. Sultan I, Lamba N, Liew A, et al. The safety and efficacy of steroid treatment for acute spinal cord injury: a systematic review and meta-analysis. Heliyon. 2020; 6(2):e03414
33. Artenstein AW, Friderici J, Holers A, Lewis D, Fitzgerald J, Visintainer P. Spinal Epidural Abscess in Adults: A 10-Year Clinical Experience at a Tertiary Care Academic Medical Center. Oxford University Press; 2016:ofw191-ofw191
34. Connor DE, Jr, Chittiboina P, Caldito G, Nanda A. Comparison of operative and nonoperative management of spinal epidural abscess: a retrospective review of clinical and laboratory predictors of neurological outcome. J Neurosurg Spine. 2013; 19(1):119–127
35. Patel AR, Alton TB, Bransford RJ, Lee MJ, Bellabarba CB, Chapman JR. Spinal epidural abscesses: risk factors, medical versus surgical management, a retrospective review of 128 cases. Spine J. 2014; 14(2):326–330
36. Khanna RK, Malik GM, Rock JP, Rosenblum ML. Spinal epidural abscess: evaluation of factors influencing outcome. Neurosurgery. 1996; 39(5):958–964
37. Alerhand S, Wood S, Long B, Koyfman A. The time-sensitive challenge of diagnosing spinal epidural abscess in the emergency department. Intern Emerg Med. 2017; 12(8):1179–1183
38. Tang H-J, Lin H-J, Liu Y-C, Li C-M. Spinal epidural abscess—experience with 46 patients and evaluation of prognostic factors. J Infect. 2002; 45(2):76–81
39. Adogwa O, Karikari IO, Carr KR, et al. Spontaneous spinal epidural abscess in patients 50 years of age and older: a 15-year institutional perspective and review of the literature: clinical article. J Neurosurg Spine. 2014; 20(3):344–349
40. Soehle M, Wallenfang T. Spinal epidural abscesses: clinical manifestations, prognostic factors, and outcomes. Neurosurgery. 2002; 51(1):79–85, discussion 86–87
41. Karikari IO, Powers CJ, Reynolds RM, Mehta AI, Isaacs RE. Management of a spontaneous spinal epidural abscess: a single-center 10-year experience. Neurosurgery. 2009; 65(5):919–923, discussion 923–924

42. Kawakyu-O'Connor D, Bordia R, Nicola R. Magnetic resonance imaging of spinal emergencies. Magn Reson Imaging Clin N Am. 2016; 24(2):325–344
43. Shantharam G, DePasse JM, Kuris E, et al. Medical malpractice following spinal epidural abscess: a 30-year, multi-database investigation. Spine J. 2017; 17(10):S102–S103
44. Screven R, Noureldine MHA, Krafft PR, Alikhani P. Expandable titanium cages in the emergent treatment of severe spinal deformity secondary to osteomyelitis: a series of three complex cases. Asian J Neurosurg. 2020; 15 (2):397–404
45. Noureldine MHA, Pressman E, Krafft PR, Smith DA, Greenberg MS, Alikhani P. Minimally invasive lateral retropleural and retroperitoneal approaches in patients with thoracic and lumbar osteomyelitis: description of the techniques and a series of 14 patients. World Neurosurg. 2020; 139:e166–e181
46. Bydon M, De la Garza-Ramos R, Macki M, et al. Spinal instrumentation in patients with primary spinal infections does not lead to greater recurrent infection rates: an analysis of 118 cases. World Neurosurg. 2014; 82(6): e807–e814

IV
Surgical Techniques

33 Occipitocervical Fusion

Amna Hussein, Esteban Quiceno, and Ali A. Baaj

Summary
The occipitocervical fusion technique holds paramount importance for spine surgeons due to its application in trauma, tumors, and degenerative and congenital pathologies. Proper patient positioning stands out as one of the most critical factors for achieving favorable clinical outcomes during the procedure. Various plates and systems are available for occipitocervical fusion, with instrumentation typically extended to C2 or below as needed. This chapter delves into the key elements of occipitocervical fusion.

Keywords: occipitocervical, fusion, occiput, C2, cranial fixation, instability

33.1 Key Points

- Main goal is solid arthrodesis across the occipitocervical junction. The key to achieve this are adequate decortication, bone graft placement, and solid fixation.
- Traction is not applied in cases of occipitocervical dislocation or significant ligamentous injury on magnetic resonance imaging (MRI).
- Computed tomography (CT) angiography of the neck may be performed to evaluate the anatomical course of the vertebral artery.
- As part of preoperative planning, make sure to review the depth of the midline suboccipital keel and the thickness of the paramedian cranium.
- It is important to verify with fluoroscopy that the occipitocervical junction is in a neutral anatomical position before application of instrumentation.

33.2 Indications

- Occipitocervical instability is most commonly a result of inflammatory diseases like rheumatoid arthritis, trauma, infection, tumor, iatrogenic injury (after transoral odontoidectomy), congenital anomalies, or cranial settling with brainstem or cord compression.[1]

33.3 Technique

- Awake fiber-optic[1] intubation is often performed, and baseline somatosensory evoked potentials (SSEPs) and motor evoked potentials (MEPs) are obtained with the patient initially in the supine position.
- Maintaining cervical alignment, rotate the patient to the prone position onto chest rolls or a Jackson frame.
- The head is secured with a Mayfield cranial fixation system (Schaerer Mayfield; Randolph, Massachusetts).
- Cervical alignment is maintained and checked with fluoroscopy to ensure a neutral relationship.
- The suboccipital area is shaved and cleansed.
- A midline incision is extended from the inion to the lowest level to be incorporated in the construct.
- Subperiosteal dissection is performed to expose the suboccipital bone and the dorsal elements of the cervical spine. Special care is taken to leave a cuff of fascia near the inion for subsequent closure. This ensures that the occipital plate will be fully covered by muscle, reducing the chances of hardware eroding through the skin.
- When exposing the arch of C1, we prefer to do blunt dissection with a Penfield 1 to avoid injury to the vertebral artery.
- Any decompression required (suboccipital or cervical) is now performed, with the bone saved for autograft.
- Occipital fixation can be performed using a variety of methods: Occipital wiring, occipital screw fixation (occipital plate), or occipital condyle screw fixation.
- For the placement of the occipital plate, first place the plate in the appropriate position and mark the midline keel with a marking pen. The plate is removed, and a handheld power drill is used to make a bicortical hole. To avoid injury to the suboccipital neural structures, drill in a progressive fashion—first to a depth of 6 mm, then slowly increasing until bicortical penetration is felt, usually around 10 to 14 mm. Then the hole is tapped. The plate is placed in the correct location and fixed with a 4.5- to 5-mm-diameter screw.
- Most occipital plates provide for at least two to three screw placements in the midline and other paramedian holes. The same steps should be followed for all screws (drilling, tapping, screw placement), with the difference that the paramedian bone is usually less thick and probably will require a shorter screw (**Fig. 33.1a, b**).
- The plate should be placed high in the suboccipital bone (closer to the inion than to the foramen magnum) to leave a small area of bone caudal to the plate for fusion surface.

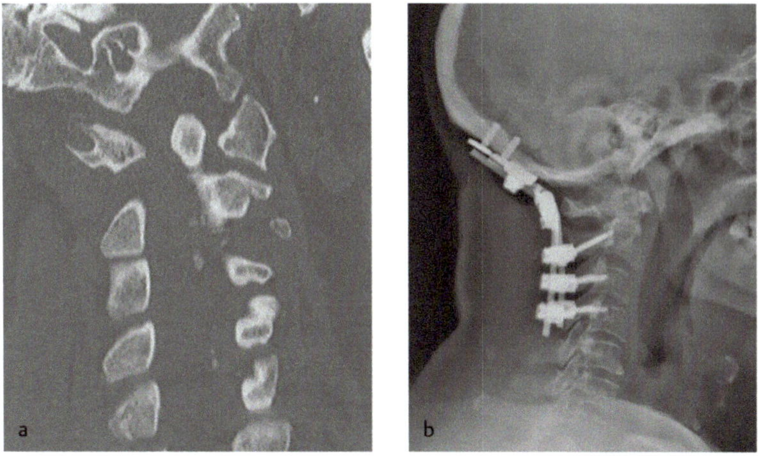

Fig. 33.1 **(a, b)** Coronal computed tomography (CT) view demonstrating atlanto-occipital dissociation (AOD). Lateral postoperative X-ray demonstrating occipitocervical fusion for AOD and subaxial injuries.

- An alternative to plate systems is occipital condyle screw fixation.[2] It is particularly useful in situations in which a suboccipital decompression is required. With this technique, a 3.5 × 20- to 22-mm effective length and 10- to 12-mm lag shank screw (30–34 mm) is placed in the center of the condyle, inferior to the hypoglossal canal. Although different techniques for its placement have been described, in general the screw has a medial trajectory (10–25 degrees) from an entry point approximately 5 mm lateral to the foramen magnum on the condyle itself. Image guidance and free-running electromyography (EMG) monitoring of the hypoglossal nerve are highly recommended with this technique.
- The occipital fixation is then anchored to cervical instrumentation that could be a combination of rod/sublaminar wires, rod/screws, or screws/plate.
- In terms of fixation points, cervical fixation may or may not include the atlas.
- Fusion is often taken down to C2.[3]

33.4 Complications[4,5]

- In contemporary series, complication rates (minor and major) range from 12 to 30%.
  - Wound infection, cerebrospinal fluid (CSF) leak, intracranial injury (sub-/epidural hematoma), spinal cord injury (instrumentation into spinal canal), vascular injury (hardware into vertebral artery).

  - Hardware failure (loosening, pullout, breakage).
  - Nonunion requiring reoperation.
  - Fixation of patient's neck in exaggerated flexion or extension.

33.5 Postoperative Care

- Cervical collar.
- Upright X-rays.
- Prophylactic antibiotics for 24 hours.
- Prompt mobilization.

33.6 Outcomes[6]

- Overall, all techniques, rod/screw, screw/plate, and rod/wiring constructs, have reported fusion rate greater than 90%.[6]
- Rod/screw construct (occipital plate/condyle screws) have highest fusion rates (94–100%[7]) and wiring/onlay graft the lowest (88.6%).
- Rod/screw constructs have highest rate of neurologic improvement and wiring/rod the lowest (81.6 versus 51.8%).[6]
- Early biomechanical studies suggest that condyle screw fixation is biomechanically equivalent to suboccipital plate systems in terms of providing craniocervical stability.[2]
- Instrumentation failure is lowest using the rod/screw technique.

33.7 Surgical Pearls

- Cervical traction is not applied in cases of occipitocervical dislocation.
- Before locking in the construct, verify that a neutral occipitocervical relationship has been achieved.

Common Clinical Questions

1. Cervical traction is contraindicated in which occipitocervical instrumentation cases?
2. Before locking the construct down, why are anteroposterior and lateral fluoroscopy views obtained?
3. Which construct has the lowest pseudarthrosis rate?

Answers to Common Clinical Questions

1. Those performed for occipitocervical dislocation or when significant ligamentous injury is suspected.
2. To ensure adequate alignment and avoid exaggerated flexion or extension.
3. Screw and rod based constructs.

References

1. Lu DC, Roeser AC, Mummaneni VP, Mummaneni PV. Nuances of occipitocervical fixation. Neurosurgery. 2010; 66(3) Suppl:141–146
2. Uribe JS, Ramos E, Youssef AS, et al. Craniocervical fixation with occipital condyle screws: biomechanical analysis of a novel technique. Spine. 2010; 35 (9):931–938
3. Pan J, Huang D, Hao D, et al. Occipitocervical fusion: fix to C2 or C3? Clin Neurol Neurosurg. 2014; 127:134–139
4. Deutsch H, Haid RW, Jr, Rodts GE, Jr, Mummaneni PV. Occipitocervical fixation: long-term results. Spine. 2005; 30(5):530–535
5. Nockels RP, Shaffrey CI, Kanter AS, Azeem S, York JE. Occipitocervical fusion with rigid internal fixation: long-term follow-up data in 69 patients. J Neurosurg Spine. 2007; 7(2):117–123
6. Winegar CD, Lawrence JP, Friel BC, et al. A systematic review of occipital cervical fusion: techniques and outcomes. J Neurosurg Spine. 2010; 13(1):5–16
7. Ahmadian A, Dakwar E, Vale FL, Uribe JS. Occipitocervical fusion via occipital condylar fixation: a clinical case series. J Spinal Disord Tech. 2014; 27(4): 232–236

34 Transoral Odontoidectomy

Karan S. Patel, Cameron Kia, Colin B. Harris, and Frank M. Phillips

Summary
Transoral odontoidectomy is a surgical technique that can be used for extradural decompression of the upper cervical spine and the brainstem. Severe anterior spinal cord compression due to anterior pathology such as an inflammatory pannus at C1–C2 can be addressed via a transoral odontoidectomy. It can be performed through a transoral and an endoscopic endonasal approach. Common complications of this technique include dysphagia, infection, airway obstruction, dural tear, instability, and vascular injury. Such complications can be avoided by proper preoperative optimization, retractor placement, and antibiotic use. Odontoid resection can often necessitate posterior instrumentation and stabilization. Case series studies have reported significant neurologic improvement in patients who have undergone an anterior transoral odontoidectomy.

Keywords: odontoidectomy, C1–C2 compression, inflammatory pannus, transoral approach, craniocervical junction, basilar invagination

34.1 Key Points

- The transoral approach allows the surgeon to gain access from the upper clivus rostrally to the top of the C3 vertebral body caudally.[1]
- The authors prefer this route for extradural pathology as dural closure can be quite difficult with this approach. When intradural pathology must be accessed, a lateral approach may be preferable.
- A thorough preoperative assessment is necessary to ensure that the patient is free from any oral or dental pathology, which may be contraindications to this approach.
- A minimum of 5 to 6 cm of dental clearance should be present to allow adequate exposure for odontoid resection.[2]
- This approach is best avoided if the compressive pathology lies above the hard palate, as this may require a more extensile approach.
- The endoscopic endonasal approach is an alternative for craniocervical junction pathology that may decrease the risk of infection, swallowing, and pulmonary issues.[3,4]

34.2 Indications

- Extradural pathology causing compression of the brainstem or upper cervical spinal cord from the clivus to the rostral extent of the C2 vertebral body.
  - Possible etiologies include rheumatoid or inflammatory pannus, os odontoideum, tumor, infection, basilar invagination, atlantoaxial dislocation, or fracture.[4]
- Continued neurologic symptoms or cord compression after C1–C2 posterior decompression and fusion.
- Severe anterior cord compression necessitating anterior decompression.

34.3 Technique

- Odontoidectomy can be performed through two approaches: the transoral approach and the endoscopic endonasal approach.
- For the transoral approach described here, patients should be able to open their mouth at least 5 to 6 cm and should have a preoperative dental evaluation if possible to rule out comorbid dental or oral pathology.[4]
- General endotracheal (ET) anesthesia with a reinforced flexible endotracheal tube is the authors' preferred method of intubation.
  - Tends to allow for easier positioning of the tube away from the midline and for its retraction inferiorly as opposed to when a nasotracheal intubation is performed.
  - Preoperative tracheostomy should also be considered for cases that require more extensive exposure as well as when ventilator dependence for several days postoperatively is anticipated.
  - Nasogastric tube is useful for gastric secretion management.
- The authors recommend the routine use of somatosensory evoked potentials (SSEPs) and, often, motor evoked potentials (MEPs) as well.
  - Baseline recordings may be indicated before final positioning of the patient.
- The patient is positioned supine on a standard operating room (OR) table. Head fixation is not necessary but the head can be secured by either a Mayfield headrest (Schaerer Mayfield; Randolph, Massachusetts) or with skull tongs/pins for greater control. Head extension is recommended.
- A preoperative dose of antibiotics is given that includes coverage for oral flora.
  - Ampicillin-sulbactam, clindamycin, cefepime, and metronidazole are potential options.
- The field is prepared by filling the oral cavity with a povidone–iodine (Betadine) solution after placing the patient into the Trendelenburg position to prevent aspiration should the ET cuff deflate.
  - The authors soak the mouth for 10 minutes before removing the solution.

- The surgeon sits at the patient's head, and a surgical microscope is used for visualization.
- A Spetzler-Sonntag transoral retractor (Integra LifeSciences; Princeton, California) is positioned over the mouth with the retractors used to form a rectangular exposure: The palate is elevated cephalad, and the tongue and endotracheal tube are retracted caudally; the tonsils and lateral oropharyngeal walls are covered in moist gauze and retracted laterally.
- The midline is identified by palpating the anterior tubercle of C1 as well as the C2–C3 disk space, which is usually prominent.
- A 3- to 5-cm full-thickness vertical incision is made in the midline with the use of the cutting current of a unipolar electrocautery, dividing the mucosa, pharyngeal constrictor musculature, and the anterior longitudinal ligament.
  - The amount of bleeding is significantly reduced by staying in the midline.
- Flaps are elevated to either side of the midline out laterally to the edge of the C2 body.
- Self-retaining retractor blades are then placed to retract the flaps laterally.
- The central portion of the anterior arch of C1 is removed using either a high-speed bur or a sharp rongeur.
  - Typically, 1 cm of bone in each direction from the midline is removed, corresponding to roughly two-thirds of the entire anterior C1 arch.
  - An effort should be made to preserve the cranial 25% of the arch to prevent lateral mass spread, as the anterior C1 arch is the load-bearing aspect of the atlas.
- Next, the odontoid is resected, which is usually performed in one of the two ways: (1) Using a high-speed side-cutting matchstick bur or (2) amputating the odontoid at its base and removing it *en bloc* by severing the soft tissue connections and working in a caudal-to-cephalad direction.
  - A variation of removing the dens with the bur is to hollow out the odontoid, leaving thin lateral and posterior cortical walls of bone. The remaining bone can then be removed using either a fine curette or micro-Kerrison rongeurs.
- To fully remove the tip of the odontoid, it is necessary to cut the remaining soft tissue attachments. Angled curettes or micro-Kerrison rongeurs can be used to detach the apical, alar, and transverse ligaments and tectorial membrane.
- In patients with rheumatoid arthritis, the retrodental soft tissue pannus is now exposed. Only loose fragments should be debulked, as complete pannus removal for dural visualization unnecessarily risks a cerebrospinal fluid (CSF) leak.[2]
- The incision is irrigated thoroughly with antibiotic solution, followed by closure of the pharynx, typically by 3–0 chromic buried sutures.

- A two-layered closure may also be performed if layered flaps were created during the initial dissection.
- The retractors are removed, and 1% cortisone cream may be applied to the mucosa and tongue to decrease postoperative edema.

34.4 Complications

- Neurologic injury:
  - SSEPs and MEPs can provide intraoperative warning of spinal cord compromise.
  - Keep mean arterial pressure (MAP) above 80 to 85 mmHg to prevent ischemic spinal cord injury.[5]
- Dural tear and CSF leak:
  - Direct dural repair is recommended (if possible), followed by fascial/fat graft or fibrin glue.
  - Placement of a subarachnoid lumbar drain postoperatively can be helpful and is recommended if a watertight dural closure is not feasible.
  - Considered a risk factor for meningitis due to a connection with the oropharynx, so broad-spectrum antibiotics (gram-positive and gram-negative coverage) should be given postoperatively.[6,7]
- Airway obstruction:
  - Avoid premature extubation as reintubation can be very difficult and require emergency tracheostomy.
  - Before extubation, evaluate for resolution of retropharyngeal swelling on lateral radiograph (usually 24–48 h postoperatively).[1]
  - Assess ability to breathe around orotracheal airway.[2]
- Other pulmonary and oral airway complications:
  - Purulent secretions, atelectasis, acute respiratory distress syndrome (ARDS).
    - Risk factors include American Society of Anesthesiologists (ASA) Grades III and greater, preoperative lower cranial nerve palsies, preoperative pulmonary involvement, and longer operative times.[8]
  - Dysphonia may occur if the soft palate is incised.[9]
  - Tongue necrosis, broken teeth, and local soft tissue edema can be caused by retractor malposition.[4]
- Infection—inherent nature of the procedure involves dissection directly through a "contaminated" field.
  - The infection rate after transoral upper cervical spine surgery has been reported to be around 2.4 to 3.6%.[6,7]
  - Direct contamination can lead to septic encephalomeningitis if the dura is compromised.

  - Can be minimized with meticulous wound closure and 24 to 48 hours of IV antibiotics.
  - In high-risk patients with a concern for an infectious etiology, preoperative oropharyngeal cultures may be useful in guiding antibiotic therapy and should be considered in high-risk patients.[6]
  - Postoperative infection or retropharyngeal abscess is considered the origin of wound dehiscence until proven otherwise.
  - Utilizing a nasogastric tube postoperatively for 5 days until evidence of mucosal healing may decrease wound contamination.
- Instability:
  - Odontoidectomy can increase range of motion in all directions and lead to instability (acute or delayed). Posterior fixation is often required to stabilize the upper cervical spine. Halo–vest immobilization can be used for immobilization prior to posterior stabilization.
- Vascular complication:
  - Preoperative computed tomography (CT) or magnetic resonance imaging (MRI) scans should be reviewed to determine the location of the vessels (i.e., an aberrant medial course of the vertebral artery).
  - Dissection of the atlas should stay within 1.5 cm of the midline, and dissection at the level of the C2–C3 disk should stay within 1 cm of the midline.[1]
  - If vertebral artery injury results in uncontrolled bleeding, vascular surgery assistance for angiography and emergent balloon embolization may be necessary.[6]

34.5 Postoperative Care

- The authors typically perform immediate posterior stabilization after odontoid resection. A hard cervical collar and manual stabilization can be used to transfer the patient from the supine to the prone position.
  - When possible, the authors recommend performing the posterior fusion before the transoral resection.
- For most transoral cases, immediate postoperative extubation is possible given that the proximal location of the surgical field within the pharynx makes airway compromise less likely.
  - Importantly, however, the tongue and soft tissues should be carefully inspected for severe swelling before extubation of the patient. If there is concern, the patient should be left intubated until the swelling resolves.
- Oral feeding can resume immediately for most patients who have short, simple procedures; however, many patients require tube feeding for several days.
- Antibiotics should be continued for 24 to 48 hours postoperatively.[10]

- Preoperatively, many patients requiring ventral decompression may be severely debilitated and malnourished. Postoperatively, there may be a need for a course of parental nutrition.

34.6 Outcomes

- No level I studies have been performed to evaluate outcomes to our knowledge.
- Based on a review of smaller case series, improvement of preoperative neurologic deficits can be expected but is dependent on chronicity of spinal cord compression.[10]
- In one 10-year review of 72 cases, there were two postoperative deaths and one pharyngeal infection requiring a repeat operation, with 100% neurological improvement seen in all patients.[6]
- A recent systematic review of transoral odontoidectomy found multiple reported complications including: arterial injury (1.9%), postoperative CSF leak (0.8%), meningitis (1.0%), pharyngeal wound dehiscence (1.7%), dysphagia (3.8%), velopharyngeal insufficiency (3.3%), tracheostomy (10.8%), and 30-day mortality (2.9%).[7]
- Similarly, improvement in neurologic symptoms were 90% based on multiple case series.[7]

34.7 Surgical Pearls

- Care should be taken to avoid entrapment of the tongue against the teeth with the retractor system.
- As an alternative to palatal retractors, a red rubber catheter can be passed through the nares and sutured to the soft palate and uvula; it can then be used as a retractor.[2]
- The soft palate and mandible can be split to provide extensile exposure in the proximal and distal directions, respectively, although the increased morbidity should be considered.
- If the dura is not visualized, the space can be filled with radiopaque dye to assess for completeness of the decompression.[4]

Common Clinical Questions

1. When performing exposure of the odontoid, the surgeon decided to remove 1 cm each side of the midline of the atlas to create a window access. What technique can help in preventing lateral mass spread and destabilization?

   A. Bur less than 0.8 cm wide from midline.

B. Leave a cephalad narrow bony bridge.

C. Remove more than anterior arch of C1, because it does not have any effect on C1 stabilization.

D. The anterior odontoid exposure does not require removal of any anterior C1 arch.

2. When removing an os odontoideum, the surgeon notices CSF leakage. On exploring the dura, a small vertical dural tear is found. What is the best technique to treat this tear during surgery and postoperatively?

   A. Repair the tear followed by placement of a subarachnoid lumbar drain postoperatively.

   B. Place a layer of fibrin glue over the tear and postoperatively place the patient on 2 weeks of broad-spectrum antibiotics.

   C. Repair the tear, follow it with a fascial/fat graft or fibrin glue and postoperatively place the patient on 2 days of broad-spectrum antibiotics.

   D. Repair the tear, follow it with a fascial/fat graft or fibrin glue, place a subarachnoid lumbar drain postoperatively, and give the patient broad-spectrum antibiotics for 2 weeks.

3. What is the preferred method for intubating a patient about to undergo transoral odontoidectomy?

   A. Nasotracheal intubation.

   B. Preoperative tracheostomy should be performed on all patients undergoing transoral odontoidectomy.

   C. General endotracheal intubation can be performed as long as the tube is retracted laterally.

   D. General endotracheal intubation can be performed as long as the tube is retracted inferiorly with the tongue.

4. How should excessive or uncontrolled bleeding from too far lateral dissection be addressed?

   A. Immediate tamponade of bleeding with bone wax.

   B. Compression, continue with decompression and hardware placement, and re-evaluate.

   C. Compression, vascular surgical consult with consideration of urgent angiography.

   D. Immediate wound closure and transfer to ICU for pressure support.

Answers to Common Clinical Questions

1. B. The surgeon can remove up to 1 cm on each side of the midline to create the access window to the odontoid.
2. D. Patients who have a dural tear are at a higher risk of developing meningitis, and broad-spectrum antibiotics should be given for at least 2 weeks.
3. D. Patients should undergo general endotracheal intubation, and the tube should be retracted inferiorly with the tongue, allowing direct visualization of operating window without the tube blocking it.
4. C. Tamponade of the bleeding with hemostatic agents or bone wax could result in a false aneurysm or late bleeding, requiring urgent surgery. Balloon embolization or ligation of the artery may be required.

References

1. Mendoza N, Crockard A. Anterior transoral procedures. In: An HS, Riley LH III, eds. An Atlas of Surgery of the Spine. London: Martin Dunitz Ltd; 1998:55–69
2. Mummaneni PV, Haid RW. Transoral odontoidectomy. Neurosurgery. 2005; 56(5):1045–1050, discussion 1045–1050
3. Goldschlager T, Härtl R, Greenfield JP, Anand VK, Schwartz TH. The endoscopic endonasal approach to the odontoid and its impact on early extubation and feeding. J Neurosurg. 2015; 122(3):511–518
4. Joaquim AF, Osorio JA, Riew KD. Transoral and endoscopic endonasal odontoidectomies—surgical techniques, indications, and complications. Neurospine. 2019; 16(3):462–469
5. Daniels AH, Hart RA, Hilibrand AS, et al. Iatrogenic spinal cord injury resulting from cervical spine surgery. Global Spine J. 2017; 7(1) Suppl:84S–90S
6. Li W, Wang B, Feng X, Hua W, Yang C. Preoperative management and postoperative complications associated with transoral decompression for the upper cervical spine. BMC Musculoskelet Disord. 2022; 23(1):128
7. Shriver MF, Kshettry VR, Sindwani R, Woodard T, Benzel EC, Recinos PF. Transoral and transnasal odontoidectomy complications: a systematic review and meta-analysis. Clin Neurol Neurosurg. 2016; 148:121–129
8. Marda M, Pandia MP, Rath GP, Bithal PK, Dash HH. Post-operative pulmonary complications in patients undergoing transoral odontoidectomy and posterior fixation for craniovertebral junction anomalies. J Anaesthesiol Clin Pharmacol. 2013; 29(2):200–204
9. Menezes AH, VanGilder JC. Transoral-transpharyngeal approach to the anterior craniocervical junction. Ten-year experience with 72 patients. J Neurosurg. 1988; 69(6):895–903
10. Elbadrawi AM, Elkhateeb TM. Transoral approach for odontoidectomy efficacy and safety. HSS J. 2017; 13(3):276–281

35 Endoscopic Endonasal Odontoidectomy

Umberto Tosi, Jeffrey P. Greenfield, and Theodore H. Schwartz

Summary
Endoscopic endonasal odontoidectomy is a valid treatment modality for pathologies of the anterior cervicomedullary junction. It is often performed along with posterior decompression and fusion, since disruption of the alar, apical, and transverse ligaments results in occipitocervical instability. The nasal corridor allows for resection of pathologies that approximate the body of C2.

Compared with transoral approaches, the endonasal corridor allows for earlier return to feeding and likely has fewer complications, albeit studies directly comparing the two remain necessary. Neurological complications are rare; CSF fistulas can be repaired directly or via temporary CSF diversion via lumbar drainage.

Keywords: cervicomedullary junction, dens, endoscopy, odontoidectomy

35.1 Key Points

- The endoscopic endonasal approach allows the surgeon access from the clivus rostrally to the inferior portion of the odontoid caudally.
- This approach allows access to anterior cervicomedullary junction (CMJ) pathologies for direct decompression. Intradural pathologies remain challenging since watertight dural closure may be difficult to achieve with this approach.
- A thorough radiographic preoperative assessment is needed to determine if this approach can safely reach the intended pathology. The naso-axial line (NAxL) and rhinopalatine line (RPL) have been proposed as good approximators of caudal extension of odontoidectomy.[1,2]
- This approach is often augmented via a posterior decompression to allow for a 360-degree release.
- Extensive odontoidectomy can result in further destabilization of the occipito-cervical junction. Posterior cervical arthrodesis is often necessary to prevent instability. This is performed either concomitantly or in a staged

fashion with odontoidectomy, generally beforehand so that the spine is never unstable.

- Compared to transoral approaches, endonasal endoscopic approaches have lower rates of complications, infections, and shorter time to extubation and feeding.

35.2 Indications

- Extradural ventral pathologies causing compression of the anterior hindbrain, cervicomedullary junction, or cervical spinal cord, from the clivus to the C2 vertebral body.
  - Common etiologies include a rheumatoid or other inflammatory, retro-odontoid pannus, basilar invagination, tumor, or trauma.
  - In pediatric patients, developmental anomalies of the craniocervical junction leading to ventral brainstem compression predominate the indications for this approach.
  - Connective tissue disorders are common in this patient population and often exacerbate ventral compression.
- Continued symptoms of brainstem and cervical cord compression despite posterior decompression.

35.3 Technique

- A preoperative CT scan that spans, at the minimum, from the frontal lobe to the posterior aspect of C3 will allow for careful surgical planning.
  - The following lines are constructed on a midsagittal cut (**Fig. 35.1**): the hard palate line (HPL—a line that joins the anterior and posterior edges of the hard palate); the nasopalatine line (NPL–a line that joins the rhinion with the posterior nasal spine of the palatine bone); the NAxL (a line that joins the midpoint between rhinion and the anterior nasal spine of maxilla with the posterior nasal spine of the palatine bone); the RPL (a line that joins a point two-thirds of the way between rhinion and the anterior nasal spine of maxilla with the posterior nasal spine of the palatine bone).
  - The extent of odontoidectomy will be overestimated by the NPL by more than 10 mm and will approximately fall between the NAxL and the RPL.
- Intraoperative CT navigation, if available, is helpful. In case of concomitant posterior cervical fusion, vascular imaging to assess for vertebral course and dominance can be performed preoperatively.
- Cervical fusion is often performed along with endoscopic odontoidectomy. In our experience, it is performed most commonly prior to odontoidectomy,

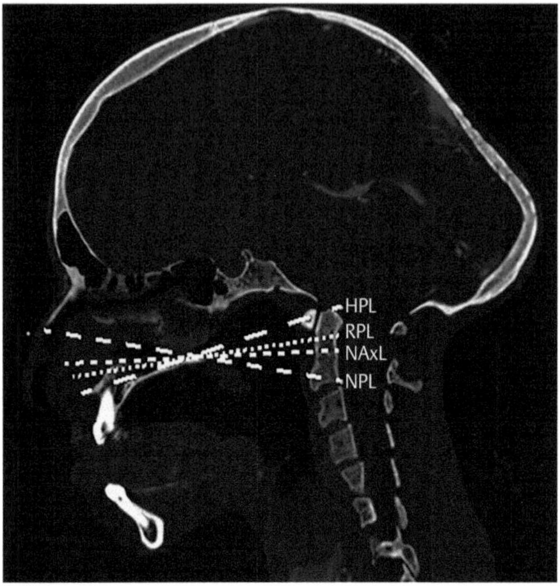

Fig. 35.1 Radiographic predictors of endonasal odontoidectomy. A preoperative image (ideally from a computed tomography [CT] or, as in this case, computed tomography angiography [CTA]) is used for radiographic analysis. On the midsagittal plane, the following lines are constructed and extended until they intersect the posterior end plate of the cervical spine: (i) hard palate line (HPL): a line that joins the anterior (anterior nasal spine of the maxillary bone) and posterior (posterior nasal spine of the palatine bone) edges of the hard palate; (ii) nasopalatine line (NPL): a line that joins the rhinion with the posterior nasal spine of the palatine bone; (iii) nasoaxial line (NAxL): a line that joins the midpoint between rhinion and the anterior nasal spine of maxilla with the posterior nasal spine of the palatine bone; (iv) rhinopalatine line (RPL): a line that joins a point two-thirds of the way between rhinion and the anterior nasal spine of maxilla with the posterior nasal spine of the palatine bone. Generally, the extent of odontoidectomy falls between the RPL and the NAxL and is overestimated by the NPL.

staging the two procedures by a few days to ensure that the patient is fused in a proper position and to allow for recovery. Operative and anesthesia time will increase if the procedures are performed together.

- If the risk of dural tear is deemed high, a lumbar drain can be placed and intrathecal fluorescein administered to assist with intraoperative determination of the presence of a leak. In low-risk cases, a lumbar drain can be placed at the end of the procedure if a CSF leak is encountered.

- Following endotracheal intubation and placement of an orogastric tube, the patient is positioned supine on a standard operating room table with the head secured in a Mayfield clamp (Schaerer Mayfield, Randolph, MA) in neutral position. The head is often already fixed in a neutral position from posterior arthrodesis.
- Following sterile prep and draping and antibiotic administration, an otolaryngologist starts the approach.[3]
  - Cefazoline is used for most cases.
- A posterior septectomy is performed and the attachment of the vomer to the hard palate is drilled flush. A linear incision is made in the basopharyngeal fascia, between the Eustachian tubes from the bottom of the clivus to the inferior limits of the odontoid.
- As shown in **Video 35.1**,[4] this is followed by removal of the anterior arch of C1 with a high-speed drill.
  - Approximately 1 cm of the arch of C1 is removed in either lateral dimension to expose the lateral limits of the odontoid.
- The odontoidectomy proper then follows through a combination of drilling, Kerrison rongeurs, and bone curettes (**Fig. 35.2**).
  - The endoscope, generally a 0-degree, can be held on a scope holder or by an assistant.
  - The alar and apical ligaments are often sacrificed. The transverse and transverse occipital ligaments are similarly often removed to gain access to dorsal structures (e.g., rheumatoid pannus).
  - The greater the extent of odontoidectomy and of ligament destruction, the higher the likelihood of instability requiring fusion.
  - The removal of the dens and associated ligaments and inflammatory material is concluded when the dura is encountered.
- Once the removal of the dens is completed, intraoperative CT scan, if available, can be used to assess the adequacy of the removal.
- Closure is performed with two 4–0 chromic sutures placed to reapproximate the basopharyngeal fascia.
- If a CSF leak is encountered, it is repaired with an onlay of autologous fat, sufficient to completely cover and plug the dural defect. This is covered with fibrin glue (e.g., Tisseel [Baxter International; Deerfield, IL]) and held in place with the chromic sutures that close the fascia as described above. A lumbar drain can be placed as well to decrease intracranial pressure (ICP) for a few days postoperatively to assist with the closure.
  - Autologous fat grafting is ideal for repairing such a leak, as it perfectly fills the anatomical defect created ventral to the dural leak.
  - Lumbar drainage at 5 to 10 cc/hour is carried out for 2 to 3 days postoperatively. Prior to lumbar drain removal, a clamp trial with patient mobilization is performed to ensure adequate closure.

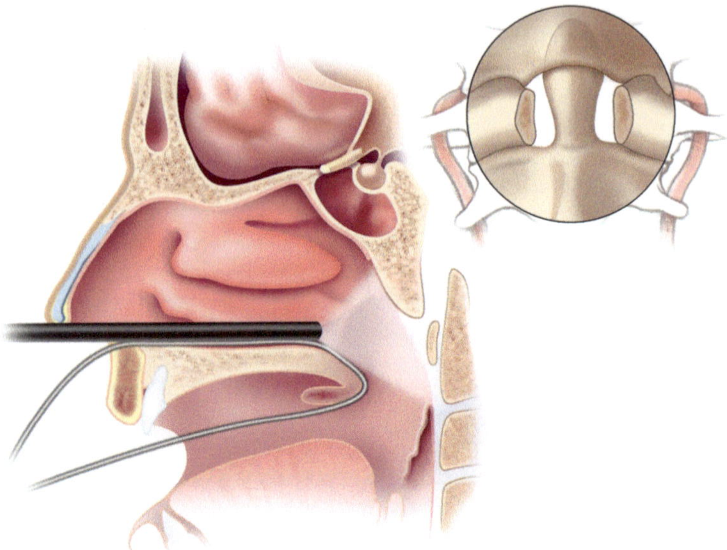

Fig. 35.2 Approach to the dens. Illustration showing an endoscopic approach to the dens. The lack of oropharyngeal trauma is important to note, especially compared to the transoral route. The inset shows an endoscopic view following removal of the anterior arch of C1. The position of the vertebral arteries relative to the lateral extent of arch removal is appreciated. (Adapted from Goldschlager T, Härtl R, Greenfield JP, Anand VK, Schwartz TH. The endoscopic endonasal approach to the odontoid and its impact on early extubation and feeding. J Neurosurg 2015;122(3):511–518.)

   - A vascularized nasoseptal flap can be attempted but is difficult to place in this location.
- Following closure, and prior to extubation, the stomach contents are aspirated with an orogastric tube to minimize postoperative nausea and vomiting.

35.4 Complications

- Neurologic injury is rare.
   - Care needs to be taken to avoid spinal cord compression during the procedure, especially toward the end of the odontoidectomy.
   - Vascular imaging is not usually necessary. If aberrant anatomy is suspected, dedicated vascular imaging with intraoperative navigation should be obtained.

- Posterior cervical fusion (discussed elsewhere) carries significant risks as well. Patients undergoing both procedures should be counseled about the risks of both.
- Velopalatal insufficiency, more common with the transoral approach, is uncommon with the endonasal approach.

- CSF fistulas: Persistent CSF leaks in the naso- and oropharynx increase the likelihood of developing meningitis.
  - Leaks should be repaired primarily as described above.
  - Patients with lumbar drains should be maintained on antibiotic prophylaxis while the drain is in place.
  - If a leak develops postoperatively, patients should be trialed with lumbar drainage first.
  - Persistent leaks that do not resolve despite prolonged drainage may require re-exploration or, ultimately, permanent CSF diversion (e.g., ventriculoperitoneal shunting).
  - In cases of meningitis, CSF sampling and culture-driven antibiosis is necessary given the extent of nasal flora. In our practice, empiric antibiotics are started immediately after CSF sampling and narrowed once culture results are obtained.
- Dysphagia: A common postoperative complaint, with incidence higher than 60% in some series, with up to 15% of patients requiring gastrostomy tubes.[5]
  - The endonasal route generally has a lower incidence of dysphagia than the transoral route due to preservation of oropharynx tissues.
  - Patients who undergo occipito-cervical fusion may have dysphagia as a consequence of an inappropriate occipito-cervical angle and may require revision.
  - Numerous patients present with pre-existing dysphagia. They should be counseled that improvements may be gradual or may not occur.
- Respiratory compromise.
  - Postoperative respiratory compromise is rare, with most patients being extubated at the end of the case.
  - The incidence of airway compromise is lower than in transoral approaches since the oropharynx is spared and the surgical corridor is smaller and yielding.
- Unforeseen complications.
  - Patients undergoing this procedure are often frail and with numerous medical comorbidities, as they are typically dichotomized in elderly patients with rheumatoid changes and in pediatric patients with congenital abnormalities.
  - A multidisciplinary approach with a team composed of, at the minimum, a skull base surgeon, a spine surgeon, and an otolaryngologist is required.
  - Postoperative antibiotics, early mobilization, and careful neuromonitoring, as necessary.

35.5 Postoperative Care

- Cervical stabilization is often concomitant with odontoidectomy and, routinely, performed a few days prior.
  - In young healthy patients who will tolerate a longer anesthesia time, surgical staging may not be necessary.
  - Following cervical fusion, a hard cervical collar should be worn at all times.
  - In patients with connective tissue disorders (e.g., osteogenesis imperfecta), longer constructs should be used to guarantee effective arthrodesis.
- Early extubation should be achieved in a majority of cases. Exception may come from significant pre-existing pathology or unusually long cases with prone positioning from the fusion leading to an increased risk of oral, tongue, and airway edema.
- Oral feeding usually resumes on the first postoperative day. Diet is advanced progressively, with liquids being introduced first.
- Antibiotics should be continued for 24 hours postoperatively or while the lumbar drain remains in place.
- Patients will have "endonasal precautions" in place—nothing will be inserted in the nose (e.g., no swabs) and noninvasive positive pressure ventilation (e.g., BiPAP) and Valsalva maneuvers will be avoided to reduce risk of CSF leak.
- Postoperative CT and MRI scans and standing anteroposterior (AP) and lateral cervical films (in cases of cervical fusion) will be needed to assess the extent of odontoidectomy, decompression, and cervical alignment.
  - Decompression improves over time as inflammation (associated both with surgery and cervical instability) subsides.
- Given often pre-existing cervical myelopathy, patients will often require inpatient physical therapy in a skilled rehabilitation center postoperatively.

35.6 Outcomes

- Although no randomized clinical trial has been performed to assess outcomes, and no Level I evidence exists, retrospective case series demonstrate excellent ventral decompression of the CMJ and rapid time to extubation and feeding with few complications.[6]
- Given its relative novelty, long-term studies are needed to assess outcomes.
- To date, the largest case series in the literature consists of 34 patients who had significant improvement in their preoperative symptoms but high incidence of dysphagia. Follow-up was limited by a frail patient population.[5]

35.7 Surgical Pearls

- Careful analysis of the preoperative imaging is necessary to determine whether a resection that will end between the NAxL and the RPL will achieve sufficient decompression. Ventral decompression often leads to instability requiring posterior fusion.
- A staged posterior decompression and fusion prior to anterior decompression may be needed to guarantee symptom resolution.
- Patient selection is essential to achieve good outcomes. Although the procedure is almost always successful with fewer morbidities than a transoral decompression, endoscopic endonasal odontoidectomy still carries risks and may not be tolerated by patients with many medical comorbidities.

Common Clinical Questions

1. What is the caudal extent of an endoscopic endonasal odontoidectomy?
2. Can endonasal odontoidectomy cause cervical instability?
3. What strategies can be employed to stop a CSF leak?

Answers to Common Clinical Questions

1. The caudal extent of an endoscopic endonasal odontoidectomy falls between the NAxL (which overestimates it) and RPL (an underestimation).
2. Yes, extensive resection of the dens and of the occipito-cervical ligaments will cause spinal instability. Posterior cervical arthrodesis is often performed concomitantly as a counterbalance.
3. Small leaks should be repaired primarily; an overlay of abdominal fat and fibrin glue should be placed in the defect and held in place with sutures that close the basopharyngeal fascia. If in doubt about the reliability of closure, a short period (1–3 days) of lumbar drainage may be carried out.

References

1. Aldana PR, Naseri I, La Corte E. The naso-axial line: a new method of accurately predicting the inferior limit of the endoscopic endonasal approach to the craniovertebral junction. Neurosurgery. 2012; 71(2) Suppl Operative: ons308–ons314, discussion ons314
2. La Corte E, Aldana PR, Ferroli P, et al. The rhinopalatine line as a reliable predictor of the inferior extent of endonasal odontoidectomies. Neurosurg Focus. 2015; 38(4):E16

3. Michael AP, Elbuluk O, Tsiouris AJ, et al. The critical importance of a vascularized flap in preventing recurrence after endoscopic repair of spontaneous cerebrospinal fluid leaks and meningoencephaloceles. J Neurosurg. 2021:1–8. Online ahead of print
4. Tosi U, Giantini-Larsen A, Mathios D, Kacker A, et al. Endoscopic odontoidectomy for brainstem compression in association with posterior fossa decompression and occipitocervical fusion. J Neurosurg. 2023; 139(4):1152–1159
5. Zwagerman NT, Tormenti MJ, Tempel ZJ, et al. Endoscopic endonasal resection of the odontoid process: clinical outcomes in 34 adults. J Neurosurg. 2018; 128 (3):923–931
6. Goldschlager T, Härtl R, Greenfield JP, Anand VK, Schwartz TH. The endoscopic endonasal approach to the odontoid and its impact on early extubation and feeding. J Neurosurg. 2015; 122(3):511–518

36 C1–C2 Fixation Techniques

Timothy Chryssikos, Nitin Agarwal, Alysha Jamieson, and Praveen V. Mummaneni

Summary

C1–C2 fixation techniques include: (1) C1 lateral mass screws in combination with C2 pars screws, pedicle screws, or translaminar screws; (2) C1–C2 transarticular screws (Magerl's technique); and (3) C1–C2 wiring techniques. Indications for C1–C2 fixation include instability, fractures, congenital malformations, inflammatory and infectious disorders, and neoplasm. Posterior C1–C2 fusion techniques are technically demanding, and caution is required to avoid vascular injury during screw placement. The vertebral arteries are vulnerable during C2 pedicle and C2 pars placement, and especially during C1–C2 transarticular screw placement. The carotid arteries can be injured if C1 lateral mass screws are placed with the screw tip too far into the retropharyngeal area. Preoperative CT (with CT angiography if feasible) is recommended to assess the position of the foramen transversarium of C1 and C2. Instrumentation of C1 and C2 is increasingly used with navigation software, which can potentially enhance safety and maximize screw size.

Keywords: C1–C2 fixation, vertebral artery, atlantoaxial instability, odontoid fracture, atlantodental interval

36.1 Key Points

- The most common method currently used for C1–C2 fixation includes independent screw placement into the C1 lateral mass and C2 pars or pedicle.
- C2 translaminar screws can be placed if there is unfavorable vertebral artery course, small pedicles, or when C2 pedicle/pars screw placement fails. Translaminar screw fixation is comparatively weak in flexion.
- Wiring methods can be used when screw placement is precluded, but wire fixation is weak in rotation and requires an intact C1 posterior arch and C2 lamina.
- C1–C2 transarticular screw fixation, when combined with wire–bone graft methods, eliminates both flexion–extension and rotational motion, but

C1–C2 transarticular screw fixation carries the highest risk of vertebral artery injury.
- C2 neurectomy can be performed to optimize exposure of the C1 lateral mass and C1–C2 joint, but dysesthetic pain may result if the C2 nerve root is not sectioned medial to the C2 ganglion.
- Viscous hemostatic agents should be avoided when there is suspected vertebral artery injury, as this may result in embolization. Use large pieces of gelfoam instead.
- If vertebral artery injury occurs during cannulation of C2 prior to screw placement, then the respective screw may be placed to tamponade bleeding. If not already placed, the contralateral C2 screw should not be placed until angiography is performed.

36.2 Indications of C1–C2 Fixation

- C1–C2 ligamentous instability (> 3 mm atlantodental interval [ADI] on flexion–extension X-rays).
- Traumatic fractures are among the most frequent indications for posterior C1–C2 fixation.
- Certain subsets of type 2 and type 3 odontoid fractures may be treated with posterior C1–C2 fixation.
  - Type 2 odontoid fracture associated with:
    - Fracture of the atlantoaxial joint.
    - Oblique fractures.
    - Jefferson (C1) fracture.
    - Ruptured transverse ligament.
    - Chronic, unhealed type 2 odontoid fracture.
    - Rotatory subluxation of C1–C2.
  - Type 3 odontoid fracture associated with:
    - Fracture of the atlantoaxial joint.
    - Jefferson fracture.
    - Chronic, unhealed type 3 odontoid fracture.
    - Rotatory subluxation of C1–C2.
- Congenital malformations of C2 (e.g., os odontoideum and odontoid agenesis with C1–C2 dynamic instability).
- Inflammatory diseases (e.g., rheumatoid arthritis with abnormal posterior atlantodental interval [PADI] < 14 mm) (**Fig. 36.1**).
- Degenerative diseases (with instability and abnormal ADI).
- Infections (with instability and abnormal ADI).
- Neoplasms (with instability and abnormal ADI).

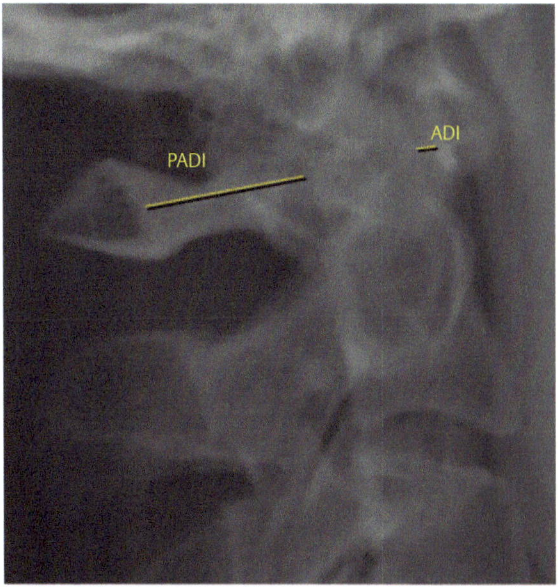

Fig. 36.1 Demonstration of atlantodental interval (ADI) and posterior atlantodental interval (PADI) on lateral X-ray.

36.3 Preparation for C1–C2 Fixation

C1–C2 fixation is technically demanding, and a three-dimensional understanding of the anatomy of the region (**Fig. 36.2**) and relationship to the vertebral arteries is mandatory (**Fig. 36.3**).

The patient is positioned prone with head fixed by a skull clamp, which is secured to the table. The neck should be placed in a neutral position. The head can be flexed in the military chin tuck position, which enables easier placement of C1 lateral mass screws. A midline posterior neck incision is made from the suboccipital area to the spinous process of C3, with subperiosteal exposure of the C2 inferior articulating processes and the posterior C1 arch. Electrocautery should be avoided more than 1 cm lateral to the posterior C1 tubercle to avoid injury to the vertebral artery as it courses within the sulcus arteriosus.

36.3.1 C1–C2 Fixation Constructs Using C1 Lateral Mass Screws with C2 Pars, Pedicle, or Translaminar Screws[1,2,3,4]

- C1 lateral mass screws connected to C2 pars/pedicle or translaminar screws provide biomechanical strength and can facilitate anatomic reduction with high rate of fusion (greater than 95%).[2]

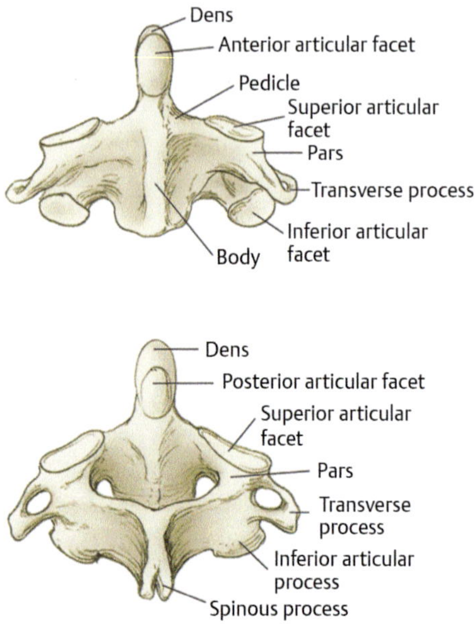

Fig. 36.2 Anatomy of the C2 vertebral body from anterior and posterior perspective. (Reproduced with permission from Fessler RG and Sekhar L, eds. Atlas of Surgical Techniques: Spine and Peripheral Nerves, Thieme; 2006.)

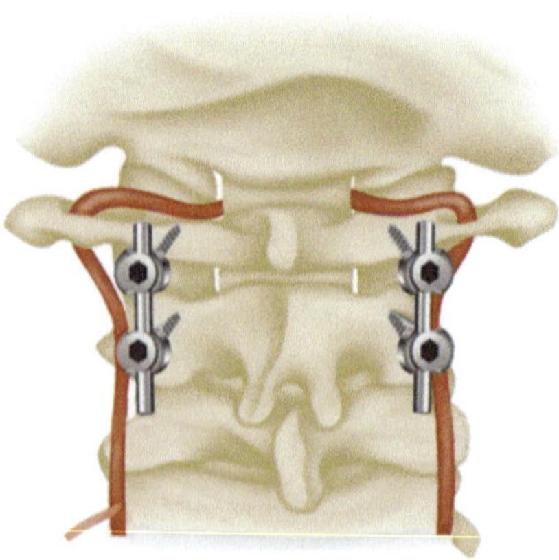

Fig. 36.3 Posterior C1–C2 screw and rod construct. Note the path of the vertebral artery which courses lateral to the pars of C2 and then loops upward into the sulcus arteriosus along the superior lateral aspect of the C1 lamina. Patients may have anomalous vertebral artery anatomy, including a vessel branch inferior to the C1 arch rather than in the normal location within the sulcus arteriosus. CT angiography may be performed before surgery to assess vertebral artery anatomy.

- C1–C2 fixation using screws placed independently into the atlas and axis and connected with rods or plates was described by Goel et al,[5] Goel and Laheri,[6] and Harms and Melcher.[7] This method represents the currently most commonly used method for C1–C2 fixation.
  - C2 neurectomy is optional but carries risk of numbness, although this is typically well-tolerated. C2 neurectomy can enhance exposure of the C1 lateral mass and C1–C2 facet joint, and enables bone graft to be placed directly along the dorsal aspect of the C1–C2 facet.
- C1 lateral mass screws:
  - Control of hemorrhage from the venous plexus between C1 and C2 can be achieved with bipolar coagulation or hemostatic agents. Exposure of the vertebral artery on the superior aspect of the C1 arch (sulcus arteriosus) is not recommended. Blunt dissection along the inferior surface of the C1 arch from medial to lateral can facilitate exposure of the superior aspect of the C1 lateral mass. Often, the C2 nerve root is mobilized caudally for exposure of the C1 lateral mass inferior to the C1 arch. Resection of the C2 nerve root can be carried out **medial** to the ganglion for enhanced exposure of the C1–C2 joint. Although this may result in scalp numbness, this is typically mild in severity and frequently patients benefit from relief of pre-existing C2 neuralgia after C2 neurectomy. We recommend placing a silk suture or small clip between the thecal sac and C2 ganglion and **sharply** sectioning the root between the clip or suture and the ganglion to prevent CSF leak.
  - The medial and lateral borders of the C1 lateral mass are carefully palpated with a blunt instrument to determine the mid-point of the C1 lateral mass. A pilot hole is created with a 2- or 3-mm drill bit at the center of C1 lateral mass, just inferior to the junction of the C1 lateral mass and the C1 arch. If the surgeon desires to drill a portion of the C1 arch to facilitate C1 lateral mass screw placement, careful examination of the anatomy of the C1 arch on preoperative CT is necessary as this technique carries a higher risk of vertebral artery injury. The screw trajectory is angled 10 degrees medial in the axial plane. On lateral fluoroscopic imaging, the drill is aimed toward the anterior tubercle of C1. The ideal depth of drilling is to the posterior aspect of the anterior C1 tubercle on lateral fluoroscopy. After tapping the cannulated tract, the C1 lateral mass screw is placed (usually 32–36 mm long). Increasingly, navigation is employed to facilitate safe cannulation of the C1 lateral masses and screw placement. We recommend placement using either navigation or fluoroscopy. With modern polyaxial screws, the C1 lateral mass screws can be easily connected with either of the three types of C2 screws described below.

- C2 pars screws:
  - The C2 pars is defined as the portions of C2 vertebra between the superior and inferior articular surfaces. The trajectory of the C2 pars screw is similar to that of a C1–C2 transarticular screw, except that it is shorter. The entry point is approximately 3 mm rostral and 3 mm lateral to the inferior medial aspect of the inferior articular surface of C2. The screw should follow a steep trajectory, 45 to 60 degrees of caudal–cranial angulation, with 10 to 15 degrees of medial angulation. The typical screw length is 16 to 18 mm. To avoid vertebral artery injury, the screw must stop short of transverse foramen which typically enters along the inferior aspect of the C2 pars. Not infrequently patients possess a "high-riding" vertebral artery, and therefore careful study of the preoperative CT or CTA is suggested. The risk of vertebral artery injury with C2 pars screws is lower than C1–C2 transarticular screws.
- C2 pedicle screws:
  - The pedicles of C2 bridge the posterior elements with the C2 vertebral body. The entry point of the C2 pedicle screw is approximately 2 mm lateral and 2 mm superior to the entry point of the C2 pars screw, and can be found in close proximity to the lateral–superior margin of the C2 lamina. Careful palpation of the lateral–superior aspect of the C2 lamina can facilitate a better understanding of the location of the C2 pedicle. The C2 pedicle screw has less steep angulation than the C2 pars screw, with 20 degrees caudal–cranial angulation and 15 to 25 degrees angulation. The mean length of the C2 pedicle screw is approximately 20 mm, notably longer than for C2 pars screws. Navigation can be used to maximize C2 pedicle screw size (potentially up to 30 mm). For those who have very narrow C2 pedicles, risk of breach into the neural canal or transverse foramen is high.
- C2 translaminar screws:
  - Translaminar screws typically serve as a salvage technique for C2 pars screws or pedicle screws in cases of high-riding vertebral artery, narrow pedicles, or when C2 pedicle/pars screw placement fails.
  - Translaminar screws do not cross to the instantaneous axis of rotation and therefore are not strong in flexion.
  - The entry point of the translaminar screw is at the junction of the spinous process and lamina. The trajectory is parallel to the slope of the lamina. Aiming too ventrally can cause breach of the spinal canal and neurologic injury.
  - If bilateral translaminar screws are used, it is necessary to offset the entry points of each screw in the cranial–caudal direction to avoid intersecting screw trajectories.

36.3.2 C1–C2 Transarticular Screws[8]

- One advantage of the C1–C2 transarticular screw technique (Magerl's technique) is interruption of axial rotation about the atlantoaxial joint. The drawbacks of this procedure are the need for anatomical reduction of C1–C2 and a higher potential for vertebral artery injury than the C2 pedicle or pars screw placement techniques. If placement of the first screw likely caused vertebral artery injury, then screw insertion into the contralateral side should not be attempted, as bilateral vertebral artery injury could result in brainstem infarction and death. It is suggested that a dedicated CTA be acquired and carefully examined to exclude a high-riding vertebral artery or destruction of bone at the site of intended transarticular screw placement.
- The screw entry point is approximately 3 to 4 mm rostral and 3 to 4 mm lateral to the inferior medial portion of the C2–C3 facet joint. A K-wire is often used for this technique. The trajectory is typically 15 degrees medial with the superior angle visualized by fluoroscopy aiming at the C1 anterior tubercle (often 60 degrees). Subtle changes in resistance may be perceived as the K-wire traverses the four cortical surfaces along the path into the C1 lateral mass: (1) the posterior C2 entry point, (2) the superior articular surface of C2, (3) the inferior articular surface of C1, and (4) the anterior cortex of the C1 ring. After the K-wire is placed, a cannulated drill bit and tap are used, followed by screw placement. The typical screw length is 36 to 46 mm.
- Transarticular screw placement is often combined with wiring methods (described below) for bone grafting. This can create a three-point fixation that completely obliterates the rotational and flexion–extension motion of the C1–C2 joint.
- C1–C2 transarticular screw fixation may facilitate an even higher rate of fusion in constructs using C1 lateral mass and C2 pars or pedicle screws. However, C1–C2 transarticular screws have a higher rate of vertebral artery injury.

36.3.3 C1–C2 Wiring Methods[3,9]

- Posterior wiring techniques represent the earliest techniques for C1–C2 fusion. Several techniques of sublaminar wiring and bone graft placement have been reported, including Brooks, Gallie, and Sonntag methods. These methods require an intact posterior arch in C1 and intact lamina of C2. In cases where screw placement is precluded, wiring techniques may be indicated. One advantage of these methods is direct placement of bone graft between the posterior elements of C1 and C2. Double-braided titanium cables are presently preferred (over steel wires), as they are more flexible and carry lower risk of spinal cord injury and dural tear during sublaminar placement of the wires. A significant drawback of C1–C2 wiring techniques is that they are weak in rotation.

- For the Gallie technique, a single bone graft is situated between the C1 arch and the C2 lamina, with a notch in the inferior midline of the graft accommodating the C2 spinous process. The graft is secured with a cable that is passed beneath the C1 arch and around the spinous process of C2.
- The Brooks technique places two separate sublaminar cables beneath the lamina of both C1 and C2, which secure two separate bone grafts on either side of the midline between C1 and C2.
- In the Sonntag technique, a single iliac crest graft is contoured and situated between the C1 arch and spinous process of C2. The graft is secured in the midline using a sublaminar cable that is passed under C1 and wrapped around the spinous process of C2, rather than passed beneath the lamina of C2.

36.4 Complications

- Vertebral artery injury (unilateral vertebral artery injury may be asymptomatic, but bilateral vertebral artery injury invariably results in a large posterior circulation infarction and possibly death). If there is a unilateral vertebral artery injury, the screw should be placed to tamponade the bleeding, and the contralateral screw should not be placed. Strong consideration should be given to acquiring catheter angiogram for evaluation of the suspected injury and assessment of the contralateral vertebral artery.
- Dural injury or spinal cord injury.
- CSF leak.
- Rod and/or screw fracture.
- Nonunion of C1 and C2.

36.5 Postoperative Care

- A rigid cervical collar is used for 6 weeks postoperatively.

36.6 Surgical Pearls

- A thorough understanding of the three-dimensional anatomy of C1 and C2 is mandatory.
- Preoperative planning is crucial. CT (with CTA if feasible) is recommended to rule out anomalous path of the vertebral arteries and to assess the anatomy of C1 and C2.

- Bipolar cautery and hemostatic agents can be used to control bleeding around from the robust venous plexus dorsal to the C1–C2 joint.
- Viscous hemostatic agents should never be used in the setting of suspected vertebral artery injury, as this can be taken up by the vertebral artery and embolized to the cerebral vasculature resulting in stroke. When vertebral artery injury is suspected during screw placement, the screw should be placed and the contralateral screw should not be placed (if not already done so), followed by catheter angiogram for further evaluation.
- Instrumentation of C1 and C2 can be performed using navigation software, which can potentially enhance safety and maximize screw size.

Common Clinical Questions

1. Where is the entry point for the C2 pars screw?
2. Where is the entry point for the C1–C2 transarticular screw?
3. Should you place a contralateral C2 pars screw if you have an ipsilateral vertebral artery laceration during insertion of the first C2 pars/pedicle or transarticular screw?

Answers to Common Clinical Questions

1. The C2 pars screw entry point is approximately 3 mm rostral and 3 mm lateral to the inferior medial aspect of the inferior articular surface of C2.
2. The screw entry point is approximately 3 to 4 mm rostral and 3 to 4 mm lateral to the inferior medial portion of the C2–C3 facet joint (approximately the same as for the C2 pars screw).
3. No. Patients may tolerate a one-sided vertebral artery injury, but a bilateral vertebral injury could be fatal.

References

1. Mummaneni PV, Haid RW. Atlantoaxial fixation: overview of all techniques. Neurol India. 2005; 53(4):408–415
2. Mummaneni PV, Lu DC, Dhall SS, Mummaneni VP, Chou D. C1 lateral mass fixation: a comparison of constructs. Neurosurgery. 2010; 66(3) Suppl:153–160
3. Wu J-C, Tu T-H, Mummaneni PV. Techniques of atlantoaxial fixation and the resection of C2 nerve root. World Neurosurg. 2012; 78(6):603–604
4. Fiore AJ, Haid RW, Rodts GE, et al. Atlantal lateral mass screws for posterior spinal reconstruction: technical note and case series. Neurosurg Focus. 2002; 12(1):E5

5. Goel A, Desai KI, Muzumdar DP. Atlantoaxial fixation using plate and screw method: a report of 160 treated patients. Neurosurgery. 2002; 51(6):1351–1356, discussion 1356–1357
6. Goel A, Laheri V. Re: Harms J, Melcher P. Posterior C1-C2 fusion with polyaxial screw and rod fixation. (Spine 2001;26: 2467–71). Spine. 2002; 27 (14):1589–1590
7. Harms J, Melcher RP. Posterior C1-C2 fusion with polyaxial screw and rod fixation. Spine. 2001; 26(22):2467–2471
8. Jeanneret B, Magerl F. Primary posterior fusion C1/2 in odontoid fractures: indications, technique, and results of transarticular screw fixation. J Spinal Disord. 1992; 5(4):464–475
9. Tran M, Wadhwa R, Ziewacz J, Mummaneni P, Chou D. Comparison between C1–2 fixation with and without supplemental posterior wiring. Evid Based Spine Care J. 2014; 5(1):12–15

37 Odontoid Screw Fixation

Rajiv Saigal and Dean Chou

Summary
Odontoid screw fixation is a surgical treatment option for stabilizing some type II dens fractures. As a motion-preserving procedure, odontoid screw placement may be considered in appropriate patients. Patient's age, bone density, and fracture age/morphology should be factored into decision-making.

Keywords: odontoid screw, C2 fracture, dens fracture, odontoid fracture

37.1 Key Points

- Odontoid fractures constitute 10 to 20% of cervical spine fractures.[1]
- The Anderson and D'Alonzo system[2] divides odontoid fractures into three categories: Type I, fracture of the odontoid tip; type II, fracture of the base of odontoid neck; type III, fracture through the odontoid base and involving the C2 vertebral body.
- Isolated type II fractures in adults should be considered for surgery (**Fig. 37.1**).[3]
- Odontoid screw fixation is a motion-preserving procedure, unlike posterior C1–C2 fusion. Approximately half of axial head rotation is generated from the C1–C2 complex. Differential effects on C1–C2 motion should be explained to the patient in the context of different operative approaches.

37.2 Indications and Contraindications

- Indications:
  - Type II odontoid fracture.
  - Fracture geometry suitable to odontoid screw reduction.
  - Acute to subacute fractures.
- Contraindications:
  - Disrupted transverse ligament.
  - Barrel chest, or short neck, or other anatomic variant that compromises desired screw trajectory.

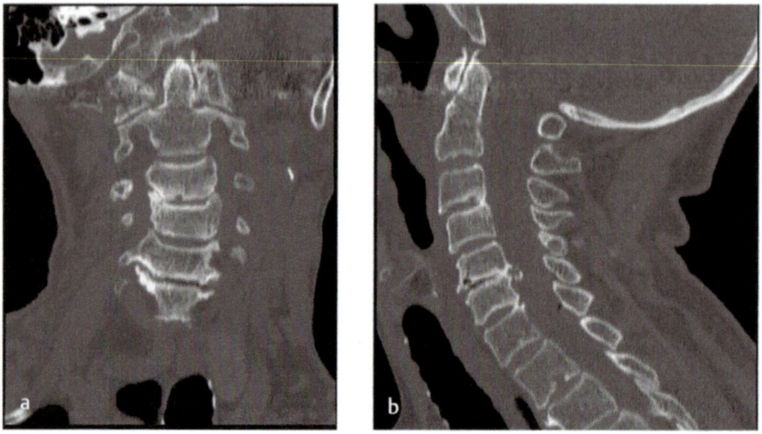

Fig. 37.1 Preoperative **(a)** coronal and **(b)** midsagittal computed tomography (CT) images showing a type II dens fracture with geometry suitable for anterior odontoid fixation.

- Fracture angulation unsuitable to anterior screw placement. If the fracture line traverses from anteroinferior to posterosuperior in the sagittal plane, the lag screw will not be able to capture the distal fragment for reduction.
- Fractures older than 6 months are associated with lower fusion rates, although the exact fracture age cutoff for surgical consideration is controversial. Most surgeons advocate odontoid screw placement soon after injury if possible.
- Os odontoideum.
- Pathologic odontoid fractures from infection or tumor.
- Fracture of the C2 vertebral body (i.e., type III fractures).
- Osteoporosis.
- Elderly patients who have osteoporosis and a severely ankylosed spine.

37.3 Technique

- The patient is placed in the supine position.
- The surgical bed is turned 180 degrees away from anesthesia. A Mayfield bar extender is also helpful in creating space for space for imaging (see **Fig. 37.2**).
- Biplanar fluoroscopy is used with two C-arms.
- A large roll of gauze or a radiolucent item is placed to keep the mouth open as wide as possible.

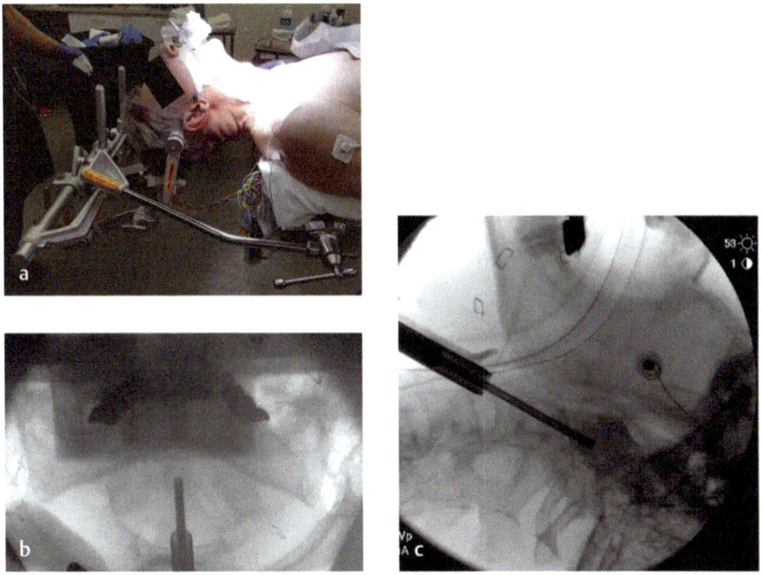

Fig. 37.2 Intraoperative **(a)** positioning with Mayfield extender to allow room for anteroposterior (AP) and lateral C-arm. Intraoperative **(b)** AP and **(c)** lateral X-rays showing the drill placed through drill guide, without use of K-wire.

- A lateral preoperative X-ray is taken to align the intended trajectory of the odontoid screw. The cervical spine is prepped and draped in the usual sterile fashion.
- A transverse skin incision is made, usually at the C5–C6 level. The skin incision should be centered several segments below the desired entry point.
- Metzenbaum scissors and bipolar cautery are used to dissect the platysma. Dissection is continued down to the spine in a similar manner as for the anterior cervical diskectomy and fusion approach. The trachea and the esophagus are mobilized medially and protected with self-retaining retractors. If two mediolateral, self-retaining retractors are used in the same manner as for anterior cervical diskectomy and fusion (ACDF) exposure, a third retractor should be used to retract cranially in order to visualize C2–C3.
- The spine is identified and dissected toward C2–C3. The level is confirmed under X-ray guidance. To properly angulate the screw, the central C2–C3 annulus should be opened. If the annulus is not opened and the drill guide is not docked within the disk space, the screw will be too anteriorly placed, possibly compromising the anterior cortex of C2.

- An entry point must be localized in both the anteroposterior and lateral planes for the correct screw trajectory. Since this starting point dictates the entire operation, it is critical that this point be precisely placed before the subsequent steps. After localizing with X-ray, the entry point can be opened with the awl or drill.
- The procedure may be done with or without a Kirschner wire (K-wire). If using a cannulated screw system, a K-wire may be applied under biplanar fluoroscopy up to the tip of the odontoid, engaging the cortex of the odontoid tip. Extreme care must be taken not to pass the point of the K-wire too deep. The brainstem and/or basilar artery could be critically injured with a deeply placed K-wire.
- The trajectory is then drilled. If using a K-wire, a cannulated drill is advanced over the wire. Multiple X-rays should be taken during drilling. It is important to ensure that the drill is advanced in the correct trajectory toward the odontoid tip. If using a K-wire, care is taken to ensure that the drill does not pass it, lest the K-wire becomes loose.
- The drill is removed, and the same trajectory is tapped.
- After tapping, a lag screw is inserted under biplanar X-ray guidance to engage the tip of the odontoid. Both cannulated and noncannulated screws are options. If using a K-wire, care should be taken to not advance it inadvertently during screw placement. The K-wire can be removed as soon as the screw is advanced into C2.
- The lag screw draws the tip of the odontoid toward the body of the odontoid. This is confirmed under fluoroscopic guidance. The screw is then tightened. The ideal screw length should be measured preoperatively on the CT, accounting for the fracture gap.
- After meticulous hemostasis is obtained, the wound is irrigated. A surgical drain may be left in place but is often not necessary. The platysma is closed with interrupted sutures. Skin is closed.

37.4 Complications

- Dysphagia.
- Hoarseness.
- Nonunion.
- Improper implant placement.
- Screw failure.
- Need for posterior C1–C2 fusion.

37.5 Postoperative Care

- After recovery in a postanesthesia care unit, patients are usually transferred to an acute care unit. Early mobilization is recommended.

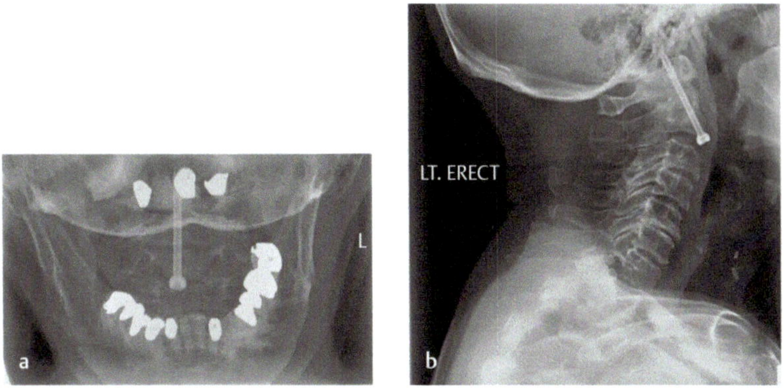

Fig. 37.3 Postoperative anteroposterior (**a**) open-mouth and (**b**) lateral X-rays show placement of odontoid screw with fracture reduction.

- The authors obtain an anteroposterior and lateral cervical X-rays prior to discharge (shown in **Fig. 37.3**) to ensure proper implant placement.
- Use of a supportive cervical collar postoperatively for 1 to 3 months is an option.
- As with other anterior cervical approaches, postoperative dysphagia is common. Diet should be advanced slowly to prevent the risk of aspiration.
- After discharge, the wound should be checked in an early postoperative visit.

37.6 Outcomes

- Fractures less than 6 months of age have demonstrated a nearly 90% fusion rate with anterior odontoid screw fixation, compared with 25% fusion rate for those over 18 months.[1]

37.7 Surgical Pearls

- Great care must be taken to avoid the tracheoesophageal groove, the anatomic location of the recurrent laryngeal nerve.
- When using a K-wire and cannulated screw system, use X-ray frequently to ensure that the wire is not inadvertently driven deeper than desired.
- If not using a K-wire, use X-ray to confirm that drill, tap, and screw follow the same trajectory.
- Sometimes, the tip of the odontoid is very difficult to see on lateral fluoroscopy. Measure the distance from the top of the C1 tubercle to the

top of the odontoid fragment by CT preoperatively. This will at least provide some idea of where the K-wire should stop if the tip of the odontoid is simply not well-visualized.

Common Clinical Questions

1. In general, should an odontoid screw be placed in an elderly patient with severe osteoporosis?
2. How long after an odontoid fracture occurs is it too late to put in an odontoid screw?
   A. 1 week.
   B. 3 weeks.
   C. 3 months.
   D. 18 months.

Answers to Common Clinical Questions

1. As a general rule, no. Most elderly patients with osteoporosis should undergo a posterior C1–C2 fusion.
2. D. The odontoid fracture fusion rate is only 25% after 18 months, but 88% within the first 6 months.[1] In general, earlier surgery leads to a higher rate of fracture healing.

References

1. Rao G, Apfelbaum RI. Odontoid screw fixation for fresh and remote fractures. Neurol India. 2005; 53(4):416–423
2. Anderson LD, D'Alonzo RT. Fractures of the odontoid process of the axis. J Bone Joint Surg Am. 1974; 56(8):1663–1674
3. Ryken TC, Hadley MN, Aarabi B, et al. Management of isolated fractures of the axis in adults. Neurosurgery. 2013; 72 Suppl 2:132–150

38 Cervical Arthroplasty

Yazid Maghrabi and Saleh Baeesa

Summary

Cervical arthroplasty, an emerging surgical option, aims to preserve segmental motion and maintain stability in managing symptomatic cervical spondylosis and central disk herniation. This chapter outlines key elements for successful outcomes, including patient selection criteria, surgical techniques, and postoperative care. It also discusses indications, contraindications, complications, outcomes, and surgical pearls associated with cervical arthroplasty.

Keywords: ACDF, cervical arthroplasty, total disk replacement, cervical spondylosis, cervical disk herniation, radiculopathy, myelopathy, radiculomyelopathy, outcome, complications

38.1 Key Points

- Anterior cervical diskectomy and fusion (ACDF) remain the gold standard in the surgical management of symptomatic cervical spondylosis and central disk herniation.
- The emerging option of cervical arthroplasty is aimed at preserving segmental motion and maintaining adequate stability.[1]
- Key elements to achieve a good result and avoid complications with cervical arthroplasty:
  - Appropriate patient selection (competent posterior elements, without spondylolisthesis).
  - Correct neck positioning during surgery (neutral to slightly lordotic cervical curvature).
  - Generous decompression with resection of the bilateral uncovertebral joints and posterior longitudinal ligament.
  - Precise end plate preparation (parallel or domed according to the device, with preservation of cortical end plates).
  - Accurate midline acquisition.
  - Proper implant sizing (footprint coverage of disk space and avoidance of over-distraction).

38.2 Indications[2]

- According to the current US Food and Drug Administration (FDA) guidelines, cervical disk arthroplasty (CDA) is indicated for the following:
  - One- or two-level symptomatic degenerative cervical disk disease at C3–C7 with symptoms and signs of intractable radiculopathy, myelopathy, or myeloradiculopathy.
  - Clinical symptoms are correlated with imaging findings.
  - Failed 6 weeks of conservative management.
  - Skeletally mature patients.
- Contraindications include the following:
  - Active infection.
  - Osteoporosis.
  - Allergy to the device material.
  - More than two affected levels requiring surgery.
  - Instability.
  - Disk height less than 3 mm.
  - Kyphotic deformity.
  - Prior surgery at the target level.

38.3 Technique

- A preoperative antibiotic is administered; however, dexamethasone and intraoperative neuromonitoring are at the discretion of the performing surgeon.
- Smith-Robinson approach is utilized for access to the anterior cervical spine, and laterality (right- or left-sided approach) depends on the surgeon's preference.
  - The patient is positioned in a neutral supine position or in slight lordosis, with shoulder retractions to enable fluoroscopic visualization.
  - Horizontal incision along the skin crease is created over the targeted level (confirmed with fluoroscopy).
  - Muscle dissection between the sternocleidomastoid and strap muscles is carried out.
  - Carotid sheath is dissected and retracted laterally; trachea and esophagus are retracted medially.
  - Index level is confirmed under fluoroscopy with the use of a spinal needle.
  - Longus colli muscle is dissected from the anterior cervical spine, and retractors are placed.
  - Distraction pins are placed, and only gentle distraction is applied.
  - Diskectomy is carried out using curette, rongeurs, and drill.

- The difference in CDA is that wide decompression has to be achieved, including the removal of bilateral uncovertebral joints.
  - Resection of the posterior longitudinal ligament (PLL) is optional, and it is left to the discretion of the performing surgeon.
- Moreover, end plates have to be prepared in accordance with the cervical arthroplasty used.
- One of the crucial steps is to identify the true midline and the perfect fitting implant sizing (footprint size and disk height).
- There are nine US FDA-approved cervical artificial disk devices for one-level use in the market, three of which are approved for one and two contiguous-level usage, namely, Mobi-C (LDR; Sainte-Savine, France), Prestige LP (Medtronic Dofamor Danek; Memphis, TN), and Simplify (Simplify Medical; Sunnyvale, CA). Even though the implantation technique varies between different prosthesis designs, it shares a common prerequisite: adequate decompression. A thorough understanding of the biomaterial and implantation techniques of the devices would enable the surgeon to select the best choice prosthesis for different case scenarios (**Table 38.1**).[3]

38.4 Complications[4]

- Complications can be divided into short-, mid-, and long-term complications.
  - Short-term complications are similar to anterior cervical diskectomy and fusion, as both procedures use the anterior cervical approach. It includes:
    - Hematoma.
    - Infection.
    - Vascular injury.
    - Horner syndrome.
    - Esophageal injury.
    - Recurrent laryngeal nerve injury.
    - Dysphagia.
  - Mid- and long-term complications are considered device-related and exclusive to cervical artificial disk replacement. It includes:
    - Heterotopic ossification.
    - Subsidence.
    - Implant migration.
    - New-onset radiculopathy.
    - Implant allergy.
    - Osteonecrosis.

Table 38.1 FDA-approved cervical arthroplasty devices in the United States

Device	Manufacturer	Classification	Biomaterials
ProDisc-C	Synthes Spine; West Chester, Pennsylvania	Semiconstrained	CCM end plates, UHMWPE core
BRYAN	Medtronic Ltd.; Memphis, Tennessee	Unconstrained	Ti end plates, PU nucleus and shell
PRESTIGE ST	Medtronic Ltd.; Memphis, Tennessee	Unconstrained	Stainless steel
SECURE-C	Globus Medical; Audubon, PA	Semiconstrained	CCM end plates, UHMWPE core
PCM	NuVasive Inc; San Diego, CA	Semiconstrained	CCM end plates, UHMWPE core
MOBI-C	LDR; Sainte-Savine, France	Unconstrained	CCM end plates, UHMWPE core
PRESTIGE LP	Medtronic Sofamor Danek; Memphis, TN	Unconstrained	Ti ceramic
M6-C	Spinal Kinetics; Sunnyvale, CA	Unconstrained	Ti end plates, PU nucleus, UHMWPE annulus
SIMPLIFY	Simplify Medical; Sunnyvale, CA		PEEK end plates, ceramic core

Abbreviations: CCM, cobalt chrome molybdenum; PEEK, polyether ether ketone; PU, polyurethane; Ti, titanium; UHMWPE, ultra-high-molecular-weight polyethylene.

38.5 Postoperative Care

- Similar to ACDF, which include:
  - Postoperative antibiotics for 24 hours.
  - Dexamethasone for 24 hours postoperatively.

- In cases of CDA:
  - Perioperative nonsteroidal anti-inflammatory drugs use for 2 weeks has shown decreased incidence of heterotopic bone formation.[5]
  - Neck collar used to be avoided, and normal motion be encouraged.

38.6 Outcomes

- To date, a large number of meta-analyses and randomized controlled trials (RCTs) with long follow-up periods exist in the literature, comparing CDA with ACDF for radiculopathy, myelopathy, one-level use, and two-level usage.[6,7,8,9,10,11]
- A recent meta-analysis by Chang and colleagues compared ACDF and CDA in terms of Neck Disability Index (NDI) and Short Form-36 (SF-36) scores. It was found that CDA was associated with better NDI scores and better SF-36 scores. However, it was noted that CDA required more surgical time, and JOA scores and neurological success were comparable between the two groups.[6]
- Another meta-analysis of 11 RCTs by Wang et al compared the long-term outcomes of CDA versus ACDF. It has shown a superior overall success of CDA compared to ACDF, NDI success, and neurological success. Regarding functional outcomes, there was no statistical difference between CDA and ACDF in terms of NDI scores; visual analog score (VAS), neck pain, and arm pain were superior in CDA. Furthermore, there is no statistical difference between the two arms (CDA and ACDF) regarding adverse events. Finally, less revision surgeries were required for the CDA group, and there was less incidence of symptomatic adjacent segment disease requiring surgery.[7]
- PRESTIGE ST cervical disk system (Medtronic Sofamor Danek; Memphis, TN) was compared to ACDF in a total of 541 patients with a follow-up of 7 years. CDA group had a higher rate of maintenance of neurological improvement and preservation of angular motion. Moreover, a lower rate of revision surgeries and symptomatic adjacent levels requiring surgery were associated with CDA group.[8]
- Radcliff and associates evaluated arthroplasty with MOBI-C cervical disk (LDR; Sainte-Savine, France) for one- and two-level disk disease. After 7 years of follow-up of 599 patients, it was found that CDA group had overall success rate in height when compared to ACDF. Improvement in NDI scores was observed in all groups. Patients in CDA group reported a higher rate of stratification when compared to ACDF group. Less rate of revision surgeries or adjacent level disease was found in CDA group.[9]
- Lavelle et al compared BRYAN cervical disk (Medtronic Sofamor Danek; Memphis, TN) with ACDF in a total of 232 patients and follow-ups of up to 10 years. It was shown that CDA group had higher overall success with

lower rate of surgeries for symptomatic adjacent levels. Moreover, CDA significantly improved NDI and VAS for neck and arm pain. They concluded that CDA preserved and maintained motion in the long term compared to ACDF.[10]

- Lanman el al compared PRESTIGE LP (Medtronic Sofamor Danek; Memphis, TN) artificial disk in two adjacent levels versus ACDF in a total of 397 patients with follow-up of up to 7 years. It was found that CDA was superior in terms of overall success, NDI success, and neurological success. However, the two groups had no statistical difference regarding overall implant/surgical procedure-related adverse events. In addition, CDA group had fewer rates of revision surgeries and maintained the range of motion (ROM) of the index level.[11]

38.7 Surgical Pearls

- Generous decompression of the neuroforamen bilaterally (including the asymptomatic side) is essential.
- Proper end plate preparation, but not disruption, is essential.
- Correct implant selection (footprint size, height) without oversizing is mandatory.
- Nine FDA-approved CDA devices are available in the market[3]:
  - PRESTIGE ST (Medtronic Sofamor Danek; Memphis, TN).
  - ProDisc-C (Centinel Spine; West Chester, PA).
  - BRYAN (Medtronic Sofamor Danek; Memphis TN).
  - SECURE-C (Globus Medical; Audubon, PA).
  - PCM (NuVasive Inc; San Diego, CA).
  - Mobi-C (LDR; Sainte-Savine, France).
  - PRESTIGE LP (Medtronic Sofamor Danek; Memphis, TN).
  - M6-C (Spinal Kinetics; Sunnyvale, CA).
  - Simplify (Simplify Medical; Sunnyvale, CA).

Common Clinical Questions

1. How many degrees of neck range of motion loss could result from a single-level ACDF?
2. What is the incidence of development of symptomatic adjacent-level disease after single-level ACDF?
3. Why should patients take oral NSAIDs and avoid neck collar use after cervical arthroplasty?

Answers to Common Clinical Questions

1. A fusion of one level of the cervical spine typically results in the loss of 7 degrees of flexion and extension motion and 6 degrees of rotational motion.[1]
2. The symptomatic adjacent-segment disease occurs at a rate of 2.9% per year during the 10 years after the operation (Hilibrand et al[12]).
3. NSAIDs and motion may reduce the occurrence of heterotopic bone formation around the artificial disk.[13]

References

1. Mummaneni PV, Haid RW. The future in the care of the cervical spine: interbody fusion and arthroplasty. Invited submission from the Joint Section Meeting on Disorders of the Spine and Peripheral Nerves, March 2004. J Neurosurg Spine. 2004; 1(2):155–159
2. Nunley P, Frank K, Stone M. Patient selection in cervical disc arthroplasty. Int J Spine Surg. 2020; 14 s2:S29–S35
3. Bydon M, Michalopoulos GD, Alvi MA, Goyal A, Abode-Iyamah K. Cervical total disc replacement: Food and Drug Administration-approved devices. Neurosurg Clin N Am. 2021; 32(4):425–435
4. Price RL, Coric D, Ray WZ. Cervical total disc replacement: complications and complication avoidance. Neurosurg Clin N Am. 2021; 32(4):473–481
5. Mummaneni PV, Burkus JK, Haid RW, Traynelis VC, Zdeblick TA. Clinical and radiographic analysis of cervical disc arthroplasty compared with allograft fusion: a randomized controlled clinical trial. J Neurosurg Spine. 2007; 6(3): 198–209
6. Chang CJ, Liu YF, Hsiao YM, et al. Comparison of anterior cervical discectomy and fusion versus artificial disc replacement for cervical spondylotic myelopathy: a meta-analysis. J Neurosurg Spine. 2022:1–10. Online ahead of print
7. Wang QL, Tu ZM, Hu P, et al. Long-term results comparing cervical disc arthroplasty to anterior cervical discectomy and fusion: a systematic review and meta-analysis of randomized controlled trials. Orthop Surg. 2020; 12(1): 16–30
8. Burkus JK, Traynelis VC, Haid RW, Jr, Mummaneni PV. Clinical and radiographic analysis of an artificial cervical disc: 7-year follow-up from the Prestige prospective randomized controlled clinical trial: Clinical article. J Neurosurg Spine. 2014; 21(4):516–528
9. Radcliff K, Davis RJ, Hisey MS, et al. Long-term evaluation of cervical disc arthroplasty with the Mobi-C© cervical disc: a randomized, prospective, multicenter clinical trial with seven-year follow-up. Int J Spine Surg. 2017; 11(4):31

10. Lavelle WF, Riew KD, Levi AD, Florman JE. Ten-year outcomes of cervical disc replacement with the BRYAN cervical disc: results from a prospective, randomized, controlled clinical trial. Spine. 2019; 44(9):601–608
11. Lanman TH, Burkus JK, Dryer RG, Gornet MF, McConnell J, Hodges SD. Long-term clinical and radiographic outcomes of the Prestige LP artificial cervical disc replacement at 2 levels: results from a prospective randomized controlled clinical trial. J Neurosurg Spine. 2017; 27(1):7–19
12. Hilibrand AS, Carlson GD, Palumbo MA, Jones PK, Bohlman HH. Radiculopathy and myelopathy at segments adjacent to the site of a previous anterior cervical arthrodesis. J Bone Joint Surg Am. 1999; 81(4):519–528
13. Tu TH, Wu JC, Huang WC, et al. Heterotopic ossification after cervical total disc replacement: determination by CT and effects on clinical outcomes. J Neurosurg Spine. 2011; 14(4):457–465

39 Anterior Cervical Diskectomy

TJ Florence, Ansley Unterberger, and Andrew C. Vivas

Summary
This chapter serves as a concise technical guide on anterior cervical diskectomy. We review indications, procedural details, and potential pitfalls. We discuss nuances for positioning, stepwise dissection, complication avoidance, and postoperative management. We conclude by reviewing outcomes and management of rare adverse events. We have attempted to create a useful framework for this versatile workhorse approach for spine surgeons at all stages of training.

Keywords: anterior cervical diskectomy, anterior cervical approach, ACDF, ADR, CDA

39.1 Key Points

- As with all spine surgeries, positioning nuances facilitate surgical goals.
- Appreciation of the surgical anatomy of vital structures (carotid, esophagus, recurrent laryngeal nerve) and intervening tissue planes is essential during approach.
- Limiting esophageal pressure (intermittent retractor relaxation, decreasing cuff pressure, and surgical efficiency) decreases the incidence and severity of dysphagia.

39.2 Indications

- Cervical spondylosis with radiculopathy or myelopathy due to anterior column degeneration.
- Symptomatic herniated nucleus pulposus.
- Cervical fracture with instability.
- Conversion of failed artificial disk.

39.3 Technique[1,2]

- Position the patient supine, arms tucked at sides.
  - May use flat-top Jackson table with rungs set to Trendelenburg position. This aligns disk space with the vertical and facilitates anteroposterior (AP)

fluoroscopy for confirming midline instrumentation placement (**Fig. 39.1**).
 - Position the head on foam donut; may use chin weight strap or Gardner-Wells tongs for gentle traction (10–15 lb).
 - A small longitudinal bump between the shoulder blades (axillary or towel roll) together with thick tape retraction of shoulders affords gentle neck extension while dropping the shoulders out of lateral radiographic plane. Care must be taken to avoid excess traction which can precipitate upper trunk brachial plexopathy and/or shoulder pain postoperatively.
 - Place neuromonitoring leads.
- Define surface anatomy and localize incision.
 - Medial border of sternocleidomastoid, thyroid, and cricoid cartilage, clavicle, sternal notch, and anatomic midline may be outlined with marker.
 - Palpable structures aid in estimating incision location: angle of mandible at C2/C3, hyoid at C3/C4, thyroid cartilage at C5, cricoid cartilage at C5/C6 (see **Fig. 39.2**).
 - Incision level is confirmed with lateral fluoroscopy.
 - For a single-level procedure, the incision is marked parallel to the disk space.

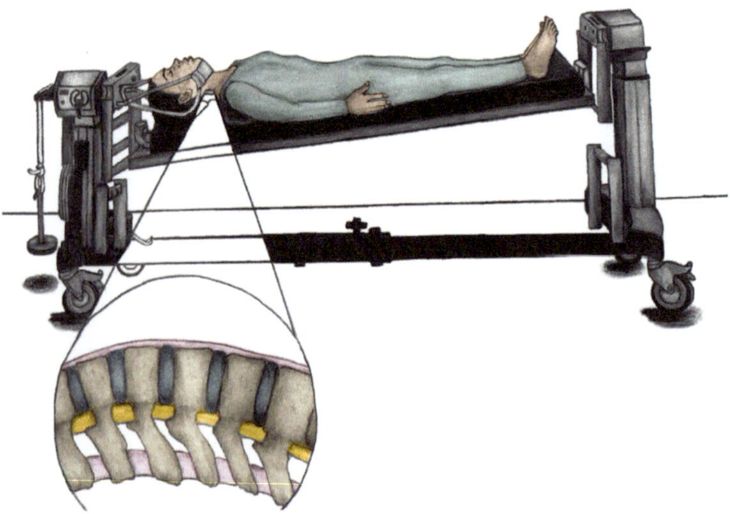

Fig. 39.1 Positioning the patient in Trendelenburg aligns disk spaces with the vertical, facilitating operative ergonomics.

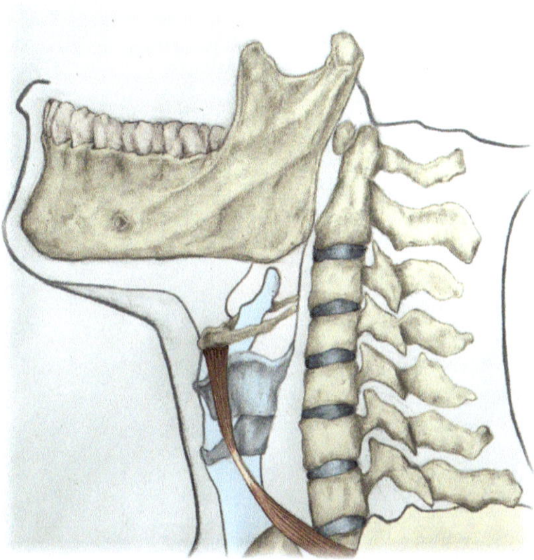

Fig. 39.2 Summary of palpable surface landmarks by cervical level. These include angle of the mandible (C2/C3), hyoid bone (C3), thyroid cartilage (C5), and cricoid cartilage (C5/C6). The omohyoid muscle begins to be encountered at lower levels. Pleura of lung apex may be encountered in C6/C7 dissections.

  - If a multilevel procedure is performed, the incision is marked at the midpoint (i.e., over the C5 body for a C4–C5, C5–C6 anterior cervical diskectomy and fusion [ACDF]).
  - A transverse incision is used for single- and two-level procedures; a longitudinal incision along the anterior border of the sternocleidomastoid can be considered for three- and four-level approaches.
  - Paradoxically, a larger incision (i.e., from medial border of sternocleidomastoid to 5 mm past midline) may provide improved cosmesis as it reduces superficial tissue stress during retraction.
- Incision is made. The platysma is defined, divided, and undermined; the plane medial to the sternocleidomastoid muscle is identified and bluntly dissected with a finger or blunt instrument in a rostral-to-caudal direction (**Fig. 39.3**). The omohyoid muscle overlies the C6 level and can be divided.[1]
  - We find early incorporation of microscope, even at the time of incision, improves surgeon ergonomics and operative efficiency.

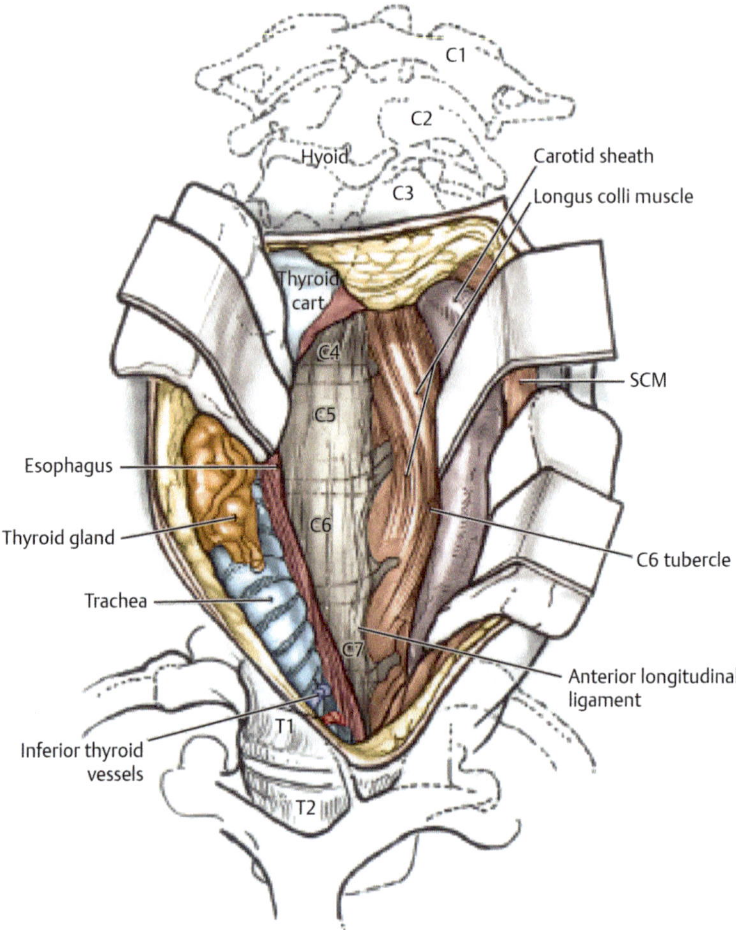

Fig. 39.3 Anterior exposure to cervical spine. SCM, sternocleidomastoid muscle. (Adapted from Haher R, Merola A, eds. Surgical Techniques for the Spine. Thieme; 2003.)

- The carotid within the carotid sheath is then palpated. The alveolar tissue plane medial to the sheath and lateral to the trachea and esophagus is developed by blunt dissection in the rostral-to-caudal direction.

- Cloward or Richardson-type retractors are used to retract and provide protection medially (the trachea and esophagus) and laterally (the carotid sheath). The spine is then palpated.
- The prevertebral fascia is entered, and the disk level is confirmed by X-ray or fluoroscopy.
  - Confirming the level with tonsil clamped to prevertebral fascia/longus colli, rather than bayonetted spinal needle, avoids disk injury if initial level estimate is wrong.
- The longus colli muscles are mobilized laterally with bipolar electrocautery. The midline is marked on the vertebral body. The sympathetic cervical trunk (specifically the middle cervical ganglia) may run longitudinally along the lateral border of the longus colli; transection of the longus colli can result in injury to the sympathetics with a resultant Horner's syndrome.
- Self-retaining retractor (Trimline [Medtronic; Memphis, Tennessee] or equivalent) is placed underneath the longus colli. The endotracheal tube cuff may be mildly depressurized at this point.
- Disk anulectomy is performed with a number 15 blade scalpel; additional disk removal is performed with a pituitary rongeur. The cartilaginous end plate is dissected away from the bony end plate with curettes or a small osteotome. Care should be taken in the lateral extent of the diskectomy to avoid inadvertent vertebral artery injury.
  - Caspar pins may be placed to assist with distraction of disk space. Pins should be placed midline, parallel to end plates, and at sufficient distance from disk space so as not to interfere with instrumentation placement.
- Osteophytes/calcified disk fragments are removed by Kerrison and precise high-speed drill down to the posterior longitudinal ligament (PLL). Care is taken to respect the bony end plate.
- The PLL is defined and first entered with a fine-angle nerve hook; it is identified by round longitudinal fibers. It is resected further with fine Kerrison punches. The dural plane is now evident. Thickened PLL can be thinned with the high-speed bur under copious irrigation and under microscopic visualization.
  - Resection of sufficient lateral extent of PLL is complete when exiting nerve roots are visualized. Venous bleeding is commonly encountered and easily addressed with hemostatic foam.
- Temporary trial sizers are introduced into the intervertebral space to assess the correct interbody spacer size. One should remove Caspar pin distraction and Halter traction when trialing to guard against over-distraction of the disk space. However, a small amount of distraction is useful when first inserting the trial.
  - An AP fluoroscopic image may be taken with temporary spacer in place. Tilt (i.e., Ferguson), orbit (oblique), and wig-wag of the fluoroscopic

plane may be rigorously aligned to the spacer insertion handle. This facilitates a precise estimate of the midline.

- Under lateral fluoroscopy, the permanent implant (allograft, autograft, or polyetheretherketone (PEEK)/carbon fiber cages filled with bone) may now be placed into the disk space.[3]
- An anterior cervical plate is placed aligning the midline with the previous mark. Alternatively stand-alone devices with inter-fixated stabilization can be utilized.
  - Ventral osteophytes may have to be drilled to afford a smooth surface to accept the plate. Prominent instrumentation contributes to delayed esophageal erosion.
- Plates can be fastened to the vertebral bodies with fixed-angle screws or variable-angle screws or a combination of the two.
  - An entirely fixed construct is useful for situations that require rigid fixation (i.e., trauma cases).
  - Variable-angle screws allow for rotational pivoting at the screw–plate interface, which allows for increased loads to be placed upon the bone graft in the disk space. This is called "rotational subsidence" and allows exploitation of Wolff's law (bone heals when subjected to loading).
  - Optimal screw trajectory subtends 90 degrees angle between caudal and rostral screws, with each screw forming a 45 degrees angle with the ventral border of the vertebral body.
- The wound is irrigated with saline.
- A small subfascial drain may be placed.
- Closure of platysma is done with interrupted 2.0 Vicryl (Ethicon, a Johnson & Johnson company; New York) and the subcutaneous layer with interrupted 3.0 Vicryl. Skin is closed with a subcuticular running 4.0 Monocryl suture.
- Steri-Strips (3M; St. Paul, Minnesota) may be used for skin.

39.4 Complications

- Dysphagia (up to 20%).[4,5]
- Nerve root injury (C5 nerve root palsy in up to 5%).[6]
- Hoarseness.
- Esophageal perforation (commonly presents in delayed fashion).
- Pseudarthrosis (2–20%).
- Wound infection (< 1%).
- Carotid or vertebral artery injury (0.3%).
- Spinal cord injury.
- Wound hematoma (higher in multilevel cases; may be mitigated by drain placement).

39.5 Postoperative Care

- Cervical collar may be used until radiographic signs of early fusion (4–6 weeks). The authors recommend cervical orthosis particularly for multilevel anterior fusions without posterior instrumentation.
- May be discharged the same day with 6-hour observation in recovery unit.

39.6 Outcomes[7]

- ACDF is a successful procedure when performed given the right indications.
- Favorable 30-day readmission rate when compared with posterior approaches.
- Adjacent-level disease occurs at a rate of around 2 to 3% per year in patients undergoing single-level ACDF.

39.7 Surgical Pearls

- Surgical fusions for neck pain are controversial. However, patients undergoing ACDF for cervicalgia or cervicogenic headaches resulting from specific, identifiable root compression (**Fig. 39.4**) may have excellent quality of life outcomes.[8]
- The surgeon must know the course of the recurrent laryngeal nerve (RLN) to avoid injury during surgery. On the right, the RLN loops around the right subclavian artery, and the left RLN loops around the arch of the aorta. It runs within the tracheoesophageal groove, where sharp dissection in the paratracheal muscles or prolonged retraction against an inflated endotracheal tube may cause injury. Injury causes hoarseness, cough, aspiration, mass sensation, dysphagia, and vocal cord fatigue.
- Contralateral approach to radicular symptoms may facilitate improved visualization of the foramen and more complete anterior foraminotomy.

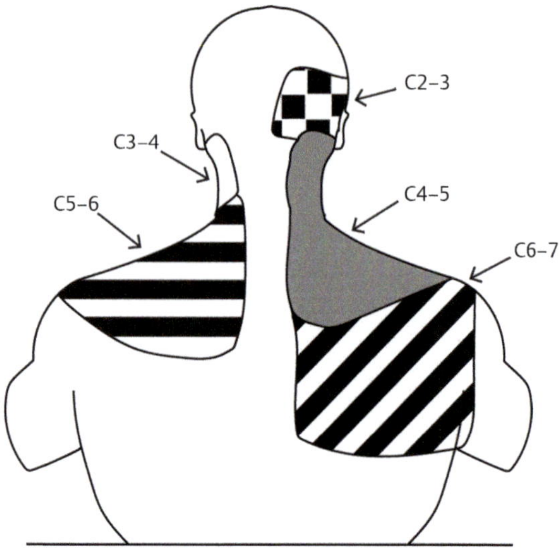

Fig. 39.4 Cervicalgia and cervicogenic headaches: Compression or irritation of cervical rami may cause pain in the illustrated dorsal distributions.

Common Clinical Questions

1. A patient recovers in PACU following a C4/C5 ACDF. The patient is at baseline strength but is noted by the PACU nurse to have a large right pupil and a drooping left eyelid. This is most likely due to
   A. Carotid pseudoaneurysm.
   B. Compression by graft or hematoma of exiting right C5 nerve root.
   C. Compression by graft or hematoma of exiting left C5 nerve root.
   D. Retractor placement on carotid sheath.
   E. Retractor placement on longus colli.
2. A patient presents to clinic for a 6-week follow-up after uncomplicated C5/C6 ACDF. Early graft incorporation is seen on visit X-rays. The patient complains of a subjective sensation of food being stuck in her throat. What is the next best step in evaluation?
   A. Consult head and neck surgery for evaluation of occult recurrent laryngeal nerve injury.
   B. Barium esophagram.

C. CT of cervical spine with contrast.

D. Observation until 3-month follow-up.

E. Flexion–extension X-rays.

3. Bony end plates are repeatedly violated with curette during diskectomy. This places the patient at an elevated risk for:

   A. Graft subsidence.

   B. Esophageal perforation.

   C. Spinal cord injury.

   D. Carotid injury.

   E. All of the above.

Answers to Common Clinical Questions

1. E. The sympathetic chain courses along the anterior surface of the longus colli. Retractor placement on top of, rather than under, these muscles can lead to a Horner's syndrome.
2. B. Delayed development of esophageal diverticula should be excluded.
3. A.

References

1. Smith GW, Robinson RA. The treatment of certain cervical-spine disorders by anterior removal of the intervertebral disc and interbody fusion. J Bone Joint Surg Am. 1958; 40-A(3):607–624
2. Cloward RB. The anterior approach for removal of ruptured cervical disks. J Neurosurg. 1958; 15(6):602–617
3. Greenberg MS. Handbook of Neurosurgery. 6th ed. New York: Thieme Medical Publishers; 2006:304–306
4. Tumialán LM, Pan J, Rodts GE, Mummaneni PV. The safety and efficacy of anterior cervical discectomy and fusion with polyetheretherketone spacer and recombinant human bone morphogenetic protein-2: a review of 200 patients. J Neurosurg Spine. 2008; 8(6):529–535
5. Ghogawala Z, Terrin N, Dunbar MR, et al. Effect of ventral vs dorsal spinal surgery on patient-reported physical functioning in patients with cervical spondylotic myelopathy: a randomized clinical trial. JAMA. 2021; 325(10): 942–951
6. Fountas KN, Kapsalaki EZ, Nikolakakos LG, et al. Anterior cervical discectomy and fusion associated complications. Spine. 2007; 32(21):2310–2317

7. Holly LT, Matz PG, Anderson PA, et al. Joint Section on Disorders of the Spine and Peripheral Nerves of the American Association of Neurological Surgeons and Congress of Neurological Surgeons. Functional outcomes assessment for cervical degenerative disease. J Neurosurg Spine. 2009; 11 (2):238–244
8. Lombardi JM, Vivas AC, Gornet MF, et al. The effect of ACDF or arthroplasty on cervicogenic headaches: a post hoc analysis of a prospective, multicenter study with 10-year follow-up. Clin Spine Surg. 2020; 33(9):339–344

40 Anterior Cervical Corpectomy

Joshua Chalif, Anran Li, Eric Chalif, and Hasan Zaidi

Summary
This chapter provides an in-depth overview of the surgical procedure used for decompressing the ventral cervical spinal cord, especially beneficial in cases where anterior cervical diskectomy is inadequate. The process involves the removal of the vertebral body and intervening disks from the cervical spine to relieve pressure on the spinal cord and nerve roots, predominantly for conditions like spondylotic myelopathy, tumor infiltration, traumatic injuries, and osteomyelitis. Despite the efficacy of the surgery, it may lead to mechanical instability, necessitating additional posterior stabilization. The chapter thoroughly covers various aspects of the surgery including indications, detailed surgical techniques, potential complications, postoperative care, and outcomes, alongside essential surgical pearls and answers to common clinical questions.

Keywords: anterior cervical corpectomy, ventral spinal cord decompression, cervical spine surgery, spinal cord compression, surgical technique, postoperative care, surgical complications, spine stabilization, neurological monitoring, cervical diskectomy

40.1 Key Points

- Anterior cervical corpectomy is a safe and effective technique for decompression of the ventral cervical spinal cord.
- The surgical approach and exposure for corpectomy are similar to the case for the more common anterior cervical diskectomy.[1]
- Corpectomy has the ability to provide more complete decompression, especially when the stenosis is from behind the vertebral body.
- Multilevel corpectomies can result in mechanical instability, therefore often requiring posterior stabilization.

40.2 Indications

- Generally, corpectomy is indicated when there is ventral spinal cord compression and diskectomy is inadequate for decompression (**Fig. 40.1**). This includes:
  - Degenerative conditions, such as spondylotic myelopathy in which ventral spinal cord compression is not restricted to the disk level and/or is complicated by cervical kyphosis and midbody osteophytes.
  - Tumor infiltration of the vertebral body causing vertebral body collapse and spinal cord compression.
  - Traumatic cervical spine injury, such as a teardrop fracture with associated spinal cord compression from retropulsion of vertebral body fragments and spinal instability.
  - Osteomyelitis with epidural abscess and concomitant ventral spinal cord compression.
  - Ossification of the posterior longitudinal ligament (OPLL).

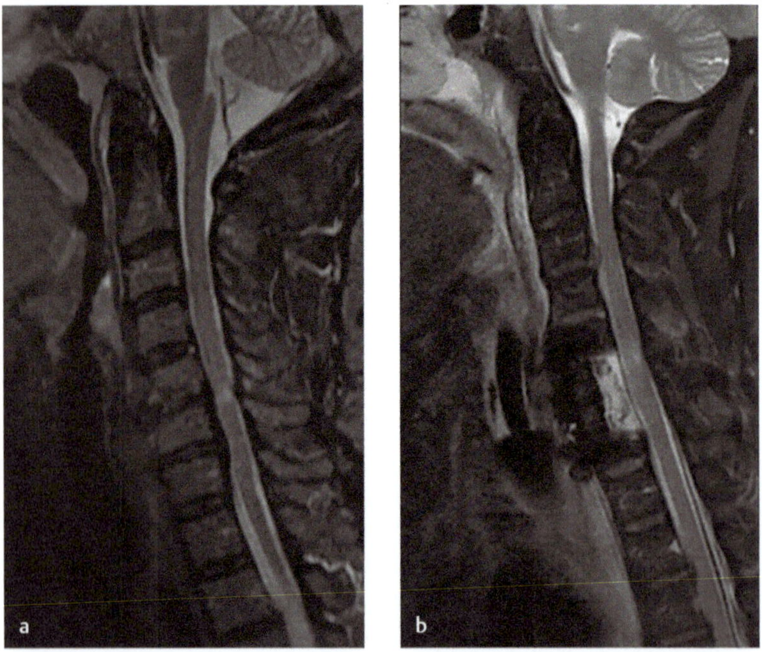

Fig. 40.1 Sagittal magnetic resonance imaging showing improvement of spinal stenosis after C6 corpectomy: **(a)** preoperative, **(b)** postoperative.

40.3 Technique

- Intubation via fiberoptic technique, whether awake or asleep, is safer in cases of significant cervical spinal cord compression, myelopathic signs, myelomalacia, and/or cervical instability.
- Awake fiberoptic intubation allows for neurologic assessment immediately after intubation to assess for changes in neurologic function.
- Endotracheal tube should be taped away from the side of surgical incision.
- Steroid administration preoperatively or intraoperatively lacks robust scientific support.
- Use of neurologic monitoring including somatosensory-evoked potentials (SSEPs) and motor-evoked potentials (MEP) is prudent during operations on myelopathic patients. Pre- and post-positioning signals may help to limit any neurologic deterioration from subtle changes encountered during positioning.
- Some surgeons use 8 to 10 pounds of traction with Gardner-Wells tongs or chin strap craniocervical traction to augment disk space distraction. Alternatively, Caspar distraction pins (Aesculap Implant Systems; Center Valley, Pennsylvania) can be placed in the adjacent vertebral bodies above and below the corpectomy site to provide direct distraction.
- Place the patient supine on the operating table.
  - Pressure points should be padded, especially the ulnar nerve.
  - A longitudinal bump between the scapulae may improve lordosis and access to the level of interest. In patients who have myelopathy, neck hyperextension must be avoided due to risk of neurological deterioration caused by hyperextension of the stenotic canal.
  - Shoulders should be taped down caudally to allow for fluoroscopic visualization of the level of interest. Care should be taken to avoid excessive traction of the shoulders to prevent injury to the brachial plexus.
  - Localize the approximate level of incision along the neck using fluoroscopy or external landmarks. The hyoid bone is at the level of C3. The thyroid cartilage is at the level of C4; the cricoid cartilage is at the level of C6.[2]
  - The surgeon may approach the anterior cervical spine from the right or left side; the left-sided approach theoretically involves less risk to the recurrent laryngeal nerve.
- The incision may be made transversely or longitudinally depending on the number of levels involved and surgeon's preference. Longitudinal incision may be preferred for multilevel approaches.
- After incision, identify the platysma muscle in the superficial layer of cervical fascia, divide it sharply in a transverse or longitudinal fashion (**Fig. 40.2**).

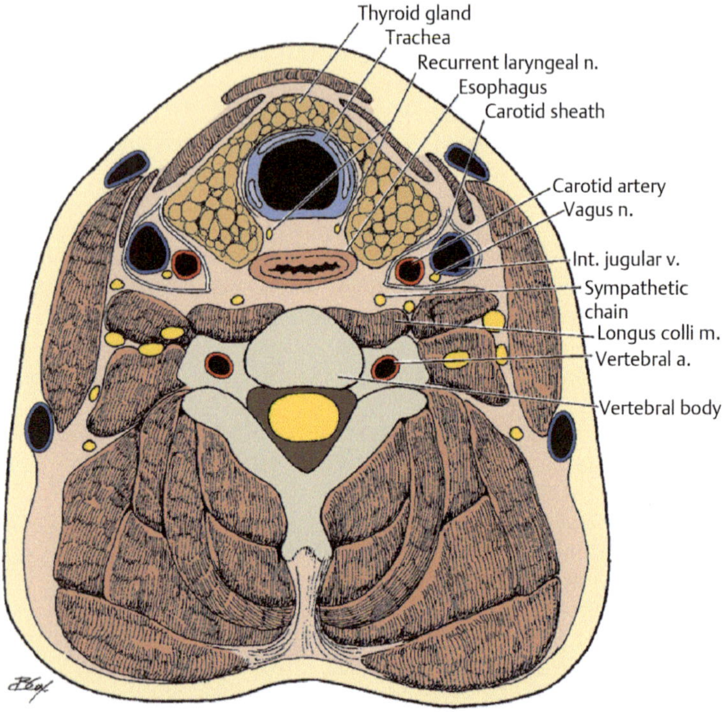

Fig. 40.2 Cross-sectional anatomy of the neck and spine at the C5 level.

  - Dissecting under the platysma superiorly and inferiorly allows for better mobilization of the tissues.
- Identify the medial border of the sternocleidomastoid (SCM).
- Using Metzenbaum scissors, dissect in the areolar plane through the deep cervical and pretracheal fascial layers, between the SCM and the medial structures (**Fig. 40.3**).
  - The carotid artery should be palpated lateral to the plane of dissection to ensure that the trajectory of dissection is correct.
  - Identify omohyoid and divide it if lower cervical approach is desired.[3]
- Using a handheld retractor, retract the medial structures from the SCM to expose the prevertebral fascia.
- Incise the fascia to expose the cervical spine; use Kittners to sweep the prevertebral fascia superiorly and inferiorly.
- Use a spinal marker in the vertebral body to confirm the level with X-ray or fluoroscopy image (avoid placing the marker in the disk space to avoid inadvertent iatrogenic injury to an adjacent level disk).

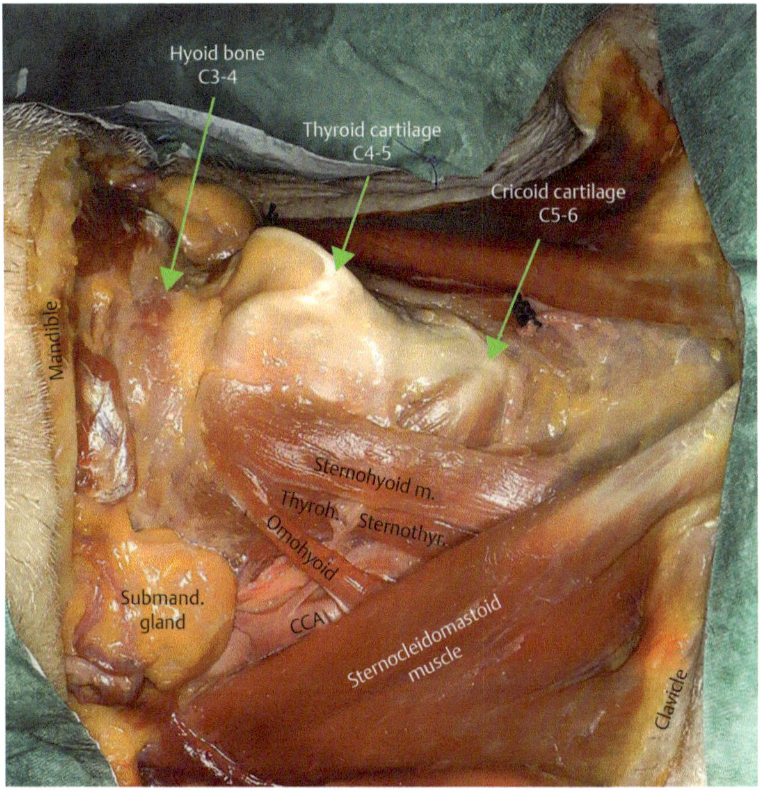

Fig. 40.3 Superficial anatomy of the right side of the neck. Common carotid artery (CCA).[4]

- With electrocautery or periosteal elevator, dissect the longus colli laterally from their midline attachments to reveal the uncinate process and ventrolateral vertebral body.
- Place self-retaining retractors deep to the longus colli and periodically deflate the cuff of the endotracheal tube to minimize esophageal/tracheal edema in prolonged cases.
- Caspar pins may be placed into the vertebral bodies above and below the level of interest, with gentle distraction applied for exposure, decompression, and alignment.
- The disks above and below the level of interest should be incised and removed with No. 11 blade, curettes, Kerrison rongeurs, and pituitary rongeurs (**Fig. 40.5a**).
- When necessary, anterior osteophytes can be removed with a rongeur.

- Leksell rongeur can be used to first begin the corpectomy and to harvest the anterior vertebral body for use as autograft if the bone is not pathologic. A high-speed bur can be used to thin the vertebral body to the posterior longitudinal ligament (PLL) or to a thin shell of posterior cortex, which can then be removed with Kerrison rongeur or drilled with a diamond bur (**Fig. 40.5b**).
- The PLL is carefully pierced with a small hook or curette.
- A small Kerrison rongeur (1 or 2 mm) can then be used to lift the PLL away from the dura and complete the decompression (**Fig. 40.5c**).
- Lateral decompression (foraminotomy) is generally completed at the level of the uncovertebral joint. The uncus can be thinned with a bur, followed by removal with a microcurette or Kerrison rongeur (**Fig. 40.4**).
- The corpectomy defect requires reconstruction for structural stability. A strut graft or expandable cage filled with autograft, allograft, or synthetic or ceramic allograft substitute can be placed into the defect after contouring of the vertebral body end plates (**Fig. 40.5d**).
- An anterior plate can be used to enhance fusion and prevent graft migration. If possible, multiple points of screw fixation should be established. However, posterior instrumentation does provide greater stability and may be required.
- Integrity of the posterior ligamentous structures and facet capsules may allow greater confidence in an anterior-only construct with plate fixation.[5]
- Some authors recommend rigid anterior fixation to enhance rigidity and reduce graft subsidence; others argue that dynamic plates and screws may enhance fusion by loading the graft (Wolff's law). Data in support of either approach are limited to theoretical considerations and retrospective studies.[6,7]
- Closure involves meticulous hemostasis, copious irrigation, and sometimes the placement of drain. The deep fascial layer and subcutaneous layers are closed separately.

40.4 Complications

- Wound infection.
- Hoarseness:
  - Reduce risk by reducing endotracheal cuff pressure and requesting that the anesthetist deflate and then reinflate the cuff once the retractors are set.
  - Avoid dissection into the carotid sheath.
  - Some surgeons advocate a left-sided approach to avoid risk of recurrent laryngeal nerve (RLN) injury, though doing so is controversial. The proponent's argument is that on the left side, the nerve consistently passes under the aortic arch and ascends to the tracheoesophageal

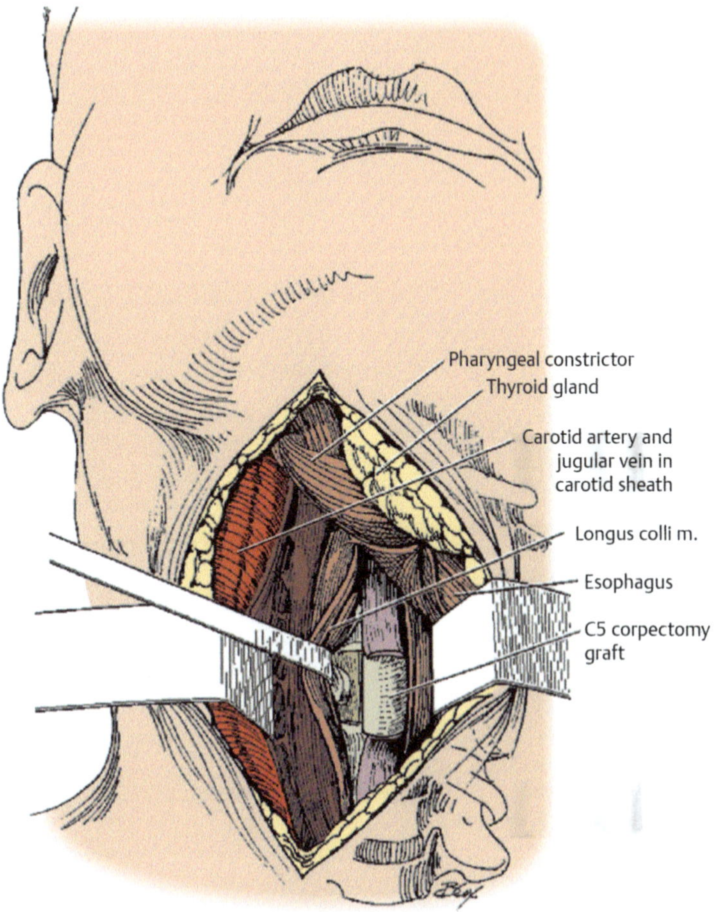

Fig. 40.4 Anterior view of the surgical field after single-level corpectomy in the cervical spine.

groove. On the right side, however, the nerve loops under the subclavian artery then proceeds cranially and medially.
- Studies have found no difference in the rates of RLN injury between corpectomy and multilevel anterior cervical diskectomy and fusion (ACDF).[8]

- Transient or permanent dysphagia, which is more common with longer operative times and greater number of operative levels.

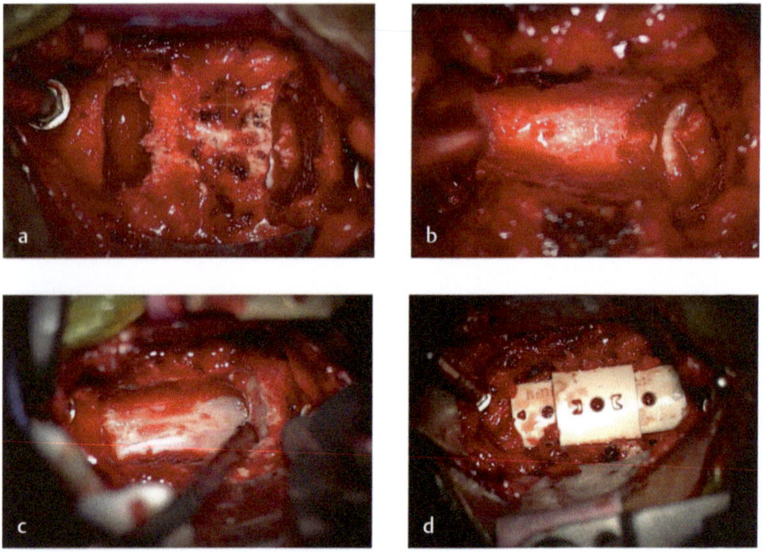

Fig. 40.5 Intraoperative images of single-level corpectomy in the cervical spine. **(a)** After removal of the disks above and below. **(b)** After removal of vertebral body. **(c)** Fully decompressed spinal cord after removal of posterior longitudinal ligament (PLL). **(d)** Insertion of strut graft.

- Nerve root or spinal cord injury.[9]
- Acute airway obstruction from swelling or hematoma:
  - Immediately stabilize the airway and intubate.
  - Open the wound at the bedside to allow for decompression of the hematoma and thereby ease intubation in an emergent setting.
  - Reintubation is difficult in this setting and emergency tracheostomy can be required.
- Cerebrospinal fluid (CSF) leak:
  - Difficult to close primarily.
  - Consider patching the defect with collagen matrix or tissue autograft and covering with fibrin glue or dural sealant. Be aware that these materials have the potential to cause neural compression, particularly after they swell.
  - Place lumbar drain to divert CSF if there is concern about the risk of persistent drainage.
- Vertebral artery injury:
  - The vertebral artery lies lateral to the uncovertebral complex and is often surrounded by a collection of veins.
  - Inadvertent injury can lead to massive bleeding.

  - In the event of injury, the surgeon must immediately tamponade the source of bleeding, usually with the aid of Gelfoam (Pharmacia & Upjohn; Kalamazoo, Michigan) or another hemostatic agent. The vessel can be repaired primarily or ligated surgically with a reported low risk of neurologic sequelae.[10,11]
  - An emergent angiogram should be considered to rule out vertebral artery dissection and may require vertebral artery embolization.
  - The artery can be sacrificed with little consequence if it is nondominant; sacrifice of the dominant vertebral artery has a higher incidence of ischemic injury to the brainstem.[10]
  - In cases involving tumor or at higher risk for aberrant vertebral artery anatomy, preoperative computed tomography (CT) or magnetic resonance (MR) angiography should be considered to determine vertebral artery dominance.
- Graft dislodgment/instrumentation failure:
  - Graft dislodgment may indicate pseudarthrosis, hardware failure, infection, or a combination of factors.
  - Primary importance is airway stabilization; if there is significant tracheal compression, emergent intubation and reoperation may be required.
  - Revision of the graft may include the use of autograft, such as iliac crest, and posterior cervical instrumentation and fusion to supplement the anterior construct.
  - Two retrospective studies have showed that incidence of graft failure is significantly higher in corpectomy versus multilevel ACDF ($n = 190$).[12,13]

40.5 Postoperative Care

- Consider external immobilization of the cervical spine.
- Patients who have myelopathy and gait unsteadiness often benefit from physical and occupational therapy evaluations.
- Ensure that the patient is tolerating oral intake and swallowing normally before discharge.
- Changes in voice quality postoperatively may reflect laryngeal nerve paresis which is typically transient.
- In cases of prolonged procedure with concern for anterior soft tissue swelling, consider keeping the patient intubated for 24 to 48 hours (until able to breathe around deflated airway cuff).

40.6 Outcomes

- The goals of decompressive corpectomy are neurologic preservation, cervical spine stabilization, and/or reduction of deformity.

- Available outcomes studies are limited in their retrospective nature but indicate excellent technical results (greater than 98% fusion rate) and improvement in radicular and myelopathic symptoms in 86%.[14]
- Even in patients with severe myelopathy resulting in a bedridden or wheelchair-bound condition, clinical outcomes showed improvement in more than 60% of patients who underwent surgery.[15]
- Outcomes are similar for both anterior and posterior approaches to cervical spondylotic myelopathy,[16] though anterior cervical corpectomy and fusion may be preferred in cases of anterior retrovertebral pathology not amenable to diskectomy alone or in cases of significant kyphosis.
- Restoration of lordosis (in cases of more severe preoperative kyphosis) with compression primarily at disk level can be performed more reliably with a multilevel anterior cervical diskectomy and fusion or hybrid approach.[17]

40.7 Surgical Pearls

- Identify the location of vertebral artery on preoperative imaging studies.
- Avoid hyperextension of the cervical spine during positioning.
- Generous dissection of the longus colli muscle allows better identification of midline, proper placement of retractor blades underneath the muscle fibers, and decreased pressure on vascular structures laterally or esophagus and trachea medially. However, avoid excessive anterior or lateral dissection to avoid possible vertebral artery injury or sympathetic nerve injury (Horner's syndrome).
- Begin decompression with diskectomy cranial and caudal to the intended corpectomy. This will assist in identification of the appropriate depth and width (uncus to uncus) of corpectomy.
- In patients with myeloradiculopathy, additional focal decompression of the nerve root(s) might be necessary.
- When the PLL is severely adherent, dissociation of the PLL from the adjacent structures, thus eliminating its constrictive effect on the spinal cord and preventing thecal sac manipulation, is the primary goal. Removing the PLL is a secondary goal if it can be safely achieved, but doing so increases risk of intraoperative CSF leak and neurologic injury.[18]

Common Clinical Questions

1. The fusion rate after anterior cervical corpectomy increases with augmented posterior fixation, especially after two- and three-level corpectomies. True or false?
2. Anterior corpectomy and fusion can achieve a greater restoration of lordosis than multilevel anterior cervical diskectomy and fusion. True or false?

Answers to Common Clinical Questions

1. True.
2. False.

References

1. Aronson N, Filtzer DL, Bagan M. Anterior cervical fusion by the Smith-Robinson approach. J Neurosurg. 1968; 29(4):396–404
2. Benzel EC. Surgical Exposure of the Spine: An Extensile Approach. American Association of Neurological Surgeons; 1995
3. Abruzzo TA, et al. Choudhri TF, McCormick PC. Anterior cervical approach. In: Connolly ES Jr., McKhann GM II, Huang J, Choudhri TF, Komotar RJ, Mocco J, eds. Fundamentals of Operative Techniques in Neurosurgery. 2nd ed. Thieme; 2010:665–673
4. Bodon G, Combalia A. Relevant surgical anatomy of the anterior cervical spine, the high retropharyngeal and the subaxial regions. In: Koller H, Robinson Y, eds. Cervical Spine Surgery: Standard and Advanced Techniques. Cham: Springer; 2019; 33–41
5. Karam YR, Dahdaleh NS, Magnetta MJ, et al. Biomechanical comparison of anterior, posterior, and circumferential fixation after one-level anterior cervical corpectomy in the human cadaveric spine. Spine. 2011; 36(7):E455–E460
6. Vaccaro A, Singh K. The role of anterior column reconstruction. In: Anterior Spinal Column Surgery. Philadelphia, PA: Hanley & Belfus; 1998:589–590
7. Ulrich C, Woersdoerfer O, Kalff R, Claes L, Wilke HJ. Biomechanics of fixation systems to the cervical spine. Spine. 1991; 16(3) Suppl:S4–S9
8. Yee TJ, Swong K, Park P. Complications of anterior cervical spine surgery: a systematic review of the literature. J Spine Surg. 2020; 6(1):302–322
9. Flynn TB. Neurologic complications of anterior cervical interbody fusion. Spine. 1982; 7(6):536–539
10. Rao R, David K. Anterior cervical surgery. In: Complications in Orthopaedics: Spine Surgery. Rosemont, IL: American Academy of Orthopaedic Surgeons; 2006:4–16
11. Daentzer D, Deinsberger W, Böker DK. Vertebral artery complications in anterior approaches to the cervical spine: report of two cases and review of literature. Surg Neurol. 2003; 59(4):300–309, discussion 309
12. Lin Q, Zhou X, Wang X, Cao P, Tsai N, Yuan W. A comparison of anterior cervical discectomy and corpectomy in patients with multilevel cervical spondylotic myelopathy. Eur Spine J. 2012; 21(3):474–481
13. Liu JM, Tong WL, Chen XY, et al. The incidences and risk factors related to early dysphagia after anterior cervical spine surgery: a prospective study. PLoS One. 2017; 12(3):e0173364

14. Eleraky MA, Llanos C, Sonntag VK. Cervical corpectomy: report of 185 cases and review of the literature. J Neurosurg. 1999; 90(1) Suppl:35–41
15. Scardino FB, Rocha LP, Barcelos AC, Rotta JM, Botelho RV. Is there a benefit to operating on patients (bedridden or in wheelchairs) with advanced stage cervical spondylotic myelopathy? Euro Spine J. 2010; 19(5):699–705
16. Lawrence BD, Jacobs WB, Norvell DC, Hermsmeyer JT, Chapman JR, Brodke DS. Anterior versus posterior approach for treatment of cervical spondylotic myelopathy: a systematic review. Spine. 2013; 38(22) Suppl 1:S173–S182
17. Liu Y, Hou Y, Yang L, et al. Comparison of 3 reconstructive techniques in the surgical management of multilevel cervical spondylotic myelopathy. Spine. 2012; 37(23):E1450–E1458
18. Sandhu H. Anterior cervical corpectomy. In: Spine Surgery: Tricks of the Trade. New York: Thieme Medical Publishers; 2003:44–45

41 Cervical Laminectomy with and without Fusion

Ian David Connolly, Muhamed Hadzipasic, and Ganesh M. Shankar

Summary

This chapter explores the surgical procedures of cervical laminectomy both with and without fusion, highlighting the scenarios where each is appropriate. It covers the fundamental concepts, indications, contraindications, surgical techniques, complications, postoperative care, and outcomes related to these procedures. Techniques for both cervical laminectomy and various fusion methods are detailed, including instrumentation techniques like the Magerl and Roy-Camille methods for lateral mass fixation. Potential complications such as postlaminectomy kyphosis, nerve root injury, and vertebral artery injury are also discussed, along with strategies for managing these risks. Postoperative care and patient outcomes are explored to provide a comprehensive view of the expected results and recovery process.

Keywords: cervical laminectomy, spinal fusion, cervical myelopathy, spinal decompression, postoperative care, cervical stenosis

41.1 Key Points

- In presence of significant central canal stenosis and cervical myelopathy, surgical treatment is appropriate.
- The goal of surgery is to decompress the neural elements and provide stabilization via instrumentation/fusion.
- Focal anterior pathology may be better treated by anterior decompression and fusion.
- Lordotic alignment of the cervical spine is needed to allow the spinal cord to "drift" posteriorly following decompression.
- Cervical laminectomy and/or fusion are not intended for the treatment of neck pain.
- Preoperative detailed history and physical examination along with radiographs, magnetic resonance imaging (MRI), and, at times, computed tomography (CT) are essential.

41.2 Indications

- Multilevel cervical spondylosis causing cervical stenosis and myelopathy.
- Cervical stenosis caused by ossification of the posterior longitudinal ligament (OPLL).
- Ligamentum flavum thickening with resultant stenosis.
- Epidural abscess.
- Tumor.
- Trauma.
- Epidural hematoma.
- Anterior neck anatomy that would preclude an anterior approach.

41.3 Contraindications

- Presence of less than 10 degrees of cervical lordosis on preoperative extension lateral radiograph, in which case inclusion of an anterior approach or multilevel facet osteotomies should be considered to restore lordosis of the cervical spine.
- Anatomy preventing safe placement of instrumentation such as aberrant course of the vertebral artery.

41.4 Technique

- Awake, fiber-optic or GlideScope (Verathon Incorporated; Bothell, Washington) intubation may be necessary in cases of severe stenosis or instability.
- Place patient in prone position (requires a team approach).
- Neural monitoring (motor-evoked potentials [MEPs], somatosensory-evoked potentials [SSEPs], electromyography [EMG]):
  - Provides real-time feedback on integrity of spinal cord and nerves.
  - Commonly used for posterior cervical operations.
  - Generally advised in select circumstances (i.e., in the setting of severe stenosis, cervical instability, intradural pathology).
  - In posterior approaches for cervical degeneration, it is controversial as to whether MEP and SSEP changes reliably predict postoperative deficits.[1]
  - Absence of MEP and SSEP intraoperative changes have high specificity and high negative predictive value (high likelihood of no postoperative neurological deficits).[1]
  - Intraoperative EMG may reduce the rate of C5 nerve root injury.[2]
  - Obtain preflip baselines in the setting of cervical instability or severe stenosis.
- Head positioning options include Mayfield head holder and ProneView (Dupaco; San Diego, California).

- In the setting of an unstable cervical spine or severe cord compression, "sandwiching the patient and spinning prone" using the Jackson table prone positioning technique is advisable.
- Assess head and neck alignment visually and fluoroscopically to ensure appropriate alignment.
- Localize with fluoroscopy and make appropriate-length midline incision.
- Use the midline avascular plane to maintain the integrity of posterior neck muscles and minimize bleeding.
- Using a Cobb and cautery, perform subperiosteal dissection to expose the spinous processes, lamina, and lateral masses.
- Avoid exposing lateral masses and violating the facet joints at levels above or below the operative levels.
- Perform lateral mass fixation.
  - Magerl technique[3]:
    - The lateral mass is divided into quadrants.
    - The entry point is at the superior medial quadrant and the trajectory is toward the superior lateral quadrant ("up and out") (**Fig. 41.1**).
    - Used for C3–C6.
  - Roy-Camille technique[4]:
    - The entry point is at the midpoint of the lateral mass.
    - The trajectory is 10 degrees lateral in the axial plane.
    - Often used at the C7 level.
  - Other described lateral mass instrumentation techniques include Anderson and An techniques.
  - If C7 is included in the fixation, options are pedicle screws versus lateral mass screw placement.
  - Technique for C7 pedicle screw placement requires additional consideration.
    - A laminotomy to palpate the medial edge of the C7 pedicle is useful.
    - The entry point is in line with the lateral mass entry points at superior levels.
    - Medial angulation is necessary to enter and traverse the pedicle (correlate/measure with preoperative cross-sectional imaging).
  - Lateral mass screw size is typically 3.5 or 4.0 mm diameter by 12 to 16 mm length.
  - C7 pedicle screw size is typically 3.5 or 4.0 mm by 16 to 24 mm.
- Insert rods of appropriate length and secure with set screws.
  - It is preferred to contour the rods to match the screw heads. (Overusing rod reduction devices such as persuaders may cause loosening or pullout of instrumentation.)
  - Assess sagittal alignment fluoroscopically before final tightening of set screws.
  - For final tightening of set screws use torque limiting screwdriver.

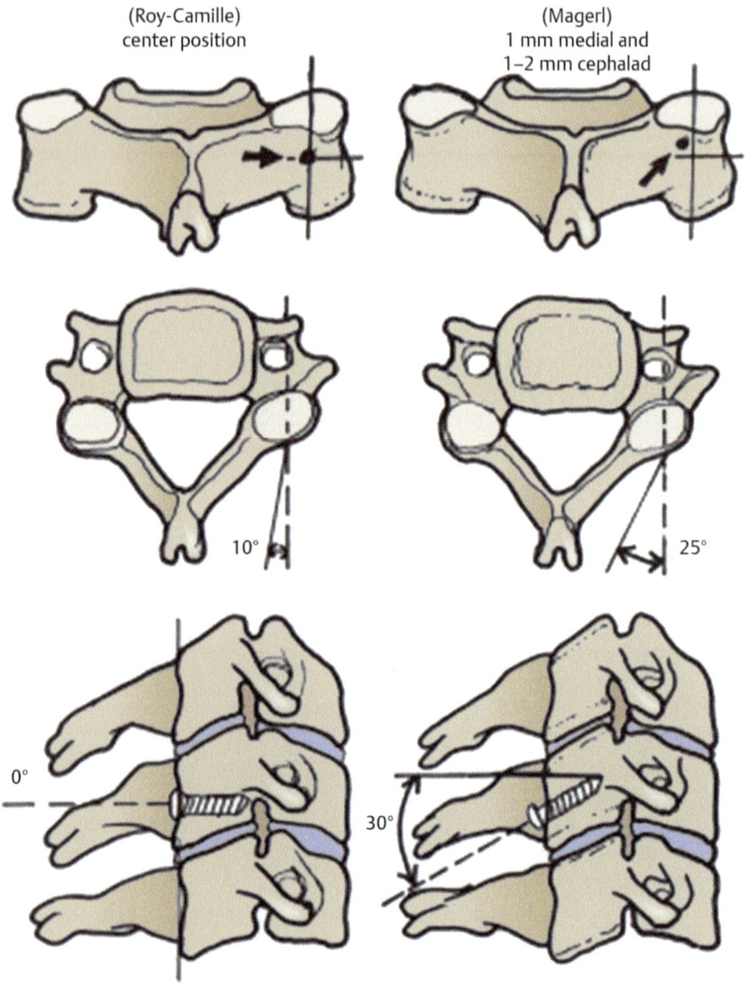

Fig. 41.1 The Roy-Camille and Magerl and An techniques for placement of lateral mass screws in the subaxial cervical spine.

- Performing posterior cervical laminectomy (three options):
  - The senior author's preferred technique is the use an AM-8 drill bit and/or a 2- to 3-mm diamond high-speed bur to create bilateral troughs at the laminar–lateral mass junction and remove the posterior elements in a "lobster tail" or "en bloc" fashion (**Fig. 41.2**).

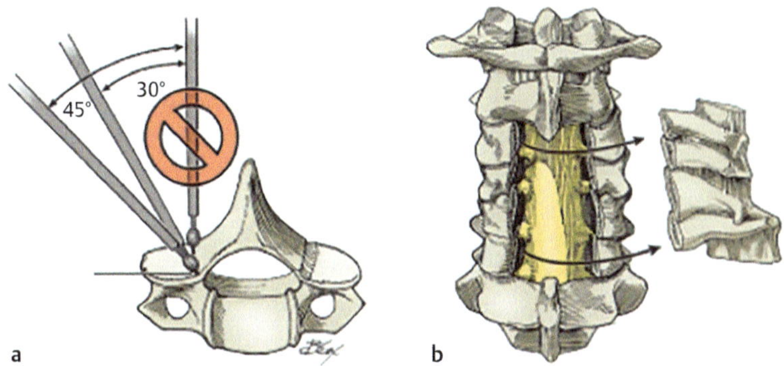

Fig. 41.2 Laminectomy. **(a)** The bur must be directed approximately 30 to 45 degrees in the sagittal plane to avoid burring into the facet joint. Doing so may risk loss of orientation and cause one to bur too deeply, endangering the dural sac or spinal cord. **(b)** En bloc ("lobster tail") removal of laminae. (Adapted from Vaccaro AR, Albert TJ, eds. Spine Surgery: Tricks of the Trade. 2nd ed. Thieme; 2009.)

- Apply clamps such as penetrating towel clips to posterior spinous process and apply gentle upward (posteriorly directed) traction while using a fine curette or Woodson to free any adherent ligamentum flavum. (Generally, the assistant applies the posteriorly directed traction.)
  - Advantage: No placement of a Kerrison under the lamina and into the spinal canal.
  - Disadvantage: Requires proficiency with the drill and places the lateral mass at risk if the troughs are too lateral.
- An alternative technique is to use a combination of a rongeur and Kerrison (manual laminectomy), similar to lumbar laminectomy technique.
  - Advantage: More familiar technique, being widely used in the lumbar spine.
  - Disadvantage: Potential risk of neural injury with Kerrison repetitively inserted deep/underneath the lamina.
- The third technique is to use a footplate craniotome to create bilateral troughs (which may carry higher risk, in the authors' opinion).
- Decortication of the facets and lateral masses is performed to create a bed for arthrodesis/fusion using a high-speed drill.
- Bone graft material (e.g., local autograft, autogenous morselized iliac crest bone graft, and/or bone graft extender) is placed along the lateral mass edges bilaterally.

- Ensure that no graft material is left in contact with the neural elements or within the spinal canal.
- Ensure hemostasis.
- Place subfascial drain and close muscle, fascia, and skin layers.
- Patients at high risk for infection may benefit from topical application of vancomycin powder to the subfascial space.

41.5 Complications

- Postlaminectomy kyphosis:
  - Occurs in 21 to 38% of uninstrumented cases at 2 years' follow-up.[5,6,7]
  - More frequent in younger patients and those who have a greater degree of facetectomy.[8]
  - High failure rates have led most authors to recommend instrumented fusion in the setting of cervical laminectomy.
- Cerebrospinal fluid (CSF) leak:
  - If possible, primary repair using nonabsorbable suture is preferred.
  - Alternatively, cover with collagen matrix and/or dural sealant (e.g., DuraSeal).
  - Maintain elevated head-of-the-bed (HOB) positioning for 2 to 5 days to decrease pressure on the dural repair.
- Nerve root injury:
  - May result either directly during foraminotomy or during screw placement.
  - C5 palsy is the most common occurrence with overall incidence ranging from 4 to 8%. Etiology is not well understood. May be caused by traction resulting from posterior drifting of the spinal cord, considering that the C5 root is shortest. Clinically evident in a delayed fashion following cervical decompression (2–3 days postoperatively). Generally resolves 6 to 12 months postoperatively.[9,10]
- Vertebral artery injury:
  - Results from misplaced lateral mass screw.
  - Screw should remain in place and postoperative angiogram obtained to assess type of injury (e.g., occlusion, dissection).
- Deep wound infection.
- Postoperative epidural hematoma with neurologic deficit.
  - Emergent return to operating room (OR) for evacuation/decompression.

41.6 Postoperative Care

- Postoperative paraspinal spasm may respond well to judicious use of muscle relaxants or low dose diazepam.
- Obtain postoperative upright anteroposterior/lateral C-spine X-rays.
- Remove drain when output becomes less than 30 to 50 mL per 8- to 12-hour shift (typically postoperative day 1 or 2).
- Mobilize the patient with physical therapy.

41.7 Outcomes

- Class III evidence shows that 70 to 95% of patients show postoperative neurologic improvement after cervical laminectomy and fusion for myelopathy.[11]
- However, the primary goal of surgery is to halt neurologic deterioration.
- Class I evidence shows no difference in 1-year patient-reported functional outcomes between dorsal (laminectomy with fusion or laminoplasty) versus ventral approaches for multilevel cervical spondylotic myelopathy.[12]

41.8 Surgical Pearls

- Preoperative cervical kyphosis and loss of lordosis are relative contraindications to posterior laminectomy without instrumentation.
- Most authors recommend performing instrumented spinal fusion in the setting of cervical laminectomy to prevent postlaminectomy kyphosis.
- Focal disk herniations and disk–osteophyte complexes should be treated by anterior approaches.
- Preoperative familiarity with the nuances of a particular instrumentation system is helpful.
- When instrumenting to C7, many authors recommend crossing the cervicothoracic junction and extending the instrumented fusion to T1 or T2 to prevent junctional disease, hypermobility/instability, and/or kyphosis. (Fixation at T1 and T2 requires pedicle instrumentation.) Evidence suggests lower reoperation rates and possibly higher fusion rate when construct extended across the cervicothoracic junction.[13,14]
- C2 is not instrumented with lateral mass fixation. Instead, C2 pars, pedicle, or translaminar fixation techniques are used.
- Study preoperative imaging to guide screw size and placement.
- Many patients who undergo posterior cervical fusion are also candidates for cervical laminoplasty.[15] It is important to consider the appropriateness of cervical laminoplasty given comparable patient-reported outcomes and favorable complication profile.[12]

Common Clinical Questions

1. When performing lateral mass instrumentation, why is the screw trajectory directed laterally and superiorly ("up and out")?
2. Which nerve root is most prone to palsy after posterior cervical laminectomy?
3. Why is preoperative cervical spine alignment an important consideration?
4. Why is instrumented spinal fusion recommended in the setting of cervical laminectomy?

Answers to Common Clinical Questions

1. To avoid the nerve root and the vertebral artery.
2. C5 nerve root.
3. Kyphotic alignment prevents posterior "drifting" of the spinal cord post decompression.
4. To prevent postlaminectomy kyphosis.

References

1. Koffie RM, Morgan CD, Giraldo JP, et al. Should somatosensory and motor evoked potential monitoring be used routinely in all posterior cervical operations for degenerative conditions of the cervical spine? World Neurosurg. 2022; 162:e86–e90
2. Jimenez JC, Sani S, Braverman B, Deutsch H, Ratliff JK. Palsies of the fifth cervical nerve root after cervical decompression: prevention using continuous intraoperative electromyography monitoring. J Neurosurg Spine. 2005; 3(2):92–97
3. Heller JG, Carlson GD, Abitbol JJ, Garfin SR. Anatomic comparison of the Roy-Camille and Magerl techniques for screw placement in the lower cervical spine. Spine. 1991; 16(10) Suppl:S552–S557
4. Ebraheim NA, Klausner T, Xu R, Yeasting RA. Safe lateral-mass screw lengths in the Roy-Camille and Magerl techniques. An anatomic study. Spine. 1998; 23(16):1739–1742
5. Kato Y, Iwasaki M, Fuji T, Yonenobu K, Ochi T. Long-term follow-up results of laminectomy for cervical myelopathy caused by ossification of the posterior longitudinal ligament. J Neurosurg. 1998; 89(2):217–223
6. Herkowitz HN. A comparison of anterior cervical fusion, cervical laminectomy, and cervical laminoplasty for the surgical management of multiple level spondylotic radiculopathy. Spine. 1988; 13(7):774–780

7. Kaptain GJ, Simmons NE, Replogle RE, Pobereskin L. Incidence and outcome of kyphotic deformity following laminectomy for cervical spondylotic myelopathy. J Neurosurg. 2000; 93(2) Suppl:199–204
8. Bell DF, Walker JL, O'Connor G, Tibshirani R. Spinal deformity after multiple-level cervical laminectomy in children. Spine. 1994; 19(4):406–411
9. Hofler RC, Frazzetta J, Zakaria J, Aziz A, Adams W, Jones GA. C5 palsy after cervical laminectomy: natural history in a 10-year series. Spine J. 2021; 21 (9):1473–1478
10. Khuyagbaatar B, Kim K, Park WM, Kim YH. Biomechanical investigation of post-operative C5 palsy due to ossification of the posterior longitudinal ligament in different types of cervical spinal alignment. J Biomech. 2017; 57: 54–61
11. Anderson PA, Matz PG, Groff MW, et al. Joint Section on Disorders of the Spine and Peripheral Nerves of the American Association of Neurological Surgeons and Congress of Neurological Surgeons. Laminectomy and fusion for the treatment of cervical degenerative myelopathy. J Neurosurg Spine. 2009; 11(2):150–156
12. Ghogawala Z, Terrin N, Dunbar MR, et al. Effect of ventral vs dorsal spinal surgery on patient-reported physical functioning in patients with cervical spondylotic myelopathy: a randomized clinical trial. JAMA. 2021; 325(10): 942–951
13. Goyal A, Akhras A, Wahood W, Alvi MA, Nassr A, Bydon M. Should multilevel posterior cervical fusions involving C7 cross the cervicothoracic junction? A systematic review and meta-analysis. World Neurosurg. 2019; 127:588–595.e5
14. Schroeder GD, Kepler CK, Kurd MF, et al. Is it necessary to extend a multilevel posterior cervical decompression and fusion to the upper thoracic spine? Spine. 2016; 41(23):1845–1849
15. Lopez WY, Goh BC, Upadhyaya S, et al. Laminoplasty—an underutilized procedure for cervical spondylotic myelopathy. Spine J. 2021; 21(4):571–577

42 Cervical Laminoplasty

Aria Jamshidi, Glen R. Manzano, and Allan D. Levi

Summary

Cervical laminoplasty is a motion-preserving decompression procedure for cervical myelopathy. It is ideal for patients with minimal to no axial neck pain and preserved sagittal alignment. In comparison to other surgical approaches for spondylotic myelopathy, laminoplasty outcomes are comparable, and in some cases superior to fusion techniques.

Keywords: cervical myelopathy, sagittal balance, motion preservation, greenstick fracture, rib allograft

42.1 Key Points

- Laminoplasty is a procedure in which the spinal canal is expanded while preserving the integrity of the posterior elements.
- Laminoplasty was developed in Japan in the 1970s as a "tissue-sparing" alternative to laminectomy to minimize its associated risk of instability and progressive kyphotic deformity and thus improve outcomes.[1]
- The procedure must be reserved for patients with neutral or lordotic alignment, as this technique relies on indirect decompression and dorsal migration of the cord from anterior compressive pathology.
- Newer laminoplasty techniques have been developed, such as the use of titanium miniplates, greatly simplifying the procedure.

42.2 Indications

- Multilevel spinal cord compression secondary to one or any combination of the following:
  - Ossification of the posterior longitudinal ligament (OPLL).
  - Cervical spondylosis.
  - Congenital canal stenosis.
- For consideration in children requiring laminectomies.

42.3 Contraindications

- Not for isolated neck pain or for patients having a significant kyphotic deformity.
- Straightening of normal cervical lordosis or fixed kyphotic deformity > 10 degrees.
- Cervical instability secondary to trauma, tumor destruction, degenerative disease, or a connective tissue disorder. Rheumatoid arthritis is a relative contraindication as these patients are at higher risk for developing postoperative instability.[2]
- Significant ventral pathology that cannot be adequately addressed via indirect decompression.

42.4 Technique

- In cases of severe stenosis, awake fiberoptic intubation should be considered to minimize the risk of hyperextension injury and allow for reexamination of the patient prior to positioning.
- Place neurophysiologic monitoring leads (including somatosensory-evoked potentials [SSEPs], motor-evoked potentials [MEPs], and electromyograms [EMGs]) and obtain baseline recordings before turning the patient.
- Secure the patient's head with pins (e.g., Mayfield three-pin headrest [Schaerer Mayfield; Randolph, Massachusetts]). Careful attention is given to neck stability during patient transfer so as to avoid spinal cord injury.
- The head is secured in a slightly flexed position so as to open the interlaminar spaces, while tensing the skin folds to facilitate exposure and closure.
- Tape superior and dorsolateral aspects of both shoulders and secure to the caudal corner of the operating table to aid in radiographic visualization of the lower cervical vertebrae.
- Place the patient in reverse Trendelenburg to facilitate venous drainage and decrease bleeding.
- Use fluoroscopy to plan an incision extending from the spinous process of C2 to that of T1 and infiltrate with 1% lidocaine with epinephrine to minimize skin bleeding.
- Make a midline incision and use a subperiosteal dissection to reflect the paraspinal muscles from the caudal end of C2 to the rostral limit of T1.
- Care is taken while dividing the ligamentum nuchae, along the midline avascular plane, so as to minimize intraoperative bleeding.
- The dissection should extend laterally to the midpoint of the lateral masses of C3 to C7, while maintaining the integrity of the facet capsule. Muscular

attachments to the C2 spinous process should be preserved to prevent instability.

- Remove the caudal third of the C2 lamina and the rostral third of the T1 lamina using the combination of a high-speed air drill and a 2-mm Kerrison punch, allowing visualization of the underlying dura at these levels.
- Remove the spinous processes from C3 to C7 with a rongeur and morselize the bone for subsequent autografting.
- Perform laminoplasty of lamina from C3 to C7 by creating an "open" side and a "hinged" side. The open side is generally the side with the greatest compression and/or the side most clinically symptomatic.
  - Use the high-speed air drill with a small drill bit to create troughs at the level of the lamina–facet junction from C3 to C7 (**Fig. 42.1**).
  - Once the "open" side has been sufficiently burred down to the inner cortical surface, a 1-mm Kerrison punch can be used to complete the bony disconnection between the lamina–lateral mass junction.
  - A Penfield #4 can be used to palpate for bony bridges and ligamentum flavum dissection to facilitate the decompression. The ligamentum must be released to open the hinge of the laminoplasty.
  - Drill through the outer and inner cortical margins of the lamina on the open side, but only through the outer cortical margin and cancellous bone (and not the inner cortex) on the hinged side. If the hinged side is inadvertently fractured, a laminectomy and fusion should instead be performed.
- Prepare the bone allografts to stabilize the canal expansion.
  - Using rib allografts and the high-speed drill, cut three separate grafts each approximately 8 to 14 mm long.
  - Make transverse grooves along the cut surfaces of the rib grafts, approximating the thickness of the cut laminae.
- Prepare to "open the door."
  - Use two small curettes placed into the trough on the open side just deep to the outer cortex.
  - Pull the curettes upward, thereby enlarging the lamina–facet gap and creating a greenstick fracture along the trough on the hinged side. Repeat the process on each successive lamina to expand the canal by approximately 4 mm (**Fig. 42.2**).
- Place the rib allografts in the gaps that have been created at the C3, C5, and C7 levels (**Fig. 42.3**).
- Place the morselized spinous process autograft over the decorticated bone surfaces of the facet and lamina on the hinged side at C3, C5, and C7 to provide for an intersegmental fusion. If the patient suffers from radiculopathy as well as myelopathy, one or more foraminotomies can be performed:

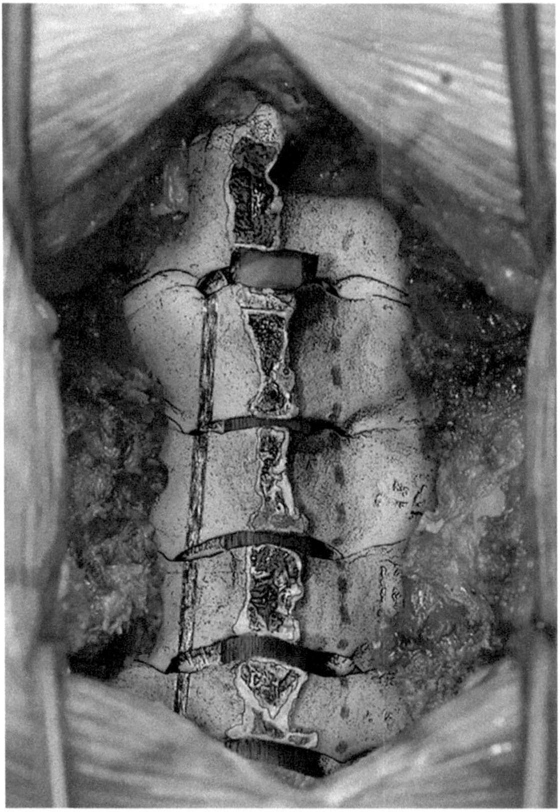

Fig. 42.1 Trough is drilled through the inner and outer cortices at the lamina–facet junction on the left (shown from C3 to C6 only). Partial laminectomy of C2 is shown. Crosshatching denotes area of drilling for closed door side.

   - After the lamina has been elevated and the ligamentum flavum excised, drill the medial third of the facet over the exiting nerve root and widen the opening as needed with 1- or 2-mm angled Kerrison punches.
- Leave the subfascial drain (e.g., Hemovac [Gohar Shafa; Tehran, Iran]) in situ to minimize hematoma formation.
- Variations in the approach:
   - Use spinous processes as autograft instead of the rib allograft.
   - Stabilize the rib allograft with titanium miniplates to the adjacent lamina and facet on the open side or sutures.

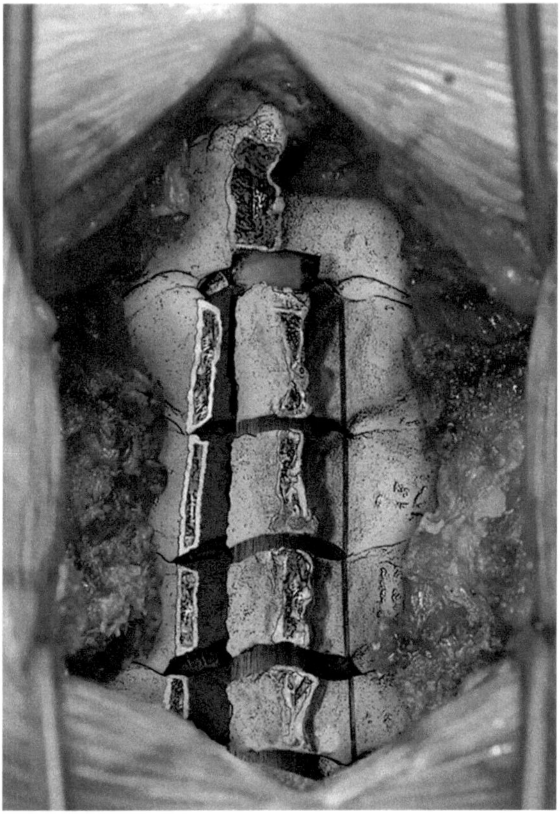

Fig. 42.2 With a trough drilled through the outer cortex only on the contralateral side (closed door side), the laminectomy door is "opened," creating a greenstick-type fracture on the closed side.

- Use titanium spacers to hold open lamina that is affixed to the lamina–facet joint on the open side.
- Perform full-thickness splitting of the lamina in the midline and create bilateral troughs, and then spread the lamina and place allograft spacers (double-door laminoplasty).
- Should rigid stabilization be required, lateral mass screws can be placed. This is best done after drilling and "opening the door," but before graft insertion.

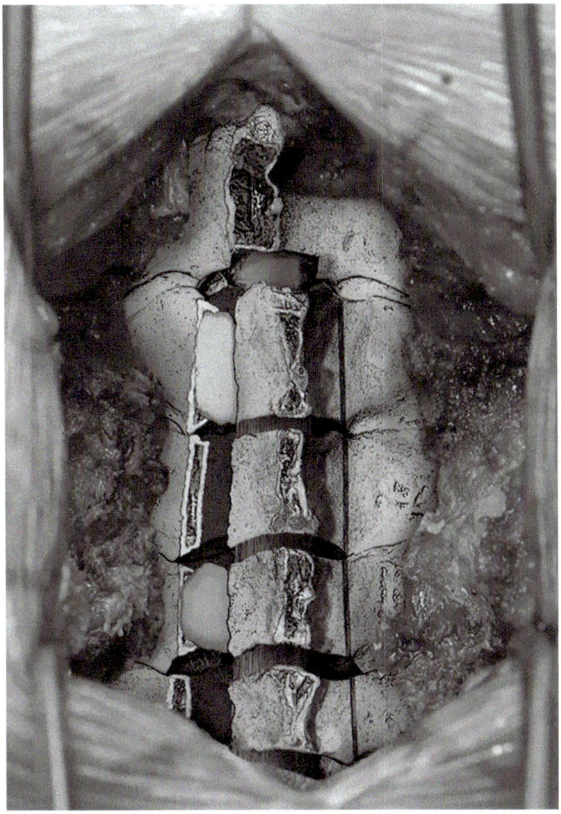

Fig. 42.3 Rib allograft is cut and secured into opening in lamina to expand the spinal canal, typically at C3, C5, and C7.

42.5 Complications

- Early:
  - Wound infection (2%).
  - Dural tear/cerebrospinal fluid (CSF) leak (< 1%).
  - Hemorrhage (< 1%).
  - Spinal cord injury (< 1%).
  - Nerve root injury.
  - Delayed C5 nerve root injury (2–13.3%).
- Late:
  - Postoperative neck pain (40–60%).
  - Reduced range of motion (20–50%).
  - New-onset kyphosis (2–15%).

42.6 Postoperative Care

- Patients are encouraged to mobilize on postoperative day 1. Patients may be placed in a rigid cervical collar; however, many surgeons now avoid immobilization, believing that it may improve range of motion and decrease neck pain.[3]
- Discharge to home once the patient is ambulating and tolerating full diet—usually 2 to 3 days postoperatively.
- To assess alignment and stability postoperatively, standing neutral and flexion–extension cervical spine X-rays are performed.
- If there is limited symptom improvement, MRI or CT scan should be considered to assess hinge stability, implant position, and canal diameter.

42.7 Outcomes

- Clinical outcome studies are drawn largely from the Japanese literature on patients with OPLL and are difficult to compare as a result of patient heterogeneity and different outcome measures used.[4]
- Long-term (5–10 years) outcome studies suggest that 50 to 70% of patients having either OPLL or cervical spondylotic myelopathy show improvement in their neurologic function after laminoplasty.[5]
- A randomized controlled[5] trial comparing laminoplasty with laminectomy and fusion for cervical spondylotic myelopathy yielded the following results:
  - Both the groups showed improvement in postoperative Nurick grade and modified Japanese Orthopaedic Association (JOA) score with overall low surgical complication rates.
  - The laminoplasty group showed statistically significant improvement in postoperative neck, interscapular and arm pain scores as well as in Neck Disability Index and SF-36 scores when compared with the laminectomy and fusion group.
  - Cervical range of motion was reduced by 75% in the laminectomy and fusion group, versus 20% in the laminoplasty group.
  - Although the patient numbers were small, there was a suggestion of increased adjacent level narrowing in the laminectomy and fusion group, noted as early as 1 year postoperatively.
- A recent randomized controlled trial comparing ventral and dorsal surgical approaches for cervical spondylotic myelopathy found laminoplasty to be associated with the lowest complication rate, improved outcomes, and less outpatient medical service utilization than ventral or dorsal fusion surgery.[6]

42.8 Surgical Pearls

- Obtain preoperative X-rays to rule out instability or kyphotic deformity.
- Ensure the provision of drilling gutters at the lamina–facet junction (and not lateral to it) and direct drill medially so as to not disrupt the facet joint.
- Lift *gently* when opening the door and ensure that drilling of the closed side (through outer cortex and some cancellous bone) is adequate to avoid creating a true fracture of the lamina. With a true greenstick fracture, some tension should remain in the opening to help maintain compression on the rib graft to hold it in place.
- If multiple foraminotomies are required, plan on making the open side the side where more foraminotomies are required.
- Visually inspect the construct and gently stress it after rib allograft is placed to ensure that you have not compromised the canal and that it remains stable.

Common Clinical Questions

1. Patients who have kyphotic deformities and symptoms of myelopathy may benefit from laminoplasty procedures. True or false?
2. List three perioperative surgical complications associated with laminoplasty.

Answers to Common Clinical Questions

1. False. Kyphotic deformities are a relative contraindication to performing this procedure.
2. Delayed C5 nerve root injury (2–13.3%), wound infection (2%), dural tear/ CSF leak (< 1%), hemorrhage (< 1%), spinal cord injury (< 1%).

References

1. Hale JJ, Gruson KI, Spivak JM. Laminoplasty: a review of its role in compressive cervical myelopathy. Spine J. 2006; 6(6) Suppl:289S–298S
2. Mukai Y, Hosono N, Sakaura H, et al. Laminoplasty for cervical myelopathy caused by subaxial lesions in rheumatoid arthritis. J Neurosurg. 2004; 100(1) Suppl Spine:7–12
3. Mandal S, Banerjee U, Mukherjee AS, Mandal S, Kundu S. Analysis of the outcome in patients with cervical spondylotic myelopathy, undergone canal expansive laminoplasty supported with instrumentation in a group of Indian population—a prospective study. Int J Spine Surg. 2016; 10:17

4. Wang MY, Shah S, Green BA. Clinical outcomes following cervical laminoplasty for 204 patients with cervical spondylotic myelopathy. Surg Neurol. 2004; 62(6):487–492, discussion 492–493
5. Manzano GR, Casella G, Wang MY, Vanni S, Levi AD. A prospective, randomized trial comparing expansile cervical laminoplasty and cervical laminectomy and fusion for multilevel cervical myelopathy. Neurosurgery. 2012; 70(2):264–277
6. Ghogawala Z, Terrin N, Dunbar MR, et al. Effect of ventral vs dorsal spinal surgery on patient-reported physical functioning in patients with cervical spondylotic myelopathy: a randomized clinical trial. JAMA. 2021; 325(10): 942–951

43 Posterior Cervical Foraminotomy

Rajakumar V. Deshpande, Murali Krishna P., Chaitanya Prabhu K., and Dhiraj Kumar Poonia

Summary

Posterior cervical foraminotomy is a method aimed at relieving compression of the cervical nerve root in patients with radiculopathy. This can be performed as an open technique as well as minimally invasive technique. It avoids ventral approach related complication while preserving range of motion.

Major indications are cervical unilateral radiculopathy often caused by foraminal soft disk herniation, lateral recess stenosis or bone spur, and focal pathologies due to ligament flavum hypertrophy or ossification, facet joint, and ligament flavum cyst. Mainstay techniques include microsurgical techniques (open microscopic procedure, tubular retractor procedure) and endoscopic techniques (full endoscopic procedure, biportal endoscopic procedure, Destandau procedure). During a posterior cervical foraminotomy, typically less than 50% of the facet joint is removed (approximately 30%), thereby maintaining stability.

Outcomes for posterior cervical foraminotomy have been reported to be effective in more than 90% of patients with cervical monoradiculopathy. Unilateral foraminotomy maintains the motion of the operated segment, thereby causing less stress on the adjacent segments. Minimally invasive techniques result in shorter surgical time and hospital stay and decreased postoperative analgesic usage.

Keywords: cervical radiculopathy, posterior cervical foraminotomy, cervical neural foramina decompression

43.1 Key Points

- Posterior cervical foraminotomy was described by Frykholm[1] and Scoville et al[2] as a method aimed at relieving compression of the cervical nerve root in patients with radiculopathy.
- The ventral approach related complications, such as postoperative dysphagia, hematoma, recurrent laryngeal nerve palsy, adjacent

segmental diseases, pseudoarthrosis, and instrument-related complications, can be avoided with posterior approach while preserving the range of motion.[3]

- Although open procedure is a well-accepted technique, it can also be performed using minimally invasive techniques (tubular retractor and endoscopy) which are advantageous due to minimal blood loss and a shorter hospital stay.

43.2 Indications and Contraindications

43.2.1 Indications

- Cervical unilateral radiculopathy, often caused by foraminal soft disk herniation, lateral recess stenosis or bone spur, and focal pathologies due to ligamentum flavum hypertrophy or ossification, facet joint cyst, and ligamentum flavum cyst.
- Failure to improve after an appropriate trial of conservative care for a minimum of 6 weeks or presence of a neurological deficit.
- When anterior approach is not suitable (recurrent surgery, difficult anterior approach, cervicothoracic levels, previous radiation, history of dysphagia).
- Patients who are at high risk for nonunion might be better candidates for laminoforaminotomy than anterior cervical diskectomy and fusion (ACDF).

43.2.2 Contraindications

- Primary axial neck pain.
- Segmental kyphosis.
- Segmental instability.
- Bilateral foraminal stenosis.
- Osteophytes ventral to the nerve root.
- Large central disk herniation and central spinal canal stenosis.
- Evidence of spinal cord compression or myelomalacia.
- Symptoms of cervical myelopathy.
- Symptoms not concordant with findings on imaging studies.

43.3 Technique

43.3.1 Patient Positioning

- After induction of general anesthesia and fiberoptic endotracheal intubation, the patient is positioned in a prone position with the head fixed in a Mayfield or Sugita head frame or positioned on a horseshoe head holder. Position the table in a reverse Trendelenburg position to reduce intraoperative bleeding.

43.3.2 Preparation and Draping

- Confirm the correct operative level with C-arm image intensifier and metallic marker.
- Draping is done in such way to expose C2 to C7.

43.3.3 Surgical Techniques

- Microsurgical techniques:
  - Open microscopic procedure.
  - Tubular retractor procedure.
- Endoscopic techniques:
  - Full endoscopic procedure.
  - Biportal endoscopic procedure.
  - Destandau procedure.

43.4 Microsurgical Techniques

43.4.1 Open Microscopic Procedure

- It is a midline posterior approach using William's retractor.
- A small 3 cm long posterior midline incision is made till the exposure of the nuchal fascia.
- The paraspinal muscles are separated only on the side of the disk prolapse. Subperiosteal dissection is carried out from spinous process to laterally up to the facet joint of the involved level with a Bovie cautery.
- Place a William's hemilaminectomy retractor and confirm level radiologically.
- Proceed to foraminotomy (see below).

43.4.2 Tubular Retractor Procedure

- It is a transmuscular approach using tubular retractor.
- Incision site is marked with initial dilator and lateral fluoroscopy.
- A 2-cm skin incision is made approximately 2 cm lateral to the midline, and the fascia is incised to enable passage of the tubular dilators.
- Introduce the initial dilator through the skin incision and advance to the inferomedial edge of the rostral lateral mass at the operative level.

- Use sequential dilators to create a working portal within the soft tissues.
- Center the final working tube over the lateral aspect of the lamina and medial facet joint of the appropriate operative level.
- The tubular retractor system of appropriate length is introduced medially and fixed using a flexible arm attached to the operating table.
- Use lateral fluoroscopy to confirm the level.
- Proceed to foraminotomy.

43.5 Foraminotomy Under Microscope

- Expose the cranial and caudal lamina of the appropriate level and expose the medial parts of the capsule of the facet joint.
- Start the laminoforaminotomy using a high-speed bur (side-cutting matchstick bur or diamond bur).
- Begin at the junction of the lamina and facet with an even amount of the cranial and caudal lamina removed, starting medially and working laterally toward the facet joints. See **Fig. 43.1** and **Fig. 43.2**.

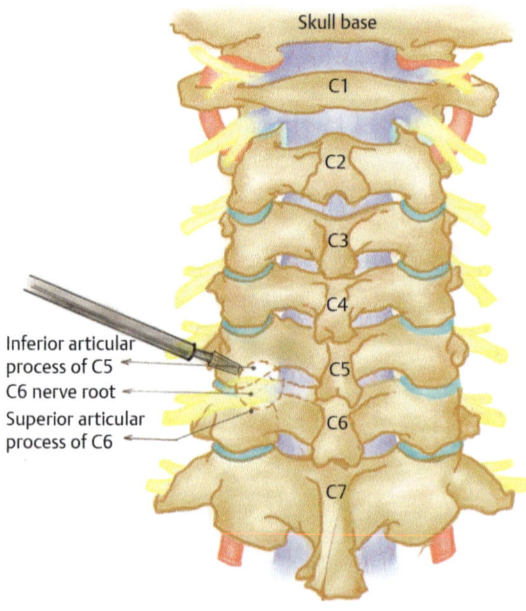

Fig. 43.1 Schematic drawing of a cervical segment (posterior view) and the amount of bone removal for foraminotomy (dotted circle).

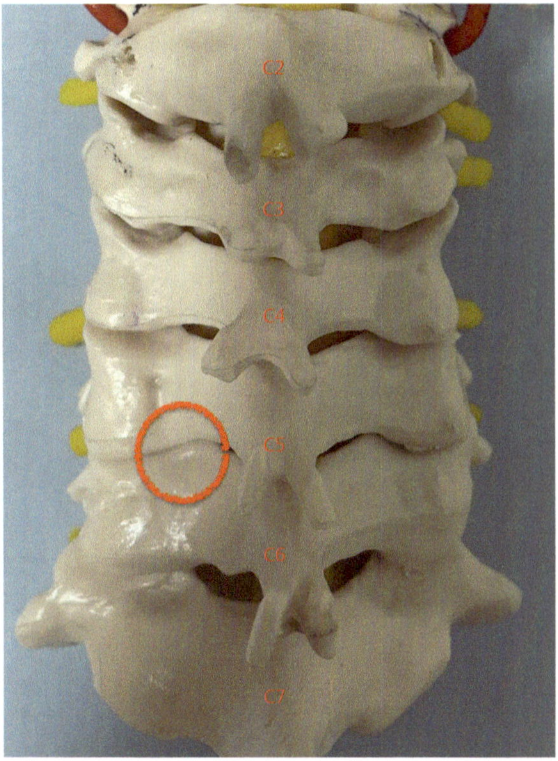

Fig. 43.2 Cervical spine model showing the small of area of bone to be removed for foraminotomy (*red circle*).

- Identify the medial and cephalad margins of the pedicle to orient with respect to the neural foramen.
- Continue the foraminotomy until the medial margin of the pedicle begins to fall away, at which point approximately one-third to one-half of the medial facet should have been removed (preserve at least 50% of the facet).
- A small laminotomy in the caudal lamina can be used to improve visualization of the nerve root.
- With a curette or nerve hook identify the superior border of the caudal pedicle. Once the top of the pedicle is identified, use a nerve hook to assess how "tight" the foramen is.
- Use a 2-mm Kerrison punch to remove bone until the amount of osseous resection and the room available to the nerve are satisfactory. Open the

ligamentum flavum with a nerve hook or a dissector, and resect it with a small Kerrison rongeur.

- Gently retract the nerve superiorly with a nerve hook to identify any disk fragments. Remove any visible, loose disk fragments with a small disk (micro-pituitary) rongeur.
- Contained disk fragments require incision of the posterior longitudinal ligament.
- Remove foraminal osteophytes with the use of a Kerrison rongeur.
- Control bleeding with hemostatic gelatin foam or flowable gelatin–thrombin matrix and bipolar cautery (use bipolar cautery on readily identifiable and discrete bleeders and avoid cautery directly on the neural structures).
- Copiously irrigate the wound with normal saline solution.
- With 1–0 Vicryl reapproximate the deep cervical fascia and close subcutaneous layer with inverted interrupted sutures.
- Close the wound with a subcuticular 2–0 Monocryl (Ethicon).

43.6 Endoscopic Techniques

43.6.1 Full Endoscopic Posterior Cervical Foraminotomy

- It is a transmuscular approach using endoscope and through "single" incision.
- Skin marking is done under guidance of anteroposterior (AP) and lateral view cervical fluoroscopy aiming the lateral margin of interlaminar space and medial border of facet joint junction (the "v" point) at appropriate level.
- An 8-mm skin incision is made at the "v" point and obturator inserted and docked, and the position confirmed fluoroscopically.
- A 7.3-mm-outer-diameter, 30-degree-viewing-angle endoscope with a 4.7-mm working channel (Joimax GmbH, Karlsruhe, Germany) is used for the procedure under continuous normal saline irrigation at the pressure of 25 mmHg.
- Soft tissue dissection is done with the radiofrequency probe and endoscopic forceps.
- V point is identified and confirmed on fluoroscopy; medial aspect of lateral mass and facet joint is drilled with a long, straight, high-speed drill to create a working window.
- About 3 mm of lateral inferior aspect of upper lamina is drilled followed by about 3 mm of the medial inferior portion of inferior articular facet and

then the medial superior aspect of superior articular facet of caudal vertebra is drilled.

- Ligamentum flavum is resected without violating the prominent venous plexus around the nerve root.
- Inspect the exiting nerve root and lateral third of the spinal cord, both of which are closely related to the pedicle of caudal vertebra ("V" point foraminotomy).
- After foraminotomy the working channel is advanced and rotated with open bevel facing away from the axilla of the spinal cord and exiting nerve root.
- Retract the exiting nerve root gently and expose the underlying prolapsed disk fragment. Use endoscopic forceps and Kerrison rongeurs to retrieve the prolapsed disk fragment.
- Uncovertebral hypertrophy is taken down with a cutter or a drill.
- Secure hemostasis with radiofrequency probe.
- Final inspection of neural elements is done to assess completeness of decompression as evidenced by pulsatile neural elements under irrigation fluid.
- The wound is closed in layers with dermabond to the skin.

43.7 Biportal Endoscopic Posterior Cervical Foraminotomy

- It is a transmuscular approach using endoscope and through "two" incisions.
- Stand on the opposite side of the lesion.
- Under the guidance of C-arm fluoroscopy, make two 0.5-cm long skin incisions vertically along lateral margin of the spinous process. The first skin incision for a cranial portal is made at the level of the upper cervical spinous process while the other skin incision for a caudal portal is made at the level of lower cervical spinous process 2 cm apart from the first one.
- Serial dilators are used to dissect the neck muscle and a 0-degree endoscope (Striker) is inserted through the cranial portal after inserting the cannula.
- A saline irrigation system is applied.
- Surgical instruments are inserted through the caudal working portal.
- Triangulation is performed with the endoscope and instrument on the "V-point."
- Bleeding is controlled with a radiofrequency probe.
- The V-point is identified and the inferolateral portion of the upper lamina, superolateral part of the lower lamina, and medial point of the facet joint (V-point) are drilled with endoscopic drills.
- Drilling around the V-point is continued till the caudocranial margin of ligamentum flavum is exposed. The boundary of decompression is

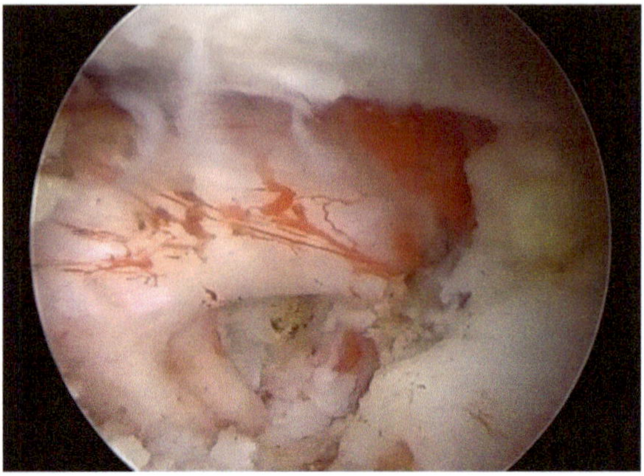

Fig. 43.3 Intraoperative endoscopic image after biportal endoscopic foraminotomy. Decompressed spinal canal and nerve root after foraminotomy. (Copyright of Saishree Hospital.)

extended to the further lateral part of the foramen by using a bendable 3.5-mm diamond bur.

- Ligamentum flavum is removed piecemeal in the direction of root from the thecal sac.
- Hemostasis around root origin is obtained by using the small radiofrequency ablator.
- Sufficient foraminal decompression is verified by passing a ball tip probe through the foraminal canal without any resistance.
- Diskectomy is done by using the hook and the pituitary forceps.
- Scope retractor is used to acquire enough space for diskectomy with the root protection.
- Additional pediculotomy is performed, in case of very narrow operative space in axilla region of root, before root manipulation for diskectomy.
- Check for complete decompression (**Fig. 43.3**) by dura pulsation and confirm meticulous hemostasis is achieved.
- The wound is closed with subcutaneous suture and skin tape.

43.8 Endoscopic Posterior Cervical Foraminotomy—Destandau's Technique

- It is an endoscopic approach using the ENDOSPINE (material designed by Destandau and manufactured by KARL STORZ USA).

- Localization is done with special localizing pin which can be moved in three different planes.
- Incision—paramedian to midline by 1 to 1.5 cm.
- Fascia is cut and muscles separated off the midline spinous process and laminae.
- The disk level is confirmed, and the ENDOSPINE is inserted and placed against the lamina. Endoscopic drill is used to thin out the cranial and caudal laminae and then 2-mm, 45-degree Kerrison punch is used to remove laminae.
- The foramen is opened till the nerve root is decompressed adequately, with one-third or half of the facet joint removed.
- Nerve hook with blunt tip is used to separate the extruded disk and then the disk fragment is pulled down off the axilla of the nerve root.
- If there is bony stenosis causing root compression then a significant part of laminae has to be removed for adequate root decompression.
- Epidural bleeding is controlled with endoscopic bipolar or Gelfoam or powdered Gelfoam.
- Ultrasonic bone rasp or knife is used to remove bone near the nerve root. This safely removes bone while the soft tissue is not at all affected.
- Muscle and fascia are closed with 2–0 taper-cutting Vicryl, and skin is closed with 3–0 Vicryl with subcuticular stitches.

43.9 Complications of Posterior Cervical Foraminotomy

- Wound dehiscence.
- Wound infection—superficial and deep (1.9 and 0.9% respectively).[4]
- Cerebrospinal fluid leak (0.6–2.5%).[5,6]
- Neurological deterioration as a result of direct trauma to the nerve root or spinal cord or to epidural hematoma (1.2–2.3%).[5,6]
- Persistence of symptoms due to residual nerve root compression, epidural scarring, early recurrent disk herniation (5.1–8%).[5,6]
- Recurrent disk herniation (7.6%).[6]
- Iatrogenic instability due to excess resection of the facet joint (4.9%).[5]
- Adjacent segment disease requiring reoperation after posterior foraminotomy estimated at 0.9% per year per level.[7]

43.10 Postoperative Care

- Mobilize the patient on the same day of surgery.
- No need for external bracing, and patients are encouraged to perform normal range of motion without restriction.

- Pain control by simple analgesics.
- Discharge patients on postoperative day 1 or 2.

43.11 Outcomes

- Outcomes for posterior cervical foraminotomy have been reported to be good in 90 to 96% of patients with cervical monoradiculopathy.[5,6,8]
- Unilateral foraminotomy maintains the motion of the operated segment and thereby causes less stress on the adjacent segments.[9]
- Minimally invasive techniques result in shorter surgical time and hospital stay and decreased postoperative analgesic usage.[10]

43.12 Surgical Pearls

- Removal of more than 50% of the facet could compromise torsional stability of the cervical spine.
- The entire length of the foramen can be enlarged safely with the use of curettes or a high-speed drill with preservation of more than 50% of the facet by initially working parallel and just inferior to the nerve root and then, as more room is gained, removing the rim just dorsal to the nerve root.
- Gentle retraction of the nerve root is a must to avoid neurological deterioration.
- Avoid placing the Kerrison rongeur between the posterior and anterior rootlets and avoid avulsion.
- Be especially vigilant about the C5 nerve root (high risk of deltoid weakness).

Common Clinical Questions

1. What are the most common indications for a posterior cervical foraminotomy?
2. When do you choose posterior cervical foraminotomy over anterior surgery?
3. What are the options for performing a posterior cervical foraminotomy?
4. How much of the facet joint can be safely removed without creating instability?
5. How will you control epidural bleeding?

Answers to Common Clinical Questions

1. Cervical unilateral radiculopathy, often caused by foraminal soft disk herniation, lateral recess stenosis or bone spur, and focal pathologies due to ligamentum flavum hypertrophy or ossification, facet joint cyst, and ligamentum flavum cyst with progressive or intractable cervical radiculopathy.
2. Posterior cervical nerve root decompression is chosen over anterior approach if an anterior approach is not suitable (recurrent surgery, difficult anterior approach, cervicothoracic levels, previous radiation, history of dysphagia).
3. Microscopic procedure with a midline incision and para midline approach using tubular retractor OR endoscopic procedures (full endoscopic, biportal endoscopic, and Destandau's technique) are the options.
4. Removal of more than 50% of the facet significantly compromises torsional stability of the cervical spine. During a posterior cervical foraminotomy, typically less than 50% of the facet joint is removed (approximately 30%).
5. Place the operating table in a reverse Trendelenburg position. Control bleeding with hemostatic gelatin foam or flowable gelatin–thrombin matrix or bipolar cautery. (Use bipolar cautery on readily identifiable and discrete bleeders and avoid cautery directly on the neural structures.)

Acknowledgments

Thanks to Dr. Ketan Deshpande for the details and figure regarding biportal endoscopic procedure. Thanks to Dr. Srinivas Rohidas for the details regarding Destandau procedure. Thanks to Dr. Vibha for the drawing.

References

1. Frykholm R. Lower cervical nerve roots and their investments. Acta Chir Scand. 1951; 101(6):457–471
2. Scoville WB, Whitcomb BB, McLaurin R. The cervical ruptured disc; report of 115 operative cases. Trans Am Neurol Assoc. 1951; 56:222–224
3. Lin GX, Rui G, Sharma S, Kotheeranurak V, Suen TK, Kim JS. Does the neck pain, function, or range of motion differ after anterior cervical fusion, cervical disc replacement, and posterior cervical foraminotomy? World Neurosurg. 2019; 129:e485–e493
4. Ng MK, Emara AK, Rajan PV, et al. Single-level posterior cervical foraminotomy associated with increased incidence of early postoperative wound infection rates relative to anterior cervical discectomy with fusion and cervical disc arthroplasty. J Spine Surg. 2023; 9(1):54–64

5. Jagannathan J, Sherman JH, Szabo T, Shaffrey CI, Jane JA. The posterior cervical foraminotomy in the treatment of cervical disc/osteophyte disease: a single-surgeon experience with a minimum of 5 years' clinical and radiographic follow-up. J Neurosurg Spine. 2009; 10(4):347–356
6. Jödicke A, Daentzer D, Kästner S, Asamoto S, Böker DK. Risk factors for outcome and complications of dorsal foraminotomy in cervical disc herniation. Surg Neurol. 2003; 60(2):124–129, discussion 129–130
7. Skovrlj B, Gologorsky Y, Haque R, Fessler RG, Qureshi SA. Complications, outcomes, and need for fusion after minimally invasive posterior cervical foraminotomy and microdiscectomy. Spine J. 2014; 14(10):2405–2411
8. Fehlings MG, Gray RJ. Posterior cervical foraminotomy for the treatment of cervical radiculopathy. J Neurosurg Spine. 2009; 10(4):343–344, author reply 344–346
9. Cho TG, Kim YB, Park SW. Long term effect on adjacent segment motion after posterior cervical foraminotomy. Korean J Spine. 2014; 11(1):1–6
10. Platt A, Gerard CS, O'Toole JE. Comparison of outcomes following minimally invasive and open posterior cervical foraminotomy: description of minimally invasive technique and review of literature. J Spine Surg. 2020; 6(1):243–251

44 Cervical Open Reduction Techniques: Anterior and Posterior Approaches

Glenn A. Gonzalez, Ahilan Sivaganesan, George M. Ghobrial, and James S. Harrop

Summary

This chapter comprehensively reviews cervical open reduction techniques, detailing both anterior and posterior approaches. It begins with an analysis of the mechanisms underlying cervical facet dislocations, typically induced by high-energy trauma. Key acute management strategies are delineated, emphasizing reduction and realignment procedures and the necessity of recreating the injury's force vectors for optimal outcomes.

The anterior approach section thoroughly discusses neuromonitoring, dissection, and diskectomy, offering a procedural guide. The posterior approach section provides insights into positioning, incision, dissection, and reduction techniques.

Complications such as wound infection, graft site pain, nerve injuries, and delayed fusion are critically examined. The chapter concludes with postoperative care guidelines, underscoring the importance of immobilization and serial radiographic evaluations to ensure stability and promote recovery.

Keywords: cervical facet dislocation, anterior reduction, posterior reduction, neuromonitoring, diskectomy, cervical spine, spinal alignment, decompression, surgical complications, postoperative care

44.1 Key Points

- Cervical facet dislocations result from high-energy traumatic forces transmitted typically through *flexion/distraction* vectors.
  - A flexion, rotational, and lateral force can result in a unilateral facet dislocation.
  - If the mechanism of injury involves *flexion/compression* forces (e.g., diving headfirst into a shallow pool), then facet and vertebral body fractures may be encountered in the form of comminuted, dislocated, and/or perched facets.

  - A very severe flexion/distraction injury with a compression component may result in a teardrop fracture which is typically accompanied by a severe neurologic injury.
- Rule of thumb: A unilateral facet dislocation results in 25% displacement (*anterolisthesis*) of one vertebral body on another (as seen on lateral plain radiographs or computed tomography [CT] scan of the cervical spine); bilateral facet dislocations are associated with a 50% or greater anterolisthesis.
- Acute management usually consists of reduction of the dislocated joints and the realignment of fractured cervical segments, through either open surgical intervention or axial cervical traction, thus decompressing the canal.
- Recreating the force vectors of the mechanism of injury can facilitate reduction of the facets or deformity and realign the spine. For example, the cervical spine is flexed and distracted to realign the facets if the mechanism of injury was flexion/distraction.
- The open anterior approach allows for the removal of extruded disk before reduction of a dislocated facet. This approach may also be effective for reducing some fractures and dislocations.
- Posterior instrumentation reestablishes the posterior tension band.

44.2 Indications

Cervical open reduction can restore spinal alignment, decompress the neural elements, and establish rigid internal fixation.

- Cervical open reduction is indicated when:
  - Decompression of neural elements is required.
  - Closed reduction fails.
  - Certain contraindications for closed reduction are present:
    - The patient has altered mental status.
    - Skull fracture precludes tong or traction device placement.
    - A relative contraindication is a rigid spine such as in ankylosing spondylitis.

44.3 Technique

44.3.1 Anterior Approach[5]

- Neuromonitoring (somatosensory-evoked potentials [SSEPs], motor-evoked potentials [MEPs]) and electromyography (EMG) allow monitoring of spinal cord function during spinal manipulation.

- Typically coordinated with a neuroanesthesiologist with the use of total intravenous anesthesia (TIVA). Avoid use of volatile inhaled anesthetics, such as
  - IV propofol: 50 to 150 μg/kg/min with IV short-acting narcotic agent (e.g., remifentanil) if using neuromonitoring.
- Localization of the cervical fracture level using fluoroscopy or plain radiographs.
- Anatomic localization:
  - C4–C5 disk space: Level of the thyroid cartilage.
  - C5–C6 disk space: Level of the cricoid cartilage.
  - C6–C7 disk space vertebrae: Carotid tubercle (the transverse process of C6).
- If a significant herniated disk is compressing the neural elements, a complete diskectomy can be performed prior to anterior or posterior reduction.

Superficial dissection:

- The use of surface landmarks, skin marking, and pre-radiologic screening help accurately determine the incision level and size required.
- Either a large transverse or longitudinal incision can provide exposure to a wide area of the spine. There may be other injuries needing to be addressed, so wide exposure is beneficial.[6]
- Once through the skin, the platysma may be split in the same direction as the skin incision or incised.
- The approach utilizes fascial planes between the sternocleidomastoid and the longus colli muscles.

Deep dissection:

- Blunt dissection: Retract the carotid sheath laterally and the trachea/esophagus medially with retractors to expose the anterior spinal column. The anterior longitudinal ligament (ALL) may be disrupted because of trauma. Typically, there is prevertebral swelling and a retropharyngeal hematoma.
- Dissect the longus colli laterally with monopolar cautery to expose the cervical vertebrae. It provides a visual guide to the midline.
- In unilateral dislocations, the superior vertebral body will be rotated away from the side of dislocation. If using Caspar pins, place the pins in the anatomic midline of the vertebral body, not the visualized midline.
- The annulus is incised with a scalpel as far laterally as possible near the uncovertebral joints.
- The disk and posterior longitudinal ligament (PLL) are removed with curettes and with Kerrison and pituitary rongeurs until the dura is visualized. The PLL is often ruptured with a bilateral dislocation.

- Caspar retractors are placed, with pins one level above and below the subluxed and dislocated segments.
  - Angulate pins divergently to place the spine in kyphotic (flexed) posture for distraction. (This is opposite of a degenerative case.)
  - Distract Caspar pins; the superior body will rotate back to its normal position and become flush with the inferior body with reduction (**Fig. 44.1**).

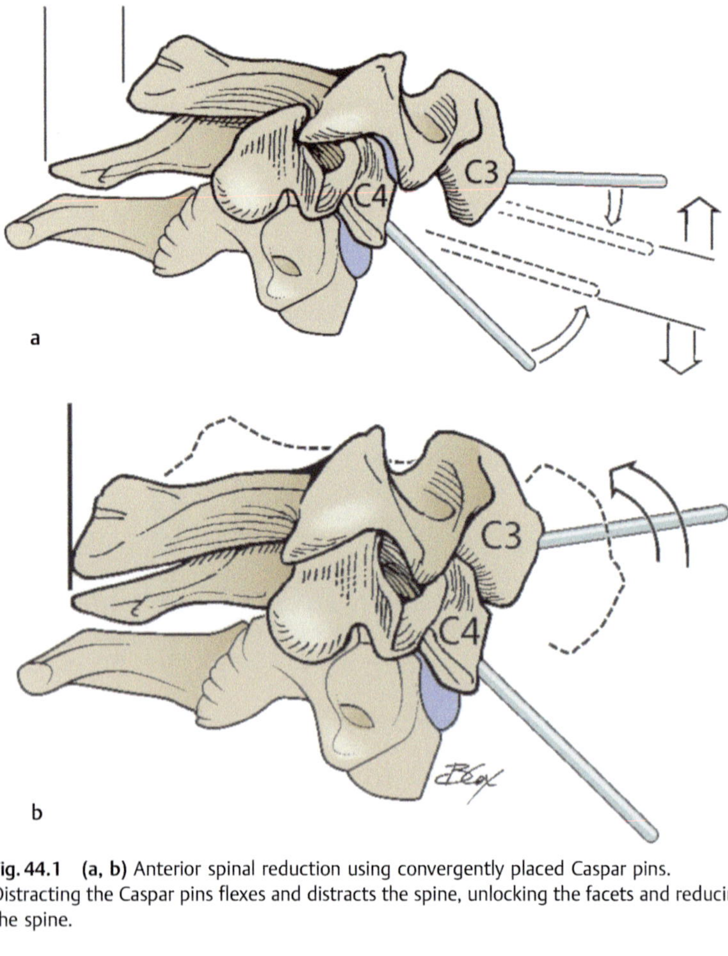

Fig. 44.1 (a, b) Anterior spinal reduction using convergently placed Caspar pins. Distracting the Caspar pins flexes and distracts the spine, unlocking the facets and reducing the spine.

- After the desired spinal alignment is achieved, a tricortical bone graft harvested from the anterior superior iliac crest or allograft may be used for arthrodesis.
- Anterior plate placement if the spine was reduced: Screws anchoring the plate should terminate by the middle third of the vertebral body to avoid violation of end plates.

44.3.2 Posterior Approach

- More commonly used when there is disruption of the posterior ligamentous complex and associated facet fractures preventing closed reduction.

Positioning:

- Prone position in Mayfield head holder (Schaerer Mayfield; Randolph, Massachusetts) or Gardner-Wells tongs, and make a midline incision.

Superficial dissection and deep dissection:

- A midline incision is made and carried down through the subcutaneous tissue and the fascia to the tips of the spinous processes.
- Often the tissue will be disrupted, and tissue planes are lost. This can result in significant bleeding.
- Localize levels with radiographs.
- Dissection of the paraspinal muscles in a subperiosteal fashion from the corresponding laminae. Be careful in that often fractures are not attached, and external forces can result in neuronal compression. Subperiosteal dissection helps to minimize bleeding. Given the distorted anatomy from fractures and displacement, there can be atypical bony defects with exposed dura. For this reason, care must be taken when using monopolar electrocautery during this exposure process.
- Reduction can be performed with direct distraction using two towel clips in opposite directions on the spinous processes, using a leveraging mechanism (**Fig. 44.2**).
- Alternatively, the superior articulating process of the inferior cervical facet can be drilled away to facilitate reduction.
- Once decompression and reduction are achieved, the spine is locked into place using either lateral mass screws and rods or posterior wiring techniques.
- Decortication of the facets and supplemental bone graft placement in the lateral gutters help with arthrodesis.

44.4 Complications

- Wound infection (increased likelihood in trauma and the neurologically injured population).

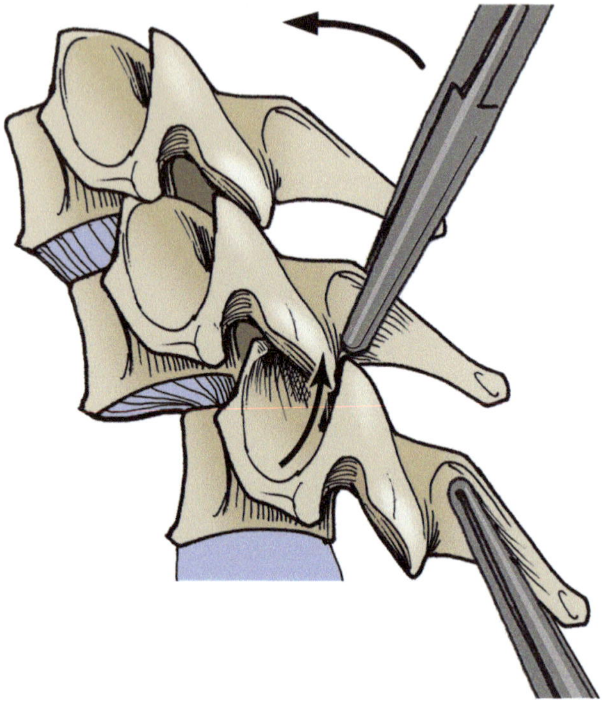

Fig. 44.2 Posterior spinal reduction using two towel clips. The inferior articulating facet of the superior vertebral body is lifted above and over the superior articulating facet of the inferior vertebral body, reducing the spine.

- Graft donor site pain from autograft, if taken. Allograft bone is an alternative but may have a lower fusion rate.
- Anterior exposure (particularly right-sided approach) may result in injury to the recurrent laryngeal nerve resulting in speech and swallowing issues.
- Esophageal perforation:
  - Maintain situational awareness of esophagus at all times.
  - Avoid drill use outside of disk space.
- Carotid injury: Carotid artery thrombosis, occlusion, or laceration most likely related to retraction. Vagal nerve injury might also occur due to violation of the carotid sheath.
- Thrombosis of internal jugular vein (IJVT) is a rare event: Pulmonary embolism incidence from IJVT is approximately 2 to 3%.[7,8,9,10]

- Thoracic duct injury in exposing lower cervical spine, primarily on the left. Thoracic duct commonly drains in the left jugulo-subclavian junction (Pirogoff's angle) where it reenters the systemic venous circulation.
- Vertebral artery injury during anterior cervical approach:
  - Evaluate preoperative imaging for anatomical deviations of the vertebral artery.
  - Avoid violation of the superior two-thirds of the uncovertebral joints.
- Vertebral artery injury during posterior fixation:
  - Maintain lateral trajectory while placing lateral mass screws in the subaxial cervical spine.
- Horner syndrome: The sympathetic chain lies adjacent and anterior to the longus colli muscles. Irritation of the sympathetic nerves or stellate ganglion is commonly associated with cervical retractors placed above the longus coli. To avoid this complication, retractors should be placed under the medial border of the longus colli muscle.
- Cerebrospinal fluid (CSF) leak (often associated with original trauma and dural injury).
- Retropharyngeal hematoma: Placement of cervical drains may reduce the risk of postoperative hematoma formation. If such a hematoma is encountered, it must be treated with emergent surgical decompression.
- Delayed fusion increases the likelihood of screw loosening, plate migration, graft migration, and ultimately construct breakage.

44.5 Postoperative Care

- Immobilization for 6 weeks: Cervical orthosis.
- Serial radiographic examination: Anteroposterior, lateral, and swimmer's views.
- Flexion–extension views for assessment of stability at 6 weeks.

44.6 Outcomes

- Kwon et al[1] conducted a prospective randomized controlled trial comparing anterior and posterior fixation for unilateral cervical facet injuries and reported equal efficacy between the two techniques. Posterior approach should be employed for end plate fractures.
- Johnson et al[2] reported a 13% incidence of loss of postoperative radiographic alignment during follow-up of cervical facet fracture-dislocations treated with only anterior decompression and fusion.
- Reindl et al[3] reported on 41 consecutive patients with unstable dislocations/subluxations, of whom 8 required anterior reduction after

failure of Gardner-Wells traction; in addition, 2 of those 8 failed, requiring posterior surgery as well.

- Fehlings et al reported on 44 consecutive patients treated with posterior cervical fusion for traumatic instability. Long-term follow-up revealed that the cervical spine was successfully stabilized in 93% of cases.[4]
- Matz et al[11] reported that anterior cervical diskectomy with fusion (ACDF) is a treatment strategy for single-level disease with regard to functional outcome (Class II). ACDF may achieve a more rapid reduction of neck and arm pain compared to ACD with a reduced risk of kyphosis, although functional outcomes may be similar. Anterior cervical plating (ACDF with instrumentation) improves arm pain (but not other clinical parameters) better than ACDF in the treatment of two-level disease (Class II). With respect to single-level disease, plating may reduce the risk of pseudarthrosis and graft problems (Class III) but does not necessarily improve clinical outcome alone (Class II).

44.7 Surgical Pearls

- Best treated anteriorly: Large disk herniation with severe cord compression so that spinal cord can be decompressed before distraction.
- Best treated posteriorly: Hyperflexion injury, including PLL injury, unilateral and bilateral facet dislocation without anterior cervical disk herniation.
- Anteriorly, avoid overdistraction of the cervical spine during placement of the interbody graft. As a result of the ligamentous laxity prevalent in spinal injury, it is often easy to overdistract.
- Posteriorly, be mindful of laminar fractures during exposure. Heat from a Bovie cautery can damage the dura and cause CSF leaks when transmitted through fractured laminae.

Common Clinical Questions

1. When should anterior reduction be used when closed reduction is not possible?
2. When should open reduction be performed?
3. Postoperatively after anterior cervical diskectomy with fusion, the patient has a hoarse voice and difficulty swallowing. What should the clinician be concerned about?

Answers to Common Clinical Questions

1. When a large anterior disk herniation is present with severe cord compression.
2. It should be performed when decompression of neural elements is required, closed reduction fails, or closed reduction is contraindicated.
3. Injury to the recurrent laryngeal nerve on exposure.

References

1. Kwon BK, Fisher CG, Boyd MC, et al. A prospective randomized controlled trial of anterior compared with posterior stabilization for unilateral facet injuries of the cervical spine. J Neurosurg Spine. 2007; 7(1):1–12
2. Johnson MG, Fisher CG, Boyd M, Pitzen T, Oxland TR, Dvorak MF. The radiographic failure of single segment anterior cervical plate fixation in traumatic cervical flexion distraction injuries. Spine. 2004; 29(24):2815–2820
3. Reindl R, Ouellet J, Harvey EJ, Berry G, Arlet V. Anterior reduction for cervical spine dislocation. Spine. 2006; 31(6):648–652
4. Fehlings MG, Cooper PR, Errico TJ. Posterior plates in the management of cervical instability: long-term results in 44 patients. J Neurosurg. 1994; 81 (3):341–349
5. Chang U, Lee MC, Kim DH. Anterior approach to the midcervical spine. In: Kim DH, Henn JS, Vaccaro A, et al, eds. Surgical Anatomy & Techniques to the Spine. Philadelphia, PA: Saunders Elsevier; 2006:45–56
6. Silber J, Albert T. Anterior and anterolateral, mid and lower cervical spine approaches: transverse and longitudinal (C3 to C7). In: Herkowitz HN, ed. The Cervical Spine Surgery Atlas. Philadelphia, PA: Lippincott Williams & Wilkins; 2003:91–98
7. Karim A, Knapp J, Nanda A. Internal jugular venous thrombosis as a complication after an elective anterior cervical discectomy: case report. Neurosurgery. 2006; 59(3):E705–E705, discussion E705
8. Ascher E, Salles-Cunha S, Hingorani A. Morbidity and mortality associated with internal jugular vein thromboses. Vasc Endovascular Surg. 2005; 39(4):335–339
9. Sheikh MA, Topoulos AP, Deitcher SR. Isolated internal jugular vein thrombosis: risk factors and natural history. Vasc Med. 2002; 7(3):177–179
10. Tajima H, Murata S, Kumazaki T, Ichikawa K, Tajiri T, Yamamoto Y. Successful interventional treatment of acute internal jugular vein thrombosis. AJR Am J Roentgenol. 2004; 182(2):467–469
11. Matz PG, Ryken TC, Groff MW, et al. Joint Section on Disorders of the Spine and Peripheral Nerves of the American Association of Neurological Surgeons and Congress of Neurological Surgeons. Techniques for anterior cervical decompression for radiculopathy. J Neurosurg Spine. 2009; 11(2):183–197

45 Surgical Resection of Spinal Vascular Lesions

James J. Zhou, Arnau Benet, Timothy D. Uschold, Alim P. Mitha, and Steve W. Chang

Summary

Early and definitive intervention for spinal vascular malformation is favored whenever feasible due to the typical malignant natural history of these lesions. Spinal angiography is a key step that must be performed preoperatively to better define each individual lesion. The appropriate type of surgical or endovascular intervention differs depending on the type of lesion being treated. Indications for surgery differ based on lesion type, such as cavernous malformations, arteriovenous malformations (AVMs), and arteriovenous fistulas (AVFs), with surgery recommended for accessible lesions and symptomatic cases. Regardless of the treatment methodology chosen, preservation of the anterior spinal artery is key to maintaining neurologic function. Open surgical treatment of spinal vascular lesions is primarily indicated for accessible cavernous malformations, symptomatic AVMs, and AVFs requiring definitive management. Surgery typically involves a posterior or posterolateral approach via laminectomy or laminoplasty. Precise dissection is necessary to avoid damaging critical structures such as the anterior spinal artery. Key techniques include linear pial openings, circumferential dissection, and intralesional coagulation. Intraoperative monitoring of somatosensory-evoked potentials and motor-evoked potentials is essential. Complications arising from intervention for spinal vascular malformations can include cerebrospinal fluid leaks, neurologic decline, and rebleeding. Postoperative angiography is essential to verify the efficacy of treatment.

Keywords: cavernous malformation, arteriovenous malformation, arteriovenous fistula, spine

45.1 Key Points

- The natural history of spinal vascular lesions is usually malignant. Depending on the eloquence of local tissue, early definitive treatment is favored whenever feasible.
- All arteriovenous (AV) lesions require preoperative spinal angiography.

- Preservation of the anterior spinal artery (ASA) is paramount during surgical treatment or embolization attempts.
- The optimal trajectory for the resection of spinal cavernous malformations is determined by the two-point method. A line connecting the center of the lesion with its most accessible margin determines the approach. Some lesions without pial contact may still be resected.
- Timing of surgical intervention after hemorrhage is controversial, although an acute hemorrhage could prompt early resection of some cavernomas.

45.2 Indications

- Cavernous malformations: Surgery is recommended for all accessible lesions that reach a pial surface. Small, deep-seated asymptomatic lesions can be treated with observation. Deep lesions with evidence of repeated hemorrhage or expansion should be considered for surgery.[1]
- Extradural–intradural AV malformations (AVMs): Palliative attempts at flow reduction and selective targeting of high-risk features are appropriate for progressive symptoms related to steal, repeated hemorrhage, mass effect, or congestion.
- Intramedullary and conus AVMs: Surgical resection, typically with preoperative embolization, is recommended if gross total excision can be achieved. Embolization alone for a cure has been demonstrated but remains controversial.
- Intradural–dorsal and intradural–ventral AV fistulas (AVFs): All require definitive treatment with either surgery or nonparticulate embolization. Surgical exploration is warranted if clinical history and imaging findings suggest an intradural–dorsal AVF despite negative angiographic findings.
- Extradural AVF: All require definitive treatment; endovascular intervention is favored. The typical goal is to use embolic agents to occlude the shunting zone, especially the proximal draining vein.[2]

45.3 Technique

- Posterior or posterolateral approach via laminectomy or laminoplasty:
  - Added costotransversectomy or facetectomy may allow further lateral exposure.
  - The dura is opened in a linear fashion, and the arachnoid is tacked to the dura.
  - If additional anterolateral visualization is necessary, the dentate ligaments may be transected and tacked contralaterally with 6–0 Prolene sutures (Ethicon Inc.; Cincinnati, Ohio) to facilitate gentle

rotation of the spinal cord. This technique can be done across several levels for maximum effect (**Fig. 45.1**).[3]
- Minimally invasive approaches using expandable tubular retractors have been described for resecting these lesions. These approaches provide the potential for complete resection while minimizing paraspinal muscle dissection. Further study is needed to determine whether these techniques are suitable for all types of spinal cavernomas.[4]

- Cavernous malformations:
  - When necessary, myelotomy is made sharply with a linear pial opening. Appropriate zones for entry into the cord include the dorsal midline and the lateral dorsal sulcus at the dorsal root entry zone. This trajectory enters the substantia gelatinosa. A third entry option is the lateral trajectory behind the dentate ligaments and between the dorsal and ventral spinocerebellar tracts (**Fig. 45.2**).[3]
  - The lesion is dissected circumferentially. Coagulation of the cavernoma may be necessary to shrink and debulk the lesion's interior. The associated venous anomaly should be preserved. Surrounding hemosiderin-stained spinal cord is not taken to avoid transgression into eloquent tissue.[1]
- Extradural AVF: Transarterial endovascular coil embolization is typically the preferred treatment modality, although transvenous routes have been described. Although less frequently used, microsurgical occlusion has also been an effective treatment for this condition.[5]

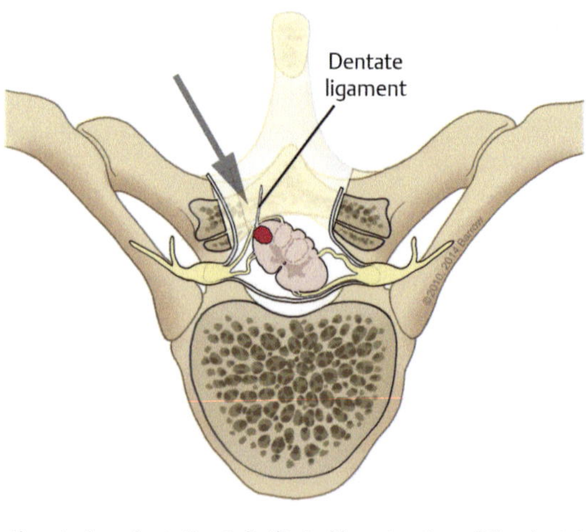

Fig. 45.1 Gentle spinal cord rotation is facilitated by retraction of the dentate ligament(s).[3] (Reproduced with permission from Barrow Neurological Institute, Phoenix, Arizona.)

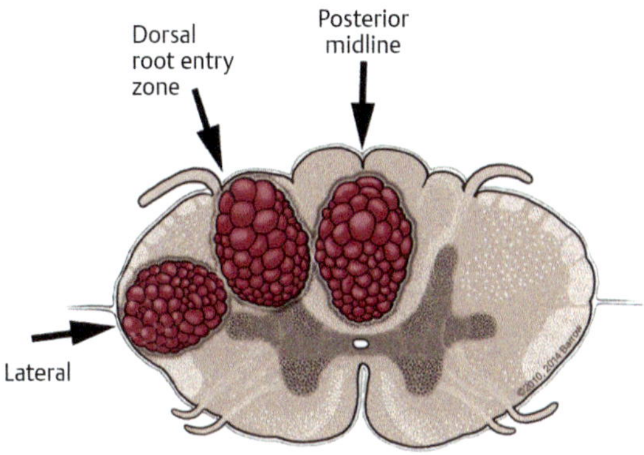

Fig. 45.2 Alternative posterior and posterolateral entry zones for a myelotomy.[3] (Reproduced with permission from Barrow Neurological Institute, Phoenix, Arizona.)

- Intradural–dorsal AVFs: After dural opening, the arterialized vein is followed to its intradural interface along the root sleeve, where the radicular artery pierces the dura. The intradural fistulous connection is clipped, cauterized, and transected. Several case series have been published in recent years detailing the successful treatment of these lesions via endovascular embolization.[6]
- Intradural–ventral AVFs: Anterior and posterolateral trajectories have been described. The fistula is cauterized and transected to preserve the arterial supply to the ASA, and the normal venous drainage is preserved. Venous varices can be further excised. Nonparticulate embolization may be useful in select cases, although surgery remains the gold standard.
- Extradural–intradural AVMs: Embolization may be the primary palliative modality for symptomatic steal, repeated hemorrhage, or vascular congestion. Surgery is typically reserved for relief of persistent, symptomatic mass effect.
- Intramedullary spinal AVMs: Arterial rather than venous feeders should be sharply dissected circumferentially, cauterized, and transected first. The largest draining vein is typically cauterized, transected, and removed last.

45.4 Complications

- Cerebrospinal fluid leak, wound complications.
- Delayed or acute neurologic decline: May be attributable to progressive venous thrombosis, especially in the setting of embolization for intradural–dorsal AVFs. Routine postprocedural heparinization is

considered in these patients. Blood pressure control is strict, and the judicious use of steroids is advised before intervention.
- Rebleeding: Can occur in incompletely resected cavernous malformations or other lesions. The estimated risk of rebleeding ranges from 1.6 to 30.7%, depending on the type of vascular anomaly and the patient population.[7]

45.5 Postoperative Care

- Postprocedural angiography or magnetic resonance angiography is essential to verify treatment effect, especially if new neurologic deficits appear.

45.6 Outcomes

- Cavernous malformations: Subtotal resection offers nominal benefit and could increase the risk of rebleeding.[8,9] Initial postoperative deterioration has been reported in 24 to 50% of cases, but long-term follow-up data suggest improved neurologic function in as many as 46 to 58%.
- Intradural–dorsal AVFs: The primary benefit of surgery over endovascular treatment is the reduced risk of recurrence. The initial success rate for surgery is as high as 98% versus 46 to 85% for successful embolization.[10] Nonetheless, endovascular capabilities are improving. Motor improvements have been reported in approximately 60% of patients, compared with 40% showing improvements in sphincter dysfunction (Aminoff-Logue scale, **Table 45.1**), irrespective of treatment modality. Numerically, improvements in Aminoff-Logue scale scores are typically modest (about 1 point).[5]
- Intradural–ventral AVFs: Available series are mostly small, but neurologic improvement or stabilization after surgery has been reported to range from 87.5 to 95% of cases. Preoperative embolization may be useful in limiting flow rate (and in some cases for cure), but incomplete occlusion has resulted in more modest improvements than surgery.[11] Certain subtypes of intradural–ventral AVFs, particularly high-flow and giant fistulas, may reasonably be treated via endovascular embolization, with obliteration rates of up to 75%.[12]
- Extradural AVFs: Outcomes reported in numerous case reports have been favorable regarding fistula obliteration and clinical improvement. For acute hematoma, surgical evacuation within 12 hours is important for favorable prognosis.
- Extradural–intradural AVMs: Most multimodality attempts are purely palliative. Rare cases may be amenable to embolization followed by operative resection.

Table 45.1 Aminoff-Logue scale

Gait dysfunction	
1.	Leg weakness or gait change without significant activity impairment
2.	Restricted walking but no DME assistance required
3.	Cane for ambulation
4.	Crutches or walker for ambulation
5.	Bed-bound, does not stand, confined to wheelchair
Urinary dysfunction	
1.	Hesitancy, urgency, or frequency
2.	Intermittent incontinence or retention
3.	Full incontinence or retention

Abbreviation: DME, durable medical equipment.
Source: Modified from Aminoff MJ, Logue V. The prognosis of patients with spinal vascular malformations. Brain 1974;(97):211–218.

- Intramedullary AVMs: Clinical improvement rates of 33 to 67% have been reported for surgery, compared with rates of 8 to 20% for clinical decline. Rates of postsurgical angiographic cure have ranged from 59 to 100%. Further endovascular data using Onyx are anticipated. The most appropriate and definitive strategy remains preoperative embolization (when technically appropriate) followed by microsurgical excision.
- Conus AVMs: Little published experience. Aggressive multimodality treatment can result in clinical improvement or stabilization in addition to angiographic cure.

45.7 Surgical Pearls

- Intraoperative electrophysiologic monitoring of somatosensory-evoked potentials (SSEPs) and motor-evoked potentials (MEPs) is essential for all cases. An 80% reduction in MEP amplitude or a 50% reduction in SSEP amplitude has been described as a threshold for significant intraoperative change. Transient changes in neuromonitoring have been found to have reduced risks for permanent postoperative neurologic deficits when compared to permanent changes during the resection of spinal cavernomas.[13]

- For AV lesions, serial indocyanine green angiography (ICG) or intraoperative spinal angiography is often useful before, during, and after resection.
- Anterior or anterolateral approaches for resecting spinal vascular lesions are seldom advised due to the risk of ASA compromise and poor dural closure.[14]
- Sharp rather than blunt dissection is favored when possible.
- If required, myelotomy should expose the entire cranial–caudal extent of the lesion to minimize parenchymal retraction and aid in visualizing feeding pedicles.
- Pressure measurements in the arterialized veins of intradural–dorsal AVFs can be transduced using a small-gauge needle. Pressure should more closely approximate central venous pressure following fistula obliteration.

Common Clinical Questions

1. Name the primary advantage of surgery (in terms of outcome) over embolization for intradural–dorsal AVFs.
2. Name three zones of entry for myelotomy from a posterior approach.
3. Name three intraoperative tools or strategies useful in guiding and confirming the treatment of AVMs and AVFs.

Answers to Common Clinical Questions

1. Decreased risk of recurrence with surgery.
2. Dorsal midline, dorsal lateral sulcus, and lateral between the nerve roots.
3. Intraoperative monitoring, ICG, and intraoperative spinal angiography.

References

1. Vishteh AG, Sankhla S, Anson JA, Zabramski JM, Spetzler RF. Surgical resection of intramedullary spinal cord cavernous malformations: delayed complications, long-term outcomes, and association with cryptic venous malformations. Neurosurgery. 1997; 41(5):1094–1100, discussion 1100–1101
2. Marcus J, Schwarz J, Singh IP, et al. Spinal dural arteriovenous fistulas: a review. Curr Atheroscler Rep. 2013; 15(7):335
3. Mitha AP, Turner JD, Spetzler RF. Surgical approaches to intramedullary cavernous malformations of the spinal cord. Neurosurgery. 2011; 68(2) Suppl Operative:317–324, discussion 324

4. Winkler EA, Lu A, Rutledge WC, et al. A mini-open transspinous approach for resection of intramedullary spinal cavernous malformations. J Clin Neurosci. 2018; 58:210–212
5. Ehresman J, Catapano JS, Baranoski JF, Jadhav AP, Ducruet AF, Albuquerque FC. Treatment of spinal arteriovenous malformation and fistula. Neurosurg Clin N Am. 2022; 33(2):193–206
6. Goyal A, Cesare J, Lu VM, et al. Outcomes following surgical versus endovascular treatment of spinal dural arteriovenous fistula: a systematic review and meta-analysis. J Neurol Neurosurg Psychiatry. 2019; 90(10): 1139–1146
7. Ren J, Hong T, Zeng G, et al. Characteristics and long-term outcome of 20 children with intramedullary spinal cord cavernous malformations. Neurosurgery. 2020; 86(6):817–824
8. Bakir A, Savas A, Yilmaz E, et al. Spinal intradural-intramedullary cavernous malformation. Case report and literature review. Pediatr Neurosurg. 2006; 42 (1):35–37
9. Santoro A, Piccirilli M, Brunetto GM, Delfini R, Cantore G. Intramedullary cavernous angioma of the spinal cord in a pediatric patient, with multiple cavernomas, familial occurrence and partial spontaneous regression: case report and review of the literature. Childs Nerv Syst. 2007; 23(11):1319–1326
10. Steinmetz MP, Chow MM, Krishnaney AA, et al. Outcome after the treatment of spinal dural arteriovenous fistulae: a contemporary single-institution series and meta-analysis. Neurosurgery. 2004; 55(1):77–87, discussion 87–88
11. Cho KT, Lee DY, Chung CK, Han MH, Kim HJ. Treatment of spinal cord perimedullary arteriovenous fistula: embolization versus surgery. Neurosurgery. 2005; 56(2):232–241, discussion 232–241
12. Gross BA, Du R. Spinal pial (type IV) arteriovenous fistulae: a systematic pooled analysis of demographics, hemorrhage risk, and treatment results. Neurosurgery. 2013; 73(1):141–151, discussion 151
13. Niedermeyer S, Szelenyi A, Schichor C, Tonn JC, Siller S. Intramedullary spinal cord cavernous malformations-association between intraoperative neurophysiological monitoring changes and neurological outcome. Acta Neurochir (Wien). 2022; 164(10):2595–2604
14. Connolly ES, Jr, Zubay GP, McCormick PC, Stein BM. The posterior approach to a series of glomus (Type II) intramedullary spinal cord arteriovenous malformations. Neurosurgery. 1998; 42(4):774–785, discussion 785–786

46 Freehand Thoracic Pedicle Screw Insertion

Kelly Chamberlin, Martin G. Piazza, and Michael Galgano

Summary
Freehand thoracic pedicle screw insertion is a valuable technique for spinal surgeons. This technique can even be employed in cases of spinal deformity. This chapter covers the indications, technique, special considerations in spinal deformity, complications, and postoperative care.

Keywords: freehand technique, pedicle screws, thoracic spine, spinal instrumentation

46.1 Key Points

- Thoracic pedicle screw fixation is the principal modality for posterior stabilization of the thoracic spine.
- Small pedicle dimensions and the proximity of the great vessels and neural elements all make placement of thoracic pedicle screws challenging.
- There are established techniques for safely and effectively placing thoracic pedicle screws using freehand techniques.
- For the experienced surgeon, freehand pedicle screws can be safely and efficiently placed even in deformity cases.

46.2 Indications

- Stabilization of the thoracic spine following traumatic or pathologic fracture.
- Stabilization after iatrogenic destabilization from decompression of degenerative, neoplastic, infectious, or inflammatory processes.
- Correction of deformity for restoration of sagittal or coronal balance.
- Freehand technique also allows for reduction in intraoperative radiation exposure to the patient, operating room staff, and surgeon.

46.3 Technique

- Preoperative considerations:
  - Overall health of the patient should be optimized as much as reasonably possible. Issues to address include, but are not limited to, smoking, obesity, cardiopulmonary status, life expectancy (especially in the setting of tumor), nutrition, narcotic or substance dependency, and mental health.
  - Preoperative imaging:
    - Standing 36-inch (long film or scoliosis) X-rays are important when considering long constructs and in instances of deformity correction.
    - Computed tomography (CT) analysis of pedicle size preoperatively is important to assist the surgeon in choosing the appropriate type and size of implant. We recommend obtaining preoperative CT scans to measure both pedicle length and width to choose appropriate screw sizes. The CT scan should include thin axial cuts through the disk space for best results.
- For deformity cases, we recommend maximizing the diameter and length of pedicle screws to withstand rotational and sagittal corrective forces.
- General (**Fig. 46.1**):
  - The authors prefer a freehand technique.[1] Other acceptable techniques include intraoperative fluoroscopy, CT, and image-based navigation.
  - Complications can be minimized by using sensory, motor, and electromyographic (EMG) neurophysiologic monitoring intraoperatively.
- Exposure:
  - A dorsal midline incision is performed with subperiosteal dissection. The lateral extent of dissection is performed until the lateral facets and transverse processes are visualized, taking care to preserve the facet capsules of the adjacent cranial and caudal levels.
  - Initial fluoroscopic localization is performed to identify the levels of fixation using either the ribs and/or the sacrum as radiographic landmarks. It is essential to identify anomalies on the preoperative imaging—assumptions cannot be made regarding these landmarks.
- Starting point:
  - In general, there is a uniform entry point that can be used for all levels: Just caudal to the junction of the lateral margin of the superior articulating process and the transverse process.
  - However, there are some very small differences in the entry point for T1–T3, which is in the midpoint to upper third of the thoracic transverse process, whereas at T4–T9 it is superior to the transverse process and at T10–T12 it is again at the midpoint of the transverse process.

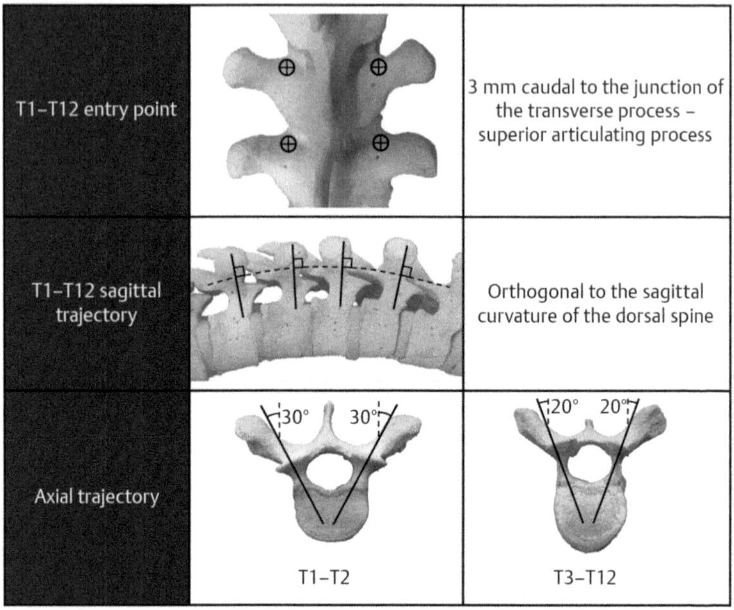

Fig. 46.1 Anatomic landmarks for placement of thoracic pedicle screws using freehand technique. (Copyright of Ali A. Baaj.)

- Dorsal cortical burring:
  - A small matchstick drill bit or awl[1] is used to create a posterior cortical breach, approximately 5 mm in depth. The pedicle "blush" can be visualized which suggests entrance into the cancellous bone of the pedicle.
- Trajectory:
  - The sagittal trajectory is orthogonal to the curvature of the dorsal spine.
  - The medial angulation generally decreases from about 30 degrees at T1 to −5 degrees at T12 as the morphology transitions to the lumbar spine.
  - Care must be taken with vertebral rotation in cases of scoliosis.
- Gearshift probing:
  - A sharp curved pedicle gearshift is used to create the trajectory through the cancellous bone of the pedicle and vertebral body to a depth determined based on preoperative imaging. In general, the length of the pedicle is reached at 20 mm and the trajectory with the gearshift is taken further into the vertebral body to about 30 mm total.
  - A thin, ball-ended feeling probe is used to assess all four walls and floor of the pedicle looking for cortical breaches. Particular attention should

be paid to the medial and inferior walls as they correspond to the spinal canal and neural foramen, respectively, and could result in cord/nerve injury without appropriate troubleshooting. Lateral breach could result in screws in the rib head or without sufficient purchase resulting in potential decreased strength in construct.

- Tapping:
  - Tapping is optional but, when performed, uses the same trajectory as the gearshift.
  - The pedicle tract is undertapped with a 1.0 mm less diameter tap than the intended screw (e.g., a 4.0-mm tap for a 5.5-mm diameter screw).[2]
- Screw placement (**Video 46.1**):
  - Screw length can be determined by measuring the depth of the bell-ended probe after tapping. Once the length has been determined, an appropriately sized screw is then slowly placed into the pedicle tract based on trajectories heretofore described.[1]
- Confirmation of accurate screw placement:
  - Final anteroposterior (AP) and lateral fluoroscopy is performed to assess for adequate screw placement. We recommend routine intraoperative (if available) or postoperative CT imaging to confirm accurate placement. However, many surgeons confirm adequate screw placement with plain AP and lateral X-rays.
- Salvage techniques:
  - A new trajectory can be created as already described. In these instances, a sequential tap may be used to ensure that the screw follows the new trajectory created in place of the previous one.
  - A combination of pedicle, laminar, and transverse process hooks or sublaminar wires may also be used when necessary.

46.4 Freehand Screws for Deformity: Special Considerations

- For the experienced deformity surgeon, freehand pedicle screws can be safely and efficiently placed. Fluoroscopic or imaging-guided techniques may increase the accuracy of pedicle screw insertion, but this must be weighed against the risk of increased radiation to the patient, operating room staff, and surgeon.
- Preoperative imaging evaluation:
  - Preoperative imaging must be studied particularly closely in deformity patients to determine:
    - Pedicle width and length at every level of planned instrumentation.
    - Coronal curvature.
    - Kyphosis.

    - Presence of hypoplastic pedicles.
    - Other anatomical abnormalities that may result in difficulty understanding unique patient anatomy intraoperatively.
- Additional techniques:
  - Funnel technique:
    - Another well-described technique is the "funnel technique" which imagines the pedicle as a funnel. This is well described by Yingsakmonkol et al.[2]
    - The top of the pedicle is visualized, the cancellous bone over it is removed, and then the posterior cortical portion of the pedicle (the part posterior to the isthmus) is used as a funnel to directly guide the pedicle probe through the pedicle isthmus into the rest of the pedicle (**Fig. 46.2**).
    - Then progressively larger taps are used to cut threads into the cortical bone of the pedicle isthmus and the appropriate size screw is placed.[2]
  - Removal of the inferior articulating process (IAP):
    - This allows the surgeon to see the starting point better and can be helpful particularly if there is significant bony overgrowth.
    - Allows for more surface area for bony fusion.

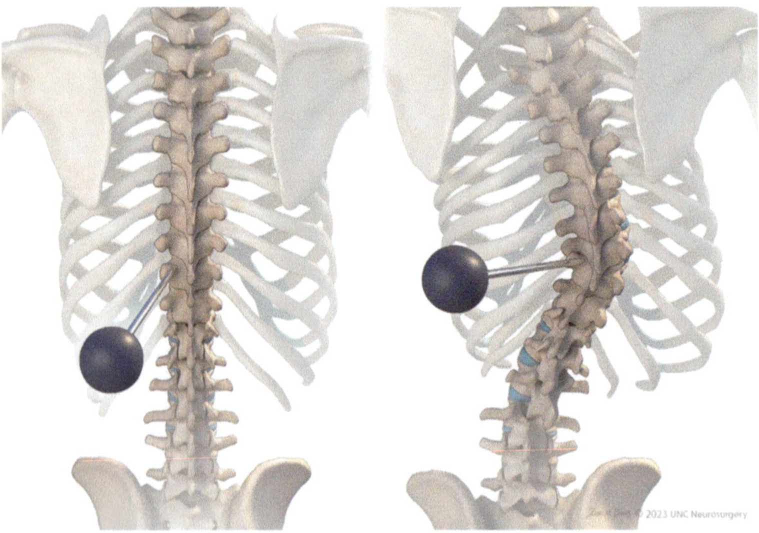

Fig. 46.2 Demonstration of the use of a pedicle probe in a patient with normal alignment (left) compared to a patient with scoliosis (right). (©2023 UNC Neurosurgery. Used by permission.)

- Different pedicle finders:
  - There are different pedicle finders, but the authors prefer a curved gearshift.
- Hypoplastic pedicles:
  - The authors recommend sequential dilation with increasing tap size for hypoplastic pedicles.
- Laminotomy:
  - Performance of a small laminotomy can assist the surgeon in pedicle screw placement as it allows one to visualize the medial wall of the pedicle and help guide the screw.

46.5 Complications

- Breach:
  - Previous studies describe safe and effective use of the freehand technique with acceptable breach rates.[1,3,4]
- Neurovascular:
  - Rare (< 1%) but can be devastating.
  - The inherently lateral trajectory described here may decrease the risk of cerebrospinal fluid (CSF) leak and significant neural injury from spinal cord impingement.[1]
- Long-term:
  - Adjacent-segment disease (ASD):
    - Rare: One study found only 1 case of radiographic ASD in a series of 123 patients.[5]
  - Postsurgical junctional kyphosis (PJK):
    - More data are needed to estimate the risk of PJK in the thoracic spine.
    - Meta-analyses have reported a wide range of incidence of PJK, anywhere from 5.6 to 62%.[5]
  - Pseudoarthrosis/Hardware failure:
    - In a series of 123 patients who had 1135 thoracic pedicle screws and 233 rods placed, 7 incidences of instrumentation failure and 8 lucencies around screws were observed.[5]

46.6 Postoperative Care

- Imaging:
  - Postoperative screw placement can be confirmed via X-ray or CT, the latter for better delineation of trajectory and potential breach.
  - Magnetic resonance imaging (MRI) may be used to evaluate neoplastic or infectious processes, though artifact from metallic hardware can significantly reduce the quality of the information received.

  - Standing 36-inch X-rays are important to assess overall sagittal and coronal balance, but these may be delayed to eliminate confounding factors such as postoperative pain and the need for bracing.
- Pain management:
  - Patients are generally hospitalized and treated with a combination of oral and intravenous narcotic medications and an aggressive bowel regimen. A strong emphasis is placed on early mobilization.
- Bracing:
  - Optional, and depends on underlying pathology, bone stock, and other variables.
- Wound care:
  - Optimization of blood sugar and nutrition status, mobilization, and avoiding extended periods of dependence on the postoperative site are paramount to adequate incision healing.

46.7 Outcomes

- Multiple clinical and cadaveric biomechanical studies have demonstrated the efficacy of thoracic pedicle screw instrumentation as advantageous for stabilization and deformity correction.

46.8 Surgical Pearls

- The freehand technique for the placement of thoracic pedicle screws is safe, effective, and efficient. It may significantly reduce operative time and radiation exposure.
- The standardized technique already described is easy to teach and implement in cases of standard posterior thoracic instrumentation.
- The extrapedicular ("in–out–in") technique is a viable option for pedicles that are too small or in the setting of revision but are biomechanically inferior to their intrapedicular counterparts.[6]
- Screws may be augmented with polymethylmethacrylate (or other similar agents) in situations of weakened cortical bone.
- Freehand thoracic pedicle screws can be safely and efficiently placed in a variety of spinal disorders, including deformity.

Common Clinical Questions

1. Which of the following demonstrates the most biomechanically advantageous technique for thoracic fusion?

   A. Transverse process hooks.

   B. Extrapedicular screw fusion (in–out–in technique).

C. Pedicle screw fixation.

D. Sublaminar wires.

2. All of the following are commonly used intraoperatively to confirm adequate pedicle screw trajectory *except* which?

   A. MRI.

   B. Stereotactic navigation.

   C. Fluoroscopy.

   D. CT.

3. Which of the following assists with correct intraoperative localization in the thoracic spine?

   A. Scout MRI showing C2 down to sacrum.

   B. CT scan of the entire thoracic spine to correctly count the ribs.

   C. Preoperative chest X-ray.

   D. All of the above.

   E. A and B only.

4. Freehand pedicle screws can be safely placed in patients with severe spinal deformity. True or false?

   A. True.

   B. False.

Answers to Common Clinical Questions

1. C.
2. A.
3. E.
4. A.

References

1. Fennell VS, Palejwala S, Skoch J, Stidd DA, Baaj AA. Freehand thoracic pedicle screw technique using a uniform entry point and sagittal trajectory for all levels: preliminary clinical experience. J Neurosurg Spine. 2014; 21(5):778–784
2. Yingsakmonkol W, Karaikovic E, Gaines RW. The accuracy of pedicle screw placement in the thoracic spine using the "Funnel Technique": part 1. A cadaveric study. J Spinal Disord Tech. 2002; 15(6):445–449

3. Kim YJ, Lenke LG. Thoracic pedicle screw placement: free-hand technique. Neurol India. 2005; 53(4):512–519
4. Kim YJ, Lenke LG, Bridwell KH, Cho YS, Riew KD. Free hand pedicle screw placement in the thoracic spine: is it safe? Spine. 2004; 29(3):333–342, discussion 342
5. Agarwal N, Heary RF, Agarwal P. Adjacent-segment disease after thoracic pedicle screw fixation. J Neurosurg Spine. 2018; 28(3):280–286
6. White KK, Oka R, Mahar AT, Lowry A, Garfin SR. Pullout strength of thoracic pedicle screw instrumentation: comparison of the transpedicular and extrapedicular techniques. Spine. 2006; 31(12):E355–E358

47 Navigation in Spine Surgery

Salah A. Alakkad and Esteban Quiceno

Summary
Computer-assisted navigation is an adjunct for the spine surgeon that is continuously under development. It offers multiple advantages for the surgical team, including more accurate placement of instrumentation and reduced radiation exposure. In this chapter, fluoroscopic and tomographic spinal navigation systems are discussed, along with the workflow for utilizing them.

Keywords: computed tomography, fluoroscopic, spinal navigation

47.1 Key Points

- Computer assisted navigation (CAN) for spine surgery was developed to improve safety and pedicle screw placement while reducing radiation exposure for the surgical team.
- CAN is useful for open and minimally invasive (MIS) instrumentation of the cervical, thoracic, and lumbosacral spine and the pelvis.
- CAN systems use an optic sensor to coordinate relevant spinal anatomy with surgical instruments, using reference markers on a fixed frame attached to bony anatomy or to the skin.
- CAN is a tool to aid in the instrumentation of the spine, but should never replace surgical experience and a detailed knowledge of anatomy.

47.2 Description

- Different CAN systems are available; an important variable is the imaging acquisition modality.
- Imaging can be acquired preoperatively or intraoperatively.
- The advantage of preoperative image (first-generation devices) was its high quality (CT), but these systems usually needed widespread bony exposure for accuracy which precluded their use in MIS surgery.
- Other issue with preoperative imaging is the change of the anatomic landmarks during positioning. Acquisition is usually in the supine position in contrast to the prone position during surgery. Additionally, the use of

Mayfield clamps and maneuvers that realign the spine during positioning may affect the accuracy of the navigation.

- Preoperative image-based navigation worked by point-by-point surface navigation with a probe, each vertebral level had to be registered separately, which was time consuming.
- CAN systems are also divided according to the imaging used, fluoroscopy or CT.
- Fluoroscopy-based navigation (second generation) is acquired intraoperatively after attachment of the reference array and is useful for MIS and open surgery.
- Fluoroscopy-based navigation is preferred for thoracic and lumbar cases, except high thoracic spine where visualization of landmarks is usually obscured by the blade and the shoulders.
- Fluoroscopy-based navigation systems have a large field of view, which can include the entire lumbar spine and up to six or seven thoracic segments. These systems had a widespread use due to accurate registrations of the patient's spinal anatomy without the need for point and surface matching technique.
- Image quality of fluoroscopy-based systems may be an issue in osteoporotic or morbidly obese patients.
- Intraoperative CT-based navigation (third generation) has the largest field of view, and the best image quality but is the most expensive one.

47.3 Indications and Advantages

- CAN increases the accuracy of pedicle screw placement.
- Shin et al published a systematic review, which included 7000 pedicle screws. The authors described an incidence of pedicle breach of 6% using CAN compared to 15% for freehand technique.[1]
- No significant difference in neurologic complications between freehand technique and CAN has been reported in systematic reviews or meta-analysis.
- Some of the most important advantages are the possibility to use larger screws, larger screw/pedicle diameter, and significantly fewer revisions.
- Baky et al reported a 1% rate of 4-mm pedicle breach with CAN versus a 3.3% rate of those placed via fluoroscopy (p: 0.27); 3.6% of the fluoroscopy cases required surgical revision versus 0 cases in the CAN group (p: 0.02).[2]
- Surgeons who use CAN for thoracolumbar instrumentation are exposed to approximately half the radiation when compared to surgeons who do not use this technology regularly.[3]
- The use of intraoperative radiation is variable among spinal surgeons, and in some cases, the radiation associated with fluoroscopy may be

comparable to the one produced by one intraoperative CT, but in general the use of CT navigation increases radiation exposure to the patient, which is an important fact when considering its use in patients with increased risks to radiation exposure such as children with congenital scoliosis or adolescent idiopathic scoliosis.[4]
- Although the equipment cost is high and the learning curve to streamline workflow is slow, these factors are mitigated by the reduction in re-interventions due to misplacement of screws.[5]
- Navigation techniques are especially useful when spinal anatomy is distorted or in cases of revision surgery.
- Modern robotic arm navigation platforms are now integrated with CAN systems, and they are able to reduce human error via increased accuracy, decreased fatigue, and tremor suppression via mechanical aid.[5]

47.4 Future of Spinal Navigation

- The most important areas in the future of spinal navigation are the development of smaller registration trackers and the widespread use of augmented reality headsets with real-time navigation and anatomic landmarks directly overlaid on the patient.
- Liu et al reported the results of 205 pedicle screws placed under augmented reality. The authors found that the screw accuracy was 98%. One of the advantages of this new technology is the ability to simultaneously visualize the actual operative field while using navigation, favoring less line-of-sight interruptions.[6]
- Co-registration with magnetic resonance imaging is not commonly available in spine navigation platforms and would allow the use of CAN in soft tissue pathologies such as tumors and disk-related diseases, particularly calcified disks in the thoracic spine.
- Making these platforms more cost-effective, especially for areas with limited resources, is another future direction.

47.5 Surgical Pearls

- The workflow for most intraoperative CT-based CAN systems is the following:
  - Once the patient is positioned, prepped, and draped, usually three reference points attached to instruments used in the system are calibrated with the camera before intraoperative scanning.
  - The intraoperative CT is performed. Temporary suspension of ventilation for 1 minute at the time of image capture plays an important role in minimizing registration errors.

- The reference points are coupled with an anatomic reference clamp that is attached to an exposed spinous process or to the iliac crest via pins in percutaneous cases.
- A real-time three-dimensional image is generated.
- When using navigation care should be taken after introducing interbody cages or after performing any maneuver that affects the alignment of the spine, because of the change in the real anatomy as a result of disk preparation and insertion of a cage and restoration of the lordosis.
- For percutaneous iliac crest pin, it can be used accurately up to L3, with cautious to L2, except for spondylolysthesis where you have to be careful with the upper segment, if bony surface is not accurately delineated by your navigated prob then repeat registration using spinous reference frame on upper segment.
- The reference clamps or pins cannot be moved after registration.
- Maximizing the accuracy of pedicle screw placement should be the first step of the procedure. Navigation should be used not only to determine anatomic landmarks, but also to determine the length and contouring of the rods and the best possible position of the heads of the screws.
- SpineMask Tracker (Stryker; Kalamazoo, MI, USA) operates with a noninvasive form of referencing, which is a rectangular adhesive tracker fixed to the patient's skin. The advantage of this system is that it avoids obstruction of the camera due to hand positioning or movement of reference points after calibration. Its drawbacks are that the size of the operative field is limited by the size of the adhesive tracker and if there is an important skin tension or deep retraction it can result in inaccurate mapping.[5]

Common Clinical Questions

1. Which of the following clinical advantages of CAN is not supported by statistically significant results in the literature?

   A. Accuracy in pedicle screw placement.

   B. Less radiation exposure for the surgical team.

   C. Less reintervention due to misplacement of pedicle screws.

   D. Less neurological complications.

2. Which of the following is a disadvantage of second-generation (fluoroscopy) CAN systems?

   A. Image quality in obese and osteoporotic patients.

   B. Each vertebral level needs to be registered separately.

   C. Price.

   D. More radiation exposure.

3. During a surgical case which of the following procedures should be performed first to maintain the best possible accuracy?
   A. Disk preparation.
   B. Pedicle instrumentation.
   C. Osteotomies.
   D. Interbody cage placement.

Answers to Common Clinical Questions

1. D.
2. A.
3. B.

References

1. Shin BJ, James AR, Njoku IU, Härtl R. Pedicle screw navigation: a systematic review and meta-analysis of perforation risk for computer-navigated versus freehand insertion. J Neurosurg Spine. 2012; 17(2):113–122
2. Baky FJ, Milbrandt T, Echternacht S, Stans AA, Shaughnessy WJ, Larson AN. Intraoperative computed tomography-guided navigation for pediatric spine patients reduced return to operating room for screw malposition compared with freehand/fluoroscopic techniques. Spine Deform. 2019; 7(4):577–581
3. Kim CW, Lee YP, Taylor W, Oygar A, Kim WK. Use of navigation-assisted fluoroscopy to decrease radiation exposure during minimally invasive spine surgery. Spine J. 2008; 8(4):584–590
4. Sielatycki JA, Mitchell K, Leung E, Lehman RA. State of the art review of new technologies in spine deformity surgery-robotics and navigation. Spine Deform. 2022; 10(1):5–17
5. Yamout T, Orosz LD, Good CR, Jazini E, Allen B, Gum JL. Technological advances in spine surgery: navigation, robotics, and augmented reality. Orthop Clin North Am. 2023; 54(2):237–246
6. Liu A, Jin Y, Cottrill E, et al. Clinical accuracy and initial experience with augmented reality-assisted pedicle screw placement: the first 205 screws. J Neurosurg Spine. 2021; 36(3):351–357

48 Robotics in Spine Surgery

Brendan F. Judy, Andrew M. Hersh, and Nicholas Theodore

Summary
This chapter provides a guide for implementing robotic platforms in the operating room for spine surgery. Robots are used to improve accuracy of pedicle screw placement and successful outcomes have been reported for all spinal levels, including the cervical spine. Robots can be used to assist with treatment of any spine pathology. Robotic surgery begins with obtaining CT imaging which can be obtained preoperatively and uploaded to the robot in advance. The system is draped, and a reference array and surveillance marker are placed on the patient. Care is taken to ensure the reference array is in line of view of the infrared camera. The patient and instruments are then registered to the robot and the trajectories for pedicle screws are planned on the platform. The robotic arm then positions itself to provide the appropriate trajectory. Complications and potential solutions are also discussed in the chapter. Robotic-assisted spine surgery has been reported to improve pedicle screw accuracy to over 98% and will remain an important asset in spine surgery with expanding capabilities.

Keywords: robotics, spine surgery, accuracy, reference array, navigation

48.1 Key Points

- Robotic assistance enables spine surgeons to accurately place hardware using navigation and minimally invasive techniques.
- In comparison to traditional freehand technique, advantages of robotic spine surgery include:
  - Improved accuracy for instrumentation.[1,2,3,4,5]
  - Decreased radiation exposure for surgeons and operating room staff.[2,5,6]
  - Decreased blood loss for patients.[2,7]
- Proposed disadvantages include cost and size of the robot.
- The learning curve for robotic spine surgery is approximately 20 to 30 cases with noted improvements in screw placement time, screw accuracy, and operative time.[8]

48.2 Indications

- Robotic assistance for spine surgery is effective in open, percutaneous, and minimally invasive approaches. It can be used for all pathologies, including: tumor, trauma, deformity, congenital anomalies, and infection. Furthermore, robotic spine surgery has been safely performed on all levels of the spine, including cervical.[9,10,11]
- Current FDA approval is for instrumentation placement and navigation; however, future iterations may prove fruitful for precise laminectomies, osteotomies, and tumor resection.
- When coupled with image guidance, this technology allows for real-time navigation in addition to robotic features.

48.3 Technique

- The exact preoperative and intraoperative workflow is dependent on the specific robot. However, listed here is a general workflow for robotic spine surgery (**Table 48.1**).[12]
  - A preoperative, thin-cut computed tomography (CT) scan is obtained and uploaded to the robot (e.g., 1-mm thin slices). The operating room is set up (**Fig. 48.1**).
  - The patient is intubated, positioned, and draped in the usual sterile fashion.
  - A reference and sometimes a secondary surveillance marker (e.g., posterior superior iliac spine for lumbar and sacral, spinous process for thoracic and cervical, and Mayfield frame clamp for high cervical) are then attached to the patient.
  - Anteroposterior and lateral radiographs using a C-arm are taken in order to register the patient and surgical instruments to the preoperative CT. The C-arm is removed from the operating room.
  - Once registration is completed and landmark check performed, the trajectory of the instrumentation is planned on the robot.
  - The robot is then draped and brought into the sterile field to perform surgery (**Fig. 48.2**).
  - Conversely, intraoperative cone-beam CT or even plain radiographs can be used to navigate in some systems.

48.4 Complications

- Pitfalls during robotic spine surgery[12] can be broken down into the following main categories and potential solutions are discussed:

Table 48.1 Key steps for robotic spine surgery workflow

Step	Details
1. Preoperative setup	• Review imaging + upload CT to robot • Confirm all personnel are trained • Set up the operating room • Ensure equipment is available
2. Case start	• Time out • Drape the patient • Drape the robot/system and dock out of field
3. Reference marker placement	• Solid bony purchase on either end of incision • In line of view of infrared camera • Does not block the surgeon
4. Registration	• C-arm moves into position for images (AP and lateral), then removed from the room • Register the patient and instruments to the robot • Confirm navigation integrity with landmark check
5. Intraoperative planning	• Trajectory for instrumentation planned on robotic system
6. Perform surgery	• Bring the robot into the field and dock • Re-confirm navigation integrity with landmark check • Perform robotic spine surgery

Abbreviations: AP, anteroposterior; CT, computed tomography.

- *Registration failure:* First, attempt to repeat registration and then call for technical support. Every surgeon must be prepared to perform surgery freehand.
- *Navigation integrity:* A landmark check should be performed at the beginning of all instrumentation placement. Ensure that the reference frame has not moved and that the imaging (e.g., preoperative CT) used for navigation is thin cut and high quality. An intraoperative O-arm spin may be performed as a second registration modality and tidal volume should be held by anesthesia during the scan. Instrumentation placement should be performed prior to osteotomies in order to avoid navigation deviation.

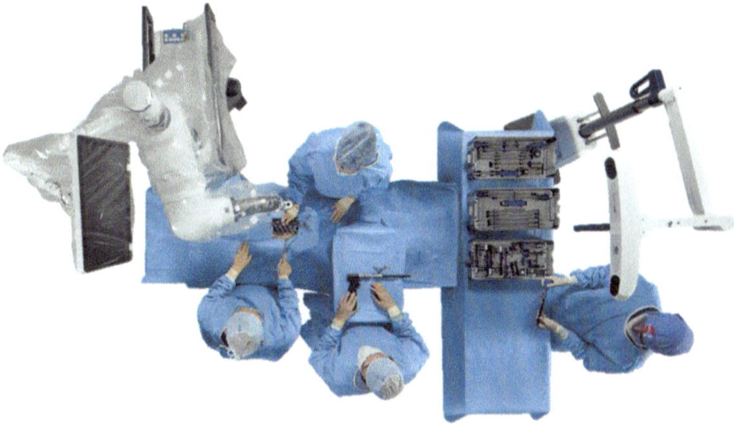

Fig. 48.1 Bird's eye view of operating room. The infrared sensor is positioned at the feet of the bed and the robot is docked out of the field until needed. (Copyright of Globus Medical, Inc.)

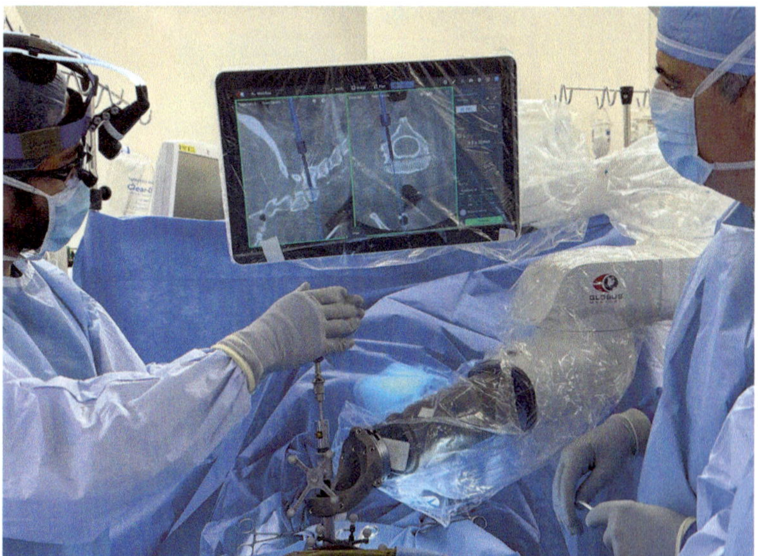

Fig. 48.2 Surgeons performing robotic cervical spine surgery. The patient is positioned prone, and the robotic arm provides guidance for precise C2 screw placement.

- *System failure:* The entire robotic system should be restarted. Registration and trajectory planning should be performed again. If necessary, convert to freehand.
- *Navigation failure due to infrared sensor:* Confirm the infrared tracker is "seeing" the reference frame and instrument fiducials. Avoid blood on the fiducials as well as obstruction of reference frame keeping the line of sight clear. Keep operating room lighting off the fiducials if feasible.
- *Deflection of instrumentation (skiving):* Tactile feedback is still needed during robotic surgery. However, certain robots do have warnings for instrumentation deflection. When necessary, use a bur to drill through cortical bone to prevent deflection.
- *Reference frame movement:* Avoid skin/tissue pressure on the post and do not inadvertently bump the reference frame. Ensure solid bony purchase prior to registration.
- *Failure to obtain trajectory:* Tilt reference frame away from the incision (e.g., caudally during lumbar surgery, rostrally in cervical surgery) to avoid obstruction. Reverse the end effector/robotic arm which may make trajectory feasible.

48.5 Postoperative Care

- Patients are cared for in the standard fashion for spine patients.
- Patients will often have one small incision for reference frame placement (< 2 cm) and bilateral incisions off midline (length dependent on levels of surgery) if decompression/decortication is not needed. The reference frame incision can be closed with 3–0 dermal suture and absorbable suture/glue on the epidermis. The lateral incisions are closed in the standard fashion: fascial stitches, a dermal layer, and absorbable suture/glue on the epidermis.
- Overall, there are no specific postoperative care requirements for patients who undergo robotic spine surgery.

48.6 Outcomes

- Clinical studies have demonstrated that in comparison to traditional freehand technique, robotic spine surgery offers:
  - Improved accuracy for instrumentation.[1,2,3,4,5]
  - Decreased intraoperative blood loss.[2,7]
  - Decreased radiation exposure for the surgeon and operating room staff.[2,5,6]
- Robotic assistance has proven safe and accurate in cervical,[9,10,11] thoracolumbar,[7,13] and sacral spine surgery.[14]

- Furthermore, some studies suggest that revision rates, length of stay, and overall complications may be reduced with robotic assistance compared to freehand surgery.[4]
- Cost is a significant concern as the robots often cost > $1 million. However, Menger et al[15] suggest that the initial investment may be returned with reduced length of stay and fewer complications.

48.7 Surgical Pearls

- Although accuracy rates may differ by robotic system and screw location, rates of over 98% accuracy have been reported using robots, particularly for newer generations.[16,17]
- New users should be aware that a learning curve exists for robotic spine surgery, usually ranging from 20 to 30 cases to develop expertise.[8]
- The location of the posterior superior iliac spine differs slightly between males and females. Accurate placement of the reference frame for lumbosacral surgery should use anatomical landmarks, palpation, and/or radiographic confirmation.[18]
- Fat and soft tissue must be dissected away in the angle of post placement to avoid post movement intraoperatively.[18]
- The reference frame can be angled laterally to prevent intersecting screw trajectory when placing S2–alar–iliac screws.[18]
- Avoid excessive force when drilling screws to prevent translation or skive.[19]
- A thorough understanding of pedicle anatomy and the specific robotic system is critical for ensuring accuracy.[20]

Common Clinical Questions

1. Which of the following is an effective method to avoid deflection (skiving) with the drill?

   A. Apply more force.

   B. Use a bur to create a trajectory through cortical bone.

   C. Increase the size of drill bit.

   D. Repeat registration.

2. Robotic spine surgery has been safely and accurately performed in which of these levels of the spine?

   A. Cervical.

   B. Thoracolumbar.

   C. Sacral.

   D. All of the above.

3. What should be done to prevent crossing the trajectory of the screw by the reference frame in the posterior superior iliac spine during S2–alar–iliac screw placement?
   A. Drive the post deeper into the pelvis.
   B. Place the post more medial.
   C. Angle the post laterally.
   D. Place the post in the sacrum.

Answers to Common Clinical Questions

1. B.
2. D.
3. C.

References

1. Li HM, Zhang RJ, Shen CL. Accuracy of pedicle screw placement and clinical outcomes of robot-assisted technique versus conventional freehand technique in spine surgery from nine randomized controlled trials: a meta-analysis. Spine. 2020; 45(2):E111–E119
2. Fu W, Tong J, Liu G, et al. Robot-assisted technique vs conventional freehand technique in spine surgery: a meta-analysis. Int J Clin Pract (Esher). 2021; 75 (5):e13964
3. Li W, Li G, Chen W, Cong L. The safety and accuracy of robot-assisted pedicle screw internal fixation for spine disease: a meta-analysis. Bone Joint Res. 2020; 9(10):653–666
4. Li J, Fang Y, Jin Z, Wang Y, Yu M. The impact of robot-assisted spine surgeries on clinical outcomes: a systemic review and meta-analysis. Int J Med Robot. 2020; 16(6):1–14
5. Chen AF, Kazarian GS, Jessop GW, Makhdom A. Robotic technology in orthopaedic surgery. J Bone Joint Surg Am. 2018; 100(22):1984–1992
6. Shahi P, Vaishnav A, Araghi K, et al. Robotics reduces radiation exposure in minimally invasive lumbar fusion compared with navigation. Spine (Philadelphia, Pa. 1976). 2022; 47(18):1279–1286
7. Jiang B, Pennington Z, Azad T, et al. Robot-assisted versus freehand instrumentation in short-segment lumbar fusion: experience with real-time image-guided spinal robot. World Neurosurg. 2020; 136:e635–e645
8. Pennington Z, Judy BF, Zakaria HM, et al. Learning curves in robot-assisted spine surgery: a systematic review and proposal of application to residency curricula. Neurosurg Focus. 2022; 52(1):E3

9. Fan M, Liu Y, He D, et al. Improved accuracy of cervical spinal surgery with robot-assisted screw insertion: a prospective, randomized, controlled study. Spine. 2020; 45(5):285–291
10. Su XJ, Lv ZD, Chen Z, et al. Comparison of accuracy and clinical outcomes of robot-assisted versus fluoroscopy-guided pedicle screw placement in posterior cervical surgery. Global Spine J. 2022; 12(4):620–626
11. Sacino AN, Materi J, Davidar AD, et al. Robot-assisted atlantoaxial fixation: illustrative cases. J Neurosurg Case Lessons. 2022; 3(25):CASE22114
12. Judy BF, Pennington Z, Botros D, et al. Spine image guidance and robotics: exposure, education, training, and the learning curve. Int J Spine Surg. 2021; 15 s2:S28–S37
13. Jiang B, Pennington Z, Zhu A, et al. Three-dimensional assessment of robot-assisted pedicle screw placement accuracy and instrumentation reliability based on a preplanned trajectory. J Neurosurg Spine. 2020; 33(4):1–10
14. Shillingford JN, Laratta JL, Park PJ, et al. Human versus robot: a propensity-matched analysis of the accuracy of free hand versus robotic guidance for placement of S2 alar-iliac (S2AI) screws. Spine. 2018; 43(21):E1297–E1304
15. Menger RP, Savardekar AR, Farokhi F, Sin A. A cost-effectiveness analysis of the integration of robotic spine technology in spine surgery. Neurospine. 2018; 15(3):216–224
16. Zhang Q, Han XG, Xu YF, et al. Robotic navigation during spine surgery. Expert Rev Med Devices. 2020; 17(1):27–32
17. Benech CA, Perez R, Benech F, Greeley SL, Crawford N, Ledonio C. Navigated robotic assistance results in improved screw accuracy and positive clinical outcomes: an evaluation of the first 54 cases. J Robot Surg. 2020; 14(3):431–437
18. Judy BF, Soriano-Baron H, Jin Y, et al. Pearls and pitfalls of posterior superior iliac spine reference frame placement for spinal navigation: cadaveric series. J Neurosurg Case Lessons. 2022; 3(9):CASE21621
19. Buza JA, III, Good CR, Lehman RA, Jr, et al. Robotic-assisted cortical bone trajectory (CBT) screws using the Mazor X Stealth Edition (MXSE) system: workflow and technical tips for safe and efficient use. J Robot Surg. 2021; 15 (1):13–23
20. Lieberman IH, Kisinde S, Hesselbacher S. Robotic-assisted pedicle screw placement during spine surgery. JBJS Essential Surg Tech. 2020; 10(2):e0020

49 Posterolateral Thoracic Approaches

Grace X. Xiong and Christopher M. Bono

Summary

Posterolateral thoracic approaches are suitable for addressing paracentral to lateral spinal pathology, including disk herniations, trauma, tumor, or infections. In the order of the least to the most invasive approach are: the transpedicular approach, in which centrolateral pathology is accessed via curettage of the ipsilateral pedicle; costotransversectomy, in which posterolateral pathology is accessed via removal of the transverse process and medial rib; and the lateral extracavitary approach, in which lateral pathology can be more thoroughly accessed via greater resection of the rib and pleural retraction. Care must be taken to select the appropriate approach as inadequate decompression may result from insufficient access. Iatrogenic instability from the approach should be addressed with instrumented stabilization, and in some cases may be performed prior to decompression to avoid iatrogenic neurologic injury. Patients should be monitored for pneumothorax, hemothorax, and chylothorax. Postoperative care should emphasize mobilization and adequate pulmonary toilet. This chapter will give a broad overview of indications, surgical technique, and postoperative care.

Keywords: spine surgery, thoracic spine, transpedicular, costotransversectomy, disk herniation, thoracic myelopathy, spinal decompression

49.1 Key Points

- Posterior and posterolateral approaches are suitable for disk herniations and pathology that are located laterally to centrolaterally. More central or extensive pathology may necessitate a combined or anterior approach.
- To minimize retraction of the spinal cord, removal of the adjacent end plates and vertebral bodies can provide a space into which the disk herniation can be delivered before removal.

- In cases of iatrogenic instability with planned fusion, pedicle screws should be placed first and rods moved from side to side as needed to prevent positional tension on the spinal cord.
- Emphasis on pulmonary toilet and chest physiotherapy (PT) is key for successful recovery postoperatively.

49.2 Indications

- Posterolateral thoracic approaches may be used for a variety of indications including:
  - Degenerative thoracic disk herniations, vertebral body osteophytes. Central calcified disks require more extensive lateral dissection such as a lateral extracavitary approach to avoid manipulation of the thoracic thecal sac.
  - Trauma: fractures requiring ventral canal decompression or anterior column support.
  - Infection: diskitis and osteomyelitis with substantial bony destruction and mechanical instability, with or without epidural abscesses necessitating decompression.
  - Neoplasm: decompression with or without stabilization for tumors.
- Indications for approach depend on the location and optimal trajectory for addressing the pathology intraoperatively. Broadly, three posterolateral approaches have been described:
  - Transpedicular approaches are suitable for single-level disease, particularly where the pathology is lateral[1] (**Fig. 49.1**).
  - Costotransversectomy is suitable for lesions of the posterolateral vertebral body and lateral disk, while lateral extracavitary approaches are suitable for lesions on the ipsilateral half of the vertebral body (**Fig. 49.2**).

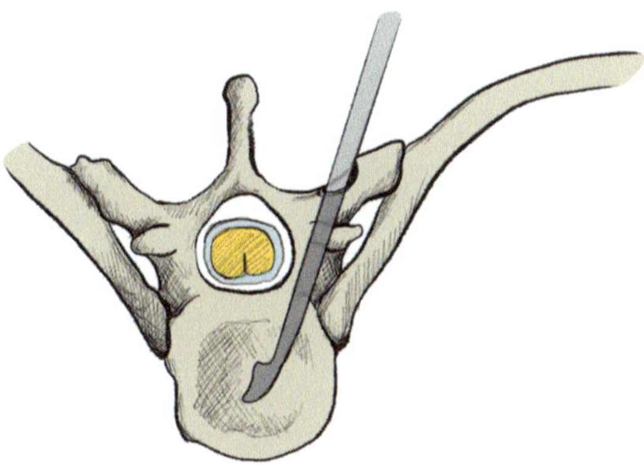

Fig. 49.1 Transpedicular approach showing "eggshell" curettage of the cancellous pedicle.

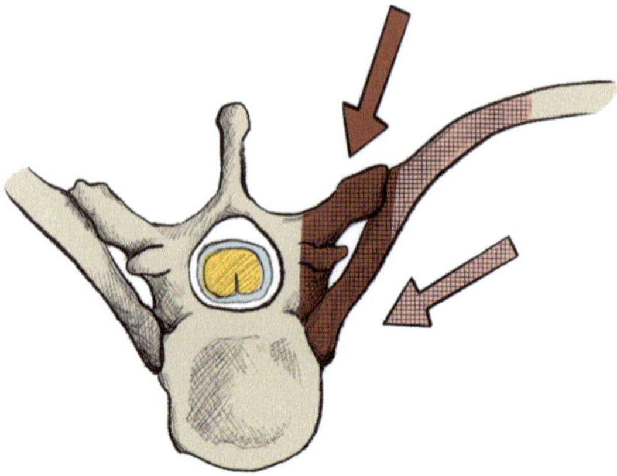

Fig. 49.2 Costotransversectomy approach allows access to the posterolateral vertebral body and disk (*dark red*), whereas the lateral extracavitary approach allow more anterior visualization (*light red*).

49.3 Technique

- Prior to positioning, ensure that adequate intravenous access and neuromonitoring including both somatosensory-evoked potentials and transcranial motor-evoked potentials are secured and functional. Prepositioning baseline potentials are measured.
- General endotracheal intubation is undertaken, with a double lumen tube used if entry of the pleural space is anticipated.
- The patient is positioned prone on a radiolucent prone table. For lateral extracavitary approaches, a semi-prone or "three-quarter" prone position can be considered.[2]
- Arms are placed on rests overhead or tucked at the patient's side as per the surgeon's preference (tucked positioned preferable for mid-thoracic or higher).
- Localization is used to approximate the incision and after dissection to confirm the operative level. The inferior tip of the scapula can be used to approximate T7. Confirm the number of rib-bearing segments on preoperative imaging and correlate with vertebral body counts from the sacrum on the lateral view, or rib counts on the anteroposterior (AP) view.
  - Thoracic facet joints are approximately in line with the intervertebral disk space.
  - Midline incision is made for a transpedicular approach or costotransversectomy, and a paramedian approach used for costotransversectomies or lateral extracavitary approaches.

- Subperiosteal dissection performed to expose lamina, facet capsule complex, transverse process, costovertebral junction, and varying amounts of rib depending on the method of exposure.
- Subperiosteal dissection of the rib can be performed with a periosteal dissector, being careful not to disrupt the parietal pleura and the neurovascular bundle, which runs at the inferior aspect of the rib.

49.3.1 Transpedicular Approach

- An ipsilateral laminotomy is performed to allow palpation of the pedicle, with extension to a laminectomy if more complete posterior decompression is needed.
- A high-speed drill is used to open the posterior pedicle cortex. The cancellous channel of the pedicle is subsequently opened into the vertebral body with a combination of probes, curettes, or a high-speed drill, maintaining the cortical pedicle walls in an "eggshell" fashion.
- A downgoing curette is used to carefully fracture the medial pedicle wall to access the lateral thecal sac. The medial portion of the adjacent facet is resected, and the superior pedicle wall removed to access the disk space.
- A thin shell of posterior vertebral wall can be maintained to protect the ventral thecal sac. A lateral annulotomy is undertaken and diskectomy achieved without retraction of the spinal cord. A cavity can be developed in the adjacent vertebral body or intervertebral space to push the disk herniation or mass into the cavity, allowing for subsequent safe removal with a pituitary rongeur.

49.3.2 Costotransversectomy

- In general, a left-sided approach is favored as the thicker-walled aorta is more resistant to injury than the thin-walled vena cava.
- Remove the transverse process and medial 3 to 5 cm of rib.
- Perform a partial laminectomy and facetectomy to identify the lateral margin of the dura. Follow the nerve roots out of the foramen after identifying the pedicle at the current level.
- Dissect the lateral aspect of the vertebral body and identify the intervertebral disk space just superior to the pedicle.
- A lateral annulotomy can be performed and diskectomy achieved by creating a cavity in the intervertebral disk space or adjacent vertebral body. Disk material can then be pushed inwards into this cavity and removed safely without manipulation of the spinal cord.

- Bilateral costotransversectomies can be considered for cases of central or bilateral pathology. If this is the case, temporary rods should be placed on the contralateral side to prevent instability-associated neurologic compromise, and the rods moved from side to side as necessary to preserve stability.

49.3.3 Lateral Extracavitary Approach

- The lateral extracavitary approach is similar to costotransversectomy. However, more extensive removal of the medial rib and pleural retraction allow for greater access to the anterolateral spinal structures.
- A curvilinear incision starts at the midline approximately two to three levels proximal to the targeted level and ends two levels caudal. The caudal extent of the incision can gently curve to the approached side to facilitate easier retraction.
- In the upper thoracic spine, approach from the right is preferred to avoid the heart and the aortic arch. In the lower thoracic spine, approach from the left is preferred to avoid the liver.
- Remove the transverse process and the rib with a combination of rib cutters and rongeurs.
- If it is necessary to sacrifice nerve roots for pathologic involvement or access, place a 2–0 silk tie proximal and distal to the dorsal root ganglion. Transect the root distal to the distal tie, leaving the ends long. These can be used to gently retract the dura for exposure.
- Access the lateral vertebral body and intervertebral disk without retraction of the spinal cord.
- Examine the lung for any air leaks and the dura for evidence of a cerebrospinal fluid leak.
- A layered closure can be performed over a red rubber catheter left in the chest, which can be removed under negative pressure to evacuate residual air or fluid in the chest.
- Obtain a chest X-ray prior to leaving the operating room to check for pneumothorax.

49.4 Complications

- Infection.
- Incidental durotomy, progressing to a pseudomeningocele if not appropriately managed.
- Pneumothorax, hemothorax, or chylothorax.
- Neurologic compromise which may occur from excessive cord-level retraction.

- Inadequate decompression from inadequate visualization of the ventral epidural space.
- Iatrogenic instability occurring with wide laminectomy, facetectomies, or bilateral transpedicular approaches.

49.5 Postoperative Care

- Consider intensive care unit admission for respiratory monitoring, hemodynamic monitoring for minimum mean arterial pressures, and frequent neurologic checks.
- Respiratory recovery is prioritized through several measures:
  - Prioritize prompt extubation.
  - Adequate pain control to avoid guarding and shallow breathing.
  - Chest PT, pulmonary toilet, and early mobilization.

49.6 Outcomes

- A systematic review from 2013 identified a mean complication rate of 17 and 14% for lateral extracavitary and costotransversectomy approaches, compared with 39% in thoracotomies.[3]
- Although outside the scope of this chapter, minimally invasive approaches such as a mini-open retropleural approach may be considered when appropriate in lieu of lateral extracavitary approaches, which may decrease complications rates and blood loss.[4]

49.7 Surgical Pearls

- Utilize preoperative magnetic resonance imaging (MRI) and computed tomography (CT) to assess for presence of calcified disk which may be adherent to dura and require more extensive lateral or anterior approaches.
- Reserve anterior column bony work and destabilization for after temporary rod fixation is placed.
- In cases of altered anatomy, the neural foramen can be located by following the neurovascular bundle immediately inferior to the rib back centrally.
- A malleable retractor may be placed anterior to the vertebral body to protect the intrathoracic structures after a subperiosteal plane has been established.

Common Clinical Questions

1. During a left-sided approach to T10, the artery of Adamkiewicz is encountered and the vessel tied off due to significant intraoperative bleeding. What postoperative neurologic deficits would you expect to find?
   A. Bilateral loss of motor function below T10 and loss of pain and temperature sensation below T11.
   B. Ipsilateral loss of motor, proprioception, and vibration below T10 and loss of contralateral pain and temperature.
   C. Greater loss of upper than lower extremity motor function.
   D. Loss of proprioception only below T10.
2. Five days following a lateral extracavitary approach you note a milky white substance being emitted from a catheter drain placed into the anterior wound. Which is the most likely diagnosis?
   A. CSF leak.
   B. Chylothorax.
   C. Wound infection.
   D. Tissue necrosis.

Answers to Common Clinical Questions

1. D.
2. B.

Acknowledgments

The authors would like to recognize contributions from previous editions of this chapter:
Chapter 48, Transpedicular Approach: Vinko Zlomislic, Steven R Garfin
Chapter 49, Costotransversectomy: Hasan Zaidi, U. Kumar Kakarla
Chapter 50, Lateral Extracavitary Approach: Marco Ferrone, Christopher M. Bono

References

1. Bilsky MH. Transpedicular approach for thoracic disc herniations. Neurosurg Focus. 2000; 9(4):e3
2. Benzel EC. The lateral extracavitary approach to the spine using the three-quarter prone position. J Neurosurg. 1989; 71(6):837–841

3. Lubelski D, Abdullah KG, Steinmetz MP, et al. Lateral extracavitary, costotransversectomy, and transthoracic thoracotomy approaches to the thoracic spine: review of techniques and complications. J Spinal Disord Tech. 2013; 26(4):222–232
4. Spiessberger A, Arvind V, Gruter B, Cho SK. Thoracolumbar corpectomy/spondylectomy for spinal metastasis: a pooled analysis comparing the outcome of seven different surgical approaches. Eur Spine J. 2020; 29(2): 248–256

50 Minimally Invasive Lateral Retropleural Approach for Thoracic Diskectomy

S. Harrison Farber, James J. Zhou, Nima Alan, and Juan S. Uribe

Summary

This chapter describes the minimally invasive lateral retropleural approach for thoracic diskectomy. The lateral retropleural approach is an important alternative to posterior approaches such as costotransversectomy or other anterior approaches including open thoracotomy or thoracoscopy. A key benefit is the ability to access and visualize the ventral spinal canal in a minimally invasive fashion without manipulating the neural elements. The patient is placed in the lateral decubitus position. A 6-cm segment of rib is removed to reveal the underlying endothoracic fascia, and a plane is developed between this fascia and the parietal pleura. Once the lateral access retractor is placed, the rib head is removed from the costovertebral joint of the caudal vertebral body. The caudal pedicle is then drilled away to reveal the lateral thecal sac. Partial corpectomies are performed of the adjacent vertebral bodies to create a ventral cavity. The posterior longitudinal ligament (PLL) attachments to the disk fragment are removed. The fragment is then pushed ventrally into the defect to complete the diskectomy. All forces must be transmitted away from the spinal cord to prevent spinal cord injury. A drain is left in the surgical cavity to prevent iatrogenic pneumothorax. Several cohort studies have demonstrated safety and good clinical outcomes of this procedure. The most common approach-related complications include respiratory or CSF-related issues.

Keywords: thoracic disk herniation, retropleural, minimally invasive, thoracic diskectomy, lateral spine surgery

50.1 Key Points

- The minimally invasive lateral retropleural approach to treat thoracic disk herniations (TDHs) is a less invasive alternative to open anterior thoracotomy that minimizes morbidity and obviates the need for the assistance of a thoracic surgeon during the approach. It also requires less

specialized equipment and enables costs savings compared to thoracoscopy.
- This approach allows ventral access to the spinal canal without manipulation of the neural elements.
- Level localization must be confirmed by combining meticulous review of preoperative and intraoperative imaging.
- Once the rib is resected, the plane between the endothoracic fascia and the parietal pleura must be developed to access the retroperitoneal corridor.
- The key steps of the procedure include removal of the rib head and the pedicle, partial corpectomies of the adjacent vertebral bodies, sectioning of the posterior longitudinal ligament (PLL), and resection of the disk fragment.

50.2 Indications

- Thoracic disk herniation causing any of the following:
  - Thoracic myelopathy with progressive neurological deficit.
  - Unilateral thoracic radiculopathy.
  - Intractable thoracic back pain.
- Thoracic disk herniations located in the lower thoracic spine below the level of T5 or T6.
- Thoracic disk herniations with any of the following characteristics:
  - Lateral and central disk herniations.
  - Small and giant herniations.
  - Soft or calcified disk herniations.

50.3 Technique

- Operating room setup:
  - Intraoperative neurological monitoring is used, and baselines are obtained prior to patient positioning.
    - The use of motor-evoked potentials (MEPs) and somatosensory-evoked potentials (SSEPs) are both recommended.
  - The surgeon stands on the posterior side of the patient. The scrub technician is set up on the surgeon's side of the room.
  - The C-arm and operative microscope are both employed during the case and are positioned on the contralateral side of the patient.
- Patient positioning:
  - The patient is placed in the lateral decubitus position with the hips flexed.
  - An axillary roll is placed under the axilla and a towel roll above the iliac crest.

- After the patient is securely taped to the table, the table is broken to open the intercostal space.
- Localization and incision marking:
  - Confirming the correct level is paramount to avoid wrong level surgery.
  - Preoperative imaging should be reviewed to count the number of ribs and assess for anatomical variations such as transitional anatomy.
  - A radio-opaque marker may be placed in the pedicle or vertebral body preoperatively to assist with localization.
  - The bed is adjusted to obtain perfect anteroposterior (AP) and lateral radiographs.
  - The target disk space and adjacent vertebral bodies are traced on the patient's flank. An incision is marked along a 6-cm segment of the overlying rib.
- Approach:
  - The skin and subcutaneous fat are opened. The muscle layer including the latissimus dorsi and the external oblique are divided to expose the underlying rib. A 6-cm segment of the rib is exposed using subperiosteal dissection and then removed. The neurovascular bundle on the inferior border of the rib should be protected. Removal of the rib creates a tear in the endothoracic fascia to reveal the parietal pleura. The retropleural plane is developed between these two layers using blunt dissection.
- Corpectomy and diskectomy:
  - The minimally invasive lateral access retractor is placed in the retroperitoneal plane, and the rib head is removed from the costovertebral joint of the caudal vertebral body.
  - The ipsilateral caudal pedicle is then drilled and removed with the ligamentum flavum to reveal the lateral aspect of the thecal sac.
  - Partial corpectomies of the adjacent vertebral bodies are performed. No more than one-third of the vertebral body typically needs to be removed (**Fig. 50.1a**).
  - The PLL above and below the herniated disk fragment is then cut and removed. A plane must first be developed between the ventral dura and the PLL. The PLL is removed using a combination of Kerrison rongeurs, microscissors, or a long knife (**Fig. 50.1b**).
  - Once the PLL has been sectioned, the diskectomy may be performed. The herniated disk fragment is pushed ventrally away from the spinal cord into the corpectomy defect. All forces must be pushed away from the spinal cord to prevent risk of injury. The deep attachments to the PLL and annulus are sharply divided to complete the diskectomy (see **Video 50.1**).
  - Morselized allograft from the resected rib segment is placed into the corpectomy cavity. Lateral interbody or posterior pedicle screw placement is not routinely performed.

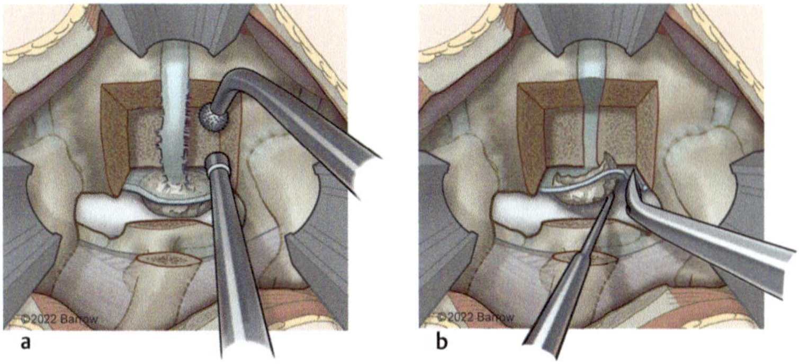

Fig. 50.1 Illustration of the surgical view in the lateral retropleural thoracic diskectomy. **(a)** After the rib head and caudal pedicle have been removed, a partial corpectomy of the two adjacent vertebral bodies is performed. **(b)** Following completion of the corpectomies, the attachments of the disk herniation to the posterior longitudinal ligament are removed and the disk is dissected off the dura into the corpectomy cavity. (Used with permission from Barrow Neurological Institute, Phoenix, Arizona.)

- Closure:
  - Once hemostasis is achieved the lateral retractor is removed. The pleura should be inspected for any tears. If a violation has occurred, primary closure is not mandatory.
  - A Hemovac drain is placed into the surgical cavity. This drain is placed in water and multiple rounds of Valsalva maneuver are performed to expel air and fluid within the retropleural cavity. This practice prevents the development of iatrogenic pneumothorax/hemothorax. Alternatively, if a lung parenchymal injury has occurred, a chest tube should be placed.
  - The muscle and fascia are closed in a layered fashion. A local intercostal nerve block may be performed to decrease postoperative pain. The dermis and skin are then closed.

50.4 Complications

- Spinal cord injury.
- Wrong level surgery.
- Pleural violation.
- Pneumothorax/hemothorax.
- Cerebrospinal fluid (CSF) leak.
  - CSF-pleural fistula.
- Abdominal pseudohernia.
- Intercostal neuralgia.

50.5 Postoperative Care

- A chest radiograph should be performed immediately in the recovery unit to exclude a large pneumothorax. A small pneumothorax may be present on this X-ray but no intervention is required if the patient remains asymptomatic.
- The patient is admitted to the intensive care unit (ICU) overnight and can typically be transferred to the floor the following day. Most patients are discharged home by postoperative day 2.
- There are no postoperative mobilization restrictions.
- The Hemovac drain is sealed, and no emptying of the drain is permitted to prevent iatrogenic air leak.
- If an enlarging pneumothorax is seen, a postoperative chest tube is required.

50.6 Outcomes

- A multi-institutional study of 75 TDHs in 60 patients showed this procedure was performed successfully in all patients. One patient experienced an adverse neurologic outcome.[1]
- Multiple subsequent patient series have demonstrated that no approach-related neurological complications occurred.[2,3,4]
- Overall, approach-related complications are rare and mainly related to respiratory or CSF-related issues.

50.7 Surgical Pearls

- A wide dissection plane between the endothoracic fascia and the parietal pleura should be achieved using blunt instruments to minimize the risk of pleural violation.
- The margins of the partial corpectomies should approximate the inferior margin of the adjacent pedicles, and the depth should approximate the medial border of the contralateral pedicle.
- We recommend use of an ultrasonic cutter as well as the coarse diamond drill bit to perform all bony work.
- The highest risk of spinal cord injury is during the dissection of the PLL and disk fragment that may be adherent to the ventral dura. All forces must be directed away from the thecal sac during this portion of the procedure. Moreover, care must be taken to avoid a sudden drop in the amount of dissection force to prevent rebounding of the disk into the spinal cord.

- If no dissection plane is possible between the calcified disk herniation and the dura, it may be circumferentially detached from its ligamentous and annular attachments and the diamond drill may be used to core out this disk until just a shell remains. This remaining free-floating fragment may be left in place to prevent CSF leak.

Common Clinical Questions

1. Benefits of the lateral retropleural approach for thoracic diskectomy include all of the following except which?
   A. This approach provides access to the ventral aspect of the spinal canal which minimizes the need for manipulation of the spinal cord during the diskectomy.
   B. The minimally invasive lateral retropleural approach does not require the use of a thoracic surgeon for access or for the lung to be collapsed during the approach.
   C. There is less approach-related morbidity with this approach compared to open anterior thoracotomy.
   D. The lateral retropleural approach provides access to treat dorsal compression such as ligamentous hypertrophy and facet arthropathy in the thoracic spine.
2. Which of the following statements is true?
   A. The lateral retropleural approach always requires the use of posterior fixation due to extensive resection of all three columns of the spine.
   B. The lateral retropleural approach may be used to treat central and paracentral thoracic disk herniations (TDHs), as well as small and giant TDHs.
   C. The lateral retropleural approach may be performed at any level in the thoracic spine.
   D. Both the rostral and caudal pedicle to the disk segment must be removed in order to access the disk herniation in the lateral approach.
3. Complications of the lateral retropleural approach for thoracic diskectomy include all of the following except which?
   A. Iatrogenic spinal cord injury.
   B. Cerebrospinal fluid (CSF)–pleural fistula.
   C. Ureteral injury.
   D. Pneumothorax.

Answers to Common Clinical Questions

1. D.
2. B.
3. C.

References

1. Uribe JS, Smith WD, Pimenta L, et al. Minimally invasive lateral approach for symptomatic thoracic disc herniation: initial multicenter clinical experience. J Neurosurg Spine. 2012; 16(3):264–279
2. Kasliwal MK, Deutsch H. Minimally invasive retropleural approach for central thoracic disc herniation. Minim Invasive Neurosurg. 2011; 54(4): 167–171
3. Yen CP, Uribe JS. Mini-open lateral retropleural approach for symptomatic thoracic disk herniations. Clin Spine Surg. 2018; 31(1):14–21
4. Farber SH, Xu DS, Walker CT, Godzik J, Turner JD, Uribe JS. Minimally invasive retropleural thoracic diskectomy: step-by-step operative planning, execution, and results. Oper Neurosurg (Hagerstown). 2022; 23(4):e220–e227

51 Lateral Approaches to the Thoracolumbar Spine

C. Rory Goodwin and Jean-Paul Wolinsky

Summary

The lateral approach to the thoracolumbar spine is an important one for the treatment of complex pathologies including trauma, tumors, and infections. A sound knowledge of the lateral spinal anatomy, including the diaphragmatic attachments, is essential. In the lumbar spine, the psoas anatomy, including the lumbar plexus anatomy, should be examined closely before surgical intervention.

Keywords: thoracoabdominal approach, lateral spine, diaphragm, thoracotomy

51.1 Key Points

- When deciding the surgical approach, the surgeon must take into account the type and location of the pathology, health status of the patient, surgeon comfort, anatomical knowledge, and goals of surgery. A case requiring extensive anterior exposure and reconstruction or a patient who is unlikely to tolerate prolonged prone positioning may favor a lateral or anterolateral approach to the thoracolumbar spine.
- The laterality of the pathology often dictates the side of the approach. However, in equivocal cases, the thoracolumbar junction may be more easily approached from the left to avoid the inferior vena cava (IVC) and to avoid retracting the liver.[1]
- Lateral access to the thoracolumbar junction can be obtained rostral or caudal to the diaphragm from a retropleural, transpleural, retroperitoneal, or combined approach.

51.2 Indications

- Lateral access to the thoracolumbar spine provides wide anterolateral exposure of the vertebral column via a retroperitoneal approach. Decompressions and reconstructions can be performed for a variety of pathologies, including trauma, degenerative disk disease, metastatic or primary spinal tumors, infections, and deformity. The lateral retroperitoneal approach allows the surgeon access to perform single-level diskectomies and fusions, disk arthroplasties, corpectomies, and lateral plating.

51.3 Technique

- The lateral approach provides access to the thoracolumbar junction (T12–L2), midlumbar region (L2–L5), and lumbosacral junction (L5–S1). The techniques for each region will be discussed separately.[2]
- Thoracolumbar junction (T12–L2):
  - All preoperative images should be carefully reviewed with special emphasis on the axial computed tomography (CT) slices. The location of the IVC and aorta is critical to avoid vascular injury. The laterality of the pathology often dictates the side of the approach. However, a left-sided approach is preferable when appropriate to avoid retracting the liver and injuring the IVC.
  - The patient is placed in the lateral decubitus position with a shoulder roll placed 4 to 5 cm below the inferior axilla to protect the brachial plexus. Preoperative X-rays are obtained to mark the incision at the correct location. Localization of pathology in the lateral position can be difficult, especially in obese or osteoporotic patients, or patients who have a variant lumbar anatomy. Accordingly, preoperative imaging is critical to understand how to count. Counting from bottom-up is usually more reliable. Preoperative marking with metallic markers or methyl methacrylate can be considered. The incision is typically made obliquely along the superior aspect of the 10th or 12th rib medially up to several centimeters onto the abdomen.
  - After the incision is made, the subcutaneous tissue, latissimus dorsi, and serratus anterior and intercostal muscles are dissected to expose the superior border of the rib. The rib is dissected off its muscular attachments, taking care to avoid injury to the neurovascular bundle on its inferior edge. The diaphragm often attaches to the 11th rib, so its dissection will allow simultaneous entry into the chest and retroperitoneal space. However, reconstruction of the diaphragm may be more complicated after resection of the 11th rib.
  - If the 10th rib is dissected, it is resected along the length of the dissection and saved for use as autograft in fusion procedures. Removal of the rib also enhances exposure and may decrease postoperative thoracotomy pain. A self-retaining DeBakey rib spreader can be placed to widen the intercostal exposure. The pleura is usually opened, but care should be taken and a retropleural dissection attempted. The benefit of the retropleural approach is that it may avoid placement of a chest tube

and can help keep the lung out of the field. The disadvantage is that it may markedly decrease the exposure. The lung is retracted anteriorly to expose the vertebral column. The caudal thoracic vertebra should be well-visualized. The diaphragm can be incised, taking care to leave a cuff for later repair for access to the upper lumbar segments.

- If the 12th rib is chosen, it is dissected and removed in similar fashion. The internal and external oblique muscles are split to expose the transversalis, which is divided. The peritoneum is bluntly dissected off the inferior surface of the diaphragm and the retroperitoneal space is opened. The diaphragm can be incised with a cuff for a combined retroperitoneal/lateral thoracic exposure of the thoracolumbar junction. There is a risk of lung injury when opening the diaphragm from the retroperitoneal space, so care must be taken. A table-mounted, self-retaining retractor is placed to aid in retraction.
- The psoas muscle overlies the lumbar spine from the lateral approach and can be dissected in a medial to lateral direction. Dissection from medial to lateral allows the lumbar plexus to rotate posteriorly with the psoas muscle and protects the muscle. A lateral to medial dissection can lead to nerve root injury. Likewise, a transpsoas approach has a higher risk to the lumbar plexus if not carefully monitored. For anterior access to the disk space or in cases requiring vertebral body resection, the segmental vessel can be found at the midposition of the vertebral body coursing in an anteromedial to posterolateral direction. This vessel can be ligated, cauterized, and cut. Care must be taken to fully cauterize these vessels a safe distance distal to the aorta, for they may retract when cut and result in copious, inaccessible bleeding.
- Injury to the artery of Adamkiewicz can lead to postoperative paraplegia. Preoperative spinal angiography can be considered for localization of this vessel. However, this is typically not an issue in conventional spine surgery, because spinal cord perfusion is not based on a single vessel, and there are multiple bilateral arterial feeders to the spinal cord.
- A blunt instrument is used to palpate the disk space(s) of interest, and confirmed with an intraoperative X-ray.
- Injury to the cisterna chyli or thoracic duct can lead to a lymphocele or chylothorax. In circumstances where injury is suspected, giving cream through a nasogastric (NG) tube and waiting for 30 minutes can help identify a lymphatic chain injury, as the chyle will become milky in color and more identifiable. If the lymphatic chain is injured, it should be ligated using a nonabsorbable suture.
- Once the goals of the surgical procedure are accomplished, a chest tube can be placed if the pleura has been violated and there is potential for

visceral pleural injury. The ribs, latissimus dorsi, and serratus anterior muscles are reapproximated with interrupted reabsorbable or permanent suture.

- Midlumbar region (L2–L5):
  - The patient is placed supine, and a left paramedian incision is marked. The left side is preferred to avoid the more prominent right common iliac vein.
  - An incision is made, and the subcutaneous dissection is carried to the external oblique fascia and the anterior rectus sheath, which are incised to expose the left rectus abdominis. The rectus is retracted medially or laterally to expose the semilunar line.
  - A space between the posterior rectus sheath and the peritoneum is created with blunt dissection caudal to the semilunar line and the rectus sheath is incised vertically.
  - The peritoneum is bluntly dissected in a lateral to medial fashion off the psoas muscle.
  - The left ureter is retracted medially along with the peritoneum until the left iliac artery and vein are identified. Above the L4–L5 disk space, ligation of the segmental vessels will allow for medial mobilization of the aorta if needed. At L4–L5, the iliac vessels are retracted medially, and a table-mounted, self-retaining retractor is inserted to aid in the exposure (**Fig. 51.1**).

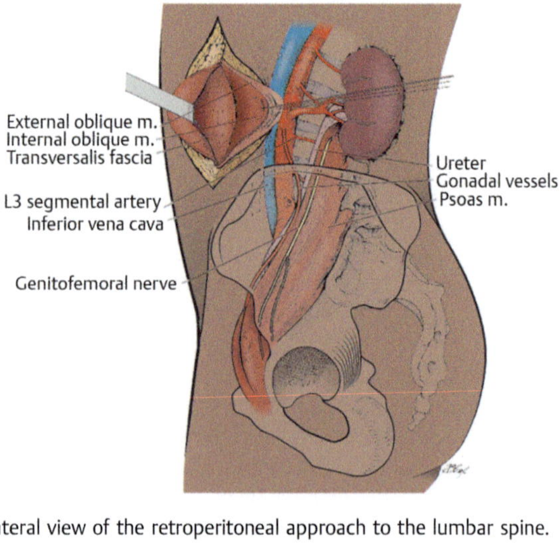

Fig. 51.1 Lateral view of the retroperitoneal approach to the lumbar spine.

  - At L4–L5, the iliolumbar vein may obscure the L5 vertebral body and limit the medial retraction of the iliac vein. At this level, it is advisable to find and ligate this vessel to improve exposure and prevent traction injury resulting in a tear in the IVC, which can result in catastrophic hemorrhage.
  - When considering instrumentation at L4–L5, a traditional lateral plate should be avoided at this level, because the contour of the L5 vertebral body is dramatically different when compared with the L4 level and will cause screws placed through the plate to preferentially have a trajectory toward the spinal canal. Posterior pedicle screw fixation or lateral screw/rod constructs are acceptable alternatives.
- Lumbosacral junction (L5–S1):
  - The L5–S1 level can be approached from a midline exposure to avoid the iliac bifurcation. A paramedian incision is made and the peritoneal contents are retracted medially.
  - The sacral promontory is exposed between the right and left iliac vessels which are retracted laterally. The median sacral vessels are ligated and cut. This allows for safe retraction of the bifurcation of the IVC superiorly and the iliac vessels laterally, enhancing the exposure of the L5–S1 disk space.
  - Care must be taken to avoid excessive electrocautery of the anterior vertebral margin as injury to the sympathetic plexus may result in retrograde ejaculation in male patients.

51.4 Complications

- Pneumothorax, lymphocele, pseudomeningocele, injury to the lung, bowel, vasculature (aorta, IVC, iliac vessels), and neural elements (nerve roots, genitofemoral nerve, lumbosacral plexus), and retroperitoneal hematomas.[3,4]
- Pseudohernias may result from incising the abdominal wall musculature and/or disruption of the nervous innervation.
- Retrograde ejaculation may result from bilateral disruption of the sympathetic chain which is unlikely in a lateral exposure to the lumbar spine. This is more likely in midline exposures of L5–S1.

51.5 Postoperative Care

- On the first postoperative day, patients are encouraged to transfer from the bed into a chair and to ambulate as tolerated. Sequential compression devices are put in place for all patients. Heparin prophylaxis for prevention of deep vein thrombosis is initiated the day after surgery.

- If surgery involved prolonged retraction of the iliac vein, then a postoperative duplex ultrasound study of the lower extremities is useful to rule out the presence of a deep vein thrombosis.
- Postoperative bowel rest is typically unnecessary after lateral retroperitoneal access. However, patients must be assessed for signs of peritoneal irritation, bowel injury being a potential, albeit infrequent, complication.
- If a chest tube is in place, it is connected to a reservoir on waterseal or −20 cm of H_2O depending on the severity of the injury. Oxygen saturation monitoring and chest X-rays are helpful in cases involving pleural injury.

51.6 Outcomes

- Few high-quality studies compare lateral and anterolateral approaches to the thoracolumbar spine with other techniques. Potential advantages of the lateral approach over a posterior based approach may include less blood loss, less retraction of nerve roots for anterior access, preservation of the posterior tension band, more thorough disk removal, and placement of larger interbody grafts.
- The anterolateral, retroperitoneal approach to the midlumbar region and lumbosacral junction avoids much of the intraperitoneal organ injury associated with an anterior transperitoneal approach, while providing similar spinal exposure. Also, the likelihood of injury to the large vessels and the sympathetic plexus is potentially reduced.

51.7 Surgical Pearls

- A true lateral decubitus position should be confirmed with intraoperative X-ray before incision, as this will aid in visualization of the lateral vertebral column.
- If the pleura is compromised, a chest tube should be placed for postoperative management.
- It is critical to leave a cuff of diaphragm during the exposure for later reapproximation.
- At L4–L5, the iliolumbar vein is ligated, and the iliac vessels are retracted medially. At L5–S1, the median sacral vein is ligated, and the bilateral iliac vessels are retracted laterally.

Common Clinical Questions

1. Retroperitoneal approaches are preferentially done on the left side of the patient for all the following reasons *except* which?
   A. It is generally safer to mobilize the aorta than the inferior vena cava.
   B. The common iliac vein may be more prominent on the right side.
   C. The presence of the liver may minimize exposure.
   D. The left ureter is less susceptible to injury than the right ureter.
2. Complications of retroperitoneal exposure include all of the following *except* which?
   A. Retroperitoneal fibrosis.
   B. Appendicitis.
   C. Ureteral injury.
   D. Femoral nerve palsy.
3. To obtain adequate exposure, which is an essential component of the thoracoabdominal approach?
   A. Incising the diaphragm along the costal margin and leaving a cuff attached at the level of the spine.
   B. Transecting the psoas to allow full retraction of the muscle.
   C. Dissection of the lumbar plexus from the overlying psoas muscle.
   D. Avoiding sacrifice of segmental arteries.

Answers to Common Clinical Questions

1. D.
2. B.
3. A.

References

1. Ronderos JF, Sonntag VKH. Approaches to the thoracic spine. Tech Neurosurg. 1996; 1(4):222–229
2. Gumbs AA, Bloom ND, Bitan FD, Hanan SH. Open anterior approaches for lumbar spine procedures. Am J Surg. 2007; 194(1):98–102
3. Vishteh AG, Apostolides PJ, Karahalios DG, Sonntag VKH. Technique of anterolateral thoracolumbar plating. Operative Techniques in Neurosurgery. 1998; 1(3):126–133
4. Gumbs AA, Shah RV, Yue JJ, Sumpio B. The open anterior paramedian retroperitoneal approach for spine procedures. Arch Surg. 2005; 140(4): 339–343

52 Open and Minimally Invasive Spinal Lumbar Microdiskectomy

Sabastian Hajtovic, Alexandra J. White, Brian Fiani, and Jonathan J. Rasouli

Summary

Both open and minimally invasive spinal lumbar microdiskectomy are safe and effective within appropriate indications. These include symptomatic herniated nucleus pulposus in patients without instability on preoperative films. The open technique: A 2- to 3-cm midline incision, subperiosteal dissection, standard laminotomy, and diskectomy, with or without an operative microscope. The minimally invasive technique: A 12- to 16-mm incision lateral to midline, serial dilators and a working tube, drilling, and diskectomy similar to the open approach with the use of an operative microscope. For both, emphasis is placed on minimal facet joint disruption. Complications of both the techniques may include durotomy, nerve root injury, infection, and hematoma. After surgery, early mobilization and discharge are recommended. Outcome data is inconsistent but points to a general lack of clinically significant differences between the approaches.

Keywords: open microdiskectomy (microdiscectomy), minimally invasive microdiskectomy (microdiscectomy), lumbar diskectomy (discectomy), MIS diskectomy (discectomy), lumbar microdisk (microdisc), facet joint preservation, facet preservation, herniated nucleus pulposus (HNP), cauda equina syndrome, radiculopathy, disk recurrence, dynamic instability

52.1 Key Points

- Conservative therapy is the initial and primary treatment modality for lumbar radiculopathy caused by a herniated nucleus pulposus (HNP).
- Lumbar microdiskectomy is a safe and effective procedure when the indication is appropriate.
- Cauda equina and conus syndromes caused by HNP in the lumbar spine constitute neurosurgical emergencies and require immediate evaluation and treatment.

52.2 Indications

- Symptomatic HNP:
  - Radiculopathy (after at least 6–8 weeks of failed conservative therapy).
  - Cauda equina syndrome (**Fig. 52.1**).
  - Conus medullaris syndrome.
- Not for isolated axial low back pain.
- No instability on preoperative dynamic plain radiographs.

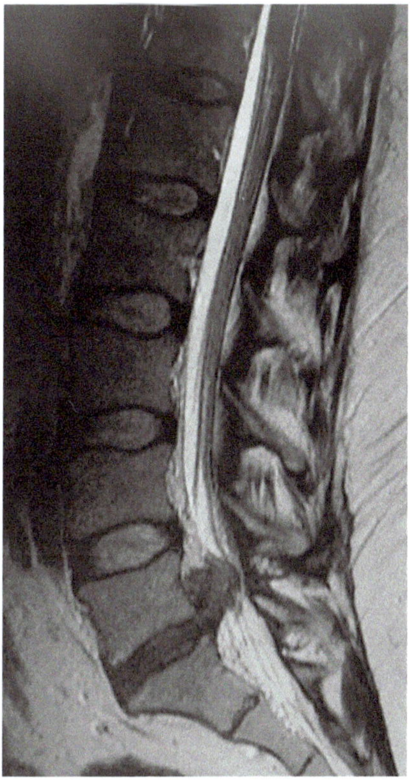

Fig. 52.1 Sagittal T2-weighted magnetic resonance imaging (MRI) demonstrating a large L5–S1 central disk herniation with extruded disk fragment causing central canal stenosis in a 32-year-old woman with cauda equina syndrome.

52.3 Technique

52.3.1 Open

- The patient is placed in the prone position in a Jackson frame.
  - Use of a Wilson frame may widen the interlaminar space and assist in access.
- Fluoroscopy is used for localization.
- A 2- to 3-cm midline incision is made with a number 10 scalpel.
- A subperiosteal dissection of tissue from spinous process and lamina on the ipsilateral side is performed.
  - Supraspinous and interspinous ligaments should be preserved.
- The medial aspect of the corresponding facet joint is the lateral limit of the dissection.
- A retractor (e.g., McCollough, Williams, or Taylor) is placed.
- The inferior lamina of the superior level and superior lamina of the inferior level are identified and confirmed with fluoroscopy.
- Using a high-speed drill, a laminotomy (usually) is performed by drilling the inferior part of the superior level and a small portion of the medial facet joint.
  - For inferior fragment migration, some of the superior lamina from the inferior level may need removing.
  - A matchstick or diamond drill bit may be used.
- Ligamentous flavum is removed using a curette and Kerrison punch.
- The operative microscope is brought in (optional).
- The nerve sleeve and dura are gently retracted medially (**Fig. 52.2**).
- The posterior longitudinal ligament (PLL) and annulus fibrosus are incised with a number 15 blade, medial to lateral (always incise away from the dura).
- Disk material is removed with a small pituitary rongeur and further mobilized with a downgoing curette (**Video 52.1**).
  - The surgeon must have an exquisite understanding of where the anterior longitudinal ligament (ALL) is to prevent inadvertent penetration into the retroperitoneal vessels with the pituitary rongeur.
- The disk space is irrigated, and loose disk tissue removed (**Fig. 52.3**).
- An instrument (e.g., Woodson or dental dissector) is passed beneath the dura to ensure that there is no residual fragment.
- A nerve hook is used to probe under the PLL superior and inferior to the disk space to check for residual.
- The fascia is closed with 0 or 2–0 absorbable suture.
- The subcutaneous layer is closed with inverted, interrupted 3–0 absorbable suture.
- The skin is closed with running suture, staples, or skin adhesive.

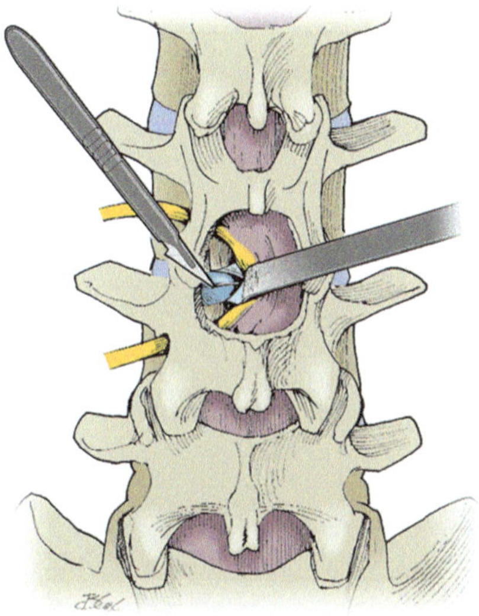

Fig. 52.2 Dorsal view of laminotomy defect showing the thecal sac, traversing the nerve root (retracted medially), and the herniated disk.

52.3.2 Minimally Invasive Technique

- After correct positioning and localization, a 12- to 16-mm incision is made 10 mm lateral to the midline on the appropriate side (**Fig. 52.4**).
- The thoracodorsal fascia is incised with blade or cautery, and serial dilators are positioned with the use of fluoroscopy.
- The final dilator and working tube should be docked over the interlaminar space with visualization of the inferior lamina of the superior level.
- It is important not to be aggressive with the initial dilators to not penetrate the interlaminar space.
- The operative microscope is brought in.
- Soft tissue is dissected, and drilling is performed until ligamentum flavum is reached.
  - If drilling is done too laterally, the pedicle or facet joint is at risk; confirm location with fluoroscopy if needed. With tubular approaches, the tube tends to "dock" more laterally; therefore, one should try to aim the tube more medially. However, an overly aggressive medial trajectory could lead to an "over-the-top" approach across the contralateral lamina. When in doubt, obtain an anteroposterior fluoroscopic shot.
- The ligament is removed and diskectomy is performed as in the open approach.

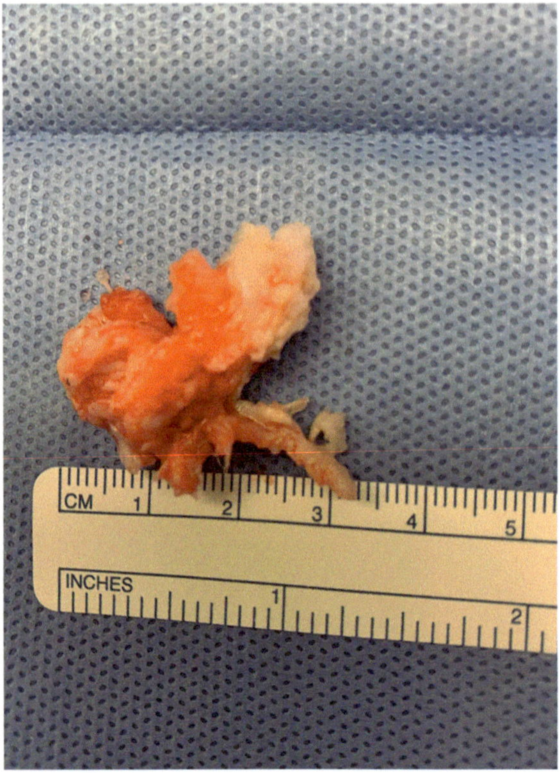

Fig. 52.3 Extruded disk fragment removed en bloc (approximately 3 cm).

- If a wider decompression is needed, the working tube may be repositioned to allow access to more lamina, and even the contralateral foramen.

52.4 Complications

- Durotomy (2.8% in open, 3.2% in microendoscopic)[1]:
  - Attempt primary repair using nonabsorbable suture (typically challenging).
  - Alternatively, cover with locally harvested fat, Gelfoam (Pharmacia & Upjohn; Kalamazoo, Michigan), and/or fibrin glue.
- Nerve root injury (0.4% in open, 0.2% in microendoscopic, 1.2% in percutaneous).[1]
- Superficial wound infection (2–3%).[2]

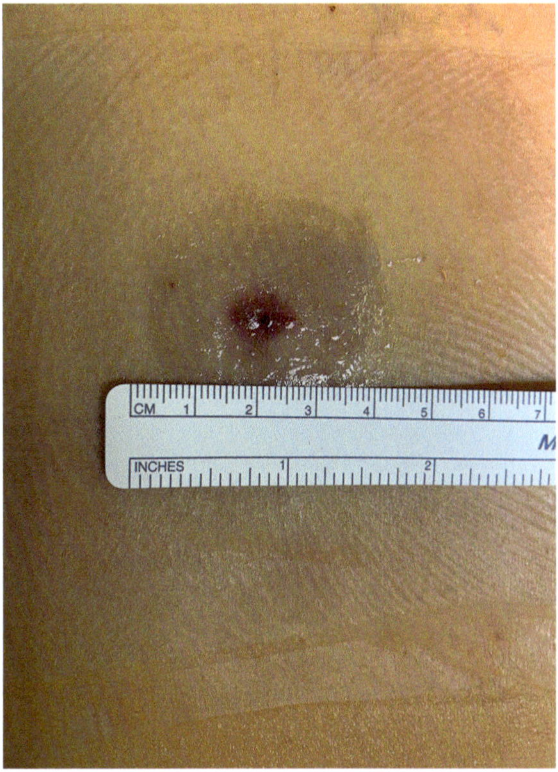

Fig. 52.4 Final image of the typical size of microdiskectomy incision when performed with a tube (skin glue was used topically).

- Disk space infection (< 1%).[2]
- Hematoma (0.7% in open, 1.2% in microendoscopic)[1]:
  - Suspected injury to the iliac vessels anteriorly (e.g., bright red blood from disk space or sudden, unexplained drop in blood pressure) requires immediate wound closure, repositioning of the patient to supine position, and immediate vascular surgery consult.

52.5 Postoperative Care

- Mobilize early; no need for bracing.
- Discharge to home when the patient meets discharge criteria (typically, ambulating, tolerating a diet, voiding, and receiving adequate pain control from oral medications—usually the same day or on postoperative day 1).

52.6 Outcomes

- With the open technique, there is an 85% chance of a good (minimal symptoms) or excellent (asymptomatic) outcome.[3]
- Moderate quality evidence suggests no difference in postoperative leg pain or functional outcomes between open and percutaneous endoscopic approaches at intermediate (3–6 months) and long-term (12 months) follow-ups.[4]
- First recurrence is usually treated with repeat microdiskectomy. Further recurrence may necessitate fusion.
- In a single-center randomized trial of 128 patients with persistent sciatica lasting 4 to 12 months and L4–L5 or L5–S1 disk herniation, microdiskectomy was found to be superior to nonsurgical management in reducing pain intensity at 6 months follow-up.[5]

52.7 Surgical Pearls

- Ensure that the HNP is the pain/symptom generator based on examination and imaging.
- Minimal disruption of medial facet (don't confuse the facet for the lamina during the initial approach).
- Overly aggressive drilling of facet may lead to instability.
- Ensure you are not in a nerve root axilla when performing diskectomy.
- Preoperative dynamic films may be necessary to rule out instability.
- May need hemilaminectomy or complete laminectomy if treating large central disk (e.g., for cauda equina or conus syndrome).

Common Clinical Questions

1. What is the best way to avoid drilling into the facet joint or pedicle during minimally invasive spine diskectomy?
2. When evaluating for recurrent lumbar herniated disk, what radiologic examination is most appropriate?
3. When evaluating a recurrent lumbar herniated disk, what radiologic examination is helpful in ruling out instability?

Answers to Common Clinical Questions

1. Obtain anteroposterior/lateral fluoroscopy images intraoperatively to confirm location.
2. MRI with and without contrast.
3. Flexion–extension X-rays.

References

1. Shriver MF, Xie JJ, Tye EY, et al. Lumbar microdiscectomy complication rates: a systematic review and meta-analysis. Neurosurg Focus. 2015; 39(4):E6
2. Kraemer R, Wild A, Haak H, Herdmann J, Krauspe R, Kraemer J. Classification and management of early complications in open lumbar microdiscectomy. Eur Spine J. 2003; 12(3):239–246
3. Tao XZ, Jing L, Li JH. Therapeutic effect of transforaminal endoscopic spine system in the treatment of prolapse of lumbar intervertebral disc. Eur Rev Med Pharmacol Sci. 2018; 22(1) Suppl:103–110
4. Gadjradj PS, Harhangi BS, Amelink J, et al. Percutaneous transforaminal endoscopic discectomy versus open microdiscectomy for lumbar disc herniation: a systematic review and meta-analysis. Spine. 2021; 46(8): 538–549
5. Bailey CS, Rasoulinejad P, Taylor D, et al. Surgery versus conservative care for persistent sciatica lasting 4 to 12 months. N Engl J Med. 2020; 382(12): 1093–1102

53 Lumbar Laminectomy

Matthew T. Carr, Frank J. Yuk, and Jeremy Steinberger

Summary
Lumbar laminectomy is a common spine surgery to decompress the central canal and lateral recesses of the lumbar spine. Diskectomy or foraminotomy can also be performed intraoperatively to provide further decompression as needed. A high-speed drill and/or rongeurs are used to remove the lamina and ligamentum flavum. Surgical outcomes are favorable. Randomized trials show significant improvement in leg and back pain following surgery compared to nonoperative treatment. Severe radiculopathy and neurogenic claudication symptoms are most likely to improve after surgery. Complication rates are low, with cerebrospinal fluid leak as the most common intraoperative complication. Postoperatively, recurrent stenosis or spondylolisthesis may develop warranting future reoperations.

Keywords: laminectomy, lumbar spine, surgical decompression, foraminotomy, spinal stenosis

53.1 Key Points

- The goal of a lumbar laminectomy is to provide decompression of the central canal and the lateral recesses, and it may provide access for further decompression of the central canal through a diskectomy and decompression of the neural foramina with foraminotomies.
- Care must be taken to avoid disrupting the bilateral facet joints and pars interarticularis, which can potentially lead to worsening of instability that may require further surgical intervention and stabilization.
- Additional care must be taken to avoid removal or fracture of the pars interarticularis, which may also result in iatrogenic instability.

53.2 Indications

- Focal or multilevel lumbar central and lateral recess stenosis resulting from lumbar degenerative disease, trauma, infections, or neoplastic conditions.

- Laminectomy without arthrodesis is discouraged if there is instability commonly seen with degenerative spondylolisthesis at the index segment, in a patient with a significant scoliosis at the index level, or if significant facet joint resection is performed.

53.3 Technique

- The patient is placed in the prone position.
  - There are two schools of thought regarding operating room (OR) table selection. If no instrumentation is used, many surgeons prefer using a Wilson frame, as the patient's lumbar spine is flexed, which opens up the posterior elements and may allow for easier access for the decompression. However, some feel that it may artificially augment the surgeon's sense of adequate decompression intraoperatively owing to the flexed position. The Wilson frame should not be used if the patient is to be instrumented, as the vertebrae will be fused in kyphosis in the flexed position.
  - Alternatively, some authors prefer using an orthopedic surgical table (e.g., Jackson four-post table) for laminectomies, and this table is used if instrumentation will be performed with the decompression. This table helps maintain the lumbar spine in its anatomic lordotic position. Accordingly, if an adequate decompression is performed in this position, then it should be adequate once the patient is mobilized.
- A spinal needle or other radiopaque marker is placed at the desired level and is confirmed with fluoroscopy or a single standard intraoperative X-ray. If a spinal needle is used to puncture the skin and palpate bone, care must be taken to avoid causing an inadvertent durotomy with the localizing needle. It is recommended to position laterally and aim for the transverse process to avoid durotomy.
- A midline incision is made at the appropriate level. A single clean incision through the fascia is helpful when the time comes to close the fascia at the end of the case. A subperiosteal dissection is performed to detach the erector spinae muscles from the lamina.
  - It is important to remain subperiosteal during the dissection, for this significantly limits the bleeding that is encountered if the paraspinal muscles are violated. Excess intramuscular dissection can also lead to increased postoperative pain.
- The dissection is carried laterally until the medial aspect of the facet joint, but every effort should be made to leave the facet joint capsule intact and avoid disrupting the joint. The bilateral pars are exposed to serve as a lateral marker for the laminectomy.

- A Horsley or Leksell rongeur is used to remove the spinous process.
  - If a fusion is also being performed, care should be taken to save the removed bone to use as fusion autograft, except in cases of abnormal bone (i.e., tumor or infection).
- A high-speed drill with either a cutting, matchstick, or diamond bur or an ultrasonic drill is used to thin or remove the lamina. Alternatively, some surgeons perform all of the bone removal with Kerrison and Leksell rongeurs.
- Alternatively, a Leksell rongeur can be used to remove the interspinous ligament above and below the desired level of laminectomy. A high-speed drill or ultrasonic drill can be used to create full-thickness troughs bilaterally on each side of the lamina. Care is taken to stay medial to the facets and pars interarticularis. The bony lamina can then be removed in a lobster-tail fashion and the ligamentum flavum is detached from the lamina using curettes. This method does not serve well during reoperation laminectomies due to scar tissue and higher risk of durotomy and subsequent cerebrospinal fluid (CSF) leak.
  - The ligamentum flavum attaches to the superior edge of the lower lamina, and runs ventral to the inferior half to two-thirds of the upper lamina. Thus, you are protected by the ligamentum flavum while drilling the lower half to two-thirds of the lamina. It is recommended to advance the decompression cranially to maximize the protection of the ligamentum, and to perform all drilling and bony removal prior to removing the ligamentum.
- Once the drilling is complete, the ligamentum flavum can be released from the lamina, and the remainder of the laminectomy is completed with Kerrison rongeurs.
- Next, lateral recess stenosis is addressed. The dura is dissected from the lateral recess using a Woodson elevator or Penfield 4, and Kerrison rongeurs are used to remove the bone (**Fig. 53.1** and **Fig. 53.2**).
  - The facets are often hypertrophied, and the medial third can be drilled or removed with Kerrison rongeurs.
  - The pars may need to be undercut to help decompress the lateral recess, but great care should be exercised, because excessive removal may lead to an iatrogenic pars defect and increase the risk of postoperative spondylolisthesis.
- A ball-tipped probe or Woodson elevator is used to inspect the foramina, as the nerve exits the spinal canal beneath the pedicle.
  - Kerrison rongeurs (generally number 2 and number 3) or foraminotomy rongeurs are used to complete foraminotomies, if necessary.

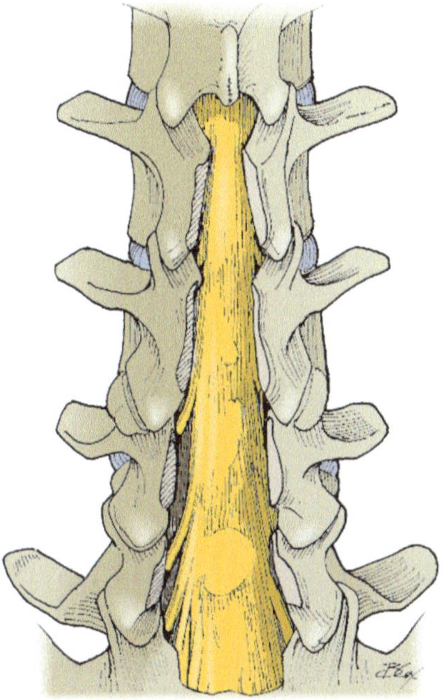

Fig. 53.1 Dorsal view of lumbar spine showing decompressed thecal sac and nerve roots with laminectomy taken to the medial facets laterally.

  - Angling the rongeur in the inferolateral direction parallel to the exiting nerve root may limit the risk of inadvertent nerve root injury.
- Know your landmarks, and be careful to avoid drilling the facet joint, pedicle, or pars.
- A subfascial drain can be used in the wound if warranted, and is often needed if multiple levels are performed, to aid with wound healing as well as help to prevent an epidural hematoma.
- Ensure a tight fascial closure and close the skin in the standard fashion.
  - Paraspinal muscles should be approximated to help close the dead space. The fascia is closed with 0 Vicryl sutures in a watertight fashion, especially if the dura is violated. Another layer of Scarpa's fascia or deep tissue may be closed especially in larger patients.
- Some alternative procedures have been proposed including laminotomy, spinous process osteotomy, and several variations of minimally invasive approaches, although significant benefits of these alternatives have not been clearly demonstrated in the literature.

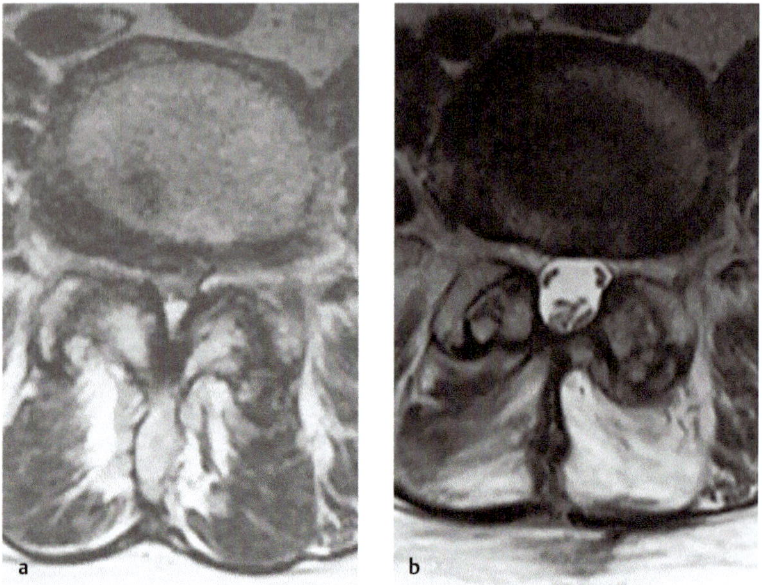

Fig. 53.2 **(a)** T2-weighted axial magnetic resonance imaging (MRI) demonstrating severe central and lateral recess stenosis from ligamentum flavum hypertrophy, disk protrusion, and facet joint hypertrophy. **(b)** T2-weighted axial MRI demonstrating thecal sac expansion following lumbar laminectomy.

53.4 Complications

- Mortality and complications are more common in elderly and patients who have multiple pre-existing comorbidities.
- Durotomy/CSF leak (8–10%)[1,2]:
  - Leads to increased operative time, blood loss, and inpatient stay, but no difference clinically at 1-year follow-up.
- Epidural hematoma requiring evacuation (0.18% rate for laminectomy and 0.09% rate for laminotomy in retrospective review of 15,000 patients).[3]
- Wound infection (1–2%).[2,4]
- Spondylolisthesis or recurrent stenosis (occurred in 1–4% at 2 years).[2]
- Inpatient mortality rate (0.2%).[4]
- Neurological deficit (0.7%).[4]

53.5 Postoperative Care

- Operative time is approximately 2 hours, with an average of 300 mL blood loss.[2]

- Approximately 10% of patients required intraoperative transfusion, and around 5% of patients required postoperative transfusion.[2]
- An average of 3-day hospital stay for standard laminectomy.[2]
- Pain control can generally be managed with oral analgesics alone, depending on preoperative narcotic usage. Use stool softeners and laxatives with narcotics to prevent postoperative ileus.
- Antibiotics are typically continued for 24 hours perioperatively.
- The patient can be mobilized on postoperative day 0 and does not require a brace.
- If a durotomy is encountered during the surgery, the patient is usually kept flat for 24 hours to minimize pressure on the lumbar dura.

In case of a durotomy, a lumbar drain can be considered to decrease the intrathecal pressure in the lumbar cistern to prevent CSF leak or decrease the formation of a pseudomeningocele or duro-cutaneous fistula. This should be a consideration with any spinal fluid leak, particularly if a watertight repair is not achievable.

- Drain removal is dependent on the individual surgeon but often ranges between < 30 mL output over 24 hours to < 50 mL over an 8-hour shift.
- Discharge home when the patient meets the discharge criteria.

53.6 Outcomes

- In a recent randomized trial, around 60 to 70% of the patients reported improvement in condition from 3 months to 2 years when treated with surgical decompression. Surgery led to greater improvement in Oswestry disability index, stenosis bothersomeness index, and leg pain bothersomeness index.[2] As reviewed previously,[4] two other randomized trials showed significant improvement in leg and back pain at 1 year compared with nonoperative treatment, though this difference decreased by 2 years.
- Recurrent/adjacent stenosis or progressive spondylolisthesis was reported in 1 to 4% of patients at 1 to 2 years.[2]
- Several cohort studies demonstrated > 80% improvement in symptoms after decompressive surgery, but at least a third of the patients reported recurrent back pain at 7 to 10 years, and 10 to 23% required reoperation by this time.[4]
- Patients with most severe radiculopathy symptoms were most likely to improve.[4]

53.7 Surgical Pearls

- With advanced degenerative disease, obtain preoperative dynamic films to rule out a dynamic spondylolisthesis and spinal instability at the index segment.

- Care should be taken to dissect the dura from the surrounding bone and ligamentum flavum with a curette, Woodson elevator, or Penfield 4 before removing the bone with a rongeur. Never take blind bites with a rongeur without visualizing that the dura is completely dissected. The "Catch and Release" method can be used to verify that the dura is not moving with the rongeur bite.
- Apply bone wax or hemostatic matrix to the bone edges to stop bleeding. Hemostatic matrix or Gelfoam (Pharmacia and Upjohn Company; Kalamazoo, Michigan) can be used to coagulate epidural venous bleeding. If minor bleeding remains or a multilevel laminectomy is performed, consider leaving a subfascial drain to mitigate the risk of postoperative hematoma requiring reoperation and to assist with wound healing.
- In reoperation laminectomies, a computed tomography (CT) scan of the lumbar spine is useful to examine the extent of bony resection from the prior laminectomy.

Common Clinical Questions

1. Why are preoperative dynamic X-rays sometimes obtained before a lumbar laminectomy?
2. During lumbar laminectomy, what location is associated with the highest likelihood of a CSF leak?
3. When should an arthrodesis be considered in combination with lumbar laminectomy?

Answers to Common Clinical Questions

1. To rule out spondylolisthesis or instability, which would indicate that a fusion procedure should be performed in conjunction with the decompression.
2. The superior aspect of the lamina as the ligamentum flavum ends at this location, and thus the dura is not protected. Additionally, this can occur in the lateral recess if there is significant stenosis. Accordingly, care should be taken to dissect the dura from the surrounding bone and ligamentum flavum with a curette, Woodson elevator, or Penfield 4 before removing the bone with a rongeur.
3. Laminectomy without arthrodesis is discouraged if there is instability or degenerative spondylolisthesis with instability at the index segment, in a patient with a significant scoliosis at the index level, and if a significant amount of the facet joint is removed. Additionally, arthrodesis should be considered if an iatrogenic pars defect is caused by extending the laminectomy too far laterally.

Acknowledgments

We would like to thank Benjamin Elder and Timothy F. Witham for their work on this chapter in previous edition of this book.

References

1. Desai A, Ball PA, Bekelis K, et al. SPORT: does incidental durotomy affect long-term outcomes in cases of spinal stenosis? Neurosurgery. 2011; 69(1): 38–44, discussion 44
2. Weinstein JN, Tosteson TD, Lurie JD, et al. SPORT Investigators. Surgical versus nonsurgical therapy for lumbar spinal stenosis. N Engl J Med. 2008; 358(8):794–810
3. Kao FC, Tsai TT, Chen LH, et al. Symptomatic epidural hematoma after lumbar decompression surgery. Eur Spine J. 2015; 24(2):348–357
4. Li G, Patil CG, Lad SP, Ho C, Tian W, Boakye M. Effects of age and comorbidities on complication rates and adverse outcomes after lumbar laminectomy in elderly patients. Spine. 2008; 33(11):1250–1255

54 Endoscopic Lumbar Techniques

Sananthan Sivakanthan and Christoph Hofstetter

Summary

Uniportal endoscopic techniques include transforaminal and interlaminar approaches to the spine. These two techniques can be utilized to approach any pathology in the lumbar spine. Although the setup and approach may be different the principles of endoscopy are the same and both the techniques employ a similar framework of positioning, trajectory, docking, decompression, and closure.

Keywords: endoscopic spine, transforaminal, interlaminar, lumbar spine

54.1 Key Points

- Full-endoscopic lumbar spine surgery is a safe and effective means to address central, foraminal, and extraforaminal pathologies.
- There are two main approach corridors: interlaminar and transforaminal.
- Functional outcomes are similar to traditional minimally invasive surgery (MIS) or open approaches and overall perioperative complications are lower.

54.2 Indications

- Transforaminal:
  - Foraminal disk herniations.
  - Central disk herniations.
  - Previous interlaminar surgery.
- Interlaminar:
  - Posterolateral disk herniations.
  - Concomitant lateral recess stenosis.
  - Central stenosis.
- Either transforaminal or interlaminar:
  - Recurrent disk herniation.
  - Synovial cysts.
  - Tumors.

54.3 Surgical Technique

- Transforaminal (**Video 54.1** and **Fig. 54.1**):
  - Positioning:
    - Either prone on a Wilson frame or in lateral decubitus position with the symptomatic side up.
  - Trajectory:
    - Mark the intended disk space on an anteroposterior (AP) end plate view.

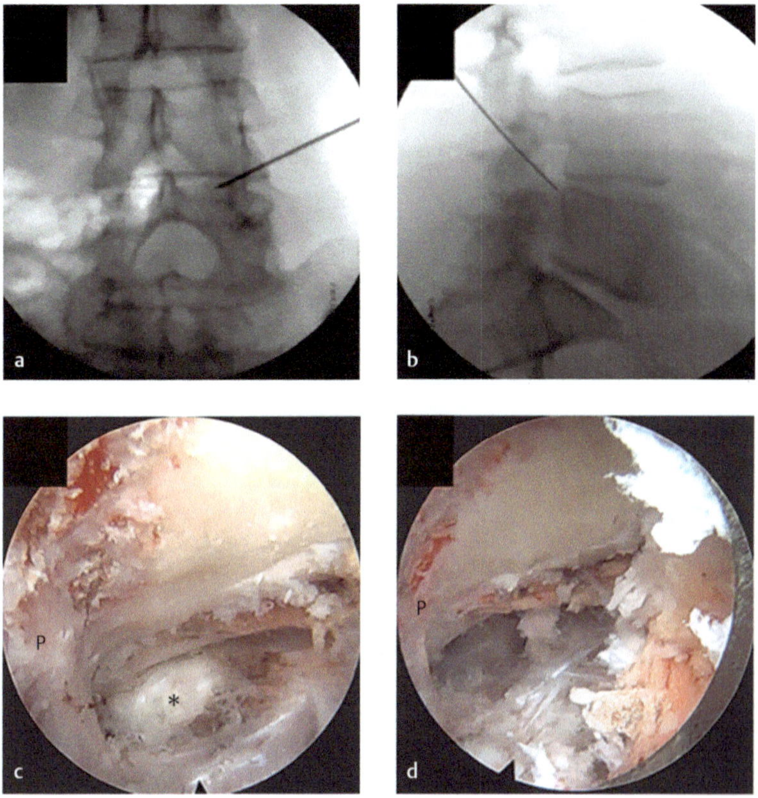

Fig. 54.1 **(a)** The tip of the needle is positioned in the inferior aspect of the intervertebral disk at the mid-pedicle line. **(b)** In the lateral projection the tip of the needle is seen just dorsal to the posterior spinal line. **(c)** The disc protrusion (*asterisk*) is seen ventral to the traversing nerve root and medial to the pedicle (*P*). **(d)** The traversing nerve root is entirely decompressed following resection of the disk herniation.

    - Mark rostrocaudal inclination to allow for a transisthmic approach by connecting the rostral aspect of the superior articular process and the medial aspect of Kambin's triangle.
    - Mark midline and three lines 8 cm (L3/L4), 10 cm (L4/L5), and 12 cm (L5/S1) away from midline.
    - Reference the entry point along this line with the lateral X-ray projection of a line drawn along the tip of the spinous process.
  - Docking:
    - Advance an 18-G spinal needle toward the superior articular process of the caudal index level (bevel facing ventrally).
    - Once reached, turn the bevel of the needle 180 degrees and advance into the medial aspect of Kambin's triangle (target area).
    - Confirm the tip of the needle at the medial pedicle line (AP) and posterior to the posterior vertebral line (lateral X-ray).
    - Place a K-wire followed by sequential dilators and a reamer to establish the trajectory.
    - Place the working channel followed by the endoscope.
  - Decompression:
    - Complete foraminoplasty using bur.
    - Identify pedicle of caudal index level (principle anatomic landmark).
    - Identify traversing nerve root and dissect free from any disk herniation.
    - Resect disk herniation.
  - Closure:
    - Achieve hemostasis using cautery and thrombin/Gelfoam.
    - Close fascia and skin in a two-layered fashion.
- Interlaminar (**Fig. 54.2**):
  - Positioning
    - Prone on a Wilson frame.
  - Trajectory:
    - Obtain AP end plate view of the caudal index level.
    - Adjust the caudal tilt of the C-arm so that the spinous processes are centered on the disk space.
    - Trajectory can be modified for caudally or cranially migrated disk spaces.
  - Docking:
    - Through a stab incision over the index level advance the trocar with a rostrocaudal motion until the inferomedial edge of the lamina can be palpated.
    - Confirm appropriate positioning at the target area with AP and lateral fluoroscopy.
    - Place sequential dilators followed by working channel.

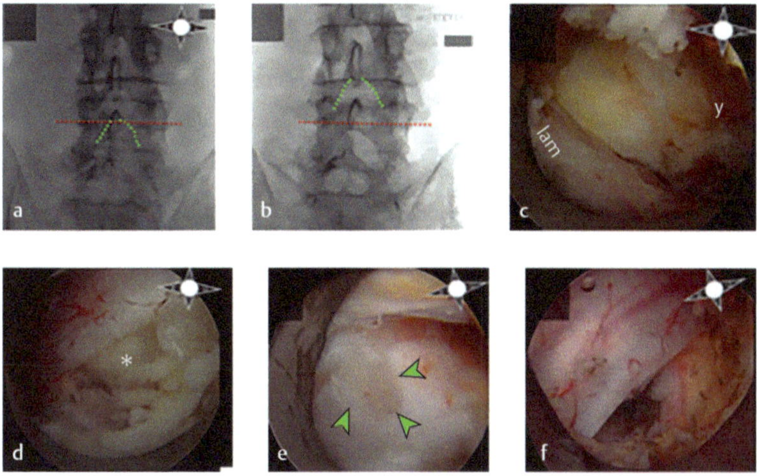

Fig. 54.2 **(a)** First an anteroposterior (AP) end plate view of the superior end plate of the caudal index level is obtained (spinous process, *green line*; index level, *red line*). **(b)** Addition of distal tilt to the rostrocaudal X-ray beam angle moves the projection of the superior spinous process (*green line*) centered over the projection of the disk space (*red line*) and an ideal rostrocaudal trajectory has been determined. **(c)** Utilizing a diamond bur the lamina is partially resected, and the yellow ligament and its lamina attachment unambiguously identified. **(d)** The lateral margin of the neural elements is exposed, and the herniated disk fragment (*asterisk*) is seen. **(e)** Upon resection of the disk sequester and retraction of the nerve root, the annular defect is identified (*green arrowheads*). **(f)** At the end of the procedure the decompressed traversing nerve root is inspected.

    - Directly visualize target area under endoscopy. Use forceps and cautery to clean bony edge if needed.
- Decompression:
    - Using a high-speed drill perform a complete laminectomy until the yellow ligament is visualized in its entirety.
    - Use a micropunch to open and resect the yellow ligament.
    - Identify the lateral edge of the neural elements and thecal sac and mobilize with a blunt dissector.
    - Medialize the thecal sac using the bevel of the working channel.
    - Disk fragments can be safely resected with the neural elements retracted.
- Closure:
    - Achieve hemostasis using cautery and thrombin/Gelfoam.
    - Close fascia and skin in a two-layered fashion.

54.4 Complications

- Durotomies can occur and will need to be addressed at the time of discovery with DuraGen inlay and Tisseal to prevent postoperative radiculopathy.
  - In the event the durotomy cannot be repaired via an endoscopic approach consider converting to open surgery for primary repair.
- Postoperative hematomas should prompt return to the operating room for evacuation if clinical presentation warrants. Generally, it is prudent to perform this via an open approach.
- Extensive intraoperative bleeding: Do not move endoscope, obliterate the egress port, cover the area of the last surgical move with the RF probe, increase the water pressure, fill the operative cavity with Gelfoam powder.

54.5 Postoperative Care

- Patients can typically be discharged the same day.
- Nonsteroidal anti-inflammatory drugs (NSAIDs) are safe to give postoperatively.
- Injection of local analgesia can help with recovery.
- Patients are to have limited mobility for 2 weeks for wound healing.

54.6 Outcomes

- Endoscopic lumbar diskectomy provides equivalent results in pain relief and functional recovery to traditional microdiskectomy.
- Endoscopic surgery, however, does result in fewer complications, shorter hospital length of stay, less postoperative pain medication requirement, and less postoperative disability.

54.7 Surgical Pearls

- Meticulous hemostasis is paramount for visualization given the small working space. Strategies to achieve hemostasis include:
  - Generous use of bipolar cautery.
  - Minimize disruption and dissection of muscle/soft tissue.

Common Clinical Questions

1. What is the target area for the interlaminar approach?
2. What is the target area for the transforaminal approach?

Answers to Common Clinical Questions

1. Inferomedial edge of the lamina.
2. Kambin's triangle.

55 Open Transforaminal Lumbar Interbody Fusion

Jose A. Canseco, Yunsoo Lee, Jeremy C. Heard, and Christopher K. Kepler

Summary

The open transforaminal lumbar interbody fusion (TLIF) involves an approach to the disk through a unilateral facetectomy, which allows wide access to the disk space with minimal retraction of the central neural elements. Recent literature suggests that TLIF procedures are associated with improved patient-reported outcome measures and reduced complication rates.

Keywords: TLIF, open, transforaminal, fusion, spondylolisthesis

55.1 Key Points

- Spinal fusion is an effective treatment for multiple spine disorders, including spinal instability, deformity, and neural element compression.[1]
- Compared to traditional posterolateral fusion, interbody fusion techniques have demonstrated improved arthrodesis rates, as well as restoration of radiographic parameters, such as lumbar lordosis, by providing anterior column support and disk height resulting in indirect foraminal decompression.[2,3,4,5,6]
- Transforaminal lumbar interbody fusion (TLIF) involves an approach to the intervertebral disk through a unilateral facetectomy, which permits wide access to the disk space with minimal retraction of the central neural elements.[7]
- Although reported complication rates are similar between TLIF and other lumbar fusion alternatives, recent literature has suggested TLIF is associated with improved patient-reported outcome measures and reduced complication rates.[2,8,9,10,11]

55.2 Indications

- Spondylolisthesis.
- Disk space collapse with vertical neuroforaminal narrowing.

- Degenerative scoliosis with coronal or sagittal imbalance.
- Revision for pseudoarthrosis.

55.3 Technique

55.3.1 Open Transforaminal Lumbar Interbody Fusion

- Approach (for example, L4–L5 TLIF):
  - The spinous processes and posterior elements, including the lamina, pars interarticularis, and transverse processes, of the levels above L4 and below L5 are exposed subperiosteally. Care should be taken to avoid damaging the facet capsules of the level immediately above the surgical target. After disk space level confirmation with fluoroscopy, the spinous process of the superior level (L4) is removed, and a superior level laminectomy (L4) is performed with thorough medial facetectomy—if the symptoms are bilateral, medial facetectomies are performed on both sides. Disk space distraction is then achieved by placing a laminar spreader between the spinous processes of the level above (L3) and the inferior level (L5). All removed bony elements are saved and morselized for use as fusion autograft.
  - The pars interarticularis of the most symptomatic side is identified and an osteotome is used to remove the remaining inferior articular process (IAP) of the superior vertebra (L4) just below the level of the pars. Once the IAP of L4 is removed, the remaining superior articular process (SAP) of the inferior vertebra (L5) is visualized. Using a Kerrison rongeur, the superior and inferior aspects of the L5 SAP are removed until the ipsilateral L4 and L5 pedicles are easily palpable with a Woodson elevator. The exiting L4 nerve root is then identified, and a foraminotomy is performed at this time by following the exiting nerve root laterally with Kerrison rongeurs. The Woodson elevator is then used to feel the inferior pedicle and then placed laterally just superior to the pedicle to protect the exiting nerve root. Any remaining SAP is removed with an osteotome, aimed in the direction of the Woodson elevator and ensuring the cut is above the superior edge of the pedicle. Alternatively, the entire SAP can be removed piecemeal using a Kerrison rongeur. This achieves a pedicle-to-pedicle exposure.
  - Bipolar electrocautery is used to achieve hemostasis from any epidural bleeding in the floor of the disk space between the exposed pedicles, and a Penfield 4 is used to clear off the disk space. Care should be taken to avoid injuring the exiting L4 nerve root, which can be visualized just superiorly exiting under the pedicle of L4. A nerve root retractor is then used to gently retract the dura and the traversing L5 nerve root medially. At this time the disk space should be fully exposed (**Fig. 55.1**).

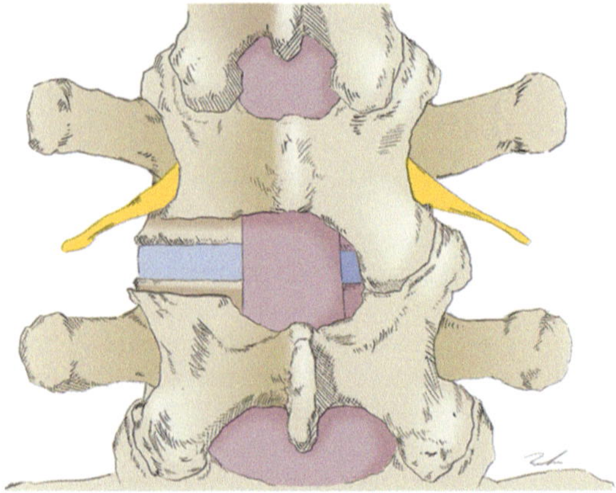

Fig. 55.1 Demonstration of the open transforaminal lumbar interbody fusion (TLIF) approach with unilateral facetectomy and exposure of the left-sided disk space.

- Diskectomy:
  - Annulotomy is performed with a #15 knife in a box cut fashion. If the disk is severely collapsed, a dilator can be used instead. Pituitary rongeurs are then used to remove as much disk as possible. If the box annulotomy needs to be enlarged, Kerrison rongeurs can be used to cut the edges of the annulus fibrosus. Dilators and shavers of increasing size are then used to remove the rest of the disk tissue and size the cage, while also preparing the end plates for fusion. The loose pieces of disk are removed with the pituitary rongeur. When using dilators and shavers, be mindful of the cranial–caudal angle of the disk and aim medially to reach the contralateral side.
  - Curettes are used to scrape the end plates to remove any remaining disk and cartilaginous tissue. Care should be taken to curette off the cartilage without damaging the bony end plate as that will increase the rate of interbody device subsidence.
- Interbody device placement:
  - Based on the dilator size, an interbody cage of the appropriate size is chosen and packed with autograft with or without additional autograft and/or fusion substrates. Nerve root retractors can be placed to protect the traversing and exiting nerve roots.
  - Prior to placing the cage, the disk space is packed with autograft, allograft, and/or other fusion substrates, and then the interbody cage is inserted and malleted in until the edge of the cage is beyond the posterior border of the cephalad and caudad vertebral bodies.

Intraoperative fluoroscopy should be used to assist in interbody cage placement to ensure the anterior edge of the end plates is not violated. Once satisfied with insertion, if the cage is expandable, the cage is then dilated at this time. The laminar spreader can be removed at this time.

- Pedicle screw placement:
  - The mammillary body is exposed and used as the landmark for the pedicle screw start site, which is found just superior to the mamillary body where the transverse process meets the superior facet in line with the lateral border of the pars interarticularis. A high-speed bur is used to decorticate the entry point and then a curved Lenke probe is used to cannulate the pedicle. The probe should be pointed medially, and radiographs should be considered for caudal–cranial angulation. If fluoroscopy or image guidance is not available, a Woodson elevator can be used through the decompression to palpate the pedicles and direct trajectory of cannulation. A ball probe is then used to confirm patency of the screw trajectory. All pedicle screw trajectory cannulations are done at this time. Bone wax or another form of hemostatic agent can be used to control bleeding from pedicle screw sites.
  - The transverse process and facet joint of the contralateral side (non-TLIF side) are then decorticated with the high-speed bur. A mix of autograft and allograft with or without additional fusion substrates is then packed onto the lateral gutter over the decorticated elements to augment the procedure with a posterolateral fusion. Care should be taken to ensure no autograft mixture fall into the decompressed neural elements.
  - Once the posterolateral bone graft is in place, the ball probe is used to find the screw start sites. Pedicle screws are placed and tested with EMG to ensure there is no bony breaching. A lordotic rod of appropriate length is inserted, and screw caps are tightened up to manufacturer specifications. During screw cap placement, compression across the screw heads can be performed if additional lordosis correction is desired.
- Closure:
  - A surgical drain may be left in place deep to fascia. The lumbodorsal fascia and subdermis are closed in a layered fashion with absorbable sutures. The skin is closed with nylon sutures.

55.4 Complications

- The main complications include nerve root injury, hardware failure, and wound infection.[12]
- Other complications include dural tear and hardware migration.[13,14]
- Use of bone morphogenetic protein (BMP) in the interbody graft has been associated with BMP-related radiculitis, as well as heterotopic ossification with osteolysis.[14,15]

55.5 Postoperative Care

- Pain management: Patient-controlled administration of narcotics, muscle relaxants, and early transition to oral medications.
- Mobilization: Early mobilization with physical therapy is essential; for patients remaining inpatient longer than 1 day, deep vein thrombosis (DVT) chemoprophylaxis is recommended starting from postoperative day 1.
- Drain management: Discontinue drain based on output (e.g., less than 50 mL in 12 h, "overnight shift").

55.6 Outcomes

- Patient-reported outcome studies show benefits in both back and leg pain.[2,11]
- Multiple studies have demonstrated an arthrodesis rate of > 90%.[2,3,6,14]

55.7 Surgical Pearls

- When planning for multilevel fusion, first proceed with the level of the TLIF to preserve adjacent spinous processes for distraction.
- When using a laminar spreader, ensure a surgical assistant maintains control of the device to avoid sudden slip and incidental durotomy.
- Use a Woodson elevator to feel the pedicle and serve as a guide for the facet osteotomies, being careful to avoid damaging the pedicles.
- Take care to curette the cartilaginous end plate without excessive curetting of the underlying bony end plate to reduce the risk of cage subsidence.
- Consider anterior positioning of cage to focus on correction of lumbar lordosis and posterior positioning for more indirect foraminal decompression. Keep in mind TLIF has been shown multiple times to maintain but not improve global lumbar lordosis. If correction of sagittal balance is an important feature of the surgical plan, an alternative surgical strategy is recommended.
- Do not neglect the contralateral facet joint. Arthrodesis often occurs through the remaining facet joint despite the intervertebral disk preparation and bone grafting.

Common Clinical Questions

1. Which side should be chosen for the TLIF approach?
2. TLIF doesn't do much for sagittal plane correction. What are some ways to adjust the TLIF procedure to optimize sagittal alignment?

3. What should you be wary of when compressing across the disk space to improve segmental lumbar lordosis?
4. Is performing TLIF better than posterior lumbar decompression and instrumented fusion without an interbody device?

Answers to Common Clinical Questions

1. As the TLIF only requires a unilateral approach, it is usually performed on the more symptomatic side for decompression of the neural elements directly.
2. Options include using a larger or expandable TLIF cage, anterior positioning of the cage, and using a TLIF cage in conjunction with bilateral facetectomies and compression across the segment.
3. As compression increases lumbar lordosis, it also reduces the neuroforaminal space and carries a risk of causing contralateral radiculopathy. Care must be taken to check the preoperative MRI to evaluate the foramen bilaterally regardless of symptoms and directly decompress the contralateral side if compression across the segment is essential to the surgical plan.
4. There is little evidentiary support for the superiority of TLIF over posterior lumbar decompression and instrumented fusion (PLDF). Although fusion rates are higher in some series, no clinical benefit in terms of patient-reported outcome measures has been shown and some series have reported a higher rate of nerve root injury.

References

1. Allen RT, Rihn JA, Glassman SD, Currier B, Albert TJ, Phillips FM. An evidence-based approach to spine surgery. Am J Med Qual. 2009; 24(6) Suppl:15S–24S
2. Levin JM, Tanenbaum JE, Steinmetz MP, Mroz TE, Overley SC. Posterolateral fusion (PLF) versus transforaminal lumbar interbody fusion (TLIF) for spondylolisthesis: a systematic review and meta-analysis. Spine J. 2018; 18 (6):1088–1098
3. Schroeder GD, Kepler CK, Millhouse PW, et al. L5/S1 fusion rates in degenerative spine surgery: a systematic review comparing ALIF, TLIF, and axial interbody arthrodesis. Clin Spine Surg. 2016; 29(4):150–155
4. Kepler CK, Rihn JA, Radcliff KE, et al. Restoration of lordosis and disk height after single-level transforaminal lumbar interbody fusion. Orthop Surg. 2012; 4(1):15–20

5. Fujimori T, Le H, Schairer WW, Berven SH, Qamirani E, Hu SS. Does transforaminal lumbar interbody fusion have advantages over posterolateral lumbar fusion for degenerative spondylolisthesis? Global Spine J. 2015; 5(2): 102–109
6. Souslian FG, Patel PD. Review and analysis of modern lumbar spinal fusion techniques. Br J Neurosurg. 2024; 38(1):61–67
7. de Kunder SL, van Kuijk SMJ, Rijkers K, et al. Transforaminal lumbar interbody fusion (TLIF) versus posterior lumbar interbody fusion (PLIF) in lumbar spondylolisthesis: a systematic review and meta-analysis. Spine J. 2017; 17(11):1712–1721
8. Lambrechts MJ, Siegel N, Heard JC, et al. Trends in single-level lumbar fusions over the past decade using a national database. World Neurosurg. 2022; S1878–8750(22)01039-7
9. Teng I, Han J, Phan K, Mobbs R. A meta-analysis comparing ALIF, PLIF, TLIF and LLIF. J Clin Neurosci. 2017; 44:11–17
10. Campbell RC, Mobbs RJ, Lu VM, Xu J, Rao PJ, Phan K. Posterolateral fusion versus interbody fusion for degenerative spondylolisthesis: systematic review and meta-analysis. Global Spine J. 2017; 7(5):482–490
11. Karamian BA, Lambrechts MJ, Mao J, et al. Adult isthmic spondylolisthesis: a radiographic and outcomes analysis comparing circumferential fusions versus TLIF procedures. Clin Spine Surg. 2022; 35(8):E660–E666
12. Hammad A, Wirries A, Ardeshiri A, Nikiforov O, Geiger F. Open versus minimally invasive TLIF: literature review and meta-analysis. J Orthop Surg Res. 2019; 14(1):229
13. Chrastil J, Patel AA. Complications associated with posterior and transforaminal lumbar interbody fusion. J Am Acad Orthop Surg. 2012; 20 (5):283–291
14. Kim CH, Easley K, Lee J-S, et al. Comparison of minimally invasive versus open transforaminal interbody lumbar fusion. Global Spine J. 2020; 10 2 Suppl:143S–150S
15. Rihn JA, Patel R, Makda J, et al. Complications associated with single-level transforaminal lumbar interbody fusion. Spine J. 2009; 9(8):623–629

56 Minimally Invasive Transforaminal Lumbar Interbody Fusion

Marisa Gandía and Jose Manuel Viñuela-Prieto

Summary

Minimally invasive transforaminal lumbar interbody fusion (MIS-TLIF) is one of the most frequent minimally invasive spine surgeries performed nowadays, achieving a successful lumbar decompression, fixation, and fusion with similar clinical results to the open approach but reducing soft tissue and muscle damage, postoperative pain, blood loss, recovery time, and hospital stay.

A comprehensive knowledge of the pathoanatomy and the landmarks under either fluoroscopy or navigation is mandatory to perform the procedure safely. Surgical skills in working through a tubular system and being familiar with instruments used in minimally invasive spine surgery are highly recommended to achieve a good result and avoid complications such as incomplete decompression or incidental durotomy.

A unilateral (or bilateral) facetectomy, decompression, diskectomy, intervertebral bone grafting, cage implantation, and placement of pedicle screws are the main steps of this technique. Osteobiologic adjuvants and bone graft application in combination with decortication of facet joints and/or transverse processes can be helpful to increase fusion rates and prevent pseudoarthrosis.

Identification of Kambin's triangle and working within the safe zone above the superior border of the inferior pedicle, lateral to the dural sac and inferior to the exiting nerve root, allows safe access to the intervertebral space. A careful localization and dissection of nervous structures is recommended to avoid the most severe complications like nerve root injury.

Single- or two-level degenerative disk disease, spondylolisthesis grade I or II, focal spinal deformity, and synovial cysts associated with spinal instability are the main indications of MIS-TLIF. Proper selection of patients is the main pearl to achieve excellent outcomes by using the technique described in the present chapter.

Keywords: minimally invasive spine surgery, transforaminal interbody fusion, surgical technique, spinal decompression, spinal fusion, safe zone, indications, complications

56.1 Key Points

- Minimally invasive transforaminal lumbar interbody fusion (MIS-TLIF) can be used to achieve lumbar spinal decompression, fixation, and fusion.
- The intent behind this approach, is to reduce soft tissue injury, postoperative pain, blood loss, recovery time, complications rate, and length of hospital stay associated with open TLIF.
- It is important to recognize the anatomic landmarks at the interpedicular space, referred to as Kambin's triangle: Medial (traversing root), lateral (exiting root), and base (inferior pedicle).

56.2 Indications

Harms and Rolinger first described the transforaminal lumbar interbody fusion (TLIF) technique for circumferential fusion in 1982 using an interbody spacer and a supplemental pedicle screw construct.[1] This procedure was a departure from the traditional posterior lumbar interbody fusion (PLIF) in that the TLIF required only a unilateral facetectomy and a single interbody cage. TLIF then became popular because of its lower rates of nerve root injury given the reduced surgical manipulation of neural elements, and it was also found to be effective for revision surgery, because the midline dural sac did not have to be exposed. A minimally invasive approach for accomplishing the TLIF procedure was subsequently developed.[2] This technique used the advantages of either expandable or sequential dilating working tubes and percutaneous pedicle screw technology to reduce the soft tissue injury that has been documented to result from open surgery.[3] Although no class I evidence exists to demonstrate the superiority of MIS-TLIF over open TLIF, comparative studies suggest comparable long-term clinical outcomes (improved quality of life, function, and pain scores)[4] and a trend toward reduced postoperative pain, hospital length of stay, infection rates, and blood loss.[5] A reduced overall complications rate and similar clinical outcomes have been reported for patients with obesity who underwent MIS-TLIF, which deserves mention as they represent a technical surgical challenge and wound size can be reduced particularly in these patients.[6,7] MIS-TLIF can generally be applied in the majority of situations where an open TLIF and a minimally invasive screw placement can be used:

- Single- or two-level degenerative disk disease with correlative clinical symptoms.
- Spondylolisthesis less than Meyerding grade III.
- Recurrent lumbar disk herniation.
- Spondylosis with radiculopathy and back pain.
- Focal spinal deformity concentrated at less than three intersegmental levels.
- Synovial cysts exhibiting spinal instability.

Recently, endoscopic TLIF techniques have been developed and proved to be an efficient alternative surgery for single-segment lumbar spondylolisthesis when compared to MIS-TLIF in at least one prospective randomized pilot study.[8]

56.3 Technique

There are several variations of the MIS-TLIF technique. Here a standard approach is described that has been successfully used by numerous surgeons:

- The patient is positioned prone on a Jackson operating room table, which offers several advantages. The location of the incision is targeted under fluoroscopy or navigation, and two paramedian skin incisions are made between 3 and 4 cm lateral to the midline. Sharp incision of the fascia allows for blunt finger dissection between the longissimus and multifidus muscles along a modified Wiltse plane (**Fig. 56.1**).[9] This not only minimizes trauma to muscular tissues, but also minimizes intraoperative bleeding and creates a natural plane that allows for efficient maintenance of the trajectory of the retractors. The approach, if unilateral, is taken from the side where decompression is most necessary.
- Tubular dilator retractors are then placed through this plane and the level confirmed with fluoroscopy or navigation. Monopolar cautery is then used to clear any muscle tissue over the facet joint, making sure to expose the lateral aspect of the joint.

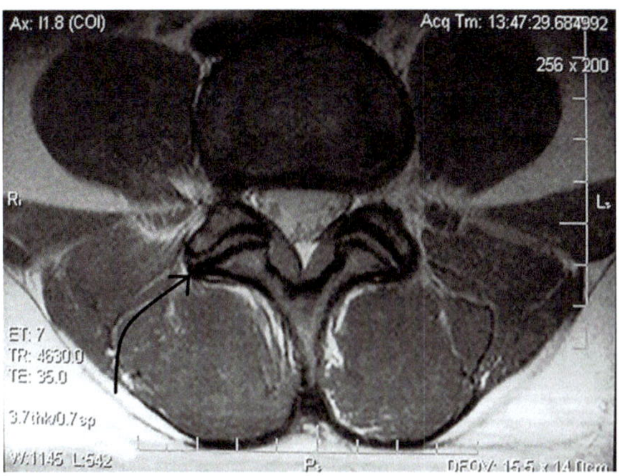

Fig. 56.1 Axial magnetic resonance imaging (MRI) showing the modified Wiltse plane between the longissimus and multifidus muscles (*arrow* showing trajectory between the abovementioned muscles). High MRI signal can be seen along this plane between the muscles, giving direct access to the facet joints.

- Once the surgeon has confirmed the location of the pars and the lower pedicle, a quarter-inch osteotome or high-speed bur is used to remove the facet joint. Either a partial or complete facetectomy can be performed, with greater bone removal for cases with more medial compression. Care must be taken not to drill into the pedicle. After facet removal, the lateral aspect of the ligamentum flavum is visualized. This is resected until the lateral thecal sac is seen (**Fig. 56.2**). Autograft bone is saved for later grafting purposes.
- Further decompression can then be performed as needed, with removal of ipsilateral ligamentum flavum, decompression under the pars, or contralateral decompression. This is best achieved by angling the retractors more medially. Alternatively, bilateral decompression can be accomplished through dual ports placed on each side.
- After palpation of the caudal pedicle and confirmation of the location of the exiting and traversing nerve roots, the annulus is incised, followed by aggressive intervertebral disk removal and endplate preparation, as with the open technique. This is followed by intervertebral cage placement.

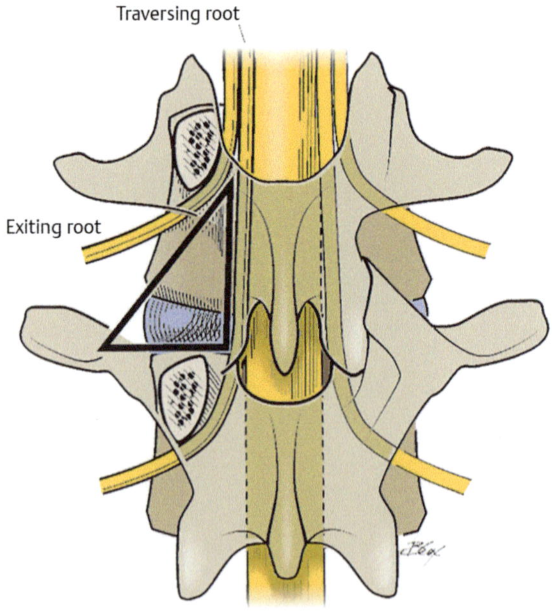

Fig. 56.2 Kambin's triangle.

- Supplemental pedicle screw placement can then be accomplished either using a mini-open technique (through the retractor with visualization) or percutaneously before or after the decompression. For the mini-open method, the screw placement is very similar to open TLIF. Various methods are used for percutaneous targeting, including (1) anteroposterior only, (2) the owl's-eye en face approach, (3) biplanar fluoroscopy, and (4) image guidance. Percutaneous methods involve placement of a jamshidi needle into the pedicle, followed by the use of a cannulated awl and tap to create a screw entry tract. Finally, screw placement and rod tunneling are used to connect the construct components. Another option is to use one step percutaneous navigated screws either under navigation or robotic assistance.
- A drain is not typically used.[10]

56.4 Complications

- Cerebrospinal fluid (CSF) leakage is uncommon with these procedures because the dural exposure is limited to those areas that are to be decompressed directly. However, when it occurs, dural repair can be difficult. Some surgeons have advocated leaving the durotomy unrepaired and applying a collagen sponge locally, which suggests that the limited dead space reduces the risk of CSF leakage postoperatively. Use of a Castro-Viejo needle holder can help the surgeon sew through a tubular retractor.
- Incomplete neural decompression is more problematic than in open surgery given the small working corridor. Care must be taken to visualize critical landmarks to ensure that any compression (such as at a far lateral disk) is adequately addressed. The critical landmarks include the caudal pedicle, pars interarticularis, and lateral ligamentum flavum.
- Nerve root injury is best avoided by maintaining an appreciation of the medial–lateral location in which the surgeon is working. Careful identification and control of the exiting and traversing nerve roots prior to diskectomy are critical.
- Cage misplacement occurs most frequently when inadequate disk material has been removed or the bony endplate has been violated. Care in endplate preparation is essential to minimize graft settling. In addition, it is desirable that the cage cross the midline, and this can be confirmed with fluoroscopy.
- Screw misplacement is most commonly the result of poor targeting technique. Thus, close familiarity with one technique for ensuring that the pedicle is not breached is essential. The anteroposterior (AP) targeting techniques are excellent for preventing neural injuries.

One meta-analysis showed that there is no significant difference between unilateral or bilateral pedicle screw fixation after MIS-TLIF in terms of postoperative pain, disability, fusion rate, or complication rate.[11]

- Pseudarthrosis can be minimized but never totally prevented. Proper endplate preparation, cage sizing, and the use of osteobiologic adjuvants will limit this complication. In addition, attention to postoperative nutrition, bracing, and external electrical bone stimulation is helpful.

56.5 Postoperative Care

Care after surgery is the same as with open TLIF. Patients should be rapidly mobilized with physical/occupational therapists, with external bracing remaining as optional.[12] Muscle spasm occurs more commonly with MIS procedures and is better treated with muscle relaxants and benzodiazepines than with narcotics.

56.6 Outcomes

Proper patient selection is vital for achieving excellent outcomes. Although MIS-TLIF has not been conclusively shown to be superior to open TLIF,[4] several reports suggest this pattern. MIS-TLIF has shown better long-term functional outcome for the treatment of single-level spondylolisthesis grades 1 and 2.[13]

In a well-selected population, radiculopathy will show meaningful improvement in 80 to 95% of cases; axial back pain will improve in 70 to 85% of cases.

Regarding fusion rates, MIS-TLIF has yielded figures ranging from 80 to 95% in meta-analysis.[4,14] The results are likely to differ because of a disparity between studies when defining fusion. Moreover, one meta-analysis showed that MIS-TLIF performed with interbody bone grafting alone has similar fusion rates to MIS or open TLIF supplemented with posterolateral bone grafting and fusion.[14]

56.7 Surgical Pearls

- In cases in which substantial muscle creeps under the edges of the retractor, consider pharmacologic paralysis. Also consider removing the retractor and making a longer fascial opening, followed by placement of a deeper retractor.
- When performing a contralateral neural decompression, leave the ipsilateral ligamentum flavum intact at first. This will push the thecal sac

ventrally, keeping it out of the way while the contralateral work is being performed.

- Intervertebral disk can be removed efficiently using an insert-and-rotate scraper. These devices allow entry into collapsed disk spaces and effectively remove any disk herniations causing neural compression.
- Self-distracting cages, usually with a "bulleted" nose, will allow the placement of larger interbody cages, as it is difficult to use pedicle screw manipulation of a laminar spreader to open the disk space in MIS surgery.

Common Clinical Questions

1. MIS-TLIF is used because it is believed to result in all of the following *except* which?
   A. Decreased soft tissue damage.
   B. Higher fusion rates.
   C. Shorter hospital stays.
   D. Reduced blood loss.
2. Which of the following is one of the critical maneuvers to reduce neural injury?
   A. Remove more lateral facet bone so that less nerve retraction is needed.
   B. Use intraoperative intravenous steroids.
   C. Use stronger pedicle screw fixation.
   D. Repair dural tears.
3. When placing intervertebral cages in an MIS-TLIF, it is important to do what?
   A. Make sure the cage is higher than 13 mm.
   B. Make sure the cage is longer than 27 mm.
   C. Use only nondegradable interbody devices.
   D. Cross the midline.

Answers to Common Clinical Questions

1. B.
2. A.
3. D.

Acknowledgments

As authors we want to express our very great appreciation to Michael Y. Wang for his contribution to this chapter with his previous work on the previous edition.

References

1. Harms J, Rolinger H. [A one-stager procedure in operative treatment of spondylolistheses: dorsal traction-reposition and anterior fusion (author's transl)]. Z Orthop Ihre Grenzgeb. 1982; 120(3):343–347
2. Schwender JD, Holly LT, Rouben DP, Foley KT. Minimally invasive transforaminal lumbar interbody fusion (TLIF): technical feasibility and initial results. J Spinal Disord Tech. 2005; 18 Suppl:S1–S6
3. Kawaguchi Y, Matsui H, Tsuji H. Back muscle injury after posterior lumbar spine surgery. Part 2: Histologic and histochemical analyses in humans. Spine. 1994; 19(22):2598–2602
4. Heemskerk JL, Oluwadara Akinduro O, Clifton W, Quiñones-Hinojosa A, Abode-Iyamah KO. Long-term clinical outcome of minimally invasive versus open single-level transforaminal lumbar interbody fusion for degenerative lumbar diseases: a meta-analysis. Spine J. 2021; 21(12):2049–2065
5. Dhall SS, Wang MY, Mummaneni PV. Clinical and radiographic comparison of mini-open transforaminal lumbar interbody fusion with open transforaminal lumbar interbody fusion in 42 patients with long-term follow-up. J Neurosurg Spine. 2008; 9(6):560–565
6. Terman SW, Yee TJ, Lau D, Khan AA, La Marca F, Park P. Minimally invasive versus open transforaminal lumbar interbody fusion: comparison of clinical outcomes among obese patients. J Neurosurg Spine. 2014; 20(6):644–652
7. Tan JH, Liu G, Ng R, Kumar N, Wong HK, Liu G. Is MIS-TLIF superior to open TLIF in obese patients?: A systematic review and meta-analysis. Eur Spine J. 2018; 27(8):1877–1886
8. Lv Y, Chen M, Wang SL, et al. Endo-TLIF versus MIS-TLIF in 1-segment lumbar spondylolisthesis: a prospective randomized pilot study. Clin Neurol Neurosurg. 2022; 212:107082
9. Wiltse LL, Bateman JG, Hutchinson RH, Nelson WE. The paraspinal sacrospinalis-splitting approach to the lumbar spine. J Bone Joint Surg Am. 1968; 50(5):919–926
10. Hung PI, Chang MC, Chou PH, Lin HH, Wang ST, Liu CL. Is a drain tube necessary for minimally invasive lumbar spine fusion surgery? Eur Spine J. 2017; 26(3):733–737
11. Wang L, Wang Y, Li Z, Yu B, Li Y. Unilateral versus bilateral pedicle screw fixation of minimally invasive transforaminal lumbar interbody fusion (MIS-TLIF): a meta-analysis of randomized controlled trials. BMC Surg. 2014; 14:87

12. Ma HH, Wu PH, Yao YC, et al. Postoperative spinal orthosis may not be necessary for minimally invasive lumbar spine fusion surgery: a prospective randomized controlled trial. BMC Musculoskelet Disord. 2021; 22(1):619
13. Qin R, Liu B, Zhou P, et al. Minimally invasive versus traditional open transforaminal lumbar interbody fusion for the treatment of single-level spondylolisthesis grades 1 and 2: a systematic review and meta-analysis. World Neurosurg. 2019; 122:180–189
14. Bevevino AJ, Kang DG, Lehman RA, Jr, Van Blarcum GS, Wagner SC, Gwinn DE. Systematic review and meta-analysis of minimally invasive transforaminal lumbar interbody fusion rates performed without posterolateral fusion. J Clin Neurosci. 2014; 21(10):1686–1690

57 Lateral Lumbar Interbody Fusion

Mohamed A.R. Soliman, Asham Khan, and John Pollina

Summary

A successful lateral lumbar interbody fusion (LLIF) technique depends on careful patient positioning, gentle retroperitoneal dissection, intraoperative electromyography (EMG) and somatosensory-evoked potentials monitoring, fusion bed preparation with release of contralateral annulus, and positioning and placement of the appropriately sized interbody implant. This chapter discusses the indications, contraindications, perioperative care, complications, outcomes, and surgical pearls.

Keywords: lateral lumbar interbody fusion (LLIF), single-position surgery, prone transpsoas interbody fusion (PTP)

57.1 Key Points

A successful lateral lumbar interbody fusion (LLIF) technique depends on the following five key steps:

- Careful patient positioning.
- Gentle retroperitoneal dissection.
- Intraoperative electromyography (EMG) and somatosensory-evoked potentials monitoring.
- Fusion bed preparation with release of contralateral annulus.
- Positioning and placement of the appropriately sized interbody implant.

57.2 Indications[1]

General indications for lumbar fusion also apply for the lateral retroperitoneal approach; this approach is utilized when accessing any level from T12–L1 through L4–L5.

- Adjacent level failure: Reduces dealing with scar tissue and previous instrumentation, which reduces the risk of durotomy.
- Axial low back pain associated with degenerative disk disease.
- Central spinal stenosis (mild to moderate only).

- Grade I or II spondylolisthesis.
- Indirect decompression for foraminal stenosis.
- Total disk replacement.
- Tumors and fractures requiring a corpectomy.
- Retrieval of malpositioned or damaged disk replacement devices.[2]
- Adult spinal deformity (specifically with anterior column release).[3]
- Correction of lumbar lordosis, sagittal vertical axis (SVA), and coronal imbalance.

57.3 Contraindications

- L5–S1 fusion: The lateral lumbar approach does not allow access due to the significant risk of injury to the lumbar plexus at that level and the fact that the iliac crest prevents an appropriate working angle.
- Requiring direct decompression:
  - Spinal canal pathology where disk space distraction will not correct the pathology, such as synovial cyst or disk herniation.
  - Severe "pinpoint" canal stenosis (may respond).
- Grade III–V spondylolisthesis.
- Disk space height > 12 mm (difficult to achieve further disk height distraction).
- Significant disk space ossification or osteophyte formation.
- Vascular anatomy anomalies that can interfere with the approach.
- Previous ipsilateral retroperitoneal surgery (can still be done either on the contralateral or ipsilateral).
- Psoas abscess.
- Relative contraindications:
  - Previous history of retroperitoneal disease or infection.
  - Osteoporosis.
  - Active infection.

57.4 Preoperative Planning

- Lumbar spine computed tomography (CT) or magnetic resonance imaging (MRI) to assess:
  - Anatomy of regional major vessels such as aorta, iliac vessels, and inferior vena cava.
  - Anatomy of segmental vessels and its relation to the disk space (risk of injury during contralateral release of the annulus).
  - Psoas muscle configuration.
- DEXA scan to assess the bone quality.

Table 57.1 Table comparing the advantages and disadvantages of approaching the spine through the concave and convex side

	Concave side	Convex side
Advantage	• Easier to access the lower disk spaces • Easier to access multiple disk spaces through the same short longitudinal incision	• Disk space closer to the surgeon • More open disk spaces
Disadvantage	• Requires a longer tube • Working on the collapsed side of the disk space	• Requires more incisions per level

- Side to approach for access in scoliosis patients (**Table 57.1**).
- Formerly, in the absence of scoliosis and the index levels of L4–L5, the side with the lower iliac crest was chosen for the approach; however, bending the table in the standard LLIF position or craniocaudally rotating the specialized prone transpsoas bolsters now allows the surgeon to access the spine from both sides.

57.5 Patient Positioning

57.5.1 Standard LLIF

- The patient is placed in true 90 degrees lateral decubitus position on a radiolucent bendable table with the iliac crest top just superior to the table break, and adhesive tapes at the chest and hips are used to stabilize the patient.
- Table flexion is required to increase the distance between the ribs and iliac crest, allowing access to the upper (above L3) and lower (L4–L5) disk spaces.
- In case of posterior supplementation, the surgeon can place the screws while the patient is in the lateral position or place them after turning the patient into prone position (**Fig. 57.1**).
- The left side is usually up, unless the side to approach is modified for scoliosis (as discussed in previous the table).

57.5.2 Prone Lateral (PL) LLIF

- The patient is placed in a prone lateral position on a Jackson table, tilted so that the disk level of interest is orthogonal with the facing

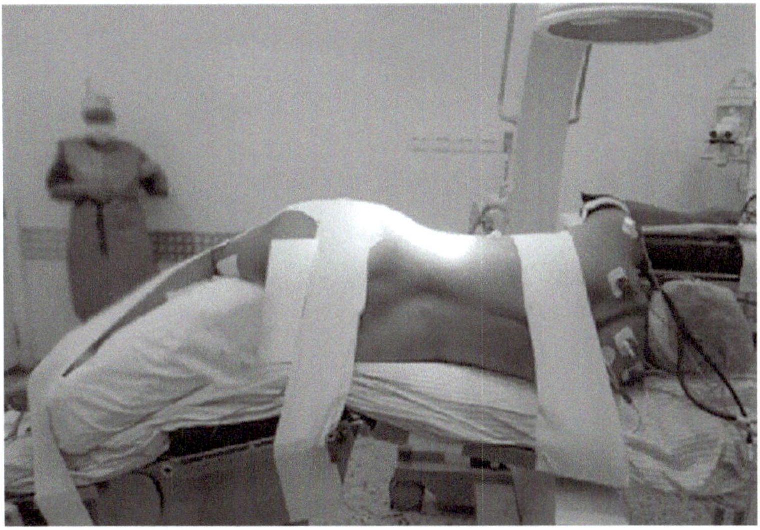

Fig. 57.1 Intraoperative photograph demonstrating the positioning of the patient for standard lateral lumbar interbody fusion (LLIF). (Reproduced from Oliveira DdA, Fernandez JS, Falcon RS, Menezes CM. Fusion via transpsoas lateral approach: considerations and initial results. Coluna/Columna. 2014; 13(3):214–218.)[4]

wall and the abdomen is freely hanging with the hips in an extended position (**Fig. 57.2**).

- Adhesive tapes across the chest and hips are used to stabilize the patient to the table followed by tape placed on the lateral chest wall aiming superiorly and the iliac crest aiming posteriorly to separate the iliac crest and ribs. This separation is aided by placement of a towel roll.

57.5.3 Prone Transpsoas (PTP) LLIF

- The patient is placed in a totally prone position on a Jackson table with the abdomen freely hanging and hips in an extended position (**Fig. 57.3**). This allows for better lumbar lordosis correction.
- The patient is secured to the table with the specially designed PTP bolsters with sticky straps that are tightly applied around the hips and chest to maintain proper positioning (ATEC Spine; Carlsbad, California). These bolsters also allow for coronal bending at the chest and hips, improving the surgeon's access to the upper (above L3) and lower (L4–L5) disk spaces.
- The table is elevated to the surgeon's eye level or the surgeon may sit for better visualization.

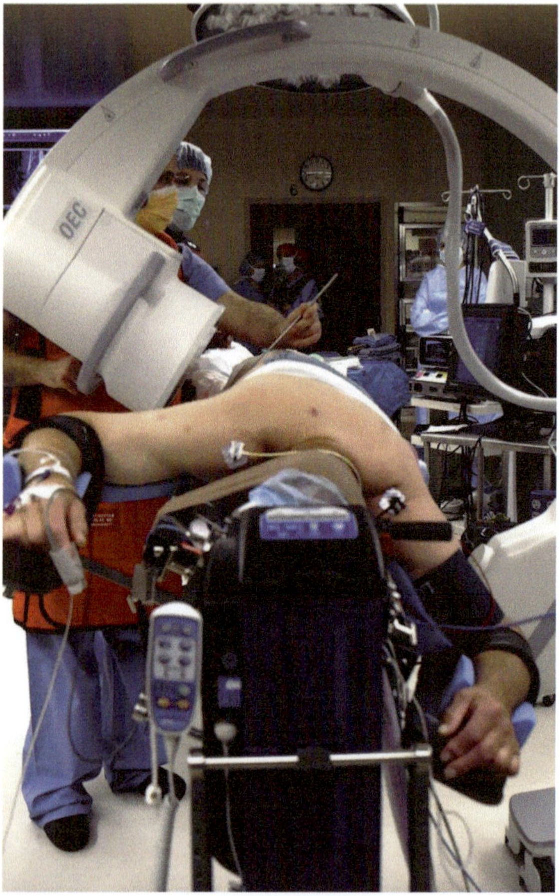

Fig. 57.2 Intraoperative photograph demonstrating the positioning of the patient in the prone lateral (PL) position for lateral lumbar interbody fusion (LLIF). (Reproduced from Martirosyan NL, Uribe JS, Randolph BM, Buchanan RI. Prone lateral lumbar interbody fusion: case report and technical note. World Neurosurg. 2020; 144:170–177.)[5]

57.6 Technique

- Localize the skin incision with lateral fluoroscopy by centering crossed K-wires over the disk's midposition. For multilevel approaches, a single longitudinal incision with individual transverse fascial openings for each level is adequate.
- Retroperitoneal access minimally invasive surgery (MIS) (single skin/fascia incision technique):

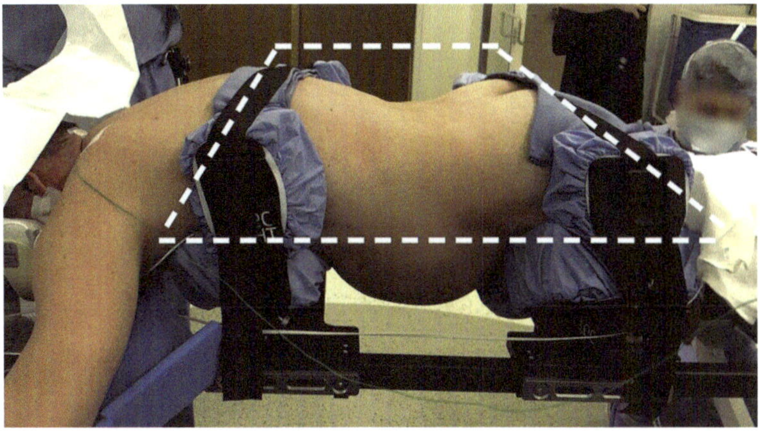

Fig. 57.3 Intraoperative photograph demonstrating the positioning of the patient in the prone transpsoas (PTP) position for lateral lumbar interbody fusion (LLIF). (Reproduced from Soliman MAR, Khan A, Pollina J. Comparison of prone transpsoas and standard lateral lumbar interbody fusion surgery for degenerative lumbar spine disease: a retrospective radiographic propensity score-matched analysis.World Neurosurg. 2022; 157:e11–e21.)[6]

- Work perpendicular to the floor while dissecting through the muscle fibers to avoid entry into the peritoneal cavity, which is anteriorly displaced in the lateral position.
- Entry into the retroperitoneal cavity is confirmed by the appearance of bright yellow fat and a loss of resistance by the muscle tissues. Finger dissection is then performed so that the surgeon can feel the psoas muscle deep in the cavity and the transverse processes posteriorly.

- Transpsoas approach and retractor placement:
  - A series of tubular dilators are placed with EMG monitoring. Intraoperative EMG and somatosensory-evoked potentials (SafeOp, ATEC Spine, Carlsbad, California; or Neurovision: NuVasive, San Diego, California) allow the location of these nerves in relation to the dilator (**Fig. 57.4**). It is essential to guide the dilators with the finger to avoid inadvertent entry into the peritoneal cavity.
  - Lateral fluoroscopy will guide dilator placement into Zone III of disk space while bluntly splitting the fibers of the psoas muscle. The exception is at the L4–L5 level, where the initial dilator should be placed at the midpoint between Zones II and III (**Fig. 57.5**). A K-wire is placed through the initial dilator and into the disk space to hold it in place. EMG monitoring is performed with each dilator before introduction of a larger dilator.
  - The retractor (2 or 3 blade) is then placed, and a shim needle is introduced to the disk space under anteroposterior (AP) fluoroscopy to secure it.

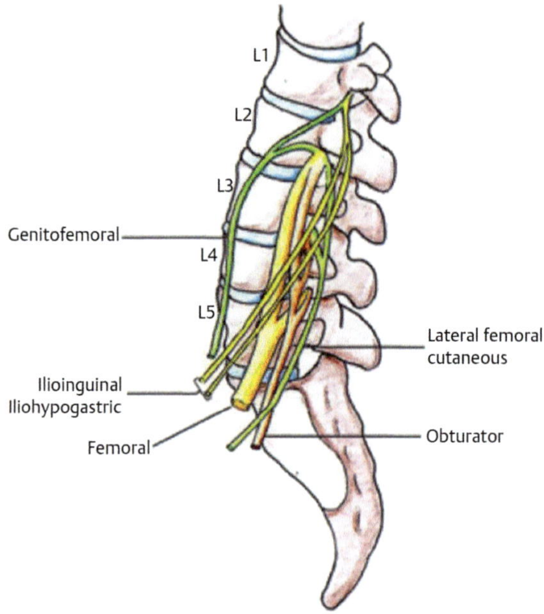

Fig. 57.4 Lateral view of the lumbar plexus. Understanding this anatomy is critical for successful implementation of the lateral transpsoas approach. (Reproduced from Uribe JS, Arredondo N, Dakwar E, Vale FL. Defining the safe working zones using the minimally invasive lateral retroperitoneal transpsoas approach: an anatomical study. J Neurosurg Spine. 2010; 13(2):260–266.)[8]

- Preparation of the disk space:
  - The disk space is incised with a knife just anterior to the shim, with a small rim of disk kept just in front of it to keep the retractor from sliding anteriorly.
  - A Cobb elevator is passed along both end plates and through the contralateral annulus under fluoroscopic guidance.
  - A series of instruments (curettes, pituitaries, rasps) are used to clean the space and prepare the end plates.
- For standard interbody fusion:
  - Interbody spacer and instrumentation are then placed.
- For anterior column release (MIS–ACR), additional steps must be performed after diskectomy[7]:
  - A curved custom retractor is inserted gently between the anterior longitudinal ligament (ALL) and the great vessels and the sympathetic plexus.
  - A knife is used to cut the ALL in sequential fashion.

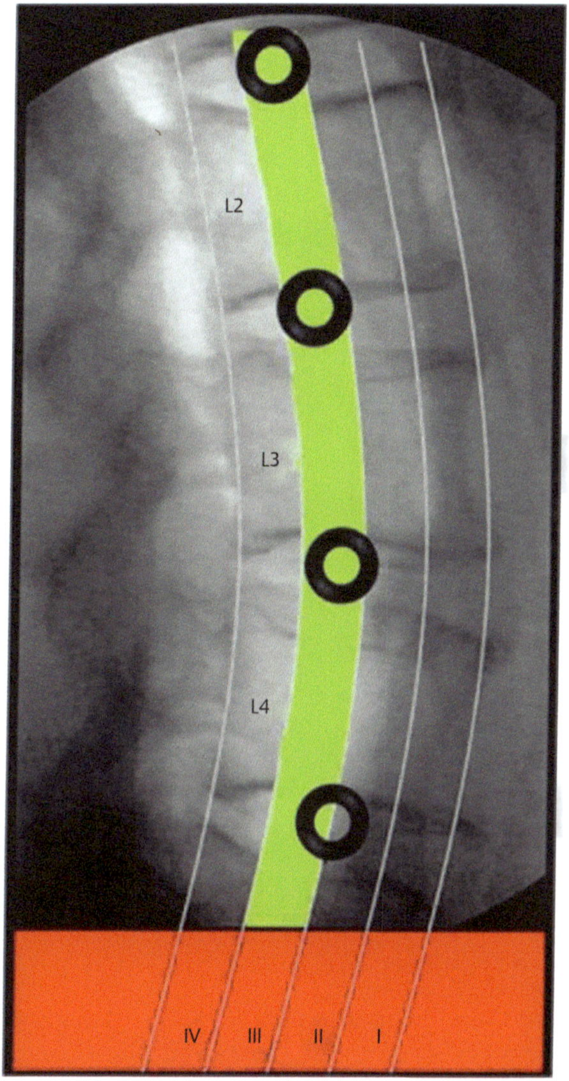

Fig. 57.5 Lateral radiograph of the lumbar spine demonstrating the division of the vertebral body into four zones (Zones I–IV) from anterior to posterior. The relatively "safe zone" (Zone III) is depicted in *green*. The recommended safe working zones to prevent direct nerve injury have been indicated with *black circles* at each level. (Reproduced from Uribe JS, Arredondo N, Dakwar E, Vale FL. Defining the safe working zones using the minimally invasive lateral retroperitoneal transpsoas approach: an anatomical study. J Neurosurg Spine. 2010; 13(2):260–266.)[8]

  - Hyperlordotic cages (20 or 30 degrees) are inserted into the disk space and fixed to an adjacent vertebra with one or two screws.
- The retractor is removed slowly in the open configuration to allow the psoas muscle to be inspected for bleeding.
- The external oblique fascia is closed with interrupted absorbable suture, and the skin is closed in a subcuticular fashion.
- Other different technique modifications include the following:
  - Transpsoas: Mini-open and open direct retroperitoneal transpsoas dissection.
  - Prepsoatic: Mini-open anterolateral retroperitoneal dissection anterior to psoas muscle.

57.7 Complications

- Hip flexor weakness[1]:
  - Incidence: Increases when more than two levels are done.
  - Etiology: Psoas muscle trauma.
  - Prognosis: Usually transient and resolves in 1 to 8 weeks.
- Thigh numbness[3]:
  - Incidence: 12 to 30%.
  - Etiology: Injury to the anterior cutaneous branch of the femoral nerve.
  - Prognosis: Usually transient and spontaneously resolves by the 3-month follow-up.
- Quadriceps weakness[1,9]:
  - Incidence: Approximately 2.6%.[10]
  - Etiology: Injury to the femoral nerve by:
    - Retracting the nerve within the psoas muscle against the transverse process (immediate postoperative weakness).
    - Psoas hematoma (delayed—1 to 2 days—postoperative weakness).
  - Prognosis: Usually transient and spontaneously resolves in 3 to 12 months.
- Lumbar plexus injury.
- Contralateral femoral nerve injury.
- Genitofemoral neuralgia.[3]
- Abdominal viscera perforation.
- Great vessel injury including common iliac artery and vein (at the L4–L5 level), aorta, and inferior vena cava (above L4–L5).[11,12]
- Kidney—ureteral injury.
- Unintended rupture of the anterior longitudinal ligament.
- Psoas/retroperitoneal hematoma, ipsilateral or contralateral.[1]
- Abdominal wall paresis or hernia.[1]
- Rhabdomyolysis.[3]
- Retrograde ejaculation (specific to ACR and prepsoatic approaches).
- Graft subsidence.[1]
- End plate fracture.

57.8 Postoperative Care

- For single-level lumbar cases, the patient is mobilized in the immediate postoperative period without a brace. No drains are placed.
- Expect hip flexion pain on the approach side during the immediate postoperative period.
- The patient is usually discharged on postoperative day 1 for single-level cases.
- Perioperative prophylactic antibiotic for 24 hours.
- In cases of significant leg weakness, CT or MRI is indicated to exclude a psoas hematoma.

57.9 Outcomes

- Fusion rates range from 91 to 100%.[3,13]
- For the standard LLIF, PL-LLIF, and PTP, outcomes scales (Oswestry Disability Index and Visual Analog Scale) are significantly improved at follow-up.[6,14,15,16]
- PL-LLIF is associated with significantly better improvement in the segmental lordosis (5.1 degrees) but not the regional lumbar lordosis (6.3 degrees) compared to the standard LLIF.[17]
- PTP is associated with significantly better improvement in the regional lumbar lordosis (9.9 degrees) compared to the standard LLIF.[6]
- In terms of MIS–ACRs, long-term follow-up is not available yet.

57.10 Surgical Pearls

- Perfect AP and lateral projections of the disk space are imperative before starting the surgery. This is best accomplished by careful patient positioning, not by adjusting the fluoroscopy machine.
- To potentially decrease the amount of tension on the lumbar plexus, minimize the amount of lateral flexion of the patient and flex the ipsilateral hip during positioning.
- To reduce the risk of direct lumbar plexus injury, it is recommended that the surgeon stay anterior to or at the safe working zone, defined as the middle of the posterior quarter of the vertebral body at the L1–L4 level and the midpoint of the vertebral body at the L4–L5 level.[8]
- Guide all dilators with finger dissection through the retroperitoneal space to prevent visceral injury.
- During triggered EMG monitoring, place the nerves *posterior* to the retractor, where they can be safely retracted away from the surgical field without the risk of root avulsion or stretch injury.

- MIS-ACR should be performed once surgeons have mastered the standard lateral transpsoas technique. Careful examination of the location of the great vessels is necessary to prevent vascular complications during the dissection of the ALL.

Common Clinical Questions

1. During the directional EMG monitoring, where should the lower numbers be located?
2. What is the most likely explanation for postoperative hip flexor weakness?
3. Retraction against which nerve at the L4–L5 level is responsible for postoperative anterior thigh numbness?
4. To reduce the risk of lumbar plexus injury at L3–L4 level, it is recommended that the surgeon stay at which zone of the vertebral body?
5. What is the degree of correction of regional lumbar lordosis after PTP and PL-LLIF?

Answers to Common Clinical Questions

1. Posteriorly.
2. Psoas muscle bruising as opposed to damage to femoral nerve branches to the psoas.
3. The femoral nerve (sensory fibers via the anterior femoral cutaneous nerve).
4. Middle of the posterior quarter of the vertebral body.
5. The degrees of correction after PTP and PL-LLIF are 9.9 degrees and 6.3 degrees, respectively.

References

1. Rodgers WB, Gerber EJ, Patterson J. Intraoperative and early postoperative complications in extreme lateral interbody fusion: an analysis of 600 cases. Spine. 2011; 36(1):26–32
2. Pimenta L, Díaz RC, Guerrero LG. Charité lumbar artificial disc retrieval: use of a lateral minimally invasive technique. Technical note. J Neurosurg Spine. 2006; 5(6):556–561
3. Dakwar E, Cardona RF, Smith DA, Uribe JS. Early outcomes and safety of the minimally invasive, lateral retroperitoneal transpsoas approach for adult degenerative scoliosis. Neurosurg Focus. 2010; 28(3):E8

4. Oliveira DdA, Fernandez JS, Falcon RS, Menezes CM. Fusion via transpsoas lateral approach: considerations and initial results. Coluna/Columna. 2014; 13(3):214–218
5. Martirosyan NL, Uribe JS, Randolph BM, Buchanan RI. Prone lateral lumbar interbody fusion: case report and technical note. World Neurosurg. 2020; 144:170–177
6. Soliman MAR, Khan A, Pollina J. Comparison of prone transpsoas and standard lateral lumbar interbody fusion surgery for degenerative lumbar spine disease: a retrospective radiographic propensity score-matched analysis. World Neurosurg. 2022; 157:e11–e21
7. Deukmedjian AR, Le TV, Baaj AA, Dakwar E, Smith DA, Uribe JS. Anterior longitudinal ligament release using the minimally invasive lateral retroperitoneal transpsoas approach: a cadaveric feasibility study and report of 4 clinical cases. J Neurosurg Spine. 2012; 17(6):530–539
8. Uribe JS, Arredondo N, Dakwar E, Vale FL. Defining the safe working zones using the minimally invasive lateral retroperitoneal transpsoas approach: an anatomical study. J Neurosurg Spine. 2010; 13(2):260–266
9. Ahmadian A, Deukmedjian AR, Abel N, Dakwar E, Uribe JS. Analysis of lumbar plexopathies and nerve injury after lateral retroperitoneal transpsoas approach: diagnostic standardization. J Neurosurg Spine. 2013; 18(3):289–297
10. Abel NA, Januszewski J, Vivas AC, Uribe JS. Femoral nerve and lumbar plexus injury after minimally invasive lateral retroperitoneal transpsoas approach: electrodiagnostic prognostic indicators and a roadmap to recovery. Neurosurg Rev. 2018; 41(2):457–464
11. Assina R, Majmundar NJ, Herschman Y, Heary RF. First report of major vascular injury due to lateral transpsoas approach leading to fatality. J Neurosurg Spine. 2014; 21(5):794–798
12. Aguirre AO, Soliman MAR, Azmy S, et al. Incidence of major and minor vascular injuries during lateral access lumbar interbody fusion procedures: a retrospective comparative study and systematic literature review. Neurosurg Rev. 2022; 45(2):1275–1289
13. Youssef JA, McAfee PC, Patty CA, et al. Minimally invasive surgery: lateral approach interbody fusion: results and review. Spine. 2010; 35(26) Suppl: S302–S311
14. Alimi M, Hofstetter CP, Cong GT, et al. Radiological and clinical outcomes following extreme lateral interbody fusion. J Neurosurg Spine. 2014; 20(6): 623–635
15. Godzik J, Ohiorhenuan IE, Xu DS, et al. Single-position prone lateral approach: cadaveric feasibility study and early clinical experience. Neurosurg Focus. 2020; 49(3):E15
16. Soliman MAR, Aguirre AO, Ruggiero N, et al. Comparison of prone transpsoas lateral lumbar interbody fusion and transforaminal lumbar interbody fusion for degenerative lumbar spine disease: a retrospective radiographic propensity score-matched analysis. Clin Neurol Neurosurg. 2022; 213:107105
17. Walker CT, Farber SH, Gandhi S, Godzik J, Turner JD, Uribe JS. Single-position prone lateral interbody fusion improves segmental lordosis in lumbar spondylolisthesis. World Neurosurg. 2021; 151:e786–e792

58 Single-Position Lateral Lumbar Interbody Fusion

James J. Zhou, S. Harrison Farber, Nima Alan, and Juan S. Uribe

Summary
Single-position lateral surgery in the lumbar spine is meant to achieve the surgical objectives with a decrease in operative time due to repositioning of the patient. Interbody work is performed laterally, and simultaneous pedicle screw fixation is performed in the same position and setting. The risks involved are similar to those with traditional lateral and/or posterior based surgery.

Keywords: LLIF, lateral interbody fusion, single position

58.1 Key Points

- Single-position lateral lumbar interbody fusion (LLIF) is a variation of the traditional LLIF approach that allows for simultaneous placement of percutaneous pedicle screws without patient repositioning.
- Potential benefits of single-position surgery are reduced surgical time, reduced blood loss, ease of access to the posterior elements, and improved lumbar lordosis due to more physiologic positioning on the operating table.
- One potential downside of single-position surgery is a steeper surgeon learning curve. Also, in the prone position there is diminished access corridor due to inability to "break" the bed and increased difficulty of accessing the retroperitoneum and abdominal cavity in case of vascular compromise.
- For appropriately selected patients, single-position LLIF surgery offers a safe and efficient alternative to traditional lateral-then-prone positioning.

58.2 Indications

- Spondylolisthesis.
- Degenerative disk disease with central or foraminal stenosis.
- Adjacent segment disease.
- Sagittal and coronal deformity.

58.3 Technique

- Prepositioning preparation:
  - Appropriate intraoperative neuromonitoring must be set up prior to positioning. These include: somatosensory-evoked potentials (SSEPs), free-run and triggered electromyography (EMG), and optionally motor-evoked potentials (MEPs).
  - The operating room must be set up to accommodate the side of approach.
    - The scrub technician and equipment should be positioned on the surgeon's side of the room, while the C-arm should be positioned on the contralateral side.
- Patient positioning:
  - Prone:
    - The patient is positioned prone on a radiolucent Jackson table with chest, hip, and thigh pads.
    - On the side of approach, the hip and thigh pads may need to be shifted toward the feet so that they are not too close to the surgical site.
    - On the contralateral side, a bolster may be placed between the ribs and the iliac crest in order to help open the contralateral side for ease of access.
    - Using X-rays, the patient's position is adjusted so that the spine is completely orthogonal to the floor. Perfect lateral and anteroposterior (AP) images for each level should be obtainable with the C-arm at 0 and 90 degrees.
  - Lateral decubitus:
    - The patient is positioned in a similar manner to a traditional lateral decubitus LLIF.
    - Positioning is adjusted until true AP and lateral X-rays can be obtained with the C-arm at 0 and 90 degrees.
    - The patient is secured to the bed with foam tape at the hips and chest.
    - Optionally, the bed can be broken to increase the interval between the last rib and the iliac crest.
    - Care must be taken to position the patient close enough to the edge of the bed to facilitate placement of the contralateral pedicle screws.
  - Once the patient has been positioned perfectly, the hips and chest are secured to the bed using foam tape. Optionally, the additional tape can be used to pull the crest toward the foot of the bed and the hips toward the head of the bed. Generally, taping until the skin over the access corridor is slightly tense provides sufficient retraction.

    - When taping, ensure that the tape does not obscure the posterior working corridor. If intraoperative navigation is being used, the posterior superior iliac spine should also be left uncovered.
- Incision planning:
  - The LLIF skin incision is localized using X-ray and a radio-opaque instrument. For single-level surgery, an incision parallel to the disk space corresponding the length between the anterior and posterior aspects of the disk space is sufficient. For multilevel surgery, an oblique incision that traverse the posterior aspect of each target disk space is appropriate.
    - In the prone position, it is helpful to err the incision slightly posterior to the disk space in order to account for the tendency of the retractor to fall anteriorly due to gravity.
  - The pedicle screw incisions can be planned in the typical fashion using either intraoperative navigation or fluoroscopy.
- Approach and retractor placement:
  - A standard approach to the retroperitoneum is performed. Blunt dissection through the layers of the abdominal wall will prevent damage to the abdominal contents when first entering the retroperitoneum.
  - Extensive finger dissection of the retroperitoneum is performed until the following structures can be palpated: the psoas muscle, the transverse processes of the spine, the lower ribs, and the iliac crest.
  - The first dilator is placed while a finger protects the abdominal contents anteriorly. Using intraoperative X-ray, the dilator is docked onto the target disk space.
    - The preferred docking location is just posterior to the midpoint of the disk space.
    - For lower levels (e.g., L4–L5) it may be helpful to dock more anteriorly and then "drag" the dilator posteriorly to help cushion the lumbar plexus.
  - A K-wire inserted halfway into the disk space is used to secure the dilator.
  - Directional triggered EMG is then used to confirm the location of the dilator anterior to the lumbar plexus.
  - Once adequate positioning of the first dilator on AP and lateral X-rays is confirmed, progressive dilation and stimulation are performed until the final retractor is replaced and secured to the OR table.
  - Several techniques of securing the retractor to the spine exist. These include: posterior disk space shims, anterior disk space shims, and anchoring K-wires in the vertebral body. We prefer using only a posterior shim for standard LLIF surgery.
    - It may be helpful to place lights in the retractor and visually confirm the absence of neural elements underneath the posterior blade prior

to placing a shim. A balltip electrode can also be used to stimulate within the opening of the retractor to confirm that no nerves are present.

- Disk space preparation and interbody placement:
  - The disk space is incised using a knife just anterior to the posterior shim. A small cuff of annulus is preserved anterior to the shim to help prevent the retractor from migrating anteriorly.
  - Cobb elevators are passed using hand pressure along the superior and inferior end plates with fluoroscopic guidance. Care should be taken not to violate the end plates. At the contralateral annulus, a mallet may be used to penetrate the annulus and achieve a contralateral release.
  - Curettes and rasps may be used to further prepare the disk space; however, in our experience this is often unnecessary and only serves to prolong retractor time.
  - Finally, the interbody is sized using templates and then placed in the standard fashion.
- Pedicle screw placement:
  - Placement of pedicle screws can be performed either before or after the LLIF, depending on the surgeon's preference.
  - Pedicle screws are placed percutaneously using intraoperative navigation, C-arm fluoroscopy, or other assistive technologies such as robot navigation.
    - Note that in the lateral position, placement of the contralateral screws requires the surgeon to approach from the floor with an upward angulation; thus, it may be helpful to either raise the bed significantly or rotate the bed away from the surgeon.
- Closure:
  - The LLIF retractor is closed and removed slowly under direct visualization to ensure no excessive bleeding is present.
  - Venous oozing can be controlled with topical hemostatic agents and pressure. The field should be completely dry prior to removing the retractor.
  - The fascia of the external abdominal oblique is closed using interrupted absorbable suture.
  - The skin over the LLIF incision and pedicle screw incisions is closed with absorbable suture in a subcuticular fashion.

58.4 Complications

- This technique is still not widely adopted; thus, data on complications compared to traditional lateral decubitus LLIF is still sparse.

- Preliminary studies demonstrate no significant differences in complication rates between the two techniques. However, most early adopters of single-position surgery are experienced lateral surgeons, thus flattening the learning curve.[1,2,3]
- Complication profile is likely to be similar to that of traditional lateral decubitus LLIF:
  - Hip flexor weakness.
  - Thigh numbness.
  - Femoral nerve injury.
  - Abdominal visceral injury.
  - Great vessel injury.
  - Retroperitoneal hematoma.
  - Ureteral injury.
  - Graft subsidence.
  - Graft migration.
  - Abdominal wall hernia or pseudohernia.

58.5 Postoperative Care

- Early mobilization is encouraged, preferably on the same day of the surgery.
- An LSO brace should be worn when the patient is out of bed and upright, but can be taken off to eat and to shower.
- Single-level cases with or without posterior fixation can often be discharged the same day.
- Multilevel cases often will need to stay overnight in the hospital, but can typically be discharged on postoperative day 1.
- Routine prophylaxis measures, including incentive spirometer use, early mobilization, sequential compression devices, and chemoprophylaxis are utilized for inpatients.

58.6 Outcomes

- Preliminary studies demonstrate no differences in complication rates between prone single-position LLIF and lateral decubitus LLIF.[1,2,3]
- Some studies suggest that lordosis restoration may be improved in single-position surgery, as the prone position maximizes the natural lumbar lordosis.[3,4]
- As the technique was only adopted recently, long-term outcome data will be essential to establish its safety and efficacy.

58.7 Surgical Pearls

- Just as in the lateral decubitus position, precise positioning of the patient such that the AP and lateral X-rays are perfectly aligned with the C-arm at 90 and 0 degrees is essential to retractor placement and subsequent diskectomy.
- The surgeon should be constantly aware of the tendency of the retractor and instruments to migrate anteriorly due to the effects of gravity, which are not present in the lateral decubitus position. Inadvertent anterior migration could lead to unintended release of the ALL, or even injury to the retroperitoneal great vessels.
- Intraoperative assistive technology such as triggered directional EMG and neuronavigation may provide an additional margin of safety and should be strongly considered for each case.
- As the learning curve for single-position surgery is high, it is recommended that surgeons achieve proficiency in traditional lateral decubitus LLIF surgery prior to attempting the prone position.

Common Clinical Questions

1. What is the primary difference between single-position surgery and more traditional techniques?
2. When using neuronavigation in single-position prone surgery, what locations can be used for tracker placement?
3. In what direction does the LLIF retractor tend to migrate during single-position prone surgery?

Answers to Common Clinical Questions

1. Single-position surgery allows for placement of percutaneous screws before or after an LLIF without patient repositioning.
2. Either the spinous process of the level immediately cranial/caudal to the construct, or the posterior superior iliac spine (PSIS).
3. Downward due to gravity; in the case of prone single-position surgery this means that the retractor migrates anteriorly.

References

1. Farber SH, Naeem K, Bhargava M, Porter RW. Single-position prone lateral transpsoas approach: early experience and outcomes. J Neurosurg Spine. 2021; 36(3):358–365
2. Lamartina C, Berjano P. Prone single-position extreme lateral interbody fusion (Pro-XLIF): preliminary results. Eur Spine J. 2020; 29(1) Suppl 1:6–13
3. Pimenta L, Amaral R, Taylor W, et al. The prone transpsoas technique: preliminary radiographic results of a multicenter experience. Eur Spine J. 2021; 30(1):108–113
4. Walker CT, Farber SH, Gandhi S, Godzik J, Turner JD, Uribe JS. Single-position prone lateral interbody fusion improves segmental lordosis in lumbar spondylolisthesis. World Neurosurg. 2021; 151:e786–e792

59 Pedicle Subtraction Osteotomy/Smith-Petersen Osteotomy

Stephen M. Bergin, Khoi D. Than, Frank La Marca, Paul Park, and Juan M. Valdivia

Summary

This chapter covers the techniques and applications of pedicle subtraction osteotomy (PSO) and Smith-Petersen osteotomy (SPO) for spinal deformity correction. PSO is primarily used for fixed sagittal imbalance, allowing for up to 30 degrees of correction per level, while SPO addresses nonfixed sagittal imbalance with up to 10 degrees of correction per level. Both the procedures can be performed on the thoracic or lumbar spine and involve precise surgical steps to resect and realign spinal structures. The chapter details the indications, surgical techniques, postoperative care, and potential complications associated with these osteotomies, emphasizing the importance of neurophysiologic monitoring and meticulous surgical execution to minimize risks and achieve optimal outcomes.

Keywords: pedicle subtraction osteotomy, Smith-Petersen osteotomy, spinal deformity correction, sagittal imbalance

59.1 Key Points

- Pedicle subtraction osteotomy (PSO) is used for correction of mainly symptomatic fixed sagittal imbalance and Smith-Petersen osteotomy (SPO) for nonfixed sagittal imbalance.[1]
- An asymmetric PSO can also be used for correction of coronal imbalance.
- SPO can aid in the correction of coronal balance via posterior column release and PSO in three-column release.
- SPO and PSO can be performed on the thoracic or lumbar spine.

59.2 Indications

- Uncompensated spinal kyphoscoliosis (thoracic and/or lumbar) with or without progression.

- Correction of fixed kyphosis requiring more than 30 degrees of correction (PSO) at one spinal segment.
- Correction of nonfixed deformity requiring 5 to 10 degrees of correction (SPO) per spinal segment.

59.3 Technique

59.3.1 Pedicle Subtraction Osteotomy

- Position the patient on Jackson frame with extended chest bolster.
- Neurophysiologic monitoring should be used (transcranial motor-evoked potentials, somatosensory-evoked potentials, electromyography) to minimize neurologic injury during correction.
- Place two to three levels of bilateral pedicle screws cephalad and caudal to the target vertebral segment (i.e., commonly L3 or L4 in the lumbar spine).
- Remove transverse process and rib head (if in thoracic spine).
- For 360-degree extrapedicular vertebral body exposure, dissect soft tissues and vascular structures from vertebral body with placement of malleable retractors to maintain separation.
- Perform Gill laminectomy of the target vertebral body and partial laminectomies of the adjacent segments (**Fig. 59.1a**).
- Decancellate and resect pedicle while contralateral temporary rod is in place.
- Resect (chisel or drill) a posterior wedge out of vertebral body (**Fig. 59.1b**).[2]
- Repeat the steps mentioned in the above two bullet points on the contralateral side.[3]
- Resect remaining posterior vertebral body cortex; impact bone into cavity previously created during wedge resection of vertebral body with angled bone tamp or downgoing curette.[3]
- Use fluoroscopy to confirm adequate resection in addition to visual inspection.[2]
- Compress across pedicle screws to close down osteotomy (**Fig. 59.1b**).
- Evaluate neurophysiologic monitoring and/or perform wakeup test to ensure absence of neurologic compromise.

59.3.2 Smith-Petersen Osteotomy

- Position the patient on Jackson frame with extended chest bolster.
- Consider using multimodal neurophysiologic monitoring to minimize neurologic complications during deformity correction.
- Place pedicle screw instrumentation across targeted segments.
- Remove interspinous ligaments with rongeur.

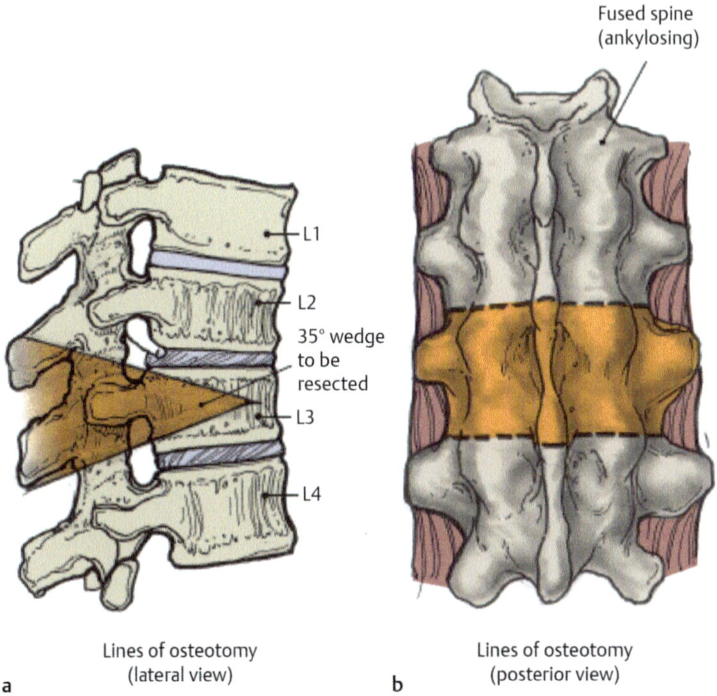

Fig. 59.1 **(a, b)** Pedicle subtraction osteotomy. (Adapted from Haher R, Merola A, eds. Surgical Techniques for the Spine. Thieme; 2003.)

- Spinous processes are removed at each targeted segment in a 45-degree angle in addition to removal of the upper and lower lamina edges.
- Bilateral facetectomies are performed with osteotomes and/or a high-speed drill[4] (**Fig. 59.2a**).
- Remove ligamentum flavum.
- Compress across the screw heads to close the osteotomy[4] (**Fig. 59.2b**).
- The patient may be placed in extension to assist in closure of the osteotomy.[4]

59.4 Complications

- Neurologic injury resulting from iatrogenic spinal stenosis upon closure of the osteotomy.
- Spinal subluxation during osteotomy.
- Durotomy.

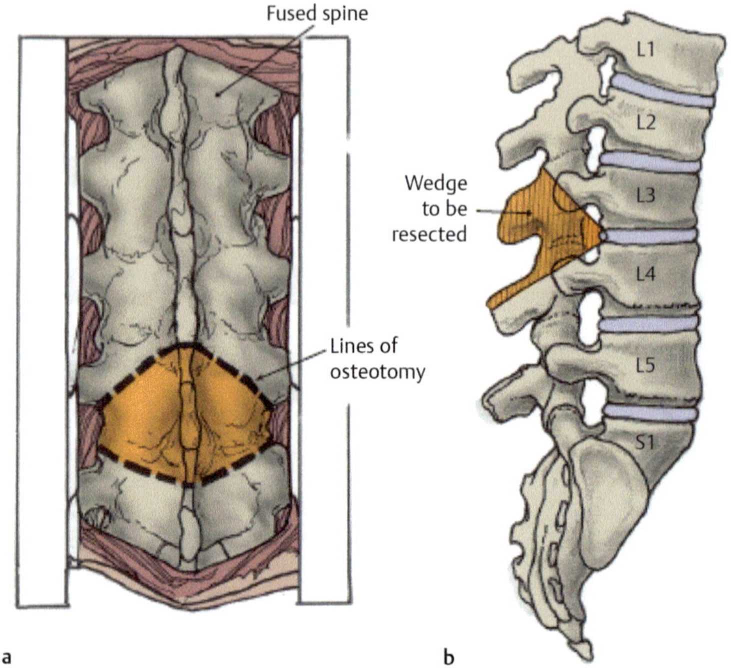

Fig. 59.2 (a, b) Smith-Petersen osteotomy. (Adapted from Haher R, Merola A, eds. Surgical Techniques for the Spine. Thieme; 2003.)

- Hypotension caused by excessive blood loss during osteotomy. Avoid hypotension, especially during correction maneuvers, lest spinal cord ischemia result.
- Epidural hematoma.
- Vascular injury.
- Pseudarthrosis.

59.5 Postoperative Care

- Immediate neurologic evaluation upon wakeup.
- For PSO patients, admission to neurologic intensive care for close monitoring.
- Maintenance of blood pressure.
- Consider postoperative computed tomography (CT) scan to evaluate adequacy of bone resection and juxtaposition of osteotomy margins.

59.6 Outcomes

- In general, a maximum of 10 degrees of sagittal correction can be accomplished with an SPO compared to 30 degrees for PSO.
- Clinical and radiographic outcomes are superior with PSO in the lumbar spine rather than in the thoracic. The lower the PSO is performed, the less the angulation is required for sagittal balance correction.[1]
- In properly selected patients, sagittal balance can be safely restored with PSO or multiple SPO.

59.7 Surgical Pearls

- Ensure that bone resection is adequate and wide enough laterally in both PSO and SPO to prevent interference upon osteotomy closure or compression of neurologic structures.
- Use thrombin powder or bioabsorbable bone wax to minimize bleeding during PSO without compromising fusion rates. Aprotinin is also an option, although controversy exists over possible associated complications.
- Do not resect the anterior vertebral wall entirely during PSO, because it will serve as a hinge during pedicle screw compression and osteotomy closure and prevent vertebral segment subluxation.
- Posterior laminectomy resection should be complete and include any epidural scar removal to assess dural sac adequately after osteotomy closure and ensure that there is no spinal canal compression.
- During SPO closure, place the patient in extension to lengthen the anterior spinal column and facilitate osteotomy closure and to minimize strain on the pedicle screw construct.

Common Clinical Questions

1. How many degrees of correction can be achieved with PSO as opposed to SPO?
2. What is the main advantage of a PSO/SPO procedure?
3. In regard to the anterior and middle columns, what is the main difference between PSO and SPO?

Answers to Common Clinical Questions

1. Up to 30 degrees per level with PSO compared with 10 degrees per level with SPO.
2. Correction of sagittal imbalance and reestablishment of lordosis or correction of kyphosis.

3. PSO is a closing wedge osteotomy involving the three columns and thus shortens the middle and posterior columns. SPO, in contrast, uses the middle column as a pivot, thus lengthening the anterior column and shortening the posterior column.

References

1. Dorward IG, Lenke LG. Osteotomies in the posterior-only treatment of complex adult spinal deformity: a comparative review. Neurosurg Focus. 2010; 28(3):E4
2. Bridwell KH, Lewis SJ, Lenke LG, Baldus C, Blanke K. Pedicle subtraction osteotomy for the treatment of fixed sagittal imbalance. J Bone Joint Surg Am. 2003; 85(3):454–463
3. Bridwell KH, Lewis SJ, Rinella A, Lenke LG, Baldus C, Blanke K. Pedicle subtraction osteotomy for the treatment of fixed sagittal imbalance. Surgical technique. J Bone Joint Surg Am. 2004; 86-A Suppl 1:44–50
4. La Marca F, Brumblay H. Smith-Petersen osteotomy in thoracolumbar deformity surgery. Neurosurgery. 2008; 63(3) Suppl:163–170

60 Vertebral Body Tethering for Scoliosis

Nuri Demirci, Altug Yucekul, Caglar Yilgor, and Ahmet Alanay

Summary
Vertebral body tethering (VBT) serves as a nonfusion alternative for treating adolescent idiopathic scoliosis, particularly in cases with growth potential. It preserves mobility and promotes growth while controlling deformity. Patient selection involves assessing growth potential, curve parameters, and considering alternative treatment modalities. A residual curve of less than 35 degrees at the end of growth or prevention of fusion has generally been accepted as successful outcomes for VBT. Nonetheless, further research is needed to fully ascertain VBT's clinical efficacy and optimal utilization.

Keywords: nonfusion, adolescent idiopathic scoliosis, vertebral body tethering, growth-friendly instrumentation, spinal deformity

60.1 Key Points

- Curve progression in scoliosis is caused by differential compressive loads acting on the spine resulting in diminished concave growth and accelerated convex growth as per the Hueter-Volkmann law.[1] Vertebral body tethering (VBT) is a growth modulation technique for treating scoliosis in patients with remaining growth potential wherein these loads are reversed. By tightening the polyethylene cord, convexity compression is applied, which decelerates growth. Curve correction, on the other hand, indirectly accelerates growth by distracting the concavity. Changes in load distribution lead to growth-dependent follow-up curve correction. Consequently, deformity correction in VBT occurs in two stages: intraoperative tethering and growth modulation.
- Spinal fusion is the gold standard procedure for correcting the deformity and improving health-related quality of life. Yet, it is not without consequences. As per the intention of the surgery, mobility is lost in the operated segments. The lever arm created by this immobile long segment can lead to adjacent disk degeneration in the long term. Another negative consequence is restricted growth in the spine as well as the chest cage.

VBT offers a nonfusion solution that would preserve the mobility and allow growth while controlling the deformity.

- As growth modulation requires remaining growth potential to work effectively, patients with skeletal maturity are considered poor candidates for VBT. Although skeletally mature children were reported to achieve satisfactory correction and stability with VBT as an alternative to fusion,[2] long-term follow-up of these patients are unknown.
- VBT's clinical value is still in question due to a lack of enough evidence. In order to identify the patients for whom VBT will be successful, it is crucial to better understand optimal remaining growth, curve size, location and flexibility, and timing of surgery.

60.2 Indications

- Due to the novel nature of this technique, currently there is no consensus on its indications. As VBT is a growth modulation technique, determination of the remaining growth potential is critical. Since remaining growth cannot be determined directly, scales and classifications such as Risser[3] and Sanders[4] are used, as well as family history, parent and child heights, secondary sex traits, and menarche status. There is no indicated specific age range.
- Sanders 2 patients with a closed triradiate cartilage and Sanders 3 patients appear to be the best candidates for VBT, while open triradiate Sanders 2 patients may be candidates for overcorrection.[5] Yet, one should not make patient selection decisions solely on a single classification scheme and evaluate all available growth determinants.
- Although there are several nuances, indications approved by the US and the EU regulatory authorities include skeletally immature patients with major Cobb angles between 30 and 65 degrees involving thoracic or lumbar curves for whom bracing has failed or who are intolerant of brace wearing (Sanders score of 2 to 5 and Risser scale of 0 to 4). Previous surgery at the same levels and T-scores of −1.5 or less were listed as contraindications.[6]
- Curve flexibility should also be evaluated. Generally, at least a 50% flexible curve is desirable. Ideally thoracic curves should bend to less than 30 degrees.
- Hyperkyphosis greater than 40 degrees is a relative contraindication since tethering the spine from the anterior portion could further exacerbate the condition.[7]

60.3 Surgical Technique

- The patient is placed on a radiolucent table in the lateral decubitus position with the convex side of the deformity pointing up. A double lumen endotracheal tube is used for selective deflation of the lung. A soft gel roll is placed under the axilla to protect the brachial plexus. The right arm is placed on an armrest with a soft gel padding to protect the ulnar nerve.
- Neuromonitoring should be performed during surgery to monitor spinal cord function.
- There are three possible approaches to the thoracic cavity: thoracoscopic, video-assisted open thoracotomy, and open thoracotomy. Approach to the retroperitoneal space can be achieved via a separate retroperitoneal incision or via a lumbar extension of a thoracic cavity approach. Thoracoabdominal combined approaches are also possible where one incision is used to approach both regions.
- The pleura is dissected from the lateral side of the vertebral bodies preceding the rib heads. Segmental vessels can either be ligated or preserved on the convex side. After dissection and exposure, staples and bicortical screws are implanted to the vertebral body, anterior to the rib head. The localization of instruments is controlled using fluoroscopy guidance and/or intraoperative navigation.
- Once the implantation has been completed, the polyethylene tether is introduced. Beginning at the most cranial end, each instrumented level is tightened. As of today, there is no consensus regarding the tension force to be applied to each segment. Generally, less tension is applied to the caudal and cranial ends to avoid overcorrection and adding-on. Maximum tension is applied to the apex to achieve desired intraoperative correction.
- Prior to closure, regular saline irrigation of the thoracic cavity is performed. The thoracic cavity is double-checked to assure proper hemostasis. A chest tube is placed, and the lung is reinflated.

60.4 Complications

- The most common and specific complications of the VBT procedure are tether breakage and overcorrection.
  - Tether breakage: Coronal angulation increasing by more than 5 degrees between adjacent screws suggests tether breakage.[8]
  - Overcorrection: Most common reason for revision surgery.[9]
  - Adding-on.
  - Progression of the untethered curve.
- Approach-related complications: pleural effusion, atelectasis, pneumothorax, and chylothorax.

60.5 Postoperative Care

- On the 1st postoperative day, patients are mobilized without restriction.
- By the 2nd or 3rd postoperative day, the chest tube is removed.
- Postoperative bracing is generally not indicated.
- The patient can generally be discharged on day 4 or 5.
- It takes approximately 2 to 3 weeks for patients to return to school after surgery.

60.6 Outcomes

- A residual curve less than 35 degrees at the end of growth or prevention of fusion has generally been accepted as successful outcomes for VBT (**Fig. 60.1**).
- Studies comparing VBT to posterior fusion reported fusion to provide better correction rates and lower revision surgery rates. Health-related quality-of-life questionnaire results, on the other hand, was similar for both techniques.[10]
- The systematic review study of Bizzoca et al[9] reveals satisfying outcomes in general.
  - In the studies, the success rate of VBT ranged from 52 to 95%. Considering the wide range of the results, this technique needs further clarification for indications.
  - Complication rates were 17.8% postoperatively, and complications were also observed in patients who achieved skeletal maturity with a successful outcome.
  - Unplanned revision surgery rate was reported to be 14.1%.

60.7 Surgical Pearls

- Positioning the patient with specialized pads is key to restoring kyphosis and achieving derotation.
- Around the apical screws, maximum or near-maximum tension should be applied, while zero tension can be applied to the caudal end of the construct, or the tether can be left slack.
- External translation and derotation maneuvers applied to the screws using T-handles should precede correction gained by tether tensioning.

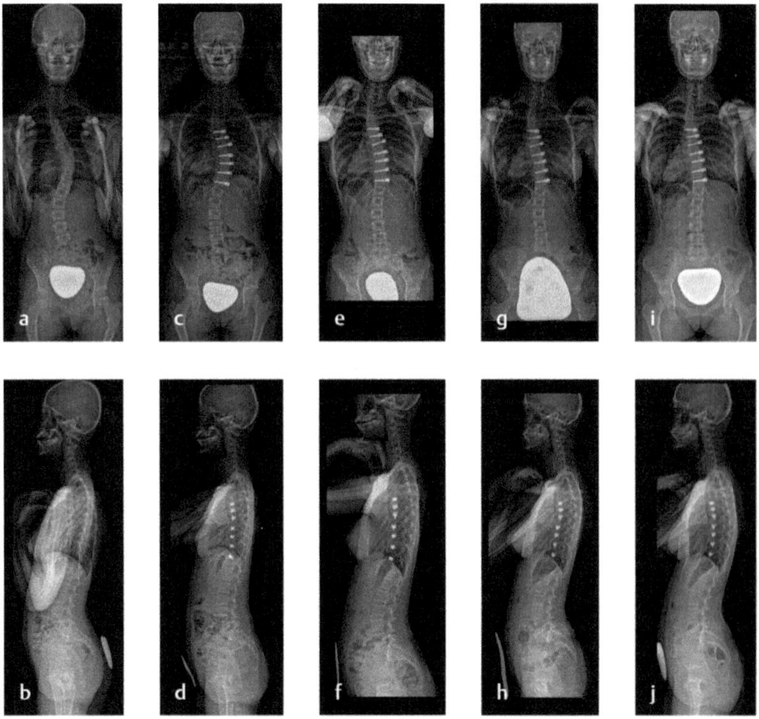

Fig. 60.1 An 11-years-and-6-months-old female patient, who was 7 months postmenarchal, measured 157 cm in height, and displayed Risser 1, Sanders 2 characteristics applied to our clinic. Her preoperative **(a)** PA and **(b)** lateral radiographs displayed a 48 degree right thoracic curve, where the compensatory proximal thoracic and thoracolumbar curves measured 31 and 35 degrees, respectively. In her pre-discharge, first-erect radiographs **(c, d)**, the main curve measured 25 degrees. During the course of the follow-up spontaneous correction was observed in all three curves, where her 1-year **(e, f)** and 2-years **(g, h)** radiographs displayed a gradual correction in all three planes where the coronal curve sizes decreased, the rib hump decreased and thoracic kyphosis increased. At her latest follow-up, at 8-years, where she measured 167 cm and displayed Risser 5 and Sanders 8 characteristics, her radiographs **(i, j)** displayed that the correction was maintained over the years.

- Due to its closer proximity to the aorta, left-sided approaches may present more technical challenges. Particularly for segmental vessel ligations, a cautious approach is needed.
- Maintaining the health of the intervertebral disks may be beneficial during this motion-preserving procedure to ensure long-term success of the construct.

Common Clinical Questions

1. Which of the following is not an absolute or relative contraindication for VBT?
   A. Hyperkyphosis > 40 degrees.
   B. Left-sided thoracic curves.
   C. T-scores < −1.5.
   D. Previous surgery at the same levels of planned VBT.
2. Which of the following is the most crucial determinant factor when VBT is planned?
   A. Age of the patient.
   B. Gender.
   C. Magnitude of rotational deformity.
   D. Remaining growth potential.

Answers to Common Clinical Questions

1. B. The left-sided curve is not a contraindication. Considering growth modulation in this group of patients involves careful assessment of the potential pathologic associations, such as syndromic conditions.
2. D. The effectiveness of growth modulation mainly depends on the remaining growth potential of the patient.

References

1. Mehlman CT, Araghi A, Roy DR. Hyphenated history: the Hueter-Volkmann law. Am J Orthop. 1997; 26(11):798–800
2. Hegde SK, Venkatesan M, Akbari KK, Badikillaya VM. Efficacy of anterior vertebral body tethering in skeletally mature children with adolescent idiopathic scoliosis: a preliminary report. Int J Spine Surg. 2021; 15(5):995–1003
3. Risser JC. The iliac apophysis; an invaluable sign in the management of scoliosis. Clin Orthop. 1958; 11:111–119
4. Sanders JO, Khoury JG, Kishan S, et al. Predicting scoliosis progression from skeletal maturity: a simplified classification during adolescence. J Bone Joint Surg Am. 2008; 90(3):540–553
5. Alanay A, Yucekul A, Abul K, et al. Thoracoscopic vertebral body tethering for adolescent idiopathic scoliosis: follow-up curve behavior according to Sanders skeletal maturity staging. Spine. 2020; 45(22):E1483–E1492

6. Samdani AF, Pahys JM, Ames RJ, et al. Prospective follow-up report on anterior vertebral body tethering for idiopathic scoliosis: interim results from an FDA IDE study. J Bone Joint Surg Am. 2021; 103(17):1611–1619
7. Samdani AF, Ames RJ, Kimball JS, et al. Anterior vertebral body tethering for immature adolescent idiopathic scoliosis: one-year results on the first 32 patients. Eur Spine J. 2015; 24(7):1533–1539
8. Newton PO, Kluck DG, Saito W, Yaszay B, Bartley CE, Bastrom TP. Anterior spinal growth tethering for skeletally immature patients with scoliosis: a retrospective look two to four years postoperatively. J Bone Joint Surg Am. 2018; 100(19):1691–1697
9. Bizzoca D, Piazzolla A, Moretti L, Vicenti G, Moretti B, Solarino G. Anterior vertebral body tethering for idiopathic scoliosis in growing children: a systematic review. World J Orthop. 2022; 13(5):481–493
10. Newton PO, Bartley CE, Bastrom TP, Kluck DG, Saito W, Yaszay B. Anterior spinal growth modulation in skeletally immature patients with idiopathic scoliosis: a comparison with posterior spinal fusion at 2 to 5 years postoperatively. J Bone Joint Surg Am. 2020; 102(9):769–777

61 Percutaneous Pedicle Screw Placement

Michael Y. Wang

Summary

Percutaneous pedicle screw placement is a critical tool in the armamentarium of spine surgeons. Various techniques exist, including fluoroscopy-based or with navigation/robotics. Obtaining the correct views and images is an absolute "must" as direct visualization is not possible. Percutaneous pedicle screws are important adjuncts in TLIF surgery, trauma, and other procedures.

Keywords: percutaneous, minimally invasive, fusion, trauma, TLIF

61.1 Key Points

- Numerous methods can be used for implanting percutaneous pedicle screws, such as image guidance, en face targeting, and biplanar fluoroscopy.
- Percutaneous screws can be safely placed in the thoracolumbar spine using a simple method based primarily on anteroposterior (AP) X-rays.
- Percutaneous screw–rod constructs are a truly minimally invasive surgical (MIS) technique for segmental fixation.

61.2 Indications

Percutaneous placement of transpedicular screws with connecting rods can find application in virtually any setting where open screw fixation might be utilized in the thoracolumbar spine. For a fusion setting, this can be employed in conjunction with interbody fusion for stabilization,[1] such as after an anterior lumbar interbody fusion (ALIF), lateral interbody fusion, transforaminal lumbar interbody fusion (TLIF), or transsacral fusion. In addition, a speculum retractor can be used to expose the lateral masses for posterolateral fusion bed preparation in conjunction with percutaneous fixation. Also, percutaneous fixation can be used for stabilization or "internal bracing" in the absence of a bony arthrodesis.[2] Thus, regardless of whether a fusion is intended, percutaneous screw–rod fixation can be used to confer spinal stability for degenerative, traumatic, neoplastic, and infectious pathologies.

61.3 Technique

There are various methods for targeting the pedicles of the lumbar or thoracic spine. These include: (1) frame-based or frameless image-guided navigation,[3] (2) biplanar fluoroscopy in the AP and lateral views, (3) "en face" or "direct down the pedicle" imaging,[4] (4) a mini-open technique with tactile feedback, and (5) an AP-based targeting method.[5] This chapter will describe the AP-based targeting method.

- The patient is positioned prone on a radiolucent operating table. Care is taken to ensure that there are no obstructions to the fluoroscopic image at the level(s) of interest; the technique being heavily dependent on intraoperative imaging.
- An absolutely precise AP view is registered at the level of screw placement. This is done by first ensuring that the axial rotation of the fluoroscope aligns the spinous process equidistant between the right and left pedicles (**Fig. 61.1**). Either the fluoroscope can be moved or the bed can be rotated to register this image, but the surgeon must compensate for any rotation depending on the method used. The sagittal (Ferguson) angle is then adjusted so that the anterior and posterior cortical rims of the upper end plate of the vertebral body are superimposed into a single line. This ensures that the X-ray beam is

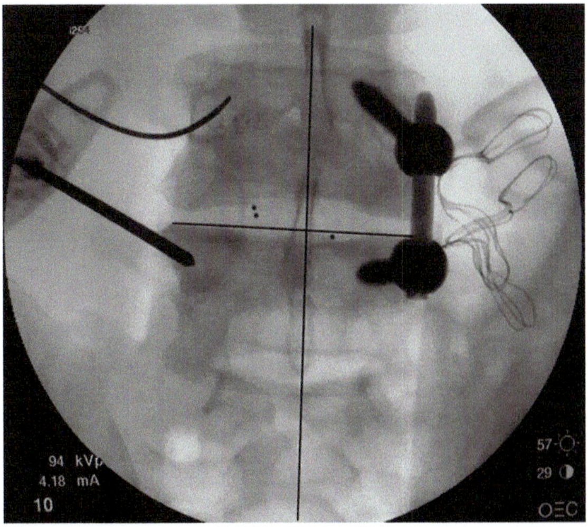

Fig. 61.1 Anteroposterior (AP) projection on the L5 vertebral body. Note that the upper end plate of the L5 body is visualized as a single line and that the spinous process is equidistant between the two pedicles.

completely aligned with the sagittal plane of the pedicles (and thus offers an ideal screw trajectory).

- The skin is then marked so that a cutaneous entry point can be made 1 to 2 cm lateral to the lateral border of the pedicle. A Jamshidi needle (MedSurge; Chennai, India) is then inserted through the skin and directed slightly medially to contact the bone surface. The needle is then docked at the junction of the transverse process and facet joint near the mammillary process (the attachment of the multifidus muscle).
- Once the Jamshidi needle has been docked on this ideal pedicle screw starting point, the needle is marked 2 cm above the skin surface with a surgical marker (**Fig. 61.2**). The needle is then hammered into the pedicle to a depth of 2 cm (where the marking meets the skin surface). The trajectory will be medialized to match the patient's anatomy (10–30 degrees). If a proper AP image has been obtained, making the Jamshidi needle parallel to the horizon and parallel to the upper end plate will place the needle in the proper sagittal orientation.
- So long as the medial wall of the pedicle is not breached at a depth of 2 cm, there will be no medial pedicle wall violation; the needle will have passed the depth of the pedicle (and spinal canal) following 2 cm of advancement. Once the Jamshidi needle has been placed, the inner stylet is removed, and a Kirschner wire (K-wire) is inserted into the vertebral body.
- The procedure is then conducted at other vertebral levels with adjustments in fluoroscopic targeting for each level. After all the K-wires have been placed, the fluoroscope is moved to a lateral position. The K-wires are then used to guide an awl and tap for pedicle preparation as with open surgery. Final pedicle screw placement is then performed followed by K-wire removal.
- During the procedure, care is taken to ensure that the K-wires do not violate the anterior vertebral body and enter the retroperitoneum, which could cause vascular or hollow viscus injury. In addition, care must be taken not to lose control of the wires or have them pull out prematurely.
- Following screw placement, a percutaneous rod is advanced subfascially through the screw extensions to connect the segmental levels (**Fig. 61.3**). Rod insertion can occur through one of the end screw incisions or through a separate incision distal to the screws.
- It is helpful to have at least some bend in the rod, because "steering" the rod medially or laterally is made easier by rotating the rod along its long axis to turn the tip medially or laterally. Finally, set screws are placed through the screw extensions to lock the rod to the individual screws.

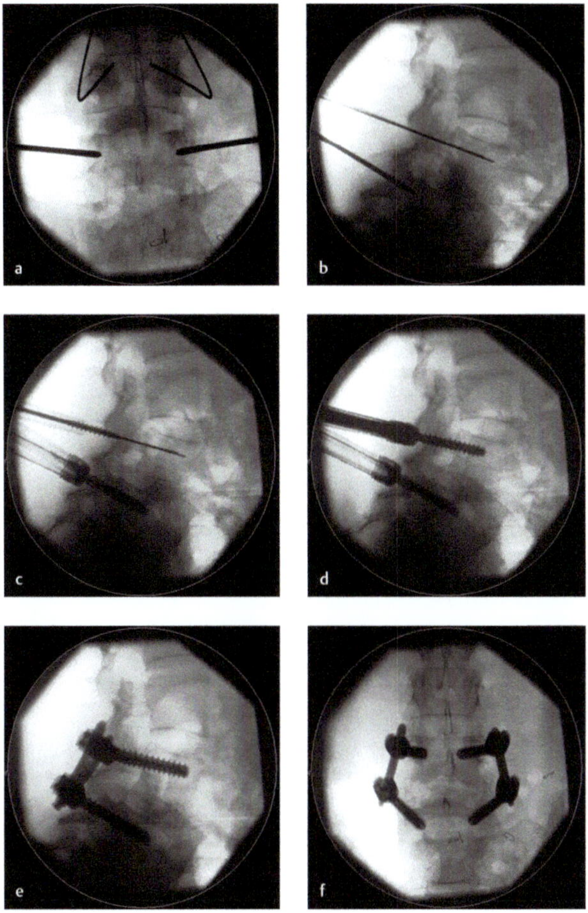

Fig. 61.2 **(a)** Anteroposterior (AP) view targeting the lower vertebral body. Note the rotation in relation to the body above (where the spinous process is not in the midline). Docking at the junction of the facet joint and transverse process is followed by 2 cm of medial needle advancement. **(b)** The needle is confirmed on lateral fluoroscopy as having passed the spinal canal, ruling out pedicle wall violation. **(c)** An insulating sheath is used to minimize soft tissue trauma while an awl and tap are advanced over the K-wire. **(d)** Final screw positioning with extension tabs attached to guide rod insertion. Final construct is visualized on **(e)** lateral and **(f)** AP views.

61.4 Complications

The complications associated with percutaneous screw placement are akin to those encountered with open surgical instrumentation procedures. In addition,

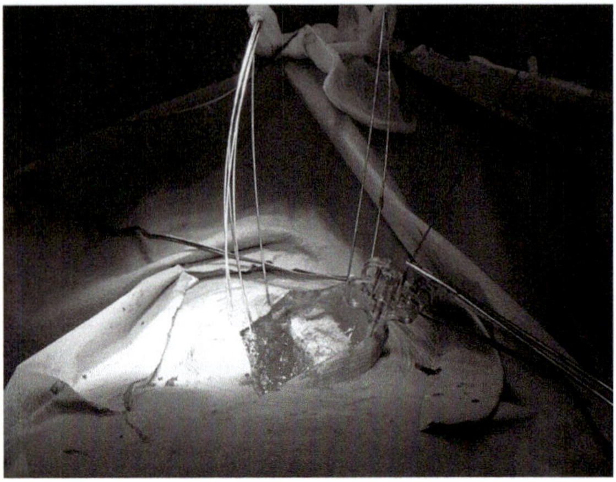

Fig. 61.3 Jamshidi needles and K-wires in place. Note the use of a long skin incision with placement of instrumentation through the exposed fascia and the use of a needle driver to control the K-wire during manipulation.

risks are associated with loss of control of the K-wires, which can result in inadvertent entry into the retroperitoneum.

Difficulties can be encountered with initial pedicle cannulation or with rod passage and screw–rod connection. Use of the AP-based technique results in a low rate of pedicle violation as long as high-quality fluoroscopic images are used for targeting the Jamshidi needles. Rod passage and connection techniques are often specific to the implant manufacturers and the instruments available for rod and screw manipulation, so they are not described here.

61.5 Postoperative Care

Care after surgery is the same as with open instrumentation. Patients should be rapidly mobilized with physical therapies, with external bracing as a treatment option. Muscle spasm occurs more commonly with MIS procedures and is best treated with muscle relaxants and benzodiazepines as opposed to narcotics.

61.6 Surgical Pearls

- In many instances the entire surgery can be accomplished by a single surgeon standing on the side opposite the fluoroscope. This improves surgical workflow and minimizes the risk of contaminating the sterile field. Because of the highly imaging-dependent nature of the method described here, standing on the same side as the pedicle screw insertion (which is typical for open surgery) is much less important.

- When a rod is passed across the thoracolumbar junction, it is usually preferable to pass the rod from cranial to caudal.
- Because the screw head heights and orientation are not immediately visible, the surgeon should be prepared to pass a prepared rod initially and then to remove it and recontour or resize the implant to achieve the optimal construct. Forcing the screw and rod to mate may result in screw pullout.

Common Clinical Questions

1. Percutaneous pedicle screws can be safely inserted using all of the following techniques *except* which?
   A. AP-guided imaging.
   B. Pure freehand technique.
   C. Biplanar fluoroscopy.
   D. Image guidance.
2. When using the AP-based technique for percutaneous pedicle cannulation, how far is the Jamshidi needle advanced before passing the medial pedicle wall?
   A. 1 cm.
   B. 2 cm.
   C. 3 cm.
   D. 4 cm.
3. Bending the rod allows what to be accomplished more easily?
   A. Cutting the rod to size.
   B. Reducing spondylolisthesis.
   C. Achieving a fusion.
   D. Medial and lateral maneuvering.

Answers to Common Clinical Questions

1. B.
2. B.
3. D.

References

1. Schwender JD, Holly LT, Rouben DP, Foley KT. Minimally invasive transforaminal lumbar interbody fusion (TLIF): technical feasibility and initial results. J Spinal Disord Tech. 2005; 18 Suppl:S1–S6
2. Jeanneret B, Jovanovic M, Magerl F. Percutaneous diagnostic stabilization for low back pain. Correlation with results after fusion operations. Clin Orthop Relat Res. 1994; 304(304):130–138
3. Wang MY, Kim KA, Liu CY, Kim P, Apuzzo ML. Reliability of three-dimensional fluoroscopy for detecting pedicle screw violations in the thoracic and lumbar spine. Neurosurgery. 2004; 54(5):1138–1142, discussion 1142–1143
4. Magerl F. Verletzungen der Brust und Lendenwirbelsaule. Langenbecks Arch Chir. 1980; 352:428–433
5. Harris EB, Massey P, Lawrence J, Rihn J, Vaccaro A, Anderson DG. Percutaneous techniques for minimally invasive posterior lumbar fusion. Neurosurg Focus. 2008; 25(2):E12

62 Awake Spine Surgery

David A.W. Sykes, Jeff Gadsden, Dhanesh K. Gupta, and Muhammad M. Abd-El-Barr

Summary

In this chapter, the topic of awake spine surgery is discussed, that is, spine surgery without the use of general anesthesia. Various anesthetic alternatives are discussed, but spinal anesthesia is more specifically illustrated. Specific indications and patient populations are discussed, as well as procedures that may lend themselves to being performed with awake techniques. Spinal anesthesia technique is described, as are its potential complications. The improved clinical outcomes associated with awake spine surgery are reviewed. Surgical pearls, common clinical questions, and their corresponding answers are also discussed.

Keywords: spine surgery, awake spine surgery, minimally invasive spine surgery, pain, anesthesia, regional anesthesia

62.1 Key Points

- In recent years, awake spine surgery under spinal anesthesia has increased in popularity.[1]
- Awake spine surgery is favorable in patients who are poor candidates for general anesthesia due to their age or medical comorbidities.[1]
- Awake spine surgery can be performed with local, epidural, or spinal anesthesia, but the most studied technique is surgery under spinal anesthesia.[1]
- Achieving spinal anesthesia is technically straightforward.
- Studies show that awake spine surgery improves patient outcomes.[2,3]
- Not all settings are appropriate for awake spine surgery.

62.2 Indications

- There are limited absolute contraindications to spinal anesthesia; these include:
  - Patient refusal.
  - Infection at proposed injection site.
  - Disturbed hemostasis.

- Many demographic factors and medical conditions make patients poor candidates for general anesthesia, and thus may be considered relative indications for awake spine surgery[4]:
  - Coronary artery disease.
  - Heart failure.
  - Respiratory dysfunction (e.g., reactive airways disease, severe chronic obstructive pulmonary disease [COPD]).
  - Advanced age.
  - History of severe postoperative nausea and vomiting.
- Several procedures have been performed under spinal anesthesia, though decompressions are the most studied setting[1,2,3]:
  - One- to three-level lumbar spine surgeries.
  - Lumbar decompression:
    - Laminectomies.
    - Diskectomies.
  - Lumbar interbody fusions:
    - Minimally invasive lumbar interbody fusion.
    - Percutaneous lumbar interbody fusion.
  - Decompression with fusion.
  - Anterior cervical diskectomy and fusion (less common).

62.3 Technique

- Place the patient in the sitting position and palpate the appropriate spinal level, generally L3–L4. A line connecting the iliac crests typically crosses the vertebral column at the L3/L4 interspace or the L4 body. Ultrasound may also be used to precisely determine the desired interspace.
- Appropriately sterilize the skin and drape the patient's lumbar region.
- Access the intrathecal space by inserting a spinal needle (**Fig. 62.1**).
  - Introduce the needle to the skin, at the interspinous space, with a slight cephalad angle.
  - Pass the needle through the skin, subcutaneous fat, the supraspinous and interspinous ligaments, and the ligamentum flavum.
  - As the needle passes through the relatively elastic ligamentum flavum (+/− dura and arachnoid mater), the operator may feel a "click" or "pop." The internal stylet is then removed from the needle and the needle hub observed for cerebrospinal fluid (CSF).
- Upon return of free-flowing CSF, local anesthetic is then injected.
- The local anesthetic and dose chosen will determine the degree of cephalad spread of the block as well as block duration. It is important that the surgeon and anesthesiologist communicate in advance about the expected duration of the case.

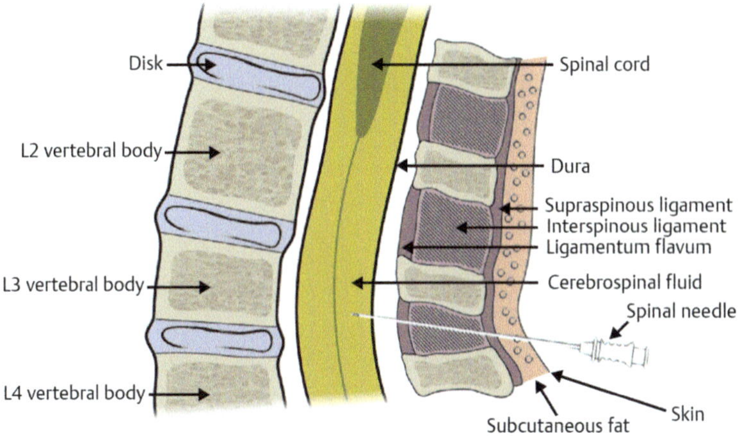

Fig. 62.1 Relevant anatomy and needle trajectory in spinal anesthesia.

62.4 Complications

- The complications associated with awake spine surgery are largely the complications associated with the procedure itself, rather than an adverse effect associated with the spinal anesthesia.
- Spinal anesthesia frequently causes a mild decrease is systemic blood pressure but this is easily treated by the administration of a low-dose vasopressor infusion (e.g., phenylephrine).
- Postoperative complications are reduced in patients receiving awake surgery, as the adverse effects associated with general anesthesia are avoided.[5]

62.5 Postoperative Care

- Much like complications associated with awake spine surgery, postoperative care is largely dictated by the nature of the procedure, rather than the effects of spinal anesthesia.
- Awake surgery is associated with reduced intensity of postoperative care, as patients are generally in less pain and able to ambulate and leave the hospital sooner.

62.6 Outcomes

- As awake surgery is a relatively new movement within the field of spine surgery, its associated outcomes have not been definitively described.

- While some early studies found awake surgery to be associated with decreased opioid utilization, others found spinal and general anesthesia to be equivalent.[2]
- Recent meta-analyses, however, have associated awake spine surgery with[2,3]:
  - Reduced blood loss.
  - Reduced intraoperative hypotension.
  - Reduced postoperative nausea and vomiting.
  - Reduced time in postanesthesia care unit (PACU).
  - Reduced hospital length of stay.
- Smaller studies have additionally described awake spine surgery's association with:
  - Reduced postoperative pain.[5]
  - Reduced opioid utilization.[6]

62.7 Surgical Pearls

- Although the current literature suggests that awake spine surgery may be associated with improved outcomes, it is worth noting that not all patients are appropriate for awake surgery.
- Awake spine surgery may be inappropriate for[1]:
  - Patients with severe anxiety.
  - Procedures of unpredictable duration.

Common Clinical Questions

1. What kinds of spine surgeries can be done awake?
2. When should I consider awake spine surgery?
3. When should I avoid awake spine surgery?
4. What type of anesthetic do you use to achieve spinal anesthesia?

Answers to Common Clinical Questions

1. Many one- to three-level spine surgeries have been performed awake, including decompressions, fusions, and decompression with fusion. Decompressions, however, are the most extensively studied.
2. You should consider performing awake spine surgery when you have a patient who is a poor candidate for general anesthesia. This includes elderly patients, as well as patients with coronary artery disease, pulmonary disease, and others.

3. There are few absolute contraindications to awake spine surgery. Consider avoiding spinal anesthesia, however, in patients who refuse due to anxiety, have an infection at the proposed injection site, or have disturbed hemostasis.
4. Although different providers may be comfortable or more experienced with certain medications, the authors have found excellent utility in administering 10-15 mg 0.5% of isobaric bupivacaine into the intrathecal space to achieve spinal anesthesia for awake spine surgery.

References

1. Fiani B, Reardon T, Selvage J, et al. Awake spine surgery: an eye-opening movement. Surg Neurol Int. 2021; 12:222
2. Urick D, Sciavolino B, Wang TY, Gupta DK, Sharan A, Abd-El-Barr MM. Perioperative outcomes of general versus spinal anesthesia in the lumbar spine surgery population: a systematic review and meta-analysis of data from 2005 through 2021. J Clin Orthop Trauma. 2022; 30:101923
3. Perez-Roman RJ, Govindarajan V, Bryant JP, Wang MY. Spinal anesthesia in awake surgical procedures of the lumbar spine: a systematic review and meta-analysis of 3709 patients. Neurosurg Focus. 2021; 51(6):E7
4. Smith G, D'Cruz JR, Rondeau B, Goldman J. General Anesthesia for Surgeons. In: StatPearls. Treasure Island, FL: StatPearls Publishing; October 12, 2021
5. De Biase G, Gruenbaum SE, West JL, et al. Spinal versus general anesthesia for minimally invasive transforaminal lumbar interbody fusion: implications on operating room time, pain, and ambulation. Neurosurg Focus. 2021; 51(6):E3
6. Waguia R, Touko EK, Sykes DAW, et al. How to start an awake spine program: protocol and illustrative cases. IBRO Neurosci Rep. 2022; 13:69–77

63 Anterior Lumbar Interbody Fusion

Cristiano Magalhães Menezes and Marlus Sérgio Borges Salomão Junior

Summary

Anterior lumbar interbody fusion (ALIF) offers several advantages, such as reduced risk during patient positioning, a minimally invasive muscle-sparing approach, and the avoidance of injury to posterior elements. Indications for ALIF include degenerative disk disease, spondylolisthesis, loss of segmental lordosis, and revisions in failed posterior approaches. The preoperative imaging considerations emphasize the importance of interpreting sagittal and axial magnetic resonance imaging (MRI) for factors like vascular anatomy and foraminal stenosis.

The surgical technique involves patient positioning, intraoperative setup, and careful exposure, including a longitudinal or transverse paramedian incision. The chapter details the step-by-step procedure, from identifying anatomical structures to disk space preparation and cage implantation. Complications associated with ALIF includes retrograde ejaculation, vascular lesions, and deep venous thrombosis. Patient-specific considerations and outcomes, such as the use of lordotic cages for restoring physiological spine shape and achieving a fusion rate of 94.5%, are also discussed. The surgical pearls provide additional insights, emphasizing precautions and considerations for successful ALIF procedures.

Keywords: anterior lumbar interbody fusion (ALIF), surgical technique, complications, patient-specific considerations

63.1 Advantages

- Less risk when positioning the patient. Allows easier airway surveillance by the anesthesiologist.
- Naturally minimally invasive for being a muscle-sparing approach.
- No injury to the posterior elements, such as the vertebral arches, muscle insertions, and ligaments.[1,2]
- Less risk of radicular lesions, durotomy, and intracanal fibrosis since there is no direct mobilization of the dural sac and nerve roots.[3]

- Allows performing wide diskectomy under direct visualization.
- Possibility of using cages with greater support surface in a compressive context.
- The release of the anterior longitudinal ligament (ALL), the main restrictor of lumbar lordosis, allows the use of larger cages, height gain, and segmental lordosis.
- Potential for indirect decompression.
- Low infection rates of up to 20 to 50 times less than in posterior approaches.

63.2 Indications

- Degenerative disk disease with or without instability and Modic changes.
- Spondylolisthesis, lithic or degenerative, especially low grade.
- Loss of segmental lordosis.
- Revision in failed posterior approaches.
- Adult spine deformities with coronal or sagittal malalignment.

63.3 Preoperative Imaging Considerations

- Interpreting sagittal and axial magnetic resonance imaging (MRI):
  - Psoas muscle.
  - Vascular anatomy.
  - Level of bifurcation and lateralization of great vessels.
  - Fatty tissue plane between vasculature and anterior disk.
  - Foraminal and central stenosis.

63.4 Technique

- Positioning and intraoperative setup:
  - The patient must be positioned in supine or lateral decubitus position on radiolucent surgical table.
  - Supine: A roll under the sacrum will allow for superficialization of lumbosacrum junction.
  - Trendelenburg maneuver associated with a slight lateral bend to allow the displacement of the abdominal contents toward right hypochondrium.
  - L5–S1 level can be accessed by planning the incision halfway between the pubis and umbilicus.
- Surgical exposure:
  - Transverse or longitudinal paramedian incision is made on either side for L5–S1.

- The anterior rectus sheath is divided longitudinally, retracted with Allis forceps, and separated from the lateral border of the rectus abdominis.
- The next plane identified is the preperitoneal, characterized by a first layer of fat.
- This plane is developed by mobilizing the peritoneum off the anterior and lateral abdominal wall. The arcuate line must be divided if approach to cranial levels other than L5–S1 is intended.
- The retroperitoneum space is reached when the second layer of fat is visualized and mobilized with blunt dissection.
- Psoas muscle is identified.
- Along the medial border of the psoas, a third layer of fat is visualized containing the ureter, which must be retracted along the peritoneal sac medially.
- Using digital palpation, the pulse of the left common iliac artery and promontory surface is felt.
- Continue medial to the vessels to create a plane between left iliac artery and peritoneum contents and ureter, until the disk space is reached, using Kittner sponge to clear adventitious tissue from the anterior disk anulus (**Fig. 63.1** and **Fig. 63.2a, b**).
- With handheld retractors equipped with fiberoptic lights, the surgeons expose the surgical field, keeping the peritoneum away from the disk space.
- The hypogastric plexus and sympathetic chain are detached from the disk using blunt dissection.[4]
- Identify and ligate/coagulate middle sacral vessels. Just after that, proceed with safe retraction of the left iliac vein.
- The manual retractors could be substituted by self-retaining table attachment.[5,6,7]
- A wide annulotomy is made and the disk material is cleared off.
- Midline is identified using C-arm visualization.
- The end plates are gently scrapped followed by trialing and cage implantation.
- The cage is properly fixed with screws or blades.
- Fluoroscopic images confirm final implantation.
- The planes are then closed starting with the rectus anterior fascia.

63.5 Complications[8]

- Retrograde ejaculation (2–2.3%).[11]
- Vascular lesion (3.03%).
- Deep venous thrombosis (1.4%).
- Hematoma formation (0.6%).

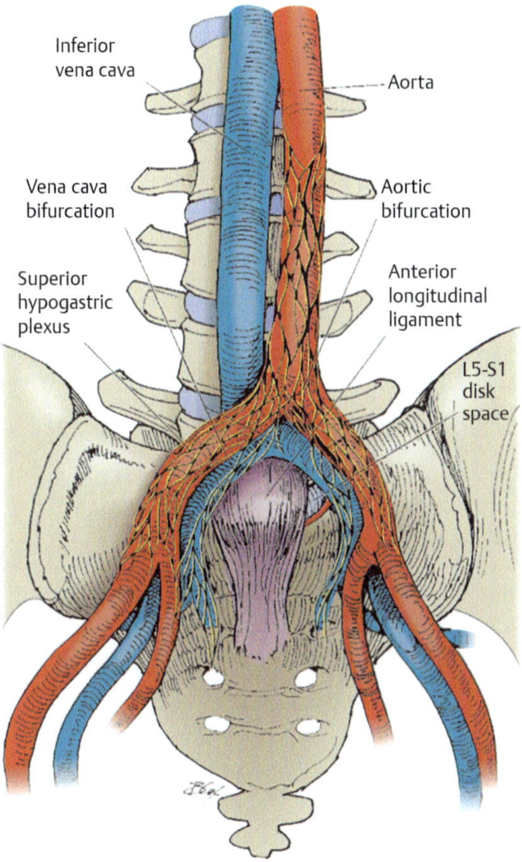

Fig. 63.1 Key structures on anterior access.

- Visceral injury (0.37%).
- Incisional hernia (1.3%).
- Wound infection (1.9%).
- Ileus (< 5%).
- Dural tears (0.04%).

63.6 Patient-Specific Considerations

- Pain history.
- Age.

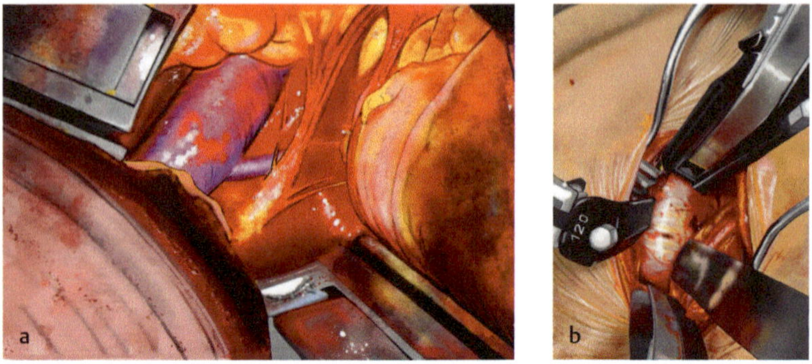

Fig. 63.2 **(a, b)** Key structures seen from the perspective of a left approach at L5–S1 with the patient positioned in lateral decubitus: left iliac vein, middle sacral vein, hypogastric plexus attached to posterior peritoneum wall **(a)**. After proper dissection and disk exposure with retractors in place **(b)**. (Copyright of Rafael Avendaño Pradel, MD.)

- Body mass index (BMI).
- Previous spine surgery.
- Previous abdominal surgery.
- Previous kidney transplant with abdominal graft.
- Previous vascular surgery.
- Previous retroperitoneal radiation.
- Comorbidities.

63.7 Outcomes[9]

- Using a lordotic or hyperlordotic cages at the lumbosacral junction reduces pelvic tilt and allows restoration of physiological spine shape.
- ALIF is an efficient technique for restoring proper sagittal alignment.
- Allows efficient indirect decompression of neural elements.
- Fusion rate 94.5 ± 5.5%.

63.8 Surgical Pearls

- Always check the level before skin incision.
- The second layer of fat visualized is the marker of reaching the retroperitoneum space.
- Lateral position enables single-position surgery for lower lumbar cases.[10]
- Approaches at the L4–L5 level are riskier because the vessels (aorta and vena cava) bifurcates at this location in two-thirds of cases.

Common Clinical Questions

1. What is the common position for patients in lateral ALIF (LatALIF)?
2. What are the benefits of LatALIF over ALIF in the supine position?
3. How retrograde ejaculation can be avoided?

Answers to Common Clinical Questions

1. In LatALIF, the patient is positioned in lateral decubitus and fixed to the surgical table with the aid of adhesive bands. The first adhesive tape should pass at the level of the patient's greater trochanter and fix it to the table. The C-arm must be used to check rotation and correct positioning.
   The next step is fixation of the patient's upper chest. Finally, an adhesive tape is positioned along the femoral axis, starting at the hip, and fixed to the table. Cushions should be positioned under bony prominences for protection.
   At the end, a new image must be taken to verify the correct positioning again. If the plan is to perform a single-position surgery, attention should be paid to the distance from the patient's back to the edge of the operating table to allow the necessary angulation for the passage of posterior pedicle screws.
2. With the aid of gravity, the lateral position allows the abdominal contents to naturally move away from the surgical path, avoiding the need for more aggressive retractions. Furthermore, in combined procedures, there is a significant difference in the reduction of surgical time allowing posterior instrumentation to be performed in the same decubitus position (single-position surgery).
3. The pathophysiology of retrograde ejaculation in anterior lumbar surgery is secondary to injury to the hypogastric plexus that traverses the prevertebral space near the L5/S1 space. Blunt and gentle dissection, from lateral to medial, avoiding elecrocautery, minimizes the occurrence. Within 3 to 48 months, 45.8% of these patients are recovered.[11]

Acknowledgment

Junyoung Ahn, Krzysztof Siemionow, Dustin H. Massel, Benjamin C. Mayo, William D. Long III, Krishna D. Modi, and Kern Singh for the previous chapter.

Rafael Avendaño Pradel, MD for the artistic illustrations used in the chapter.

References

1. Jarrett CD, Heller JG, Tsai L. Anterior exposure of the lumbar spine with and without an "access surgeon": morbidity analysis of 265 consecutive cases. J Spinal Disord Tech. 2009; 22(8):559–564
2. Brau SA. Mini-open approach to the spine for anterior lumbar interbody fusion: description of the procedure, results and complications. Spine J. 2002; 2(3):216–223
3. Goz V, Weinreb JH, Schwab F, Lafage V, Errico TJ. Comparison of complications, costs, and length of stay of three different lumbar interbody fusion techniques: an analysis of the Nationwide Inpatient Sample database. Spine J. 2014; 14(9):2019–2027
4. Sasso RC, Kenneth Burkus J, LeHuec JC. Retrograde ejaculation after anterior lumbar interbody fusion: transperitoneal versus retroperitoneal exposure. Spine. 2003; 28(10):1023–1026
5. Guiroy A, de Andrada-Pereira B, Camino-Willhuber G, et al. Setting for single position surgery: survey from expert spinal surgeons. Eur Spine J. 2022; 31 (9):2239–2247
6. Malham GM, Wagner TP, Claydon MH. Anterior lumbar interbody fusion in a lateral decubitus position: technique and outcomes in obese patients. J Spine Surg. 2019; 5(4):433–442
7. Davis TT, Hynes RA, Fung DA, et al. Retroperitoneal oblique corridor to the L2-S1 intervertebral discs in the lateral position: an anatomic study. J Neurosurg Spine. 2014; 21(5):785–793
8. Feeley A, Feeley I, Clesham K, Butler J. Is there a variance in complication types associated with ALIF approaches? A systematic review. Acta Neurochir (Wien). 2021; 163(11):2991–3004
9. Formica M, Quarto E, Zanirato A, et al. ALIF in the correction of spinal sagittal misalignment. A systematic review of literature. Eur Spine J. 2021; 30(1):50–62
10. Menezes CM, Alamin T, Amaral R, et al. Need of vascular surgeon and comparison of value for anterior lumbar interbody fusion (ALIF) in lateral decubitus: Delphi consensus. Eur Spine J. 2022; 31(9):2270–2278
11. Body AM, Plummer ZJ, Krueger BM, et al. Retrograde ejaculation following anterior lumbar surgery: a systematic review and pooled analysis. J Neurosurg Spine. 2021; 35(4):427–436

64 Sacroiliac Joint Fusion

Kalaventhan Pathinathan, Ashish D. Diwan, Joseph Maalouly, and Prashanth J. Rao

Summary

The sacroiliac (SI) joint dysfunction is an underrecognized source of low back pain/sciatica. Diagnosis with thorough physical examination and positive responses to diagnostic SI joint injections can identify the source of pain as SI joint dysfunction. Nonsurgical management include physical therapy, injections, radiofrequency ablation, and platelet-rich plasma (PRP) injections. Traumatic disruption of the SI joint is now replaced by degeneration as the main reason for SI joint fusion. Minimally invasive surgical (MIS) procedures have overtaken open surgeries due to reduced surgical morbidity. Novel MIS techniques include navigated and robotic SI joint fusion. Short- and medium-term results of MIS fusion techniques are very encouraging. Despite the reduced morbidity with the use of MIS techniques, long-term success of SI joint fusion for degenerative conditions still needs to be determined.

Keywords: sacroiliac joint, back pain/sciatica, minimally invasive SIJ fusion, robotic fusion

64.1 Key Points

The sacroiliac (SI) joint dysfunction is underrecognized source of low back pain and its diagnosis can be challenging. Careful workup with thorough physical examination and positive responses to diagnostic SI joint injections can identify a surgical candidate, but only after conservative approaches are truly exhausted.

- Traumatic disruption of the SI joint is now replaced by SI joint dysfunction and painful degeneration as the main reason for SI joint stabilization and fusion procedures.
- Such procedures could be considered as stabilization (when no bone graft is used) or SI joint fusion when either an implant-based (nonbone graft) intra-articular arthrodesis is achieved, or an intra-articular or extra-articular bone graft is utilized.
- Fixation choices and fusion technique options have increased from 2010 to 2022 with the advent of minimally invasive surgery (MIS) techniques to fuse the SI joint.[1]

- Novel MIS techniques are now used to treat painful degenerative conditions of the SI joint.
- Despite the reduced morbidity with the use of MIS techniques, long-term success of SI joint fusion for degenerative conditions still needs to be determined.

64.2 Indications

- Degeneration of the SI joint characterized by upper buttock pain just below the level of the posterior superior iliac spine (PSIS), pain with positional changes (sitting to standing), climbing or descending stairs or single-leg stance, refractory to nonoperative care, after all other pain sources are ruled out. There is evidence of good diagnostic validity utilizing at least three provocation tests of the five with a sensitivity of 77 to 91% and 78% specificity for positive responses to controlled comparative SI joint blocks in identifying SI joint pain.[2,3,4]
- Traumatic SI joint injuries[5] with angular, superior–inferior, or rotational instability of the joint in connection with pelvic ring disruption. Postpartum instabilities make a subgroup.
- Theories of pain generation include ligamentous or capsular tension, extraneous compression, shear forces, hypomobility or hypermobility, aberrant joint mechanics, and myofascial or kinetic chain imbalances resulting in pain.[6] These theories exclude SI joint involvement of spondyloarthropathies associated with systemic inflammation like ankylosing spondylitis or psoriatic arthropathy which are uncommon compared to degenerative cases.
- Intra-articular sources of SI joint pain include osteoarthritis and infection.
- Extra-articular sources of SI joint pain include enthesis/ligamentous sprain and osseous sources such as a sacral insufficiency fracture. It may also be caused by primary enthesopathy, hip joint cam impingement,[7] or long-construct lumbar spinal fusion (more than three levels) resulting in stress transfer to the SI joint.[8,9]
- Neoplasm with SI joint instability.
- Ehlers-Danlos syndrome with SI joint instability; hypermobility of the ligaments around the SI joint potentially destabilize the SI joint, inducing increased and thereby pathologic movement of the joint causing pain.[10]

64.3 Techniques (Fig. 64.1)

- Direct open reduction of a traumatically disrupted SI joint is occasionally necessary but requires large, bloody exposures. Indirect reduction using intraoperative imaging (fluoroscopy or navigation) and traction is more

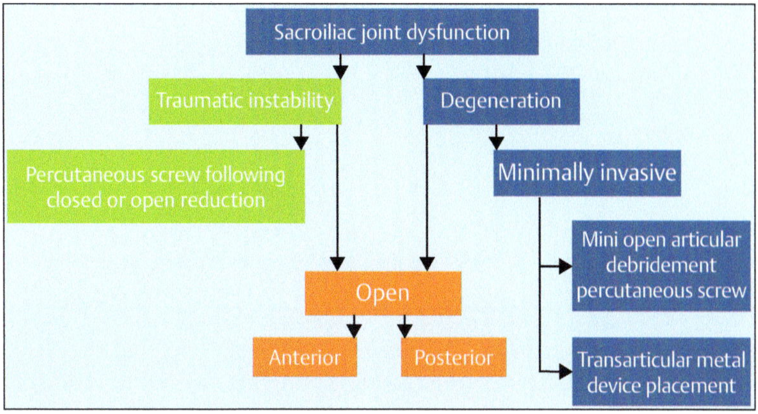

Fig. 64.1 Summary of surgical management options.

appealing, followed by compression lag screw fixation from lateral to medial, aiming for the S1 promontorium to improve screw pullout strength. Bone grafts are rarely used, because scarring and ligamentous healing stabilize the joint over time.

- High-energy sacral fractures involving the SI joint will require sacro- or spinopelvic fixation with medial-to-lateral iliac screw placement and crosslinking, with the possibility for wider dissection when performed open, especially when associated with degloving injuries of the soft tissues (**Fig. 64.2a–c**).
- Open approach can be performed anteriorly or posteriorly. The commonest approach is posterior using Smith-Petersen approach with a curved incision on the posterior two-thirds of the iliac crest. The joint is approached subperiosteally, and the cartilage of the joint is denuded. The joint is compressed and fused with plate, and[5,11] anterior approach is carried out through the same incision. The external oblique fascia is identified and the external oblique and gluteus medius muscles separated. The external oblique muscle and iliacus are elevated subperiosteally until the SI joint is visualized. The cartilage is denuded, and the joint is compressed and fixed with plate and screws.[11]
- Minimally invasive sacral pedicle screw placement and iliac teardrop targeting have decreased the morbidity of this procedure by making it a percutaneous procedure.
- For degenerative conditions, the open approach to SI joint fusion used to be technically demanding; it required the creation of a true bony window through the iliac wing into the SI joint from direct lateral. This could also be accomplished via an (often bloody) wide-open anterior or a more

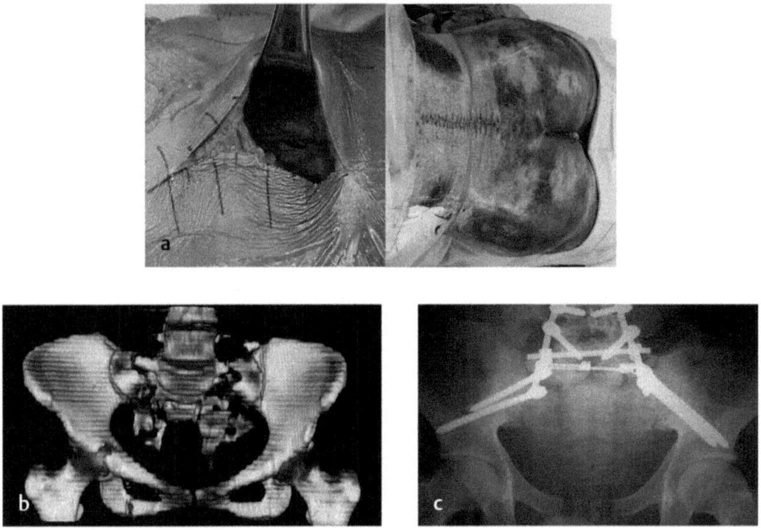

Fig. 64.2 **(a)** Degloving injury associated with **(b)** complex bilateral sacral fractures, severely disrupting lumbopelvic stability with (often) neurologic injury. **(c)** After fixation to the lower lumbar levels.

limited posterior approach through the posterior fascial reinforcements over the joint, connecting the osseous structures to the gluteus minimus, maximus, iliotibial band, and erector spinae.[6]

- After decortication and bone grafting, fixation was accomplished with lateral-to-medial screws for compression across the joint.
- MIS techniques have become increasingly more popular with the use of percutaneous screw/implant placement, often without true bone grafting of the joint itself. Multiple techniques have been described, including using direct lateral fluoroscopic, navigational (https://youtu.be/Efc7GBdHckI), or robot-assisted techniques (https://youtu.be/QJcVNUbVeeY) for visualization of the SI joint. The major MIS surgical techniques for operative treatment of degenerative SI joint pain are as follow:
  - Placement of (ideally three) semiparallel triangular metal bars from lateral to medial across the SI joint (SI Bone iFuse Implant System; San Jose, California) (**Fig. 64.3a, b**). They can also be placed from medial to lateral during a Bedrock technique along with the S2AI screw in spine constructs (**Fig. 64.4a, b**).
  - Motion-free stabilization is anticipated to occur over time via bony on-growth to the plasma-sprayed roughened bars on either side of the joint within the cortex, inside the trabecular bone of the ilium and sacrum

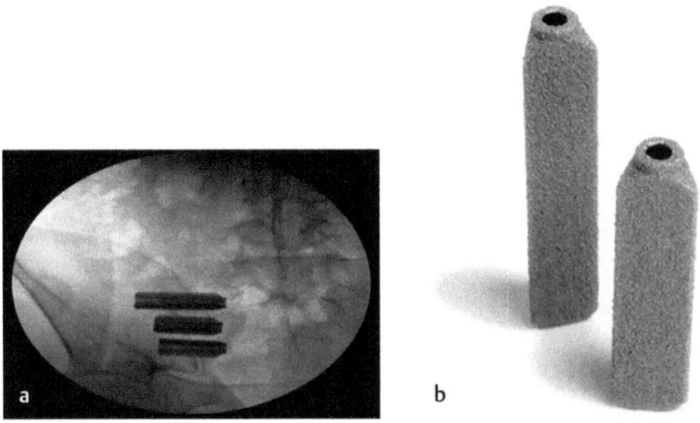

Fig. 64.3 (**a**) Radiographic image of bar stabilization across the sacroiliac (SI) joint, (**b**) with representation of the SiBone coated fusion bars for minimally invasive surgical (MIS) SI joint stabilization.

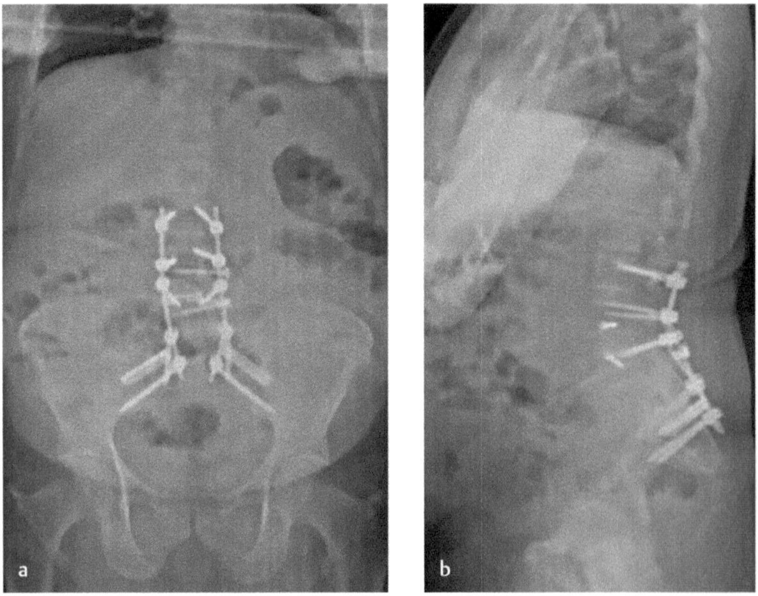

Fig. 64.4 Extension of fusion for sagittal imbalance with anterior column reconstruction and Bedrock technique (S2 alar screws and inside-out iFuse implants parallel to the S2 alar screws). (**a**) Coronal and (**b**) axial EOS scans.

without true decortication or bone grafting of the joint itself. Preliminary data have shown that bony bridging adjacent to the bars across the joint can occur over time.[12,13]

- Compression screw placement after percutaneous decortication of the joint via specialized tools to accomplish a solid arthrodesis (SImmetry SI Joint Fusion System: Zyga Technologies, Inc.; Minnetonka, Minnesota). The SI joint is targeted from lateral, and after creation of a window through the ilium, specialized scrapers and expandable 90-degree reamers are advanced into the joint (**Fig. 64.5a–d**). These allow for a 5 cm^2 area of

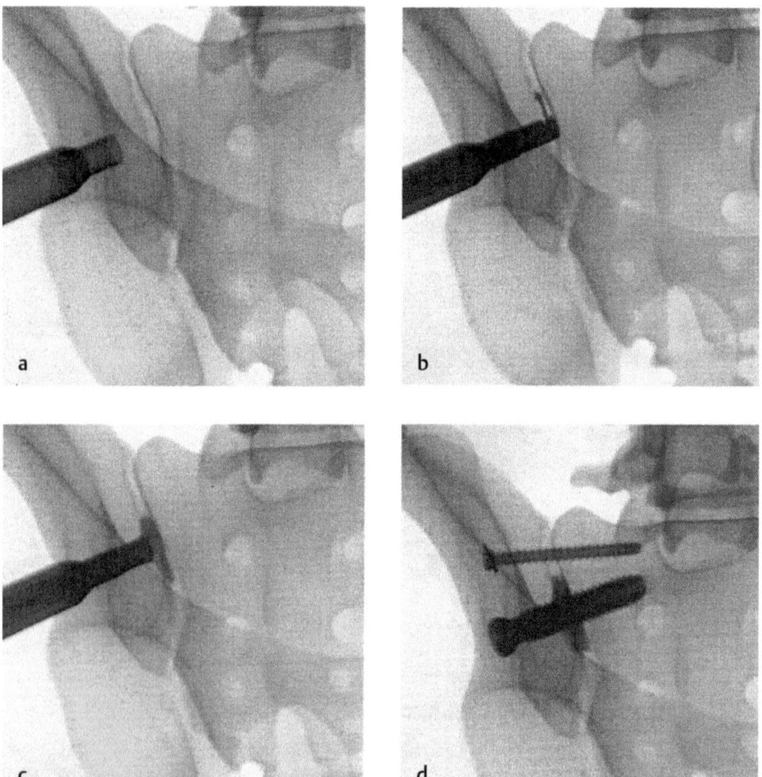

Fig. 64.5 Schematic representation of the Zyga SImmetry system for sacroiliac (SI) joint fusion stabilization. **(a)** After perpendicular access to the SI joint, **(b)** decortication of the joint surfaces is made possible by special 90-degree "rasps." **(c)** Bone graft can be placed in between the decorticated joint surfaces first, after which **(d)** compression lag screw fixation is used for stabilization.

decortication and impaction bone grafting around a large compression screw subsequently introduced through the same access portal across the joint into the sacrum. At least one additional screw needs to be placed (typically superiorly to this) to provide for rotational stability.

- Large-diameter, cannulated compression screws from a variety of companies are placed across the SI joint, either from a lateral (e.g., **Fig. 64.6a, b**; slotted and coated screws: Globus Medical Inc.;

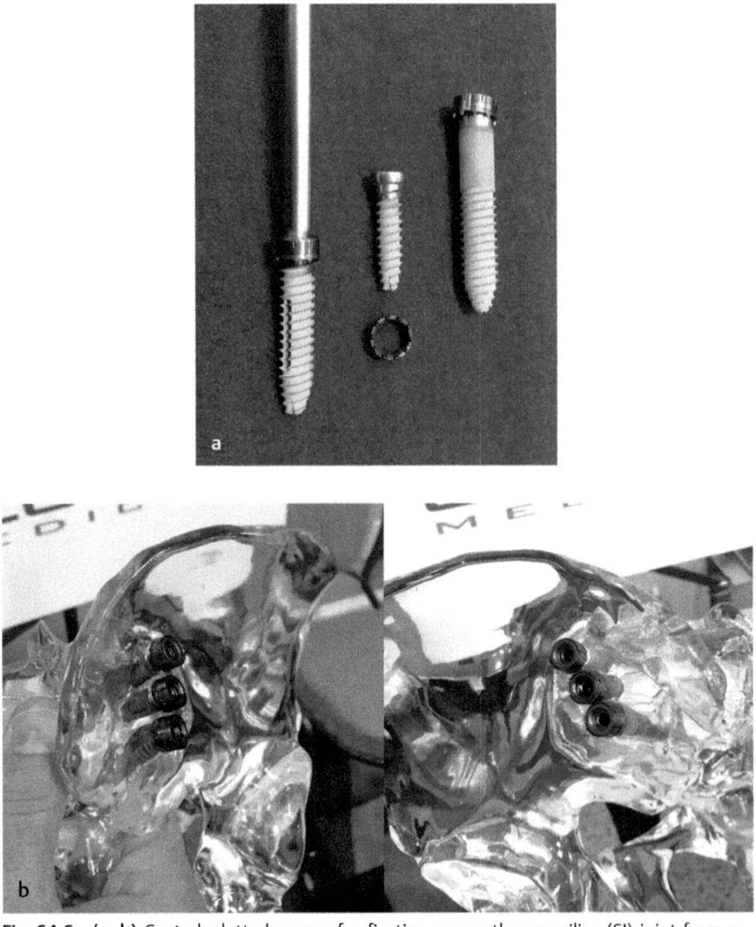

Fig. 64.6 (a, b) Coated, slotted screws for fixation across the sacroiliac (SI) joint from a lateral approach with the ability to allow for bone grafting and bone growth *inside* the large lag screw for SI joint fusion.

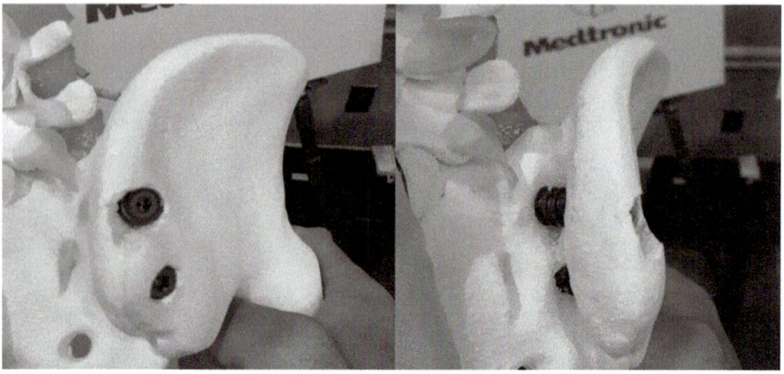

Fig. 64.7 Sacroiliac (SI) joint stabilization with lag screw fixation from a posterolateral angle.

Parsippany, New Jersey) or posterolateral approach (e.g., **Fig. 64.7**; compression screws: Medtronic, Inc.; Memphis, Tennessee), using interference stability by high-pressure lag technique compression to prevent motion of the SI joint.

64.4 Complications

- Vessel or nerve root injury resulting from improper guidewire, drill, or implant positioning, often caused by compromised SI joint visualization.
- Wound healing complications after wide dissection for open treatment of sacral fractures with exposed hardware through an area of wound breakdown.
- Pseudoarthrosis or implant loosening, as there is often no direct arthrodesis possible, or even attempted, across the joint with the percutaneous techniques (**Fig. 64.8a, b**).

Complications after SI joint fusion can be categorized according to the method of fusion[14] (open techniques versus minimally invasive techniques).

- Nonunion rates following arthrodesis has not been evaluated in many studies. It varies from 10 to 41% in open methods and 0 to 11% in minimally invasive methods.[5]
- Other complications following open fusion are prominent and painful hardware, deep surgical site infection, nerve root irritation, peroneal nerve entrapment, and iliac crest fracture at the site of fusion. In addition to these, deep vein thrombosis and pulmonary embolism, and autograft site complications also occur.[5,14]

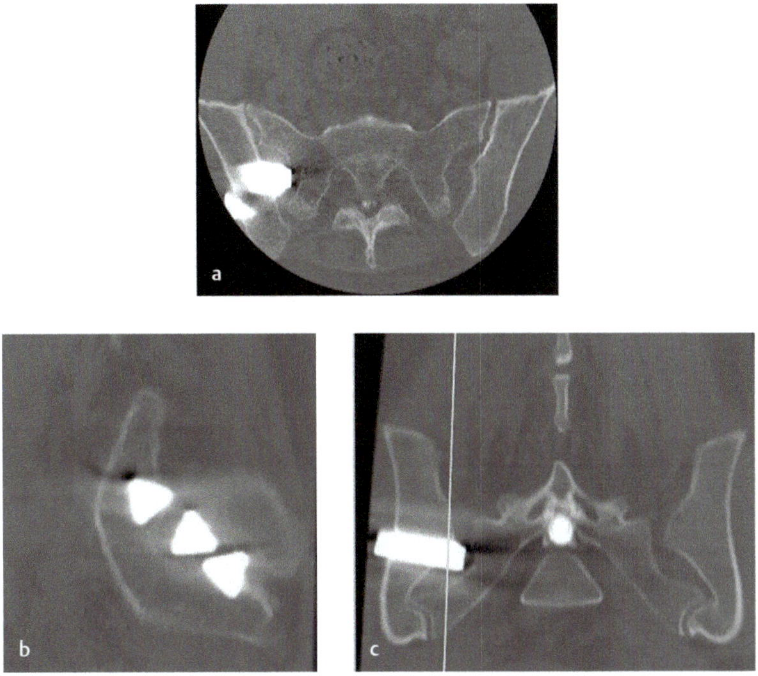

Fig. 64.8 (a) Sacroiliac (SI) joint stabilization attempt with triangular bars without crossing into the sacrum due to location of the bar compared with the joint. This plays a significant role in failure of this minimally invasive surgical (MIS) "fusion" procedure. MIS fusion on (b) parasagittal and (c) axial computed tomography (CT) images in another patient showing inadequate stabilization, leading to ipsilateral lumbar plexus irritation and foot dorsiflexion weakness.

- Minimally invasive methods also have recognized complications such as new onset of facet joint pain, trochanteric bursitis, surgical site infection, adjacent joint pain (e.g., hip or knee), hematoma at the operative site, implant penetration into the sacral foramina, avascular necrosis of the femoral head, piriformis syndrome, deep venous thrombosis, and pulmonary embolism.[5,11]

64.5 Postoperative Care

64.5.1 Open Technique

- Routine assessment of hemoglobin and serum electrolyte levels should be undertaken on the first postoperative day.[5,15]

- Following an extensile open approach to the SI joint, paralytic ileus is common. Patients may need to be nil per oral until they recover from the ileus.[5,15]
- Prophylaxis for deep venous thrombosis should be initiated unless contraindicated. The duration of prophylaxis is for 4 to 6 weeks.[5]
- Adequate analgesics should be provided to alleviate pain and its consequences (e.g., constipation).[5]
- Drains should be removed in 48 hours and dressing should be changed in 48 hours.[5]
- Mobilization and physiotherapy should be adapted according to the stability of the fixation, patient's factors, and surgeons' preferences. Breathing exercises, chest physiotherapy, bed mobility exercises, and upper limb mobility exercises should be initiated early as possible.[5]
- If stable fixation is achieved, no external immobilization is required for traumatic SI joint disruptions. Depending on the degree and direction of preoperative instability, weightbearing on the injured side may need to be reduced temporarily.
- For the unstable fixations, the mobilization starts with touch-down weightbearing. Progressive weightbearing can be encouraged according to the healing or union at the joint/the site of the fusion. Fracture healing or the evidence of fusion can be monitored with serial radiographs and the weightbearing can be increased according to it. Pelvic fracture heals in 6 to 8 weeks while ligaments heal in 3 to 4 months.[5]
- Guarded weightbearing is typically advised after operative stabilization of the SI joint for degenerative conditions, for no longer than 6 weeks postoperatively.
- For bilateral unstable SI joint fractures/dislocations, upper limb and lower limb exercises can be commenced as early as possible. Initial mobilizations are done with the wheelchair. Walking exercises are commenced after 3 to 4 weeks in a pool. Supported weightbearing can be commenced after 6 weeks after the pain is settled. Full weightbearing is allowed after 12 weeks postoperatively.[5]

64.5.2 Minimally Invasive Technique

- In many centers these are done as day surgery cases with minimal blood loss and hence no major postoperative care is required.
- Guarded weightbearing can be advised (some do not) after minimally invasive operative stabilization of the SI joint for degenerative conditions, for no longer than 6 weeks postoperatively.[16]

64.6 Outcomes

- Pelvic ring disruptions involving the SI joint(s) are high-energy injuries rendering the patients forever "different" from their state before the trauma, regardless of the surgical procedure or approach. If the soft tissue injury did not lead to wound breakdown and hardware exposure/failure of fixation and infection with osteomyelitis, the outcomes are fair to good. If wound breakdown occurs, the outcome can be unsatisfactory to disastrous.
- An abundance of recent literature (including randomized control studies) describes impressive positive outcomes up to 4 years after SI joint "fusion" surgery for degenerative conditions.[17]
- Most of these studies, however, have small series, and many of the authors are SI joint fusion company–endorsed; although trials not sponsored by company have still found good results, they are not as impressive as the company-sponsored ones.[18]
- Placement of percutaneous non-lag compression bars across the joint should be carefully considered regarding whether the anatomy might not allow for adequate stabilization using this technique (**Fig. 64.8a–c**).

Blood loss, operative time, hospital stay, and outcome measures reported by patients are better with MIS technique than the open technique.[11,14]

64.7 Surgical Pearls

- Fixation of traumatic SI joint disruption is often complex and should be performed in specialized centers by surgeons well versed in the technique.
- Preoperative workup and planning are crucial for operative treatment of degenerative SI joint disease. All other sources of pain need to be excluded, and a thorough understanding of the three-dimensional anatomy is essential when performing the first MIS SI joint "fusion" surgeries.
- Keep the possibility of failure of addressing the pain generator effectively with this technique, and counsel the patient of not meeting this expectation of complete pain relief.
- Salvage of nonhealing MIS SI joint fusion surgery (if confirmed to be the pain generator) is challenging and requires at least *two* iliac wing screws for rotational stabilization of the hemipelvis. Fixation into the lower lumbar spine, superior to the sacrum, is recommended to achieve adequate stability. Placement of iliac bolts between screws or bars crossing the nonfused SI joint is challenging and requires modification of Ferguson angle fluoroscopy to visualize a safe corridor or stereotactic navigation (**Fig. 64.9a, b**). After stable fixation has been achieved (**Fig. 64.9c**), open posterior bone grafting in between the remaining joint surfaces is the authors' preferred method for fusion (**Fig. 64.9d**).

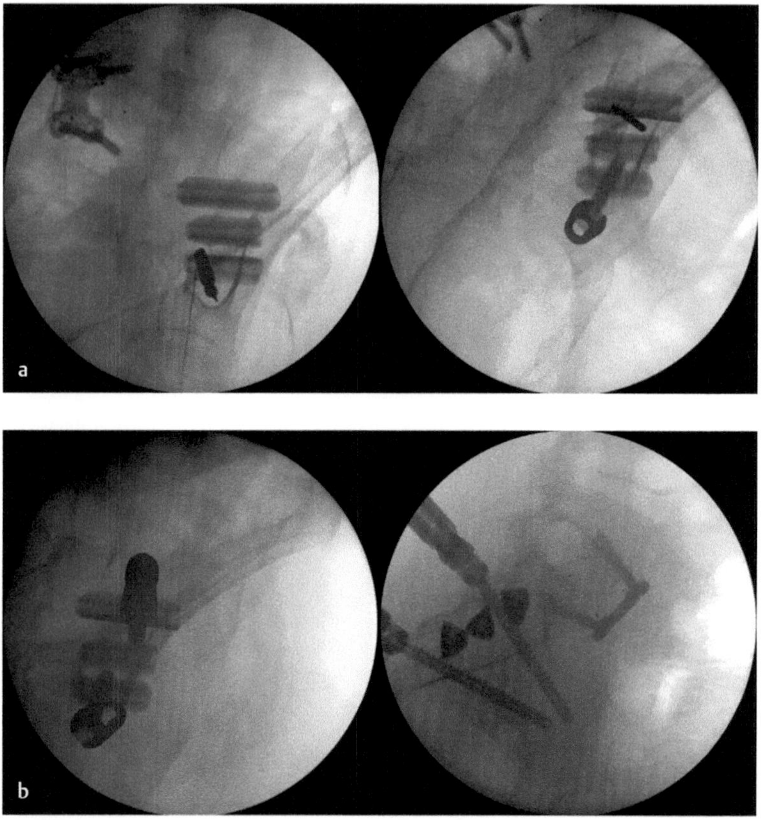

Fig. 64.9 Salvage procedure in a 41-year-old female with prior sacroiliac (SI) joint stabilization failure and confirmation of the SI joint as her pain generator after lidocaine infiltration of the joint space: **(a)** Modified Ferguson view with fluoroscopy to access a safe corridor between the greater sciatic notch (below) and the most posterior triangular bar across the SI joint using a Jamshidi needle. **(b)** A second screw should be placed into the iliac wing where possible for rotational stability; here performed through another "open" corridor, visualized with Ferguson angle modification.

(Continued)

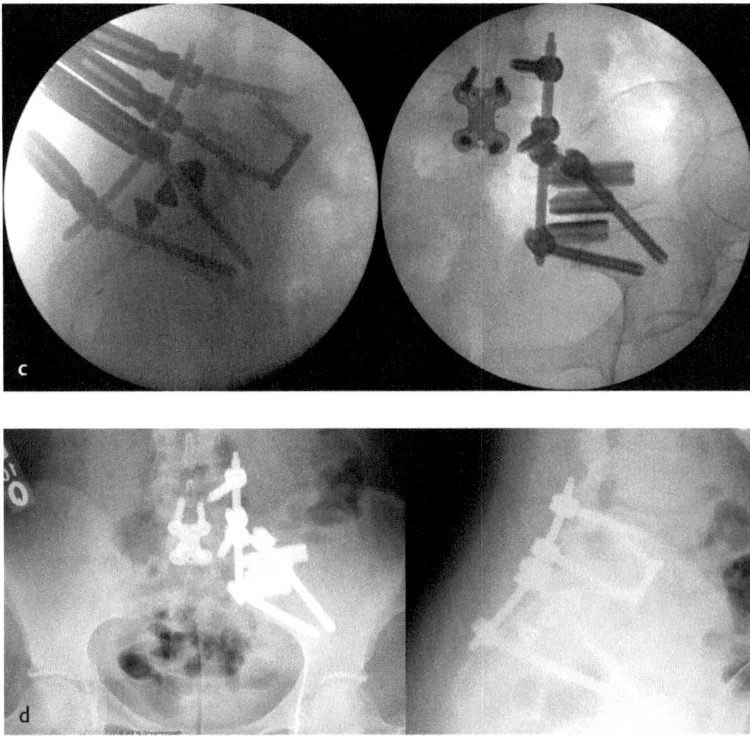

Fig. 64.9 (*Continued*) **(c)** Ultimately, a minimally invasive surgical (MIS) posterior construct was created across the stable L5–S1 fusion with two points of fixation above and below the SI joint. **(d)** This was followed by SI joint decortication and bone graft insertion from posterior, leading to excellent stability on standing radiographs. Clinical success is now more likely but is certainly not guaranteed.

Common Clinical Questions

1. What are pathognomonic signs and symptoms to look for while working up a patient for symptomatic SI joint degeneration?
2. What is the ideal fluoroscopic "view" for percutaneous iliac screw placement to stabilize a traumatically disrupted SI joint?
3. In what position do you position the fluoroscopy machine when placing percutaneous lateral bars or screws across the SI joint?

Answers to Common Clinical Questions

1. Patients complaining of maximal pain below L5 together with sacral sulcus tenderness upon palpation and pain originating lateral to the midline around the posterior superior iliac spine have the highest positive predictive value (60%) of causalgia with SI joint–generated discomfort.
2. Start with placing the fluoroscopy machine parallel to the superior part of S1 (promontorium) and the inner and outer tables of the iliac wing to be instrumented in approximately "30-degree Ferguson" and "30-degree Rainbow" view. The goal is to aim parallel to the teardrop as visualized in **Fig. 64.10**. The inferior margin of the teardrop (A) is the sciatic notch (B), and this needs to be in line with the superior lateral part of the acetabulum (C) called the "Sourcele." The view needs to be parallel to the inner and outer table. The bony column visualized can accept at least one screw—if needed, two screws—measuring 7.5 to 10 mm in diameter by 8 to 10 cm in length.
3. Initial SI joint visualization needs to be conducted with a "perfect" lateral view to the joint, overlapping the sciatic notches and aiming parallel to the superior end plate of the S1 vertebral body. This identifies the starting point for entry into the SI joint from lateral.

A pelvic outlet view (Ferguson view), obtained in straight midline anterior–posterior and parallel position to the S1 superior end plate, allows the visualization of the sacral neuroforaminae. The straight midline anterior–posterior inlet view (90 degrees perpendicular to the outlet view) shows the ventral cortex of the sacrum, identifying the safe direction and depth for lateral-to-medial screw placement.

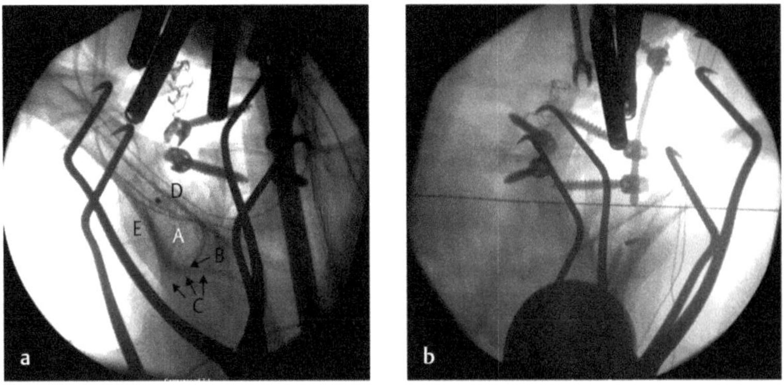

Fig. 64.10 **(a)** Intraoperative visualization of the teardrop is possible, even in complex surgery with wires and retractors in the way, and **(b)** after a total hip arthroplasty. A shows the teardrop. B shows inferior margin on the immediate teardrop is the greater sciatic notch. C shows the sciatic notch that needs to be aligned with the superior–lateral margin of the acetabulum, visualized as the sclerotic densification of the sourcele (or "eyebrow"). D shows the medial wall of the teardrop is the inner table of the iliac wing. E shows the lateral margin is the lateral wall of the iliac wing. Both the medial and lateral walls need to be parallel to the fluoroscopy beam. Choosing a starting point in the teardrop and staying, with a Jamshidi needle, within the medial and lateral walls and above the greater sciatic notch and the sourcele will ensure a safe trajectory of at least 100 mm and will prevent penetration into the hip joint.

References

1. Al-Khayer A, Hegarty J, Hahn D, Grevitt MP. Percutaneous sacroiliac joint arthrodesis: a novel technique. J Spinal Disord Tech. 2008; 21(5):359–363
2. Bogduk N. Pain provocation tests for the assessment of sacroiliac joint dysfunction. J Spinal Disord. 1999; 12(4):357–358
3. Laslett M. Evidence-based diagnosis and treatment of the painful sacroiliac joint. J Manual Manip Ther. 2008; 16(3):142–152
4. Gartenberg A, Nessim A, Cho W. Sacroiliac joint dysfunction: pathophysiology, diagnosis, and treatment. Eur Spine J. 2021; 30(10):2936–2943
5. ORIF - Anterior fixation SI Joint: SI-joint fractures. Accessed July 14, 2022 at: https://surgeryreference.aofoundation.org/orthopedic-trauma/adult-trauma/pelvic-ring/si-joint/orif-anterior-fixation-si-joint
6. Dreyfuss P, Dreyer SJ, Cole A, Mayo K. Sacroiliac joint pain. J Am Acad Orthop Surg. 2004; 12(4):255–265
7. Morgan PM, Anderson AW, Swiontkowski MF. Symptomatic sacroiliac joint disease and radiographic evidence of femoroacetabular impingement. Hip Int. 2013; 23(2):212–217
8. DePalma MJ, Ketchum JM, Saullo TR. Etiology of chronic low back pain in patients having undergone lumbar fusion. Pain Med. 2011; 12(5):732–739

9. Ha KY, Lee JS, Kim KW. Degeneration of sacroiliac joint after instrumented lumbar or lumbosacral fusion: a prospective cohort study over five-year follow-up. Spine. 2008; 33(11):1192–1198
10. Shirley ED, Demaio M, Bodurtha J. Ehlers-Danlos syndrome in orthopaedics: etiology, diagnosis, and treatment implications. Sports Health. 2012; 4(5): 394–403
11. Heiney J, Capobianco R, Cher D. A systematic review of minimally invasive sacroiliac joint fusion utilizing a lateral transarticular technique. Int J Spine Surg. 2015; 9:40
12. Smith AG, Capobianco R, Cher D, et al. Open versus minimally invasive sacroiliac joint fusion: a multi-center comparison of perioperative measures and clinical outcomes. Ann Surg Innov Res. 2013; 7(1):14
13. Sachs D, Capobianco R. One year successful outcomes for novel sacroiliac joint arthrodesis system. Ann Surg Innov Res. 2012; 6(1):13–17
14. Zaidi HA, Montoure AJ, Dickman CA. Surgical and clinical efficacy of sacroiliac joint fusion: a systematic review of the literature. J Neurosurg Spine. 2015; 23(1):59–66
15. Yson SC, Sembrano JN, Polly DW. Sacroiliac joint fusion: approaches and recent outcomes. PM&R John Wiley and Sons Inc.; 2019;11:S114–S117
16. Miller LE, Block JE. Minimally invasive arthrodesis for chronic sacroiliac joint dysfunction using the SImmetry SI Joint Fusion System. Med Devices (Auckl). 2014; 7:125–130
17. Darr E, Cher D. Four-year outcomes after minimally invasive transiliac sacroiliac joint fusion with triangular titanium implants. Med Devices (Auckl). 2018; 11:287–289
18. Wise CL, Dall BE. Minimally invasive sacroiliac arthrodesis: outcomes of a new technique. J Spinal Disord Tech. 2008; 21(8):579–584

65 Sacrectomy

Jean-Paul Wolinsky and Ziya Gokaslan

Summary

The sacrectomy procedure is an invasive one that is typically reserved for en bloc resection of primary bony tumors. Various approaches are employed depending on the extent of bony and neural element involvement. Both posterior-only and anterior–posterior approaches are utilized for the resection of tumors affecting the sacrum. Postoperative complications, including wound infection and nonunion, are common and patients are to be advised accordingly.

Keywords: sacrectomy, tumor, chordoma, chondrosarcoma, sacral tumor, spinal tumor

65.1 Key Points

- Sacrectomy is a technique reserved for en bloc resection of tumor.
- As the consequences of a sacrectomy are significant, a preoperative biopsy is critical to establish the diagnosis prior to embarking on a sacrectomy.
- The level of the sacrectomy (total, high, mid, and low) is determined by the most caudal nerve root that can be spared to achieve a negative margin resection.[1]
- Lumbo-pelvic reconstruction is required after a total sacrectomy and should be considered in high sacral amputations, particularly in osteopoenic patients or patients receiving radiation therapy who have a high fracture risk.
- An anterior and posterior approach should be considered in patients with prior radiation exposure, rectal involvement, or need for vascularized tissue for the complex plastic surgery closure.
- A complex plastic surgery closure should be considered in all en bloc sacral tumor resections. If the superior gluteal artery supply is preserved, local advancement flaps can be used. If this vascular supply is not available, plans should be made for a vertical rectus abdominis myocutaneous (VRAM) rotational flap, omental flap, or free flap with an AV loop.[2,3,4,5]

65.2 Indications

- Malignant primary tumors of the sacrum (e.g., chordoma, osteosarcoma, Ewing's sarcoma, primitive neuroepithelial tumor [PNET]).
- Tumors of the pelvis (e.g., osteosarcoma, chondrosarcoma, Ewing's sarcoma, radiation-induced sarcomas) or pelvic viscera (locally advanced adenocarcinoma of the rectum) invading the sacrum or sacroiliac (SI) joint.
- Benign tumors of the spine with aggressive invasion of local structures (e.g., osteoblastoma, giant cell tumors, osteochondromas, aneurysmal bone cysts).
- Rare situations of metastatic tumors of the sacrum causing significant destabilization or pain.

65.3 Preoperative Considerations/ Management

- A computed tomography (CT) of the chest/abdomen/pelvis or whole-body positron emission tomography computed tomography (PET CT) is useful to screen for metastatic disease. In instances of metastatic disease, it is less likely to consider a sacral amputation.
- A preoperative biopsy is critical to establish the diagnosis prior to embarking on a sacrectomy. This usually is a CT-guided biopsy. The entry point and trajectory of the biopsy is planned so that the biopsy tract can be excised with the tumor.
- Parasagittal MRI scans of the sacrum are useful to determine the most caudal uninvolved nerves. This will allow prediction of the neurologic sacrifice required. The lowest preserved nerve root will also guide the sagittal osteotomies.
- A low-residue diet for several days preoperatively and mechanical cleaning of the bowel with a bowel prep will help decrease the risk of infection if the bowel is inadvertently injured.
- As there can be considerable blood loss, good vascular access with large-bore intravenous catheters and central venous monitoring is necessary.
- Because the lower extent of posterior sacral incisions is very near to the anus and risk of infection is high, prophylactic antibiotics must be used preoperatively and postoperatively.

65.4 Anatomic Considerations

- Parasagittal MRI scans of the sacrum are useful to determine the most caudal uninvolved nerve. The most caudal uninvolved nerve will determine the functional classification of the sacral amputation (total, high, mid, low).

Postoperative functional deficits can be predicted based on the nerves that are sacrificed.[1,6]

- Sacrifice of S1 can result in plantar flexion weakness.
- Bilateral sacrifice of S2, S3, and S4 (forming the pudendal nerve) results in loss of all bowel, bladder, and sexual functions.
- Bilateral sacrifice of S3 and S4 nerves with preservation of bilateral S2 nerves results in some bowel, bladder, and sexual functions. Usually, patients will be able to feel when their bladder is full but they will not be able to empty the bladder.
- Bilateral sacrifice of S4 nerves with preservation of bilateral S2 and S3 nerves usually results in preservation of the bowel, bladder, and sexual functions.
- Unilateral sacrifice of S2, S3, and S4 nerves will usually provide enough innervation from the contralateral side for normal bowel, bladder, and sexual functions although sensation will be unilateral.

65.5 Technique

- Sacrectomy may be performed as a standalone operation or in the context of complex sacropelvic resection (e.g., extended internal or external hemipelvectomy) (**Fig. 65.1**).
- Determine whether a partial or total sacrectomy is required and, if a partial sacrectomy is required, whether the osteotomies will be done in the axial or sagittal plane (**Fig. 65.2** and **Fig. 65.3**).[1]
- Depending on the tumor location, extent of invasion, and tumor type, a posterior or a combined ventral and posterior approach may need to be used.[1]
- The posterior trans-sacral approach can be used for low-sacral, mid-sacral, and high-sacral amputations. Total sacrectomies can be approached from an entirely posterior approach as well.[7,8] A relative contraindication for an entirely posterior approach is in patients with prior radiation exposure, rectal involvement, or in cases with a need for vascularized tissue for the complex plastic surgery closure.
- Frameless stereotactic navigation can be useful to assist in understanding the anatomy of the tumor and planning osteotomies and resection of soft tissue around the tumor.[9] Additionally, navigation can be useful for instrumentation. Proper understanding of the principles of navigation is critical as after a sacrectomy, the remaining pelvic structures can be quite mobile potentially amplifying inaccuracies in navigation.
- The incision is midline or transverse depending on the exposure requirements and incorporates the biopsy tract. The biopsy tract will be left in continuity with an ellipse of soft tissue including the entry point through the skin.

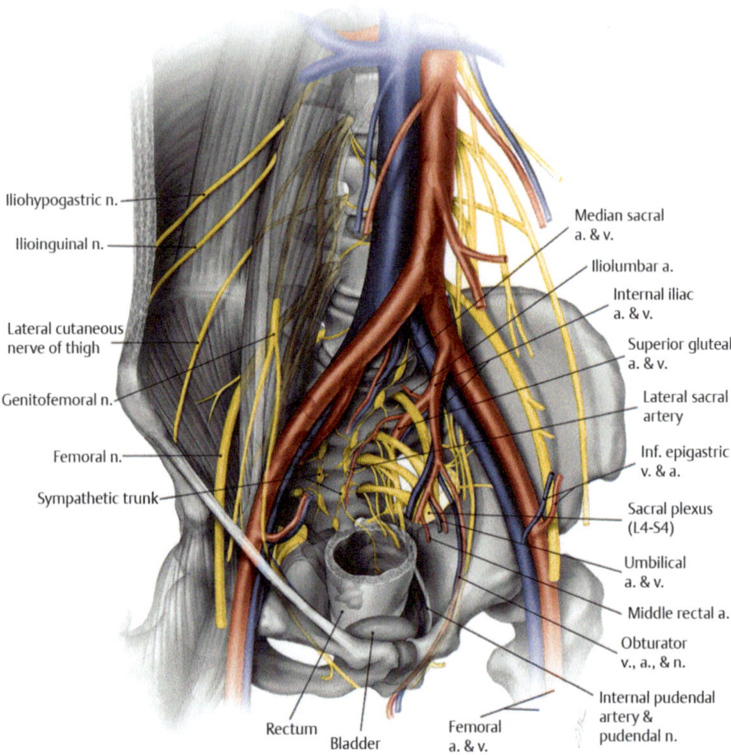

Fig. 65.1 Relationship of the ventral surface of the sacrum to the major pelvic structures, arteries, veins, and neural structures.

- Sacrifice of dorsal rami may be necessary but does not cause significant functional sequelae.
- Laminectomy is performed rostral to the extent of tumor with the standard technique.
- The sagittal osteotomies are preformed bilaterally by creating osteotomies from the dorsal foramen of the most caudal nerve root preserved on either side to the respective sciatic notch along the course of the nerve.[10,11]
- The cauda equina is ligated with double O-silk sutures below the axilla of the most caudal nerve root being preserved and then cut.

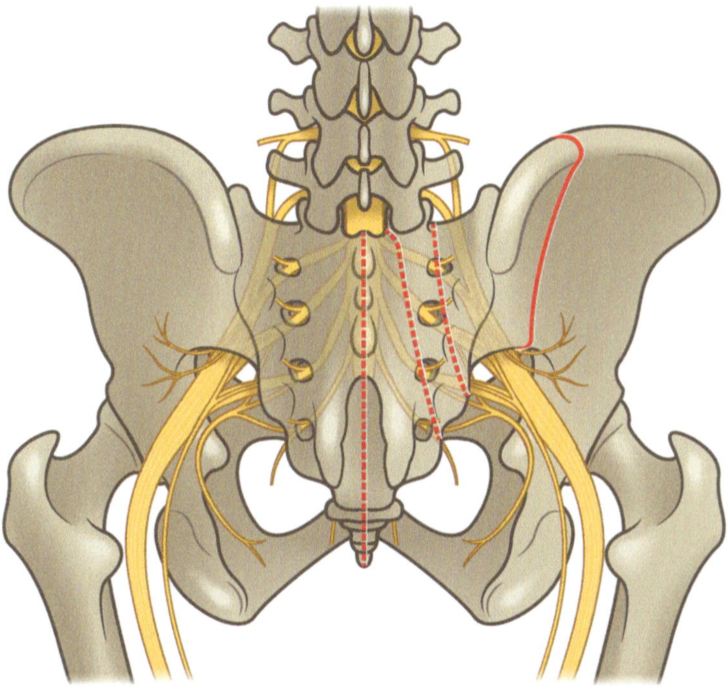

Fig. 65.2 The solid line demarcates the osteotomy for a standard lateral internal hemipelvectomy. *Dotted red lines* demarcate osteotomies for progressively larger resections of the sacroiliac joint and hemisacrectomy.

- An axial osteotomy is performed by connecting the lateral osteotomies through the midline rostral to the extent of tumor in the bone.
- The sacral mass is now more mobile and is dissected and freed from surrounding structures. Beware, as significant hemorrhage may occur if vasculature ventral to the sacrum is injured.
- The rostral aspect of the specimen is rotated posteriorly and the mesorectum is dissected away from the ventral aspect of the sacrum or the capsule of the tumor.
- The sacrospinous and sacrotuberous ligaments are cut. If the pudendal nerve is to be preserved, it is identified and protected as it courses between these ligaments.
- The annococcygeal ligaments are cut and then the specimen is delivered.

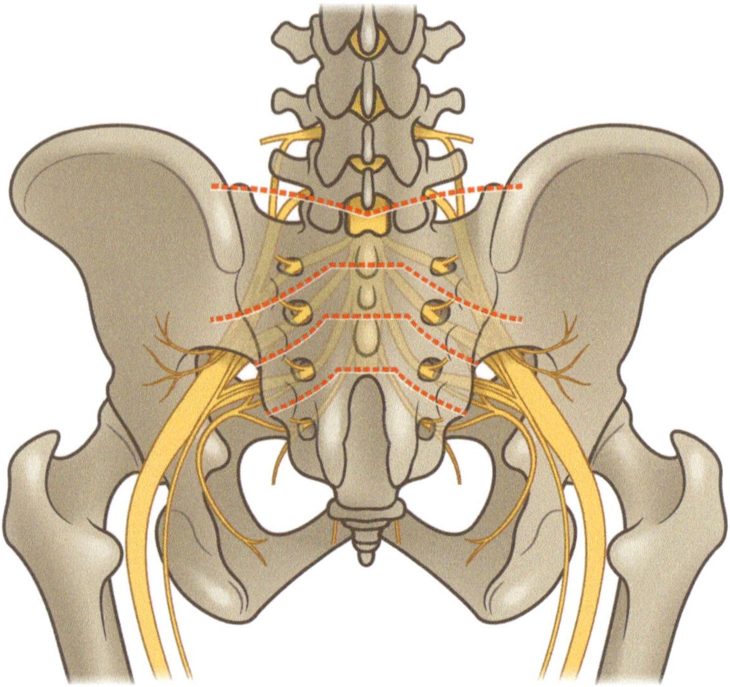

Fig. 65.3 Osteotomies for the low, middle, high, and total sacrectomy.

65.5.1 Combined Anterior–Posterior Approach

- Indications include patients with prior radiation exposure, rectal involvement, or need for vascularized tissue for the complex plastic surgery closure.
- Most often, the anterior approach is performed first, followed by the posterior approach on separate days.
- Anterior access is obtained via trans-abdominal or retroperitoneal approach in the supine position.
- The trans-abdominal approach is more familiar and is easier. The retroperitoneal approach has the advantage that the peritoneal sac is left intact and may decrease the occurrence of a postoperative ileus and may reduce the chance of a small bowel hernia into and through the sacral defect. The retroperitoneal exposure is through the midline and may need to be performed bilaterally to visualize and dissect the vasculature on either side of the rectum.

- Anterior access allows exposure of the upper and middle sacrum, facilitating dissection and mobilization of the rectum and other pelvic contents (e.g., iliac vessels) from the tumor surface as well as providing early access to the tumor vascular supply.
- Diskectomy and osteotomies are performed at the desired level, and an anterior osteotomy may be performed lateral to the SI joint if needed.
- A VRAM flap can be harvested and placed in the pelvis ventral to the great vessels and dorsal to the rectum to be retrieved during the second-stage operation for closure of the sacral wound defect. The VRAM pedicle is based on the inferior epigastric artery and vein. If these are compromised, the contralateral VRAM may be an option, or another option (omental flap, free flap) must be considered. It should be recognized that patients who have had previous inguinal hernia repairs may have had asymptomatic injuries to these vessels during their hernia repair.
- The subsequent posterior stage proceeds as described for an entirely posterior approach.

65.5.2 Reconstruction

- The goal is to restore the pelvic ring to facilitate axial load transfer from the spinal column to the pelvis.[10,11]
- Resection of lesions that are distal to S1 vertebra often does not require subsequent reconstruction. Lesions involving S1 may alter the biomechanics at the lumbosacral junction significantly requiring reconstruction. However, some believe that reconstruction has no role in sacrectomy operations.
- SI stability is not significantly affected if more than 50% of the SI joint is intact (i.e., at least the S1 segment). The pelvis becomes unstable if more than 50% of the SI joint is compromised.
- Several constructs have been proposed, many involving two to four rod constructs interconnected with sacral bars, pedicle screws placed from the mid-lumbar region and caudally, and the pelvic/iliac screws anchoring the pelvis.
- In the modified Galveston technique,[12,13] distally the vertical Galveston L-rods are directed laterally into the ilium to establish a bilateral connection between the lumbar spine and ilia. Each Galveston rod creates a bridge between the lumbar spine and ilium, and a transiliac rod completes the pelvic ring.
- Another reconstruction involves a triangular frame. Two fibular grafts are placed between L5 and the supra-acetabular region bilaterally along the force transmission lines, increasing resistance to failure.[14]

- Newer techniques are using both anterior and posterior instrumentation, including expandable cages to reconstruct the anterior column (attached inferiorly to the trans-iliac rod and superiorly to the end plate of intact vertebra) and pedicle and iliac screws as posterior instrumentation.[15]

65.6 Complications

- Injury or bleeding of the internal iliac, superior gluteal, iliolumbar, and other sacropelvic vessels.
- Visceral damage to the pelvic contents including ureters or rectum.
- Chances of motor, sensory, bowel/bladder, and sexual dysfunction increase the higher the resection is done (**Table 65.1**). Motor loss occurs if the S1 nerve root is ligated. Saddle anesthesia is common. Preservation of at least one S3 nerve root preserves bowel/bladder function in two-thirds of patients.[6,16] Similar trends have been seen for sexual function where unilateral sacral resection (recall that the pudendal nerve originates from S2–S4) still preserves overall function (albeit with numbness on the side of the resection).[17]
- Wound healing problems and infection (25–46% and even higher after radiation).[6]
- Sacral insufficiency fractures.
- General medical complications (ileus, pneumonia, deep vein thrombosis, etc.).

Table 65.1 Bowel and bladder function after sacral resection[9]

Resection and spared level	Normal bowel (%)	Normal bladder (%)
Bilateral S2–S5 resection with both S1 spared	0	0
Bilateral S3–S5 resection with both S2 spared	40	25
Bilateral S4–S5 resection with both S3 spared	100	69
Variable with unilateral S3 root spared	67	60
Unilateral S1–S5 resection and contralateral S1–S5 spared	87	89

65.7 Postoperative Care

- Because significant blood loss can often occur during surgery, fluid and blood replacement postoperatively is essential; for these patients are initially managed in the intensive care unit.
- Special air beds or routine position changes help prevent wound breakdown.
- Antibiotics are continued until all suction drains have been removed.
- Considering the proximity to the anus, special care is taken to keep wounds clean at all times.
- Denervation of the distal GI tract (S2–S4 autonomics) during high sacral resections can result in a significant postoperative ileus, requiring an aggressive bowel regimen in all patients and intravenous nutrition for a prolonged period in some patients. Studies have found higher wound infection rates in patients with postoperative bowel incontinence.[8]
- Bladder training is gradually attempted, and in some circumstances patients need to learn to self-catheterize.
- In patients who had tumor invasion of the rectum requiring resection, colostomy training is necessary.
- Patients should be mobilized as soon as possible, depending on their functional reserve and the stability of the dorsal pelvic ring.

65.8 Outcomes

- Survival depends on tumor type, tumor location, and prior surgeries. Chordoma is the most common tumor treated with sacrectomy, with 5- and 10-year survival rates of 59 and 35%, respectively, after surgery.[18]

65.9 Surgical Pearls

- Tumor vascularity, encroachment of the anterior pelvic fascia, and tumor location relative to S1 must be carefully assessed.
- Wide resection ensuring negative margins throughout is essential to minimize the chances of recurrence and significantly improve survival.

Common Clinical Questions

1. Which nerve roots should be preserved, if possible, to maintain bladder/ bowel function?
2. When is it advisable that a combined anterior–posterior approach be done for sacrectomy?

Answers to Common Clinical Questions

1. Preservation of at least one of the S3 nerve roots has been associated with good bowel/bladder function in about two-thirds of patients.[6,18]
2. Indications include patients with prior radiation exposure, rectal involvement, or need for vascularized tissue for the complex plastic surgery closure.

References

1. Fourney DR, Rhines LD, Hentschel SJ, et al. En bloc resection of primary sacral tumors: classification of surgical approaches and outcome. J Neurosurg Spine. 2005; 3(2):111–122
2. Sciubba DM, Nelson C, Gok B, et al. Evaluation of factors associated with postoperative infection following sacral tumor resection. J Neurosurg Spine. 2008; 9(6):593–599
3. Dasenbrock HH, Clarke MJ, Bydon A, et al. Reconstruction of extensive defects from posterior en bloc resection of sacral tumors with human acellular dermal matrix and gluteus maximus myocutaneous flaps. Neurosurgery. 2011; 69(6): 1240–1247
4. Kim JE, Pang J, Christensen JM, et al. Soft-tissue reconstruction after total en bloc sacrectomy. J Neurosurg Spine. 2015; 22(6):571–581
5. Reynolds JJ, Khundkar R, Boriani S, et al. Soft tissue and bone defect management in total sacrectomy for primary sacral tumors: a systematic review with expert recommendations. Spine. 2016; 41 Suppl 20:S199–S204
6. Guo Y, Palmer JL, Shen L, et al. Bowel and bladder continence, wound healing, and functional outcomes in patients who underwent sacrectomy. J Neurosurg Spine. 2005; 3(2):106–110
7. McLoughlin GS, Sciubba DM, Suk I, et al. En bloc total sacrectomy performed in a single stage through a posterior approach. Neurosurgery. 2008; 63(1) Suppl 1:ONS115–ONS120, discussion ONS120
8. Clarke MJ, Dasenbrock H, Bydon A, et al. Posterior-only approach for en bloc sacrectomy: clinical outcomes in 36 consecutive patients. Neurosurgery. 2012; 71(2):357–364, discussion 364
9. Fourney DR, Rhines LD, Hentschel SJ, et al. En bloc resection of primary sacral tumors: classification of surgical approaches and outcome. J Neurosurg Spine. 2005; 3(2):111–122
10. Wolinsky JP, Gallia GL, Bagley CA, Witham TF, Gokaslan ZL, Vacarro AR. Chapter 12: Sacrectomy and Suggested Reconstruction Techniques. In: Approaches for Spinal Fusion and Instrumentation. Riyadh, Saudi Arabia: Pan Arab Neurosurgical Society; 2006

11. Gottfried ON, Omeis I, Mehta VA, Solakoglu C, Gokaslan ZL, Wolinsky JP. Sacral tumor resection and the impact on pelvic incidence. J Neurosurg Spine. 2011; 14(1):78–84
12. Gokaslan ZL, Romsdahl MM, Kroll SS, et al. Total sacrectomy and Galveston L-rod reconstruction for malignant neoplasms. Technical note. J Neurosurg. 1997; 87(5):781–787
13. Jackson RJ, Gokaslan ZL. Spinal-pelvic fixation in patients with lumbosacral neoplasms. J Neurosurg. 2000; 92(1) Suppl:61–70
14. Dickey ID, Hugate RR, Jr, Fuchs B, Yaszemski MJ, Sim FH. Reconstruction after total sacrectomy: early experience with a new surgical technique. Clin Orthop Relat Res. 2005; 438(438):42–50
15. Gallia GL, Suk I, Witham TF, et al. Lumbopelvic reconstruction after combined L5 spondylectomy and total sacrectomy for en bloc resection of a malignant fibrous histiocytoma. Neurosurgery. 2010; 67(2):E498–E502
16. Todd LT, Jr, Yaszemski MJ, Currier BL, Fuchs B, Kim CW, Sim FH. Bowel and bladder function after major sacral resection. Clin Orthop Relat Res. 2002 (397):36–39
17. Gunterberg B, Petersén I. Sexual function after major resections of the sacrum with bilateral or unilateral sacrifice of sacral nerves. Fertil Steril. 1976; 27(10):1146–1153
18. Schwab JH, Healey JH, Rose P, Casas-Ganem J, Boland PJ. The surgical management of sacral chordomas. Spine. 2009; 34(24):2700–2704

66 Vertebral Body Augmentation

Tarek P. Sunna', Charbel Moussalem, Mohamad Nabih El Houshiemy, and Sarah Kawtharani

Summary

Vertebral body augmentation is used to treat nonhealing vertebral body fractures from trauma, osteoporosis, or tumors. Several techniques exist including creating a cavity for cement to fill or directly injecting cement to permeate through the affected vertebral body. Real-time imaging, i.e., fluoroscopy, is typically utilized to ensure cement flow is not penetrating the posterior cortex and entering the spinal canal.

Keywords: cement augmentation, kyphoplasty, vertebroplasty

66.1 Key Points

- Vertebral augmentation is commonly employed in treating compression fractures in patients who have osteoporotic or pathological compression fractures.
- Two different percutaneous vertebral augmentation methods for cement application into the vertebral body have been documented: Vertebroplasty (VP) and kyphoplasty (KP).
- In VP, polymethylmethacrylate (PMMA) cement is injected percutaneously into the collapsed vertebral body.
- KP involves placing inflatable temporary balloons percutaneously into a vertebral body. The inflation of the balloons allows some restoration of vertebral height and creation of a cavity. After deflation, the cavity that has been produced is filled by injection of PMMA.
- Previously, two randomized clinical trials showed that improvement in patients with painful osteoporotic vertebral fractures was similar between those treated with VP and those treated with a simulated procedure at 1-month follow-up.[1,2] Newer literature review has revealed that balloon KP/VP provided greater pain relief and less adjacent fractures than nonsurgical treatment.[3,4]
- One retrospective review study of 80 patients suffering from pathologic vertebral body fractures showed that both the techniques are effective in

providing pain relief, but KP is associated with lower rate of cement leakage than VP.[5]

- The CAFÉ study is the first randomized trial showing that in patients who have cancer, KP is an effective and safe treatment for vertebral fractures.[6]
- Compared with nonsurgical management, balloon KP resulted in improvements in quality of life and disability measures and reduction of back pain in patients who have acute painful vertebral fractures.[2,3]
- There is no difference in clinical outcomes between unilateral or bilateral KP.[3,7]

66.2 Indications

- Severe pain or progressive collapse as a result of vertebral body compression fractures in patients with osteoporosis (primary or secondary) or osteopenia.
- Severe pain or progressive collapse as a result of vertebral body metastasis or multiple myeloma. Treatment algorithm for painful thoracic or lumbar vertebral body fractures in cancer patients.
- Contraindications to vertebral augmentation include asymptomatic lesions, patients who are improving on conservative care, ongoing local or systemic infection, retropulsed bone fragment or epidural tumor causing myelopathy, neurological deficits, or spinal instability.

66.3 Diagnosis

- Initial diagnosis of vertebral body collapse can be established via X-rays or computed tomography (CT) scan of the cervical, thoracic, or lumbar spine.
- To verify and confirm the acuteness of the vertebral fracture, a magnetic resonance imaging (MRI) scan of the spine (T1 and short T1 inversion recovery [STIR] sequences) is used to detect vertebral body edema and associated impending fractures.
- CT scan of the fractured vertebral body with sagittal reconstruction to evaluate posterior vertebral wall integrity.
- Bone scan in some cases to assess acuity of fracture and exclude metastasis in different levels.
- According to the recommendations of the Working Group of the International Osteoporosis Foundation, surgical intervention, be it KP or VP, should go hand in hand with appropriate endocrinological workup to optimize medical treatment.[8]

66.4 Technique

- Procedures can be performed under general or local anesthesia.
- The patient is placed in prone position on Jackson radiolucent table, with postural reduction of kyphosis if present (using a mobile chest bed or additional pillows).
- Biplanar fluoroscopy is used.
- Both the techniques start with the percutaneous insertion of (11 gauge) Jamshidi needle or guide pin into the fractured vertebra via the pedicle of the corresponding vertebra, and end with the injection of PMMA.
- This can be achieved through a transpedicular approach in nearly every case.
- In the thoracic spine the needle can be inserted extrapedicularly, between the rib head and lateral aspect of the pedicle (**Fig. 66.1**).
- Unipedicular or bipedicular approach can be used to inject PMMA, with a goal of filling the center of the vertebral body.

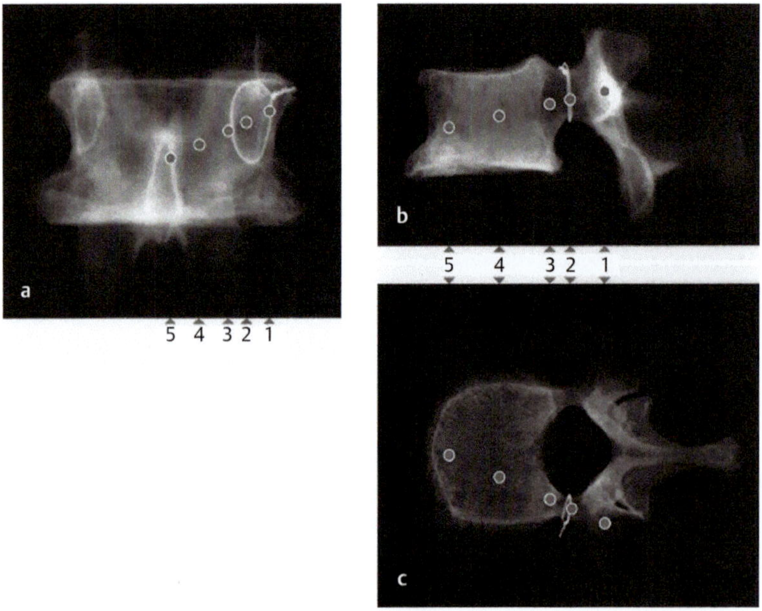

Fig. 66.1 **(a–c)** Entry points and trajectories for the transpedicular approach during kyphoplasty. (Reprinted with the permission of Medtronic, Inc.)

66.4.1 Vertebroplasty

- After correct positioning of the needle, the inner stylet is removed.
- Contrast material is then injected to ensure that the needle is not positioned in the venous flow path (optional).
- Cement, in thin liquid form, is injected into the vertebra using multiple small syringes or continuous injection system.
- The flow of the cement should be followed on the image intensifier.

66.4.2 Kyphoplasty

- After proper needle positioning, a series of tools (drill, curette) are used to create a working channel/cavity. Once inserted, the balloons are inflated using volume and pressure controls (digital manometer) to create a cavity within the vertebra.
- Once this has been achieved, the balloons are deflated and removed.
- Thick cement can be fed through the cannula under low pressure to fill the cavity created by the balloon tamp.
- In cases involving the upper thoracic spine, the shoulders can interfere with the lateral view, so a stack of pillows of appropriate height should be placed under the chest to lower both the shoulders. Alternatively, the arm and the shoulder are left hanging down parallel to the trunk.

66.5 Complications

- Procedure related: Cement leakage can result from fracture clefts or improper instrument position and can occur in the spinal canal, neuroforamen, or disk space.[2,9,10]
- Medical: Pulmonary embolism, hemo- or pneumothorax, soft tissue hematomas.[10,11]
- New adjacent vertebral fracture due to leakage of cement into the disk.[11]
- Pedicle fracture.[7,10,11]

66.6 Postoperative Care

- Conduct an immediate postoperative examination, ensuring that there is no new neurologic deficit compared with preop.
- Mobilize early, with no need for bracing.
- Clinical evaluation and plain spinal radiographs. Use a chest X-ray to rule out pneumothorax in thoracic VP/KP (optional).
- Discharge home when the patient meets discharge criteria (usually the same day).

66.7 Outcomes

- All studies reported significant improvements in pain score and functional outcome.[1,9]
- The risk of neurologic sequelae ranges from 0.4 to 4.0% according to various reports.[2,9,12]
- However, previously, a study by Kallmes et al[1] showed that improvements in pain and pain-related disability associated with osteoporotic compression fractures in patients treated with VP were similar to those for the control group, without treatment.
- Results of six randomized controlled studies (525 treated levels and a total of 424 patients) were evaluated by Bouza et al[10] to evaluate the safety of KP in treatment of osteoporotic vertebral compression fractures.
  - Cement leakage was detected in 18.3%.
  - Only 0.5% of fracture leakages proved to be symptomatic.
  - Clinical complications were recorded in 11.5%, with several cases requiring intensive treatment or postoperative surgery.
  - New vertebral fractures were noted in 20.7%.
- A randomized trial by Dohm et al showed a shorter operation time with VP but fewer risk of cement leakage and a trend toward longer fracture-free survival in the KP group.[13,14]
- A meta-analysis published in 2015 including 29 studies with total of 3000 patients comparing KP and VP showed that there is no difference in the short- and long-term disability outcomes, and postoperative pain between the two procedures.[15]

66.8 Surgical Pearls

- The possibility of cement leakage can be overcome through the use of high-quality imaging and slow application of PMMA in a viscous state.
- In cases of focal kyphosis caused by index fracture, the levels above and below the fracture should also be considered in the treatment plan. No more than three to four levels should be treated at one sitting. This policy minimizes the risk of microembolization (cement and fat emboli).[12] Impending fractures should also be treated.
- Another meta-analysis including 12 studies of 1328 patients showed no evidence of an increased risk of adjacent vertebral body fracture following augmentation with either method compared with conservative treatment.[16]

Common Clinical Questions

1. Contraindications to vertebral augmentation include all of the following *except* which?
   A. Asymptomatic lesions.
   B. Retropulsed bone fragment.
   C. Epidural tumor causing myelopathy.
   D. Severe pain due to vertebral body compression fractures in patients with osteoporosis.
2. Procedure-related complications include all of the following *except* which?
   A. Cement leakage.
   B. Pulmonary embolism, hemothorax, or pneumothorax.
   C. New adjacent vertebral fracture.
   D. Cement in the pedicle.

Answers to Common Clinical Questions

1. D.
2. D.

References

1. Kallmes DF, Comstock BA, Heagerty PJ, et al. A randomized trial of vertebroplasty for osteoporotic spinal fractures. N Engl J Med. 2009; 361(6): 569–579
2. Wardlaw D, Cummings SR, Van Meirhaeghe J, et al. Efficacy and safety of balloon kyphoplasty compared with non-surgical care for vertebral compression fracture (FREE): a randomised controlled trial. Lancet. 2009; 373(9668):1016–1024
3. Papanastassiou ID, Aghayev K, Berenson JR, Schmidt MH, Vrionis FD. Is vertebral augmentation the right choice for cancer patients with painful vertebral compression fractures? J Natl Compr Canc Netw. 2012; 10(6):715–719
4. Papanastassiou ID, Phillips FM, Van Meirhaeghe J, et al. Comparing effects of kyphoplasty, vertebroplasty, and non-surgical management in a systematic review of randomized and non-randomized controlled studies. Eur Spine J. 2012; 21(9):1826–1843
5. Li Z, Ni C, Chen L, et al. Kyphoplasty versus vertebroplasty for the treatment of malignant vertebral compression fractures caused by metastases: a retrospective study. Chin Med J (Engl). 2014; 127(8):1493–1496

6. Berenson J, Pflugmacher R, Jarzem P, et al. Cancer Patient Fracture Evaluation (CAFE) Investigators. Balloon kyphoplasty versus non-surgical fracture management for treatment of painful vertebral body compression fractures in patients with cancer: a multicentre, randomised controlled trial. Lancet Oncol. 2011; 12(3):225–235
7. Papanastassiou ID, Eleraky M, Murtagh R, Kokkalis ZT, Gerochristou M, Vrionis FD. Comparison of unilateral versus bilateral kyphoplasty in multiple myeloma patients and the importance of preoperative planning. Asian Spine J. 2014; 8(3):244–252
8. Boonen S, Wahl DA, Nauroy L, et al. CSA Fracture Working Group of International Osteoporosis Foundation. Balloon kyphoplasty and vertebroplasty in the management of vertebral compression fractures. Osteoporos Int. 2011; 22(12):2915–2934
9. Lee MJ, Dumonski M, Cahill P, Stanley T, Park D, Singh K. Percutaneous treatment of vertebral compression fractures: a meta-analysis of complications. Spine. 2009; 34(11):1228–1232
10. Bouza C, López-Cuadrado T, Almendro N, Amate JM. Safety of balloon kyphoplasty in the treatment of osteoporotic vertebral compression fractures in Europe: a meta-analysis of randomized controlled trials. Eur Spine J. 2015; 24(4):715–723
11. Robinson Y, Tschöke SK, Stahel PF, Kayser R, Heyde CE. Complications and safety aspects of kyphoplasty for osteoporotic vertebral fractures: a prospective follow-up study in 102 consecutive patients. Patient Saf Surg. 2008; 2:2
12. Mendel E, Bourekas E, Gerszten P, Golan JD. Percutaneous techniques in the treatment of spine tumors: what are the diagnostic and therapeutic indications and outcomes? Spine. 2009; 34(22) Suppl:S93–S100
13. Dohm M, Black CM, Dacre A, Tillman JB, Fueredi G, KAVIAR investigators. A randomized trial comparing balloon kyphoplasty and vertebroplasty for vertebral compression fractures due to osteoporosis. AJNR Am J Neuroradiol. 2014; 35(12):2227–2236
14. Wang B, Zhao CP, Song LX, Zhu L. Balloon kyphoplasty versus percutaneous vertebroplasty for osteoporotic vertebral compression fracture: a meta-analysis and systematic review. J Orthop Surg Res. 2018; 13(1):264
15. Gu CN, Brinjikji W, Evans AJ, Murad MH, Kallmes DF. Outcomes of vertebroplasty compared with kyphoplasty: a systematic review and meta-analysis. J Neurointerv Surg. 2016; 8(6):636–642
16. Zhang H, Xu C, Zhang T, Gao Z, Zhang T. Does percutaneous vertebroplasty or balloon kyphoplasty for osteoporotic vertebral compression fractures increase the incidence of new vertebral fractures? A meta-analysis. Pain Physician. 2017; 20(1):E13–E28

Index

Note: Page numbers set **bold** or *italic* indicate headings or figures, respectively.

A

D

M

N

P

R

S

W

X

Z